Critical Thinking in Clinical Research

Applied Theory and Practice Using Case Studies

Edited by

Felipe Fregni, MD, PhD, MMSc, MPH

Associate Professor of Epidemiology, Harvard T.H. Chan School of Public Health
Associate Professor of Physical Medicine and Rehabilitation
Harvard Medical School
Director, Collaborative Learning in Clinical Research Program
Principles and Practice of Clinical Research (PPCR) Program
Harvard T.H. Chan School of Public Health
Boston, MA

Ben M. W. Illigens, MD

Department of Neurology
Beth Israel Deaconess Medical Center
Harvard School of Medicine
Boston, MA

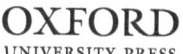

OXFORD
UNIVERSITY PRESS

Oxford University Press is a department of the University of Oxford. It furthers
the University's objective of excellence in research, scholarship, and education
by publishing worldwide. Oxford is a registered trade mark of Oxford University
Press in the UK and certain other countries.

Published in the United States of America by Oxford University Press
198 Madison Avenue, New York, NY 10016, United States of America.

© Oxford University Press 2018

All rights reserved. No part of this publication may be reproduced, stored in
a retrieval system, or transmitted, in any form or by any means, without the
prior permission in writing of Oxford University Press, or as expressly permitted
by law, by license, or under terms agreed with the appropriate reproduction
rights organization. Inquiries concerning reproduction outside the scope of the
above should be sent to the Rights Department, Oxford University Press, at the
address above.

You must not circulate this work in any other form
and you must impose this same condition on any acquirer.

Library of Congress Cataloging-in-Publication Data
Data Names: Fregni, Felipe, editor. | Illigens, Ben M. W., editor.
Title: Critical thinking in clinical research : applied theory and practice
using case studies / edited by Felipe Fregni, Ben M.W. Illigens.
Description: New York, NY : Oxford University Press, [2018] |
Includes bibliographical references and index.
Identifiers: LCCN 2017028658 | ISBN 9780199324491 (alk. paper)
Subjects: | MESH: Clinical Studies as Topic | Statistics as Topic |
Biomedical Research | Research Design | Ethics, Research
Classification: LCC R853.C55 | NLM W 20.55.C5 | DDC 610.72/4—dc23
LC record available at https://lccn.loc.gov/2017028658

5 7 9 8 6
Printed by Webcom, Inc., Canada

This material is not intended to be, and should not be considered, a substitute for medical or
other professional advice. Treatment for the conditions described in this material is highly
dependent on the individual circumstances. And, while this material is designed to offer
accurate information with respect to the subject matter covered and to be current as of the
time it was written, research and knowledge about medical and health issues is constantly
evolving and dose schedules for medications are being revised continually, with new side
effects recognized and accounted for regularly. Readers must therefore always check the
product information and clinical procedures with the most up-to-date published product
information and data sheets provided by the manufacturers and the most recent codes of
conduct and safety regulation. The publisher and the authors make no representations or
warranties to readers, express or implied, as to the accuracy or completeness of this material.
Without limiting the foregoing, the publisher and the authors make no representations or
warranties as to the accuracy or efficacy of the drug dosages mentioned in the material.
The authors and the publisher do not accept, and expressly disclaim, any responsibility for any
liability, loss or risk that may be claimed or incurred as a consequence of the use and/or
application of any of the contents of this material.

To Lucca Fregni, the light of our lives.

Felipe Fregni

To my wife Seung-Kyung Cecilia Lee, who will always
be in my heart, and our daughter Clara Eun-Bee Illigens.
You are my love and inspiration
and made me the person I am.

Ben M. W. Illigens

CONTENTS

Contributors ix

Unit I: Basics of Clinical Research

1. Basics of Clinical Research: Introduction to Clinical Research 3
   Rui Nakamura, Faiza Khawaja, Laura Castillo-Saavedra, Felipe Fregni, and Steven D. Freedman

2. Selection of the Research Question 26
   Keiko Ueda and Lotfi B. Merabet

3. Study Population 45
   Sandra Carvalho and Felipe Fregni

4. Basic Study Designs 68
   Alexandra Gomez-Arteaga, Felipe Fregni, and Vera Novak

5. Randomization 87
   Juliana C. Ferreira, Ben M. W. Illigens, and Felipe Fregni

6. Blinding 105
   Rita Tomás and Joseph Massaro

7. Recruitment and Adherence 129
   Timo Siepmann, Ana Isabel Penzlin, and Felipe Fregni

Unit II: Basics of Statistics

8. Basics of Statistics 151
   Claudia Kimie Suemoto and Catherine Lee

9. Parametric Statistical Tests 181
   Ben M. W. Illigens, Fernanda Lopes, and Felipe Fregni

10. Non-Parametric Statistical Tests 206
    Felipe Fregni and Fernanda Lopes

11. Sample Size Calculation 225
    Mohammad Azfar Qureshi and Jessica K. Paulus

12. Survival Analysis 243
Jorge Leite and Sandra Carvalho

13. Other Issues in Statistics I: Missing Data, Intention-to-Treat Analysis, and Covariate Adjustment 257
Tamara Jorquiera and Hang Lee

14. Other Issues in Statistics II: Subgroup Analysis and Meta-analysis 284
Jorge Leite and Munir Boodhwani

Unit III: Practical Aspects of Clinical Research
15. Non-Inferiority Design 307
Raquel Ajub Moyses, Valeria Angelim, and Scott Evans

16. Observational Studies 324
Minou Djannatian and Clarissa Valim

17. Confounders and Using the Method of Propensity Scores 362
Chin Lin

18. Adaptive Trials and Interim Analysis 377
Priscila Caldeira Andrade, Nazem Atassi, and Laura Castillo-Saavedra

Unit IV: Study Designs
19. Integrity in Research: Authorship and Ethics 397
Sandra Carvalho and Gustavo Rivara

20. The Business of Clinical Research 417
Lívia Caroline Mariano Compte, and Jorge Leite

21. Design and Analysis of Surveys 434
Ana R. Martins and Inês C. R. Henriques

22. Assessing Risk and Adverse Events 457
Laura Castillo-Saavedra, Suely Reiko Matsubayashi, Faiza Khawaja, John Ferguson, and Felipe Fregni

23. Manuscript Submission 470
Alma Tamara Sanchez Jimenez and Felipe Fregni

Index 493

CONTRIBUTORS

Priscila Caldeira Andrade, PharmD, MPH
Health Economics & Market Access Manager-Northern Region (Latin America)
Johnson & Johnson Medical
Sao Paulo, Brazil

Valeria Angelim, PhD
Alphacor Cardiologia Clinica e Diagnostica
Universidade de Sao Paulo (USP)
Sao Paulo, Brazil

Nazem Atassi, MD
Department of Neurology
Harvard Medical School
Massachusetts General Hospital
Boston, MA

Munir Boodhwani, BSc, MD
University of Ottawa Heart Institute
Ottawa, Canada

André Brunoni, MD, PhD
Universidade de Sao Paulo (USP)
Medical School
Sao Paulo, Brazil

Sandra Carvalho, MSc, PhD
Neuromodulation Center
Spaulding Rehabilitation Hospital
Harvard Medical School
Boston, MA

Laura Castillo-Saavedra, MD
University of Chicago Medicine
The Pritzker School of Medicine
Chicago, IL

Lívia Caroline Mariano Compte, MD
Universidade de Sao Paulo (USP)
Medical School
Sao Paulo, Brazil

Minou Djannatian, MD, MSc
Institute of Neuronal Cell Biology
Technische Universität München
Munich, Germany

Scott Evans, PhD
Director of the Statistical and Data Management Center (SDMC)
Antibacterial Resistance Leadership Group (ARLG)
Department of Biostatistics
Harvard T.H. Chan School of Public Health
Boston, MA

John Ferguson, MD
Sanofi Pharmaceutical
Boston, MA

Juliana C. Ferreira, MD, PhD
Respiratory Intensive Care Unit
Hospital das Clinicas
Universidade de Sao Paulo (USP)
Medical School
Sao Paulo, Brazil

Steven D. Freedman, MD, PhD
Chief, Division of Translational Research
Department of Medicine
Beth Israel Deaconess Medical Center
Boston, MA

Felipe Fregni, MD, PhD, MMSc, MPH
Associate Professor of Epidemiology, Harvard T.H. Chan School of Public Health
Associate Professor of Physical Medicine and Rehabilitation, Harvard Medical School
Director, Collaborative Learning in Clinical Research Program, Principles and Practice of Clinical Research (PPCR) Program
Harvard T.H. Chan School of Public Health
Boston, MA

Alexandra Gomez-Arteaga, MD
Universidad de Los Andes
Bogota, Colombia

Inês C. R. Henriques, MD
Faculty of Medicine of the University of Coimbra
Coimbra, Portugal

Ben M. W. Illigens, MD
Department of Neurology
Beth Israel Deaconess Medical Center
Harvard School of Medicine
Boston, MA

Rui Imamura, MD
Universidade de Sao Paulo (USP) Medical School
Sao Paulo, Brazil

Tamara Jorquiera, MD, MSc
Department of Medicine
University of San Martín de Porres
Lima, Peru

Faiza Khawaja, MD
Department of Clinical Pharmacology and Internal Medicine
The Michener Institute for Applied Health Sciences
Toronto, Canada

Catherine Lee, PhD
Department of Biostatistics
Harvard T.H. Chan School of Public Health
Boston, MA

Hang Lee, PhD
Department of Medicine
Massachusetts General Hospital
Harvard Medical School
Boston, MA

Jorge Leite, PhD
Laboratory of Neuromodulation
Spaulding Rehabilitation Hospital
Harvard Medical School
Boston, MA

Chin Lin, MD, PhD
University of Sao Paulo
Hospital das Clinicas (ICESP)
Sao Paulo, Brazil

Fernanda Lopes, PhD
Neuromodulation Center
Spaulding Rehabilitation Hospital
Harvard Medical School
Boston, MA

Ana R. Martins, RN
PPCR Program, ECPE
Harvard T.H. Chan School of Public Health
Boston, MA
Universidade de Coimbra
Coimbra, Portugal

Joseph Massaro, PhD
Professor of Biostatistics
Boston University School of Public Health
Boston, MA

Suely Reiko Matsubayashi, MD
PPCR Program, ECPE
Harvard T.H. Chan School of Public Health
Boston, MA

Lotfi B. Merabet, OD, PhD, MPH
Associate Professor
Department of Ophthalmology
Harvard Medical School
Boston, MA

Raquel Ajub Moyses, MD
Hospital das Clínicas
Universidade de Sao Paulo (USP)
  Medical School
Sao Paulo, Brazil

Rui Nakamura, MD
Principles and Practice of Clinical
  Research (PPCR) Program, ECPE
Harvard T.H. Chan School of
  Public Health
Boston, MA

Vera Novak, PhD, MD
Department of Neurology
Beth Israel Deaconess Medical Center
Harvard School of Medicine
Boston, MA

Jessica Paulus, ScD
Investigator, Institute for Clinical
  Research and Health Studies
Assistant Professor of Medicine
Tufts University School of Medicine
Medford, MA

Ana Isabel Penzlin, MD
University Hospital Carl Gustav Carus
Dresden, Germany

Mohammad Azfar Qureshi, MBBS
Department of Nephrology
King Abdulaziz Medical City
Saudi Arabia

Gustavo Rivara, MD, MSc
Pediatrician and Neonatologist
Universidad San Martín de Porres
Facultad de Medicina Humana Clinica
Delgado Lima, Perú

Timo Siepmann, MD
Departments of Neurology, Internal
  Medicine, Clinical Pharmacology
Universitätsklinikum Dresden
Dresden, Germany

Claudia Kimie Suemoto, MD, PhD
Division of Geriatrics
University of Sao Paulo Medical School
Sao Paulo, Brazil

Alma Tamara Sanchez Jimenez, MD
PPCR Program, ECPE
Harvard T.H. Chan School of
  Public Health
Boston, MA

Rita Tomás, MD
Adjunct Professor
Escola Superior de Tecnologia da Saúde
  de Lisboa
Instituto Politécnico de Lisboa
Clínica CUF Alvalade
Portugal Football School,
  Portuguese Football Federation
Lisbon School of Health Technology
Polytechnic Institute of Lisbon
Lisbon, Portugal

Keiko Ueda, MD
Principles and Practice of Clinical
  Research (PPCR) Program
Harvard T.H. Chan School of
  Public Health
Boston, MA

Clarissa Valim, MD, MSc, ScD
Department of Immunology and
  Infectious Diseases
Harvard T.H. Chan School of
  Public Health
Boston, MA

UNIT I
Basics of Clinical Research

1

BASICS OF CLINICAL RESEARCH
INTRODUCTION TO CLINICAL RESEARCH

Authors: *Rui Nakamura, Faiza Khawaja, Laura Castillo-Saavedra,[*] Felipe Fregni, and Steven D. Freedman*

Case study authors: *Felipe Fregni, Fabio Pinna, and André Brunoni*

The whole history of science has been the gradual realization that events do not happen in an arbitrary manner, but that they reflect a certain underlying order, which may or may not be divinely inspired.
—Stephen W. Hawking

INTRODUCTION

The search for knowledge about ourselves and the world around us is a fundamental human endeavor. Research is a natural extension of this desire to understand and to improve the world in which we live.

This chapter focuses on the process of clinical trials, ethical issues involved in the history of clinical research, and other issues that may be unique to clinical trials. As clinical trials are, perhaps, the most regulated type of research—subject to provincial, national, and international regulatory bodies—reference will be made to these regulations where appropriate.

The scope of research is vast. On the purely physical side, it ranges from seeking to understand the origins of the universe down to the fundamental nature of matter. At the analytic level, it covers mathematics, logic, and metaphysics. Research involving humans ranges widely, including attempts to understand the broad sweep of history, the workings of the human body and the body politic, the nature of human interactions, and the impact of nature on humans—the list is as boundless as the human imagination.

CLINICAL RESEARCH

Clinical research is a branch of medical science that determines the safety and effectiveness of medications, devices, diagnostic products, nutrition or behavioral changes,

---
[*] The first three authors contributed equally to the work.

and treatment regimens intended for human use. Clinical research is a structured process of investigating facts and theories and exploring connections. It proceeds in a systematic way to examine clinical conditions and outcomes, to establish relationships among clinical phenomena, to generate evidence for decision-making, and to provide the impetus for improving methods of practice.

Clinical trials are a set of procedures in medical research and drug development that are conducted to allow safety and efficacy data to be collected for health interventions. Given that clinical trials are experiments conducted on humans, there is a series of required procedures and steps for conducting a clinical trial. There are several goals tested in clinical trials, including testing whether the drug, therapy, or procedure is safe and effective for people to use. The overall purpose of a clinical trial is acquisition of new knowledge, not the treatment of patients per se.

A clinical trial, also known as patient-oriented research, is any investigation involving participants that evaluates the effects of one or more health-related interventions on health outcomes. Interventions include, but are not restricted to, drugs, radiopharmaceuticals, cells and other biological products, surgical procedures, radiologic procedures, devices, genetic therapies, natural health products, process-of-care changes, preventive care, manual therapies, and psychotherapies. Clinical trials may also include questions that are not directly related to therapeutic goals—for example, drug metabolism—in addition to those that directly evaluate the treatment of participants.

Clinical trials are most frequently undertaken in biomedical research, although research that evaluates interventions, usually by comparing two or more approaches, is also conducted in related disciplines, such as psychology. The researcher leading a clinical trial is often (but not always) a clinician, that is, a health-care provider (e.g., physician, dentist, naturopath, physiotherapist, etc.). Although various types and forms of clinical trials have methodological differences, the ethical principles and procedures are the same and are applicable to all.

History of Experimentation in Clinical Research

Clinical research has a long and rich history, dating back to as early as 2737 BCE; the first clinical trial is documented in the Old Testament. Since this first trial, the field has changed and progressed immensely, with the refinement of research methodology and practice. The most progress in the methodology and use of clinical trials has occurred in the past 50 years, changing significantly the landscape of clinical research.

2737 BCE

Shen Nung, legendary emperor of China, is considered the father of Chinese medicine. In addition to being credited for the technique of acupuncture, he purportedly experimented with and classified hundreds of poisonous and medical herbs, which he tested in a series of studies on himself.

Approximately 600 BCE

The first experiment that could be considered a trial can be found in the Old Testament. The book of Daniel describes how under King Nebuchadnezzar II, children of royal blood and certain children from the conquered Israel were recruited to be trained as the king's advisors over a period of three years during which they would be granted to eat from the king's meat and wine. Daniel, however, requested from the officer in charge of the diet that he and three other Hebrew children would be allowed to have only legumes and water. When the officer expressed concerns about the "inferior" diet, Daniel suggested a 10-day trial period, after which the officer would assess both groups of children. At the end of this "pilot study," Daniel's group was noticeably healthier than the group of children who were relegated to the diet of wine and meat. Therefore Daniel and the other three children were permitted to continue with their diet for the entire training period, after which they displayed superior wisdom and understanding compared to all other advisors of the king (Old Testament, Daniel 1:5–20).

1537

Ambroise Paré, a French surgeon during the Renaissance, accidentally carried out a clinical study when he ran out of elderberry oil, which after being boiled was used as the standard treatment for gun wounds at that time. He then used a mixture of egg yolk, turpentine (a pine tree–derived oil), and rose oil instead, and he soon noticed that patients treated with this mixture had less pain and better wound healing than those patients who had received the standard treatment [1].

1747

The first reported systematic experiment of the modern era was conducted by James Lind, a Scottish physician, when he was sailing on the Salisbury. After many of the seamen developed signs of scurvy, Lind selected 12 similar sick sailors and split them into six groups of two. All groups were given the same diet, but each group was treated differently for scurvy: group 1 received cider, group 2 vitriol (sulfuric acid), group 3 vinegar, group 4 seawater, group 5 oranges and lemon, and group 6 nutmeg and barley water (British herbal tea). The group that had the fruits recovered from scurvy within just six days. Of the other treatments, vinegar "showed the best effect" [Dr. James Lind. "Treatise on Scurvy." Published in 1753, in Edinburgh]. (Lind's experiment had little short-term impact; he was reluctant to believe in fruits being a sole remedy for scurvy, and citrus fruits were difficult to preserve and also expensive. It wasn't until 1790 that the Royal Navy made fresh lemons a standard supplement. In 1932 the link between vitamin C and scurvy was finally proven.)

In 1747, Dr. James Lind tested several scurvy treatments on crew members of the British naval ship Salisbury and discovered that lemons and oranges were most effective in treating the dreaded affliction.

1863

Austin Flint (US physician, graduate of Harvard Medical School, class of 1833) is revered for having conducted the first study with a placebo. A placebo is considered a substance or procedure with no therapeutic effect. In 1863 Flint tested a placebo on prisoners with rheumatic fever and compared their response to the response of patients who had received an active treatment (although not in the same trial). (Austin Flint murmur is a murmur associated with aortic regurgitation. This trial is somewhat problematic ethically [research conducted on a vulnerable population] and methodically [placebo and active treatment were not tested at the same time, and active treatment for rheumatic fever was questionable to be active]).

1906

The 1906 Pure Food and Drug Act imposed purity standards on products and drugs and mandated accurate labeling with content and dose.

1923

The idea of randomization was introduced to clinical trials in 1923. Randomization involves participants randomly receiving one of the treatments, one being a placebo and one being the new drug.

1938: The Federal Food, Drug, and Cosmetic (FDC) Act

This act required that new drugs be shown to be safe before marketing, thus starting a new system of drug regulation. It also provided that safe tolerances be set for unavoidable poisonous substances.

1943

Blind clinical trials—in which neither group knows which treatment they are receiving—also emerged in the twentieth century. The first double-blind controlled trial—Patulin for the common cold—was conducted, and the first widely published randomized clinical trial was conducted on Streptomycin as a treatment for pulmonary tuberculosis [2].

1944

Multicenter clinical trials were introduced, in which multiple studies were conducted at various sites, all using the same protocol to provide wider testing, generalization, and better statistical data.

1947

The Nuremberg Code was developed, which outlines 10 basic statements for the protection of human participants in clinical trials.

1964

The Declaration of Helsinki was developed, which outlines ethical codes for physicians and for the protection of participants in clinical trials worldwide.

1988

The US Food and Drug Administration (FDA) was given more authority and accountability over the approval of new drugs and treatments.

1990

The International Conference on Harmonization (ICH) was assembled to help eliminate differences in drug-development requirements for three global pharmaceutical markets: the European Union, Japan, and the United States. The ICH initiatives promote increased efficiency in the development of new drugs, improving their availability to patients and the public.

2000

A Common Technical Document (CTD) was developed. The CTD acts as a standard dossier used in Europe, Japan, and the United States for proposing data gathered in clinical trials to respective governing authorities.

THE HISTORY OF ETHICS IN CLINICAL RESEARCH
Disasters in Clinical Research

A significant part of the ethical regulations in clinical research was catalyzed by disastrous events that took place at the beginning of the new era of clinical research, when experimentation and the development of novel treatments began to take place in a more systematic way. We review these events in the context of US and global changes in ethical regulations. Although changes in ethical regulations had a similar pathway worldwide, there have been some differences between US and global changes in ethical regulations for clinical research.

US Disasters and Responses
Sulfanilamide Cold Syrup

The months of September and October of 1937 served as the tragic background for one irreparable clinical disaster. The medication responsible for this disaster was known as "Elixir sulfanilamide," and was commonly and safely used for the treatment of streptococcal infections for several years, mainly in the form of powder and tablets. On June 1937, the S. E. Massengill Company, located in Bristol, Tennessee, created and distributed 633 doses of the same compound but in liquid form, by dissolving the existing powder into ethylene glycol. The distributing laboratory controlled the new substance by testing its flavor, appearance, and fragrance and decided that it was satisfactory. Nonetheless, as safety testing was not a legal requirement by the FDA at the time, the new preparation was not tested for safety. The company then failed to understand that ethylene glycol was a toxic compound, used frequently as antifreeze.

Approximately 1 month after the distribution of the new liquid preparation of Elixir sulfanilamide, the first report of associated deaths was made public. The

American Medical Association (AMA) was the first to publicly announce the toxicity of the new compound and to warn physicians and patients against its lethal effects. The S. E. Massengill Company was also notified; the company then sent telegrams to distributors, pharmacists, and physicians, asking them to return the product, but failed to explain the reason for the request, thus undermining the urgency of the situation and the lethal effects of the product. At the request of the FDA, the company was forced to send out a second announcement, which was clear about the toxicity of the product and the importance of the situation.

The next step taken by the FDA was to make sure all of the products were returned safely; to do so, they had to locate all of the stores, dispensers, pharmacists, physicians, and buyers. This proved to be a difficult task: many of the company's salesmen were not willing to help by providing the information required to locate the recipients of the Elixir; pharmacies had no clear record of buyers; and many physicians didn't keep documentation of the patients to whom the compound was prescribed, nor their addresses. Some physicians decided to abstain from helping authorities and lied about their prescription trail, afraid that they could be held liable for prescribing the medication. In spite of these circumstances, the relentless efforts of the FDA and local authorities, as well as the help of the AMA and the media, allowed for the recovery of 234 of the 240 gallons of the drug that had been distributed. In several cases, legal action through federal seizure was required. The FDA had to refer to the compound's branding name "Elixir" to file federal charges that would allow them to complete their task. The misbranding charge was brought to the company for distributing a compound as an elixir, meaning it was dissolved in alcohol, when it was actually dissolved in ethylene glycol.

The victims were many, including young children—most sick with throat infections—young workers, older patients, mothers, and fathers. Most of the victims would suffer the lethal effects of the substance for 10–21 days before succumbing to death. The symptoms were mainly associated with severe renal failure and included oliguria, edema, nausea, vomiting, abdominal pain, and seizures.

The Response: The Federal Food, Drug, and Cosmetic Act of 1938

Given these unfortunate events and other disasters associated with medications that had not been properly tested, the FDA emphasized the need for stricter control of the production and distribution of new drugs that could ensure the welfare of patients and consumers. The enactment of the Federal Food, Drug, and Cosmetic Act of 1938 provided a new system for drug control and safety, which not only solidified the conditions required for the release of new medications, but also stimulated medical research.

Thalidomide

Thalidomide is considered a derivative of glutamic acid, first synthesized unsuccessfully in Europe by Swiss Pharmaceuticals in 1953. A German company, Chemie Grunenthal, then remarketed it in 1957 as an anticonvulsant. Given its sedative effects, it was also commercialized as a sleeping aid. It became a very popular medication, considered effective and safe, and was highly sought and prescribed due to its lack of hangover effect, as supported by small clinical studies conducted in Europe and in which the subjects were unaware of the medication being tested [3,4]. By the end of the decade, more than 10 pharmaceutical companies in all five continents were selling the drug. It was even said that the medication became nearly as famous as aspirin [5]. Its use became widespread and unregulated; it was prescribed for treatment of almost every condition, from simple colds to anxiety and asthma. Some even went as far as to attribute to the medication some beneficial effects on diabetes, cancer, and autoimmune diseases [6].

Soon after, some doctors started to recommend the off-label use of thalidomide for the relief of morning sickness in pregnant women. This use also became widespread in the late 1950s and early 1960s. After this unprecedented success in Europe, the company William S. Merrel made a formal application to the FDA for marketing thalidomide as an over-the-counter medication, which could be used for the treatment of many ailments, from anorexia and poor school performance, to asthma and tuberculosis.

The petition was assigned for review to a new FDA reviewer, Dr. Frances Kelsey. After her initial review of the available information, she became concerned with some of the initial reports of adverse effects associated with the use of thalidomide and the lack of well-designed safety studies [7]. The initial reports released regarding safety concerns were associated with irreversible peripheral neuropathy in chronic users of thalidomide [8]. At the time, previous research had shown that medications associated with peripheral nerve irritation could lead to growth retardation and birth defects, shown mainly in rabbit fetuses. These concerns were dismissed by the company's CEO, who claimed that the peripheral neuropathy was associated with isolated cases and was reversible upon discontinuation of the drug [6,9].

Given this information, Dr. Kelsey put a hold on the approval of the request by Merrel's company and asked for further data regarding safety studies and data on the effects of the biologically active compound in pregnant patients, as one of the indications for the new drug would be morning sickness. The data were not available, which led to a significant delay in the approval process. At the same time, tragedy struck as new reports of adverse events were made public [7].

It was a bittersweet surprise for both the American public and lawmakers when they found out that the only thing that kept the ill-proved drug from being commercialized in the United States was a cautious FDA agent. She had reported the safety proofs provided by the company as testimonial and not as the result of well-designed and executed studies, rendering the application incomplete and withdrawing it from approval. After the studies made clear that there was a causal association between thalidomide and severe birth defects, there was a clear urgency in recapitulating in the face of such tragedy.

The thalidomide disaster brought to light the conditions of a still ill-equipped regulatory process on drug synthesis and marketing, accounting for the weakness of the FDA in regulating efficacy, safety, test conduction, and accountability. The way in which the agency operated at the time rendered the process ineffective and left almost all of the responsibility and control in the hands of drug manufacturers. The FDA had a 60-day period to prove that a new drug was not safe and contradicted the studies conducted by the pharmaceutical company; otherwise the product would be approved. The companies controlled the conduction of clinical tests, so they could complete new studies without FDA approval or even subjects' consent, and even worse, after approval, all new data regarding the drug were considered private. All of these situations clearly showed that pharmaceutical companies had an upper hand in the game.

Response: The Kefauver-Harris Drug Amendments of 1962

At around the same time as the thalidomide disaster started to spark, Democratic Senator Estes Kefauver proposed a bill to the Senate that included price control on the products of pharmaceutical companies and tougher safety controls. The bill was widely discussed and debated, but was never passed. Well after the disaster became clear, interest in the bill revived, and Senator Kefauver modified it to include only the changes to safety control, including some of the weakness that were brought to light by Dr. Kelsey's story. The new bill made important modifications to the existing system, including the abolishment of the approval time period, which then shifted the weight of accounting for drug safety and efficacy from the FDA to the pharmaceutical companies. It also mandated that such proofs be based on well-designed and conducted clinical studies using up-to-date techniques and practices. All clinical trials had to be approved by the FDA, and all participants had to be properly informed and consented. Also, all information regarding efficacy and safety was to be shared with the FDA during all stages of the marketing process, and the agency had the freedom to make new sets of rules and limitations regarding the approval process, including immediately removing drugs from the market [10–12].

Tuskegee Study

This study, also known as the "The Tuskegee Study of Untreated Syphilis in the Negro Male," was conducted in Alabama by the United States Public Health Service (USPHS) and the Tuskegee Institute between 1932 and 1972 [13]. During this period of time, hundreds of African-American males did not receive proper and standard care for syphilis, with the intention to document the natural course of syphilis infection if it was left untreated. During the 40 years that the study took place, many of the enrolled subjects, who came from a poor, rural area in Alabama, died of syphilis, and many of their descendants were born with congenital syphilis. Directors, researchers, and collaborators of the study observed the tragic effects of the disease, completely indifferent to the suffering of their subjects, and even decided to continue their study after penicillin was proven to effectively treat and cure the infection [13,14].

In 1928, scientists from Oslo published a study conducted in white males with untreated syphilis that refuted the long-lived belief that the effects of syphilis depended on the race of the affected. It was thought that this infection had more severe neurologic effects on people of Caucasian descent, while it produced more severe cardiovascular effects in population of African-American descent, but the study from Oslo showed that most of the infected white males had severe affectation of their cardiovascular system, but very few ever developed neurosyphilis [15]. This finding amazed physicians and researchers in the United States, which led them to plan and execute a similar study, which would be carried out in a population with high prevalence of the infection. American scientists chose the city of Tuskegee because 35%–45% of the population in the area was seropositive for syphilis. The initial design proposed observing the untreated subjects for a period of 6–8 months, after which the subjects would be treated with the standard care: salvarsan and bismuth, both fairly effective but toxic. The initial purpose of the study was to benefit the health of the poor population enrolled, as well as to understand and learn more about the disease, its prevention, and its cure. This led to the support of many of the local hospitals and physicians, including African-American doctors and organizations [14,16].

Researchers initially enrolled 600 men, 201 as healthy controls and 399 seropositive for syphilis but not yet aware of their diagnosis. The subjects proceeded from Macon County in Alabama, where the city of Tuskegee was located; they were mostly illiterate men, lured into the study by the promise of free medical care, free daily meals, and US$50 for burial expenses for their participation. Throughout their participation in the study, the participants were not informed of their infection status, nor did they receive treatment. In many instances, researchers used deception to assure cooperation and avoid dropouts, including making the burial policy contingent to their previous authorization for an autopsy. After the initial allotted time for the study was completed, many of the participating researchers decided it was necessary to continue the study and obtain more clinical information. As the study continued, the great economic crisis of 1929 was gestating, which led to withdrawal of the main funding source. Researchers thought this would mean the end of the experiment, as it would be impossible to afford treatment for all participants, but soon they proposed continuing the study without offering standard care to patients, leading to a complete deviation from the initial proposal and to the resignation of one of the initial creators of the study, Dr. Taliaferro Clark [13,17].

It is important to note that during the 40 years of the Tuskegee experiment, the study was never kept secret, and many articles were published in medical journals describing initial discoveries and important information obtained from the research [18–21]. Despite its controversial and irregular techniques, many argued that the contribution of this study to science far outweighed its detrimental effects on the health of the studied population. One of the main contributions of the experiment was the development of the Venereal Disease Research Laboratory (VDRL), a non-treponemal diagnostic test now widely used. This sign of research and medical progress was instrumental for establishing a renowned position for the United States in the international research scenario, which served as an impetus for the ambition of many of the participating researchers [13,17].

By 1947, penicillin had long been established as the most effective treatment for syphilis and it was widely used for such purpose, leading to a significant decrease in the prevalence of the disease. Its efficacy was so clear that many even argued that syphilis would be completely eradicated in the near future. Nonetheless, researchers of the Tuskegee study continued to deny proper treatment to their subjects, and they were specifically warned against the use of penicillin and carefully shielded from receiving any information regarding its benefits. By the end of the study period, only 74 of the original 399 men were alive; 128 of them had died of syphilis and related complications, 40 of their wives had contracted the disease, and 19 children were diagnosed with congenital syphilis [16,22]. The relentless ambition of the Tuskegee researchers continued in spite of the establishment of the Nuremberg Code in 1947, the declaration of Helsinki in 1964, and the position of the Catholic Church urging physicians and scientists to always respect patients, superseding all scientific or research objectives [16,23].

In 1966, Peter Buxtun was the first researcher to speak publicly about his ethical concerns for the Tuskegee study. He warned the Division of Venereal Diseases about the practices and techniques being used in the study, but the Centers for Disease Control (CDC), now in charge of the experiment, argued for the importance of completing the study and obtained the support of local and national medical associations. In 1972, Buxtun took the story to the national press, which led to widespread outrage [16]. Congressional hearings were held, many researchers and physicians testified, and the deplorable objectives and practices of the study were exposed. The CDC appointed a review committee for the study, which finally determined that it was not justifiable from an ethical and medical standpoint, leading to its termination.

The Response: Belmont Report—Ethical Principles and Guidelines for the Protection of Human Subjects of Research, Report of the National Commission for the Protection of Human Subjects of Biomedical and Behavioral Research

The aftershocks of these revelations highlighted some of the main issues that afflicted the medical and scientific community of the time. As a response, the United States Congress passed the National Research Act in 1974. Its main concern was to guarantee stricter regulation and control of clinical trials. Now studies would always be required to pass through an Institutional Review Board, obtain inform consent from all study participants, and always inform and counsel participants regarding their diagnosis and study practices and techniques [24].

The National Research Act also created a Commission within the Department of Health and Human Services, destined to shape bioethics within the United States. The National Commission for the Protection of Human Subjects of Biomedical and Behavioral Research issued and published the Belmont Report in 1979. This report established three core principles that should always guide the design and review of clinical trials: respect for persons, beneficence, and justice. The first refers to one of the critical issues of the Tuskegee study—autonomy—and includes the mandatory need to obtain an informed consent from every study participant. This consent would be based on the truth, and not deception or misinformation. Beneficence refers to the basic principle of "do no harm," based on the conception of minimizing risk and maximizing benefits for the research participants. And finally, justice assures safe procedures that do not intend to exploit the participants, while arguing for a fair distribution of costs and benefits [25].

Global Disasters and Responses

Nazi Human Experimentation

The twentieth century was the background for spectacular international advances in the medical and scientific field, but some of them were associated with troubling events taking place against the international backdrop of a deadly war. The atrocities and horrendous experiments that took place during this time led to the death of most of the participants, but the few survivors were able to narrate their suffering and leave a record for history.

This period of science should be discussed and described in the light of the historical and sociopolitical events that took place at the time. Mainly, we need to point out two determining factors in order to understand the beginning of this period of Nazi experimentation and the nature of such experiments: (1) the political structure of Nazi Germany, based on a totalitarian system, and (2) the racial hygiene paradigm that arose from both political and social movements at the time. The origin of the latter preceded by roughly two decades that of the Nazi government; nonetheless, it was the totalitarianism of the time that allowed for such an ideology to flourish and to give rise to the scientific questions that were later addressed by researchers and physicians of the Nazi regime. All of them took place in a setting in which no legal or ethical boundaries existed, leading to the ideal conditions for such experimentation to take place [26].

Based on these ideas, many German scientists and physicians, mainly geneticists, found in the newly formed Nazi government the opportunity to put into practice their theories and discoveries, while at the same time, the government found in the researchers an opportunity to legitimize its political and social beliefs of racial superiority. The research scenario was further darkened by the complete violation of the civil rights of the Jewish population, which was then rendered as freely available "guinea pigs" for any research agenda. Resources were redistributed to any scientific quest that would improve the health of the superior race, and the focus of most research programs became heredity and fitness [27]. The most striking aspect of all of the experimentation that took place in the Nazi Germany is that there is no direct proof that any of the researchers involved were forced to participate, or that any of the research techniques and practices were merely imposed by the government [28,29].

The idea of biological inferiority led to unimaginable cruelty and disrespect for the unconsenting subjects. It is impossible to name and include all of the examples of such cruelty for the purpose of this review, but it is important to mention that most of the experiments conducted in the concentration camps followed the strict guidelines of clinical research of the time, some of them pursuing questions in accordance with the scientific progress of the time, though some of them used obsolete or outdated practices [26]. Some of the methods and results could even be considered innovative and helpful, as certain experiments were later continued by the conquering armies, aided by the same German physicians, but following the newly established laws of ethical research. It is fair to say, however, that regardless of the results or objectives of each study, their methods were always brutal, and researchers had a complete disregard for human life and suffering [28]. The main justification for their actions was based on the ideal of preserving the health and well-being of the population, at the same time that new critical knowledge was gained from such endeavors.

Response: The Nuremberg Code

After the end of World War II, all of the participants and collaborators of the Nazi government were brought to trial. The judgment of Nazi physicians in Nuremberg, known as the Nuremberg trial, is considered the precipitating event for the start of modern research ethics. From this trial, the founding principles of ethical research were established under the Nuremberg Code. It outlined 10 critical aspects for the conduction of experimentation with humans [30]:

- Obtaining voluntary consent from all participants, which should be based on complete and sufficient knowledge of the purpose, methods, and duration of the experiment.
- The main objective was to render fruitful results for the health and well-being of society, which could not be accomplished by any other method.
- Prior knowledge and animal research should be used as the base for any new research development.
- Researchers should avoid all unnecessary mental or physical suffering to participants.
- Experiments should not incur in any permanent injury or death, unless physicians were also considered participants in the study.
- Risk:benefit ratio should be evaluated, and risk should never be greater than possible benefits.
- All necessary tools and facilities should be available and provided to prevent injury, suffering, or death of subjects.
- Only highly trained and skilled personnel should conduct the research.
- Subjects are free to withdraw their participation if they reached their maximum point of physical and/or mental tolerance.
- Researchers should be willing and able to end any experiment if they believed that there was a risk to subjects' integrity.

Thalidomide in the International Context

As previously mentioned, the thalidomide disaster was of international magnitude. The initial reports of adverse events in both adults and newborns originated in Europe and Australia. Most of the affected patients were outside the United States. The first reports of the possible teratogenic effects of thalidomide came from Dr. William McBride, an Australian obstetrician, and Dr. Widuking Lenz, a German pediatrician, who proposed an association between the increase in birth defects and the use of thalidomide in pregnant women [31].

By 1958 the drug was sold as an over-the-counter medication in West Germany, and by 1961 46 countries were doing the same. One of the biggest concerns of its early distribution is that the medication was marketed as "completely safe," and it took several years before this claim would start crumbling. The pharmaceutical company initially dismissed the reports of irreversible peripheral neuropathy caused by long-term use of the drug. These reports were only considered serious on 1961, when West Germany restricted the market of thalidomide to only by prescription and forced the company to remove the "non-toxic" argument from the label. The second hit to the reputation of thalidomide started when doctors prescribing the medication to pregnant women noted a congruent increase in birth deformities, reaching an unprecedented incidence, with physicians delivering several cases of phocomelia per month. The reports suggested that the use of thalidomide during the first trimester of the pregnancy, probably even before the mother knew she was pregnant, could be associated with the problem. Again, the company denied the reports and qualified them as a cheap intent to murder a perfectly safe drug. Due to public pressure, the distribution of the medication was halted in Germany, but continued in other countries. Only when the news arrived of birth deformities did each country establish restrictions on the medication. Canada was the last country to stop the sale of thalidomide in 1962.

It is estimated that from the late 1950s to the early 1960s, over 13.000 babies were born with several deformities, including phocomelia, secondary to use of thalidomide during pregnancy. Many of them died soon after birth, but many lived long lives, with many surviving until 2010.

Response: Declaration of Helsinki in 1964

This document, prepared by the World Medical Association, consisted of an authoritative attestation of the importance of conducting previous concise and serious review of any research protocol with human experimentation, encouraging every researcher to apply the principles promulgated by the declaration. The initial document established clear boundaries for the conduct of clinical research, but left certain freedom for the investigator to decide if there were special circumstances for the experiment that allowed subjects to participate without previous informed consent.

In 1975, a revision was made that included the need for the review of research protocols by independent review boards. This declaration recognized that medical progress was based on research that will eventually include experimentation with human subjects, but clarified that the goal of gaining new knowledge should never surpass the need to protect the rights and health of the patients, including those participating in medical research. (For more information, see: the Declaration of Helsinki, World Medical Association; http://www.wma.net/en/30publications/10policies/b3/.)

THE PROCESS OF TESTING NEW INTERVENTIONS: STUDY PHASES

Based on the lessons learned from the major disasters in creation and commercialization of novel therapeutic drugs, the process for the development of a new drug or device has been systematized, and safety has become a major issue. The importance of safety evaluation is such that it is currently the first issue to be assessed during the development process, and it is also measured throughout the other phases of development.

Let us quickly summarize the drug development phases:

Preclinical study: Consists in completing a rigorous animal testing previous to application before the FDA for an investigational new drug (IND). Most drugs that undergo animal testing do not make it to human experimentation.

Phase I: Its main goal is to determine the pharmacokinetic and pharmacodynamics parameters of the drug and its safety in human subjects. It is mostly conducted in a group of 20–80 healthy volunteers. The main parameter to determine progression to Phase I is proof of safety (mainly no severe toxic effects).

Phase II: Its main goal is to obtain preliminary data on the efficacy of the medication on a given population. Usually, the study will be conducted in a group of diseased patients, which can range from a dozen to 300. The study should be controlled, meaning that the diseased population receiving the new drug being studied has to be compared to a control diseased population receiving either placebo or any standard medication available. This phase continues to evaluate for drug safety and short-term side effects.

Phase III: If evidence of effectiveness is shown in phase II studies, then the process can continue to phase III. The main goal of this phase is to assess effectiveness and safety. For this purpose, larger study populations should be evaluated and "real-life" conditions emulated, in order to assess the behavior of the drug when given at different doses, in heterogeneous populations or compared against the standard of care. The number of patients can range from several hundred to 3,000–10,000.

Phase IV: This phase is also known as post-marketing survey. It takes place after the drug has been approved by the FDA and has been put in the market. Post-marketing surveillance and commitment studies allow the FDA to collect further information on safety, efficacy, and tolerability profile of any given drug.

CASE STUDY: THERE IS NO FREE LUNCH—THE COST AND BENEFIT OF SEEKING THE CURE OF HIV INFECTION

Fabio Pinna, André Brunoni, and Felipe Fregni

Introduction

John Geegs is a PhD researcher form Pennsylvania University. He is one of the most prominent researchers in gene therapy, having published several influential articles in prestigious journals. Despite having a brilliant career with a solid position in academia, he has big dreams. As he describes himself, he is a "dreamer" who pursues nothing more than the final cure for HIV infection.

Since earning his PhD in Molecular, Cell, and Developmental Biology in one of the most competitive programs at UCLA, he has been dedicating his career to translational research. As a scientist, he has a passion for basic laboratory research, but also has an urgent need to apply these findings to clinical situations. In fact, he fits well with the NIH (National Institutes of Health) profile of a clinical translational scientist. As defined by this agency, "Translational research . . . is the process of applying discoveries generated during research in the laboratory, and in preclinical studies, to the development of trials and studies in humans [32]." It is also commonly known as taking knowledge from "bench to bedside." As a matter of fact, like most basic science research, Prof. Geegs's scientific breakthroughs have not yet been translated into major changes in medical therapy for humans. Truly, he deeply believes that gene therapy will be used in the near future in the treatment of severe conditions, such as cancer or HIV.

At his laboratory at UPenn, he mentors five brilliant young doctors—one of them, Dr. Ryan Stevenson, has the same dreams and passion for gene therapy as Prof. Geegs. Dr. Stevenson was born in Sweden but moved at a young age to the United States. His mother had a terrible condition—Li-Fraumeni syndrome (a rare autosomal dominant disorder associated with the *CHEK2* and the *TP53* genes that greatly increases the risk of developing several types of cancer, particularly in children and young adults, including breast cancer, brain tumors, sarcomas, leukemia, adrenocortical carcinoma, and others)—and she died at a very young age of a brain tumor. Luckily, Dr. Stevenson did not have the mutation of the p53 suppressor gene, but one of his sisters did, and she died at age 18 of adrenal carcinoma. He then decided to devote his life to medicine, and soon after he graduated with a degree in medicine in Chicago, he moved to UPenn for a PhD in molecular biology. His initial plans were to do a master's program and thereafter to start his residency in Oncology, but the outstanding reputation of Prof. Geegs and the belief that he could do more for patients as a researcher made him decide to follow this pathway. He felt that all the suffering that he had been through with his family's disease could bring something positive in the future.

Dr. Stevenson knows that although gene therapy is still in its infancy, it has been showing satisfactory results in the treatment of several hereditary diseases. As he likes to explain to the graduate students of Prof. Geegs (Dr. Stevenson is his teaching assistant in his course, Applied Molecular Biology) "gene therapy is based on the idea of gene insertions into one's cells and tissues in order to replace a mutant allele.

The replacement of non-functional genes can be done by insertion of multiple vectors being the use of different types of viruses—probably the most effective method!"

A Cold Winter in Pennsylvania and the Jesse Gelsinger Case

It was a late afternoon of a cold winter in Pennsylvania. Although Prof. Geegs does not enjoy cold weather, as he lived most of his life in Southern California, for him, winter is a particularly productive season, as students are often busy with final exams and grant deadlines are usually in the spring. On one of these cold days, in a staff meeting, Prof. Geegs and his team were having a pleasant chat while having coffee and talking about designing a new HIV phase I study using gene therapy. Although the conversation was collegial and pleasant, suddenly there was a moment of awkwardness in the room, and Prof. Geegs with a sad look said to his staff, "OK—let us discuss the "elephant in the room"—we shall never forget the Gelsinger case!" and he started talking about it:

"As not all of you know, let me narrate again this important ethical case. Jesse Gelsinger was an 18-year-old patient who suffered from onithine transcarbamilase defciency, an X-linked genetic disease of the liver that is characterized by the liver's inability to metabolize ammonia, a byproduct of protein breakdown. Indeed, the disease is usually fatal at birth. However, Jesse Gelsinger had the non-severe form of the disease, as some of his cells were normal, which enabled him to survive on a restricted diet and special medications. Gelsinger was really excited to join a UPenn phase I trial that aimed at developing a new drug for children born with the severe form of the disease. He was the last subject of his group. During the phase I study, Gelsinger was injected with adenoviruses carrying a corrected gene to test the safety of the procedure. Four days later, he died by immune response triggered by the use of the vector used to transport the gene into his cells. Consequently, this led to multiple organ failure and brain death. Afterward, the FDA (Food and Drug Administration) ran an investigation on this case and concluded that this phase I trial broke several rules of conduct, such as:

1. Inclusion of Gelsinger as a substitute for another volunteer who dropped out, despite having high ammonia levels that should have led to his exclusion from the trial;
2. Failure by the university to report that two patients had experienced serious side effects from the gene therapy; and
3. Failure to mention the deaths of monkeys given a similar treatment in the informed consent documentation.

After this terrible incident, which shot down human research at UPenn for several months and led to a detailed investigation, UPenn paid the parents an amount of money in settlement. Both the university and the principal investigator (PI) had serious financial stakes."

Finishing his thoughts, Prof. Geegs concluded, "The Gelsinger case was an important setback for phase I studies in gene therapy."

Dr. Stevenson, thinking about his family with Li-Fraumeni syndrome, said, "The thought of benefits at any cost has brought up terrible lessons for humankind such as the Tuskegee Study in 1932 [a syphilis experiment conducted between 1932 and 1972 in Tuskegee, Alabama, by the US Public Health Service in which impoverished African-Americans with syphilis were recruited in order to study the natural progression of the untreated disease] or the thalidomide case in 1959 in Germany [a drug that was used to inhibit morning sickness during pregnancy and resulted in thousands of babies being born with abnormalities such as phocomelia]. We should not disregard the issue of ethics and regulatory requirements in any phase of a drug trial, especially phase I!"

Prof. Geegs looked at his watch and realized he was late to meet a group of researchers from Japan who had come to visit his laboratory. He then wrapped up the discussion, "Guys, let us continue this discussion tomorrow; and I also want you to do a bit of research on the phases of a trial, so we can continue our discussion."

Phases of a Trial

In the investigation of a new drug, sequences of clinical trials must be carried out. Each phase of a trial seeks to provide different types of information about the treatment in relation to dosage, safety, and efficacy of the investigational new drug (IND).

Preclinical research: Before using an IND in humans, tests should be taken in the laboratory usually using animal models. If an IND shows good results in this phase, then researchers are able to request permission to start studies in humans.

Phase I trial: The aim of this phase is to show that the IND is safe. Data are collected on side effects, timing, and dosage. Usually dosage is increased until a maximum dosage (predetermined) or development of adverse effects are found. It usually requires a small sample size of subjects and it helps researchers to understand the mechanism of action of a drug. Much of the pharmakocinetics and pharmacodynamics of INDs are researched in this phase. Also during this phase, the drug is usually tested in healthy subjects, except for some drugs such as oncologic and HIV drugs.

Phase II trial: Once an IND is found to be safe in humans, phase II trials focus on demonstrating that it is effective. This is also done in relatively small sample sizes, in studies often referred to as "proof-of-principle" studies. The response rate should be at least the same as standard treatment to encourage further studies. These small trials are usually placebo-controlled.

Phase III trial: Also referred to as pivotal studies, they represent large studies with large samples and are usually (but not always) designed as a randomized, double-blinded trial comparing the IND to the standard treatment and/or placebo. Successful outcomes in two phase III trials would make a new drug likely to be approved by the FDA.

Phase IV trial: Also referred to as post-marketing studies, in phase IV trials, approved drugs are tested in other diseases and populations and usually in an open-label fashion.

Early Morning Meeting and Gene Therapy in HIV

The next morning, Prof. Geegs arrived in the lab's small conference room. Prof. Geegs started the meeting, saying, "Because Dr. Wang is our new post-doctoral fellow from Beijing, China, I want someone to explain our preliminary HIV study to her." Dr. Stevenson, the senior post-doc, quickly volunteered: "It will be a pleasure to do so.

Our team at the University of Pennsylvania School of Medicine has recently reported the first clinical test of a new gene therapy based on a disabled AIDS virus carrying genetic material that inhibits HIV replication. In this first trial, we studied five subjects with chronic HIV infection who had failed to respond to at least two antiretroviral regimens, giving them a single infusion of their own immune cells that had been genetically modified for HIV resistance. In the study, viral loads of the patients remained stable or decreased during the study, and one subject showed a sustained decrease in viral load. T-cell counts remained steady or increased in four patients during the nine-month trial. Additionally, in four patients, immune function specific to HIV improved." Prof. Geegs, who was extremely excited about these findings (and the approval for the paper's publication in Proceedings of the National Academy of Sciences (PNAS)), could not resist interrupting and added, "Overall, our results are significant, because it is the first demonstration of safety in humans for a lentiviral vector (of which HIV is an example) for any disease." Although Dr. Wang was still jet-lagged from her long trip to the United States, she added, "Thank you so much, Dr. Stevenson. In fact, we appreciate the work of Prof. Geegs in Beijing and it is a wonderful opportunity to be here in the lab. What is the next step now?" Prof. Geegs responded, "Our results are good, but they are preliminary—meaning that we shall replicate it in a larger population. We have much more work to do. In the study we are planning, each patient will now be followed for 15 years."

Stevenson completed with the details of this new study, "The new vector is a lab modified HIV that has been disabled to allow it to function as a 'Trojan horse,' carrying a gene that prevents new infectious HIV from being produced." He continued, "Essentially, the vector puts a wrench in the HIV replication process. Instead of chemical- or protein-based HIV replication blockers, this approach is genetic and uses a disabled AIDS virus which carries an anti-HIV genetic payload. This approach enables patients' own T-cells, which are targets for HIV, to inhibit HIV replication—via the HIV vector and its anti-viral cargo."

Dr. Cameron, an extremely educated research fellow from Australia, then made a comment, "I believe that it is wonderful to go in this direction instead of drugs only as they have significant toxicity, but in the first trial, patients were still taking the drug. Do you think patients would be able to stay off drugs with this gene therapy, Prof. Geegs?"

Prof. Geegs liked to stimulate his fellows to think, and he asked Stevenson to respond—which he quickly did, with a subtle smile, "That is an excellent point, which is why, in this second trial using the new vector with HIV patients, we will select a group of patients who are generally healthier and use six infusions rather than one—we therefore want to evaluate the safety of multiple infusions and test the effect of infusions on the patients' ability to control HIV after removal of their anti-retroviral drugs. The hope is that this treatment approach may ultimately allow patients to stay off antiretroviral drugs for an extended period. This would be a great breakthrough for this laboratory."

Prof. Geegs quickly concluded, "But we should never forget the Gelsinger case as, you know, *fool me once, shame on you; fool me twice, shame on me* . . .. Our group should then reflect on the ethical implications in this case. I want you guys thinking about this subject tonight and send an email to the group with your conclusions. Looking forward to hearing back from you!"

Dr. Cameron—The First Email: Email Subject, "Too Risky for Subjects"

He starts the message with his usual politeness:

Greetings my dearest colleagues,
We obviously cannot predict or control all the possible side effects that can occur—or will probably occur, considering the risks of our investigational therapy. Although the pilot trial was OK, it had only a few patients and we do not know very well what the long-term effects of gene therapy may be. In addition, we cannot even submit our study to a grant; reviewers would kill our proposal very quickly. I would respectfully suggest to go back to our lab and think again about the next steps.

Warmest regards,
Cameron

Dr. Stevenson—The Quick Emotional Reply: Email Subject, "Risks Are Justified Based on Potential Individual Benefits"

Stevenson, thinking about his family, goes directly to the point:

Thanks Cameron—Remember our first study! We saw a significant decrease in viral load in two patients, and in one patient, a very dramatic decrease. There is hope here . . . . Imagine that you have HIV, you would like to enroll in a trial that could make you stop taking medications and perhaps be cured . . . . *No pain, no gain!* . . . we should go on with our trial!

Dr. Wang—The Late Response: Email Subject, "Risks Are Justified Based on the Knowledge Being Produced—Benefits for Society"

Dr. Wang had not been sleeping well due to problems adjusting. She then replied at 3 a.m. to the group:

Dear All,
Thank you for sharing so much knowledge. One point that I believe we should consider is the potential benefit for society. In fact I have reservations of having a trial that might benefit individuals. This is called "therapeutic misconception"—when subjects interpret a clinical trial as therapy rather than producing knowledge. But in this case as this study might benefit future patients, I think there is a reasonable justification for this trial.

Best wishes,
Sleepless Wang :)

The Next Morning

After reading all the emails, Prof. Geegs called all the fellows into his office, "OK! I enjoyed the discussion. Now I want everyone to rest and perhaps enjoy the last winter weekend and next Monday we will discuss this ethics issue again. By now, I just ask you to reflect on combining ethics, benefits, and minimizing risks."

CASE DISCUSSION

This case illustrates how ethical dilemmas can influence the design of any given study. Particularly, the readers should pay special attention to the study phases of a given study and how to design a study of a novel intervention while keeping the safety of subjects as a main concern. The readers need also to identify that a clinical goal should not be applicable to a design of a given study; the clinician-scientist needs to use a different "hat" when designing and conducting a clinical study.

CASE QUESTIONS FOR REFLECTION

The following questions can be used to reflect on this case:

1. What challenges does Prof. Geegs face in choosing the next steps for his HIV study?
2. What are Prof. Geegs's main concerns?
3. What should he consider in making this decision?

FURTHER READING

Articles

Azeka E, Fregni F, Auler Junior JO. The past, present and future of clinical research. *Clinics.* 2011; 66(6): 931–2. [PMCID: PMC3129946] (Outstanding article in order to grasp the outline of clinical research)

Bhatt A. Evolution of clinical research: a history before and beyond James Lind. *Perspect Clin Res.* 2010 Jan–Mar; 1(1): 6–10. [PMCID: PMC3149409]

Blixen CE, Papp KK, Hull AL, et al. Developing a mentorship program for clinical researchers. *J Contin Educ Health Prof.* 2007 Spring; 27(2): 86–93. [PMID: 17576629]

Drucker CB. Ambroise Paré and the Birth of the Gentle Art of Surgery. Yale J Biol Med. 2008 December; 81(4): 199–202. [PMCID: PMC2605308]

Glickman SW, McHutchison JG, Peterson ED, et al. Ethical and scientific implications of the globalization of clinical research. *N Engl J Med.* 2009 Feb 19; 360(8): 816–823. [PMID: 19228627]

Goffee R, Jones G. Managing authenticity: the paradox of great leadership. *Harv Bus Rev.* 2005 Dec; 83(12): 86–94, 153. [PMID: 16334584]

Herzlinger RE. Why innovation in health care is so hard. *Harv Bus Rev.* 2006 May; 84(5): 58–66, 156. [PMID: 16649698]

Kottow MH. Should research ethics triumph over clinical ethics? *J Eval Clin Pract.* 2007 Aug; 13(4): 695–698. [PMID: 17683317]

Murgo AJ, Kummar S, Rubinstein L, Anthony JM, et al. Designing phase 0 cancer trials. *Clin Cancer Res.* 2008 Jun 15; 14(12): 3675–3682. [PMCID: PMC2435428]

Umscheid CA, Margolis DJ, Grossman CE. Key concepts of clinical trials: a narrative review. *Postgrad Med.* 2011 Sep; 123(5): 194–204.

Wilson JM. Lessons learned from the gene therapy trial for ornithine transcarbamylase deficiency. *Mol Genet Metab.* 2009 Apr; 96(4): 151–157. [PMID: 19211285].

Books

Beauchamp TL, Childress JF. *Principles of biomedical ethics*, 7th ed. New York: Oxford University Press; 2012. (7th edition of the first major American bioethics textbook, written by co-author of the Belmont Report)

Gallin JI, Ognibene FP. *Principles and practice of clinical research*, 3rd ed. Burlington, VT: Academic Press; 2012.

Groopman J. *How doctors think*. Boston, MA: Mariner Books; 2008.

Robertson D, Gordon HW. *Clinical and translational science: principles of human research*. Burlington, VT: Academic Press; 2008.

Online

FDA CFRs for regulations in details. www.fda.com
http://cme.nci.nih.gov/
http://firstclinical.com/journal/2008/0806_IIR.pdf
http://ohsr.od.nih.gov/
http://www.availclinical.com/clinical-study/clinical-trials-history/
http://www.cioms.ch
http://www.fda.gov
http://www.james.com/beaumont/dr_life.htm
http://www.niehs.nih.gov/research/resources/bioethics/whatis/
http://www.wma.net
https://web.archive.org/web/20131021022424/http://www.innovation.org/index.cfm/InsideDrugDiscovery/Inside_Drug_Discovery
https://web.archive.org/web/20120526134445/http://www.nihtraining.com/cc/ippcr/current/downloads/HisClinRes.pdf
https://web.archive.org/web/20160401233046/http://www.cancer.org/treatment/treatmentsandsideeffects/clinicaltrials/whatyouneedtoknowaboutclinicaltrials/clinical-trials-what-you-need-to-know-phase0

REFERENCES

1. Bull JP, A study of the history and principles of clinical therapeutic trials. MD Thesis, University of Cambridge, 1951. Available at http://jameslindlibrary.org/wp-data/uploads/2014/05/bull-19511.pdf
2. Streptomycin Treatment of Pulmonary Tuberculosis. *BMJ.* 1948; 2(4582): 769–782.
3. Burley DM, Dennison TC, Harrison W. Clinical experience with a new sedative drug. *Practitioner.* 1959; 183: 57–61.
4. Lasagna L. Thalidomide: a new nonbarbiturate sleep-inducing drug. *J Chronic Dis.* 1960; 11: 627–631.
5. Ghoreishni K. Thalidomine. In: *Encyclopedia of toxicology*. Burlington, VT: Academic Press; 2014: 523–526.
6. Rice E. Dr. Frances Kelsey: Turning the thalidomide tragedy into Food and Drug Administration Reform. 2007. Available at http://www.section216.com/history/Kelsey.pdf
7. Kelsey FO. Inside story of a medical tragedy. *U.S. News & World Report.* 1962; 13: 54–55.

8. Fullerton PM, Kremer M. Neuropathy after intake of thalidomide (distaval). *Br Med J.* 1961; 2(5256): 855–858.
9. Mintz M. *By prescription only*, 2nd ed. Boston: Houghton Mifflin; 1967.
10. Tighter rein on drug testing. *Business Week.* January 12, 1963.
11. The Kefauver Hearings: the drug industry finally has its day and does quite well. *Science.* 1961; 134(3494): 1968–1970.
12. The drug hearings: to no one's surprise, Kefauver and the AMA do not agree on what should be done. *Science.* 1961; 134(3472): 89–92.
13. Cuerda-Galindo E, Sierra-Valentí X, González-López E, et al. Syphilis and human experimentation from World War II to the present: a historical perspective and reflections on ethics. *Actas Dermosifiliogr.* 2014; 105(9): 847–853.
14. Jones, J. *Bad blood: The Tuskegee syphilis experiment—a tragedy of race and medicine.* New York: The Free Press; 1981.
15. Gjestland T. The Oslo study of untreated syphilis: an epidemiologic investigation of the natural course of the syphilitic infection based upon a re-study of the Boeck-Bruusgaard material. *Acta Derm Venereol Suppl (Stockh).* 1955; 35(Suppl 34): 3–368; Annex I–LVI.
16. Heller J. Syphilis victims in U.S. study went untreated for 40 years: syphilis victims got no therapy. *New York Times.* July 26, 1972. Associated Press.
17. Carmack HJ, Bates BR, Harter LM. Narrative constructions of health care issues and policies: the case of President Clinton's apology-by-proxy for the Tuskegee syphilis experiment. *J Med Humanit.* 2008; 29(2): 89–109.
18. Edmundson WF, Ackerman JH, Gutierrez-Salinas E, et al. Study of the TPI test in clinical syphilis. 1. Untreated early symptomatic syphilis. *AMA Arch Derm Syphilol.* 1954; 70(3): 298–301.
19. Olansky S, Simpson L, Schuman SH. Environmental factors in the Tuskegee study of untreated syphilis. *Public Health Rep.* 1954; 69(7): 691–698.
20. Peters JJ, Peers JH, Olansky S, et al. Untreated syphilis in the male Negro; pathologic findings in syphilitic and nonsyphilitic patients. *J Chronic Dis.* 1955; 1(2): 127–48.
21. Schuman SH, Olansky S, Rivers E, et al. Untreated syphilis in the male negro; background and current status of patients in the Tuskegee study. *J Chronic Dis.* 1955; 2(5): 543–558.
22. Katz RV, Kegeles SS, Kressin NR, et al. The Tuskegee Legacy Project: willingness of minorities to participate in biomedical research. *J Health Care Poor Underserved.* 2006; 17(4): 698–715.
23. Yoon C. Families emerge as silent victims of Tuskegee syphilis experiment. *New York Times,* May 12, 1997.
24. Stuart H. *History of medical ethics.* Oxford: Elsevier; 1998: 3: 165–175.
25. Van Valey T. *Ethical guidelines and codes of conduct in social and behavioral research.* Oxford: Elsevier; 2015: 37–43.
26. Weindling P. *Nazi medicine and the Nuremberg trials.* New York: Houndmills; 2004.
27. Lopez-Munoz F, Alamo C, García-García P, et al. The role of psychopharmacology in the medical abuses of the Third Reich: from euthanasia programmes to human experimentation. *Brain Res Bull.* 2008; 77(6): 388–403.

28. Roelcke V. Nazi medicine and research on human beings. *Lancet*. 2004; 364(Suppl 1): s6–7.
29. Roelcke V, Maio G. *Twentieth century ethics of human subjects research*. Sttugart: Steiner; 2004.
30. Guraya SY, London NJM, Guraya SS. Ethics in medical research. *Journal of Microscop and Ultrestructure*. 2014; 2: 121–126.
31. Lenz W, Knapp K. Thalidomide embryopathy. *Arch Environ Health*. 1962; 5: 100–105.
32. National Institutes of Health. RFA-RM-07-007: Institutional Clinical and Translational Science Award (U54). Mar 2007, Available at http://grants.nih.gov/grants/guide/rfa-files/RFA-RM-07-007.html.

2

SELECTION OF THE RESEARCH QUESTION

Authors: *Keiko Ueda and Lotfi B. Merabet*

Case study authors: *André Brunoni and Felipe Fregni*

The difficulty in most scientific work lies in framing the questions rather than in finding the answers.
—Arthur E. Boycott (Pathologist, 1877–1938)

The grand aim of all science is to cover the greatest number of empirical facts by logical deduction from the smallest number of hypotheses or axioms.
—Albert Einstein (Physicist, 1879–1955)

INTRODUCTION

The previous chapter provided the reader with an overview of the history of clinical research, followed by an introduction to fundamental concepts of clinical research and clinical trials. It is important to be aware of and to learn lessons from the mistakes of past and current research in order to be prepared to conduct your own research. As you will soon learn, developing your research project is an evolutionary process, and research itself is a continuously changing and evolving field.

Careful conceptual design and planning are crucial for conducting a reproducible, compelling, and ethically responsible research study. In this chapter, we will discuss what should be the first step of any research project, that is, how to develop your own research question. The basic process is to select a topic of interest, identify a research problem within this area of interest, formulate a research question, and finally state the overall research objectives (i.e., the specific aims that define what you want to accomplish).

You will learn how to define your research question, starting from broad interests and then narrowing these down to your primary research question. We will address the key elements you will need to define for your research question: the study population, the intervention (x, independent variable[s]), and the outcome(s) (y, dependent variable[s]). Later chapters in this volume will discuss popular study designs and elements such as covariates, confounders, and effect modifiers (interaction) that will help you to further delineate your research question and your data analysis plan.

Although this chapter is not a grant-writing tutorial, most of what you will learn here has very important implications for writing a grant proposal. In fact, the most important part of a grant proposal is the "specific aims" page, where you state your research question, hypotheses, and objectives.

HOW TO SELECT A RESEARCH QUESTION

What Is a Research Question?

A research question is an inquiry about an unanswered scientific problem. The purpose of your research project is to find the answer to this particular research question. Defining a research question can be the most difficult task during the design of your study. Nevertheless, it is fundamental to start with the research question, as it is strongly associated with the study design and predetermines all the subsequent steps in the planning and analysis of the research study.

What Is the Importance of a Research Question?

Defining the research question is instrumental for the success of your study. It determines the study population, outcome, intervention, and statistical analysis of the research study, and therefore the scope of the entire project.

A novice researcher will often jump to methodology and design, eager to collect data and analyze them. It is always tempting to try out a new or "fancy" method (e.g., "Let's test this new proteomic biomarker in a pilot study!" or "With this Luminex assay we can test 20 cytokines simultaneously in our patient serum!"), but this mistake all too often makes the research project a "fishing expedition," with the unfortunate outcome that a researcher has invested hours of work and has obtained reams of data, only to find herself at an impasse, and never figuring out what to do with all the information collected. Although it is not wrong to plan an exploratory study (or a hypothesis-generating study), such study has a high risk of not yielding any useful information; thus all the effort to have the study performed will be lost. When planning an exploratory or pilot study (with no defined research question), the investigator must understand the goals and the risks (for additional discussion on pilot studies, see Lancaster et al. 2002).

It is important to first establish a concept for your research. You must have a preset idea or a working hypothesis in order to be able to understand the data you will generate. Otherwise, you will not be able to differentiate whether your data were obtained by chance, by mistake, or if they actually reflect a true finding. Also, have in mind ahead of time how you would like to present your study at a conference, in a manuscript, or in a grant proposal. You should be able to present your research to your audience in a well-designed manner that reflects a logical approach and appropriate reasoning.

A good research question leads to useful findings that may have a significant impact on clinical practice and health care, regardless of whether the results are positive or negative. It also gives rise to the next generation of research questions. Therefore, taking enough time to develop the research question is essential.

Where Do Research Questions Come From?

How do we find research questions? As a clinical research scientist, your motivation to conduct a study might be driven by a perceived knowledge gap, the urge to deepen your understanding in a certain phenomenon, or perhaps to clarify contradictory existing findings. Maybe your bench research implies that your findings warrant translation into a study involving patients in a clinical setting. Maybe your clinical work experience gives you the impression that a new intervention would be more effective for your patients compared to standard treatment. For example, your results could lead you to ask, "Does this drug really prolong life in patients with breast cancer?" or, "Does this procedure really decrease pain in patients with chronic arthritis?"

Once you have identified a problem in the area you want to study, you can refine your idea into a research question by gaining a firm grasp of "what is known" and "what is unknown." To better understand the research problem, you should learn as much as you can about the background pertaining to the topic of interest and specify the gap between current understanding and unsolved problems. As an early step, you should consult the literature, using tools such as MEDLINE or EMBASE, to gauge the current level of knowledge relevant to your potential research question. This is essential in order to avoid spending unnecessary time and effort on questions that have already been solved by other investigators. Meta-analyses and systematic reviews are especially useful to understand the combined level of evidence from a large number of studies and to obtain an overview of clinical trials associated with your questions. You should also pay attention to unpublished results and the progress of important studies whose results are not yet published. It is important to realize that there likely are negative results produced but never published. You can inspect funnel plots obtained from meta-analyses or generated from your own research (see Chapter 14 in this volume for more details) to estimate if there has been publication bias toward positive studies. Also, be aware that clinical trials with aims similar to those of your study might still be ongoing. To find this information, you can check the public registration of trials using sites such as clinicaltrials.gov.

HOW TO DEVELOP THE RESEARCH QUESTION: NARROW DOWN THE QUESTION

Once you have selected your research topic, you need to develop it into a more specific question. The first step in refining a research question is to narrow down a *broad research topic* into a specific description (*narrow research question*) that covers the four points of *importance, feasibility, answerability,* and *ethicality.*

Importance: Interesting, Novel, and Relevant

Your research can be descriptive, exploratory, or experimental. The purpose of your research can be for diagnostic or treatment purposes, or to discover or elucidate a certain mechanism. The point you will always have to consider when making a plan for your study, however, is how to justify your research proposal. Does your research question have scientific relevance? Can you answer the "so what" question? You need to describe the importance of your research question with careful consideration of the following elements:

- *The disease (condition or problem)*: Novelty, unmet need, or urgency are important. What is the prevalence of this disease/condition? Is there a pressing need for further discoveries regarding this topic because of well-established negative prognoses (e.g., HIV, pancreatic cancer, or Alzheimer's disease)? Are existing treatment options limited, too complex or costly, or otherwise not satisfactory (e.g., limb replacement, face transplantation)? Does the research topic reflect a major problem in terms of health policy, medical, social, and/or economic aspects (e.g., smoking, hypertension, or obesity)?

- *The intervention*: Is it a new drug, procedure, technology, or medical device (e.g., stem-cell derived pacemaker or artificial heart)? Does it concern an existing drug approved by the Food and Drug Administration (FDA) for a different indication (e.g., is Rituximab, a drug normally indicated for malignant lymphoma, effective for systemic lupus erythematosus or rheumatoid arthritis)? Is there new evidence for application of an existing intervention in a different population (e.g., is Palivizumab also effective in immunodeficiency infants, not only in premature infants to prevent respiratory syncytial virus)? Have recent findings supported the testing of a new intervention in a particular condition (e.g., is a β-blocker effective in preventing cardiovascular events in patients with chronic renal failure)? Even a research question regarding a standard of care intervention can be valuable if in the end it can improve the effectiveness of clinical practice.

Feasibility

In short, be realistic: novel research tends to jump right away into very ambitious projects. You should carefully prove the feasibility of your research idea to prevent wasting precious resources such as time and money:

- *Patients*: Can you recruit the required number of subjects? Do you think your recruitment goal is realistic? Rare diseases such as Pompe or Fabry's disease will pose a challenge in obtaining a sufficient sample size. Even common diseases, depending on your inclusion criteria and regimen of intervention, may be difficult to recruit. Does your hospital have enough patients? If not, you may have to consider a *multicenter* study. What about protocol *adherence* and *dropouts*? Do you expect significant deviations from the protocol? Do you need to adjust your sample size accordingly?
- *Technical expertise*: Are there any established measurements or diagnostic tools for your study? Can the outcome be measured? Is there any established diagnostic tool? Do we have any standard techniques for using the device (e.g., guidelines for echocardiographic diagnosis for congenital heart disease)? Is there a defined optimal dose? Can you operate the device, or can the skill be learned appropriately (e.g., training manual for transcutaneous atrial valve replacement)? *A pilot study or small preliminary study* can be helpful at this stage to help answer these preliminary questions.
- *Time*: Do you have the required time to recruit your patients? Is it possible to *follow up* with patients for the entire time of the proposed study period (e.g., can you follow preterm infant development at 3, 6, and 9 years of age)? When do you need to have your results in order to apply for your next grant?
- *Funding*: Does you budget allow for the scope of your study? Are there any research grants you can apply for? Do the funding groups' interests align with those of your study? How realistic are your chances of obtaining the required funding? If there are available funds, how do you apply for the grant?

- *Team*: How about your research environment? Do your *mentors* and *colleagues* share your interests? What kind of specialists do you need to invite for your research? Do you have the staff to support your project (technicians, nurses, administrators, etc.)?

Answerability

New knowledge can only originate from questions that are answerable. A broad research problem is still a theoretical idea, and even if it is important and feasible, it still needs to be further specified. You should carefully investigate your research idea and consider the following:

- Precisely define what is known or not known and identify what area your research will address. The research question should demonstrate an understanding of the *biology, physiology,* and *epidemiology* relevant to your research topic. For example, you may want to investigate the prevalence and incidence of stroke after catheterization and its prognosis before you begin research on the efficacy of a new anticoagulant for patients who received catheter procedures. Again, you may need to conduct a *literature review* in order to clarify what is already known. Conducting *surveys* (*interviews* or *questionnaires*) initially could also be useful to understand the current status of your issues (e.g., how many patients a year are diagnosed with stroke after catherization in your hospital? What kind of anticoagulant is already being used for the patients? How old are the patients? How about the duration of cauterization techniques? etc.).
- The standard treatment should be well known before testing a new treatment. Are there any established treatments in your research field? Could your new treatment potentially replace the standard treatment or be complementary to the current treatment of choice? *Guidelines* can be helpful for discussion (e.g., American College of Cardiology/American Heart Association guidelines for anticoagulant therapy). Without knowing the current practice, your new treatment may never find its clinical relevance.
- We also need information about clinical issues for *diagnostic tests and interventions*. Are you familiar with the diagnoses and treatment of this disease (e.g., computerized tomography or magnetic resonance imaging to rule out stroke after catherization)? Do you know the *current guidelines*?

Ethical Aspects

Ethical issues should be discussed before conducting research. Is the subject of your research a controversial topic? The possible ethical issues will often depend largely on whether the study population is considered vulnerable (e.g., children, pregnant women, etc.; see Chapter 1) [1]. You must always determine the possible *risks and benefits* of your study intervention [1].

Finally, you may want to ask for *expert opinions* about whether your research *question is answerable* and relevant (no matter how strong your personal feelings may be about the relevance). To this end, a presentation of your idea or preliminary results at a study meeting early on in the project development can help refine your question.

HOW TO BUILD THE RESEARCH QUESTION

The next step of formulating a narrow research question is to focus on the primary interest (*primary question*): What is the most critical question for your research problem? You will define this primary question by addressing the key elements using the useful acronym PICOT (population, intervention, control, outcome, and time), while keeping in mind the importance, feasibility, answerability, and ethicality. Although PICOT is a useful framework, it does not cover all types of studies, especially some observational studies, for instance those investigating predictors of response (E [exposure] instead of I [intervention] is used for observational studies). But for an experimental study (e.g., a clinical trial), the PICOT framework is extremely useful to guide formulation of the research question.

Building the Research Question: PICOT

P (Population or Patient)

What is the *target population* of your research? The target population is the population of interest from which you want to draw conclusions and inferences. Do you want to study mice or rabbits? Adults or children? Nurses or doctors? What are the characteristics of the study subjects, and what are the given problems that should be considered? You may want to consider the pathophysiology (acute or chronic?) and the severity of the disease (severe end stage or early stage?), as well as factors such as geographical background and socioeconomic status.

Once you decide on the target population, you may select a sample as the *study population* for your study. The *study population* is a subset of the target population under investigation. However, it is important to remember that the *study population* is not always a perfect representation of the target population, even when sampled at random. Thus, defining the *study population* by the inclusion and exclusion criteria is a critical step (see Chapter 3).

Since only in rare cases will you be able to study every patient of interest, you will have to identify and select whom from the target population you want to study. This is referred to as the study sample. To do this requires choosing a method of selection or recruitment (see Chapter 7).

A specific study sample defined by restricted criteria will have a reduced number of covariates and will be more homogeneous, therefore increasing the chance of higher internal validity for your study. This also typically allows for the study to be smaller and potentially less expensive. In contrast, a restricted population might make it more difficult to recruit a sufficient number of subjects. On the other hand, recruitment can be easier if you define a broad population, which also increases the generalizability of your study results. However, a broad population can make the study larger and more expensive [2].

I (Intervention)

The *I* of the acronym usually refers to "intervention." However, a more general and therefore preferable term would be "independent variable." The independent variable is the explanatory variable of primary interest, also declared as x in the statistical analysis. The independent variable can be an intervention (e.g., a drug or a specific drug dose), a prognostic factor, or a diagnostic test. I can also be the exposure in an observational study. In an experimental study, I is referred to as the fixed variable (controlled by the investigator), whereas in an observational study, I refers to an exposure that occurs outside of the experimenter's control.

The independent variable precedes the outcome in time or in its causal path, and thus it "drives" the outcome in a cause-effect relationship.

C (Control)

What comparison or control is being considered? This is an important component when comparing the efficacy of two interventions. The new treatment should be superior to the *placebo*, when there is no standard treatment available. Placebo is a simulated treatment that has no pharmaceutical effects and is used to mask the recipients to potential expectation biases associated with participating in clinical trials. On the other hand, *active controls* could be used when an established treatment exists and the efficacy of the new intervention should be examined at least within the context of non-inferiority to the standard treatment. Also the control could be baseline in a one-group study.

O (Outcomes)

O is the dependent variable, or the outcome variable of primary interest; in the statistical analysis, it is also referred to as y. The outcome of interest is a random variable and can be a clinical (e.g., death) or a surrogate endpoint (e.g., hormone level, bone density, antibody titer). Selection of the primary outcome depends on several considerations: What can you measure in a timely and efficient manner? Which measurement will be relevant to understand the effectiveness of the new intervention? What is routinely accepted and established within the clinical community? We will discuss the outcome variable in more detail later in the chapter.

T (Time)

Time is sometimes added as another criterion and often refers to the follow-up time necessary to assess the outcome or the time necessary to recruit the study sample. Rather than viewing time as a separate aspect, it is usually best to consider time in context with the other PICOT criteria.

What Is the Primary Interest in your Research?

Once you have selected your study population, as well as the dependent and independent variables, you are ready to formulate your primary research question, the major specific aim, and a hypothesis. Even if you have several different ideas regarding your research problem, you still need to clearly define what the most important question of your research is. This is called your *primary question*. A research project may also contain additional secondary questions.

The primary question is the most relevant question of your research that should be driven by the hypothesis. Usually only one primary question should be defined at the beginning of the study, and it must be stated explicitly upfront [3]. This question is relevant for your sample size calculation (and in turn, for the power of your study—see Chapter 11).

The specific aim is a statement of what you are proposing to do in your research project.

The primary hypothesis states your anticipated results by describing how the independent variable will affect the dependent variable. Your hypothesis cannot be just speculation, but rather it must be grounded on the research you have performed and must have a reasonable chance of being proven true.

We can define more than one question for a study, but aside from the primary question, all others associated with your research are treated as *secondary questions*. Secondary questions may help to clarify the primary question and may add some information to the research study. What potential problems do we encounter with secondary questions? Usually, they are not sufficiently powered to be answered because the sample size is determined based on the *primary question*. Also, type I errors (i.e., false positives) may occur due to multiple comparisons if not adjusted for by the proper statistical analysis. Therefore, findings from secondary questions should be considered exploratory and hypothesis generating in nature, with new confirmatory studies needed to further support the results.

An *ancillary study* is a sub-study built into the main study design. Previous evidence may convince you of the need to test a hypothesis within a sub-group ancillary to the main population of interest (e.g., females, smokers). While this kind of study enables you to perform a detailed analysis of the subpopulation, there are limitations on the generalizability of an ancillary study since the population is usually more restricted (see Further Readings, Examples of Ancillary Studies).

Variables

It is important to understand thoroughly the study variables when formulating the study question. Here we will discuss some of the important concepts regarding the variables, which will be discussed in more detail in Chapter 8.

We have already learned that the *dependent variable* is the outcome, and *the independent* variable is the intervention. For study design purposes, it is important to also discuss how the outcome variables are measured. A good measurement requires reliability (precision), validity ("trueness"), and responsiveness to change. Reliability refers to how consistent the measurement is if it is repeated. Validity of a measurement refers to the degree to which it measures what it is supposed to measure. Responsiveness of a measurement means that it can detect differences that are proportional to the change of what is being measured with clinical meaningfulness and statistical significance.

Covariates are independent variables of secondary interest that may influence the relationship between the independent and dependent variables. Age, race, and gender are well-known examples. Since covariates can affect the study results, it is critical to control or adjust for them. Covariates can be controlled for by both planning (inclusion and exclusion criteria, placebo and blinding, sampling and randomization, etc.)

and analytical methods (e.g., covariate adjustment [see Chapter 13], and propensity scores [see Chapter 17]).

- *Continuous (ratio and interval scale), discrete, ordinal, nominal (categorical, binary) variables*: Continuous data represent all numbers (including fractions of numbers, floating point data) and are the common type of raw data. Discrete data are full numbers (i.e., integer data type; e.g., number of hospitalizations). Ordinal data are ordered categories (e.g., mild, moderate, severe). Nominal data can be either categorical (e.g., race) or dichotomous/binary (e.g., gender). Compared to other variables, continuous variables have more power, which is the ability of the study to detect an effect (e.g., differences between study groups) when it is truly present, but they don't always reflect clinical meaningfulness and therefore make interpretation more difficult. *Ordinal and nominal data* may better reflect the clinical significance (e.g., dead or alive, relapse or no relapse, stage 1 = localized carcinoma, etc.). However, ordinal and categorical data typically have less power, and important information may be lost (e.g., if an IQ less than 70 is categorized as developmental delay in infants, IQs of 50, 58, and 69 will all fall into the same category, while an IQ of 70 or more is considered to be normal development, although the difference is just 1 point). This approach is called categorization of continuous data, where a certain clinically meaningful threshold is set to make it easier to quickly assess study results. It is important to note that some authors differentiate between continuous and discrete variables by defining the former as having a quantitative characteristic and the latter as having a qualitative characteristic. This is a somewhat problematic classification, especially when it comes to ordinal data.
- *Single* and *multiple variables*: Having a *single variable* is simpler, as it is easier for clinical interpretation. Multiple valuables are efficient because we can evaluate many variables within a single trial, but these can be difficult to disentangle and interpret. *Composite endpoints* are combined multiple variables and are also sometimes used. Because each clinical outcome may separately require a long duration and a large sample size, combining many possible outcomes increases overall efficiency and enables one to reduce sample size requirements and to capture the overall impact of therapeutic interventions. Common examples include MACE (major adverse cardiac events) and TVF (target vessel failure: myocardial infarction in target vessel, target vessel reconstruction, cardiac death, etc.). Interpretation of the results has to proceed with caution, however (see section on case-specific questions) [9].
- *Surrogate variables (endpoints) and clinical variables (endpoints)*: Clinical variables directly assess the effect of therapeutic interventions on patient function and survival, which is the ultimate goal of a clinical trial. Clinical variables may include mortality, events (e.g., myocardial infarction, stroke), and occurrence of disease (e.g., HIV). A clinical endpoint is the most definitive outcome to assess the efficacy of an intervention. Thus, clinical endpoints are preferably used in clinical research. However, it is not always feasible to use clinical outcomes in trials. The evaluation of clinical outcomes presents some methodological problems since they require long-term follow-up (with problems of adherence, dropouts, competing risks, requiring larger sample sizes) and can make a trial more costly. At the same time, the clinical endpoint may be difficult to observe. For this reason, clinical scientists often use alternative outcomes to substitute for the clinical outcomes. So-called *surrogate*

endpoints are a more practical measure to reflect the benefit of a new treatment. Surrogate endpoints (e.g., cholesterol levels, blood sugar, blood pressure, viral load) are defined based on the understanding of the mechanism of a disease that suggests a clear relationship between a marker and a clinical outcome [8]. Also, a biological rationale provided by epidemiological data, other clinical trials, or animal data should be previously demonstrated. A surrogate is frequently a continuous variable that can be measured early and repeatedly and therefore requires shorter follow-up time, smaller sample size, and reduced costs for conducting a trial. Surrogate endpoints are often used to accelerate the process of new drug development and early stages of development, such as in phase 2 [10]. As a word of caution, too much reliance on surrogate endpoints alone can be misleading if the results are not interpreted with regard to validation, measurability, and reproducibility (see Further Reading) [4].

HOW TO EXPRESS A RESEARCH QUESTION
Hypothesis

Once a narrow research question is defined, you should clearly specify a hypothesis in the study protocol. A *hypothesis* is a statement about the expected results that predicts the effect of the independent on the dependent variable. A research hypothesis is essential to frame the experimental and statistical plan (statistics will be discussed in Unit II of this volume) and is also important to support the aim of the study in a scientific manuscript.

Types of Research Questions

To refine the research question and form the research hypothesis, we will discuss three types of research questions that investigate group differences, correlations, or descriptive measures. This classification is particularly important in discussing which statistical analysis is appropriate for your research question [5].

- *Basic/complex difference (group comparison) questions*: Samples split into groups by levels associated with the independent variable are compared by considering whether there is a difference in the dependent variable. If you have only one independent variable, the question is classified as a *basic difference question* (e.g., drug A will reduce time to primary closure in a 5-mm punch biopsy vs. placebo) and you would rely on a t-test or one-way analysis of variance (ANOVA) for the analysis. If you have two or more independent variables (e.g., drugs A and B led to a 15-mg/dl reduction in LDL cholesterol versus placebo, but there was no reduction with only drug A), this then becomes a *complex difference question* and is analyzed by other statistical methods, such as a factorial ANOVA.
- *Basic/complex associational (relational/correlation) questions*: The independent variable is correlated with the dependent variable. If there is only one dependent variable and one independent variable (e.g., is there a relationship between weight and natriuretic peptide levels?), it is called a *basic associational question,* and in this

situation, a correlation analysis is used. If there is more than one independent variable associated with one dependent variable (e.g., smoking and drinking alcohol are associated with lung cancer), it is called a *complex associational question*, and multiple regression is used for statistical analysis.
- *Basic/complex descriptive question*: The data are described and summarized using measures of central tendency (means, median, and mode), variability, and percentage (prevalence, frequency). If there is only one variable, it is called a *basic descriptive question* (e.g., how much MRSA isolates occur after the 15th day of hospitalization?); for more than one variable, a classification of *basic/complex descriptive question* is used.

Where Should You State Your Research Question?

Finally, where should you state your hypothesis? You may be writing for a research grant, research protocol, or manuscript. Usually, research questions should be stated in the introduction, immediately following the justification ("so what") section. Research questions should be clearly stated in the form of a hypothesis, such as "We hypothesize that in this particular population (P), the new intervention (I) will improve the outcome (O) more than the standard of care (C)."

A Research Question Should Be Developed over Time

It is important that the investigator spend a good amount of time developing his or her study question. During this process, everything we discussed in this chapter needs to be reviewed and the research question then needs to be refined as this process takes place. A good planning, starting with the research question, is one of the key components for a study's success.

Related Topics for Choosing the Research Question
Selecting the Appropriate Control in Surgical Studies or Other Challenging Situations

Let's think about various situations. Can we use placebo (sham) or another procedure as a control in a surgical trial? What exactly can be considered a placebo in surgical studies? How do we control for a placebo effect in surgical procedures?

Placebos can be used for the control group in clinical studies in comparison to a new agent if no standard of care is available. In order to fully assess the placebo effect in the control arm, participants have to be blinded. The control group could either have no surgery at all or undergo a "sham" procedure, but both options might be unethical depending on the given patient population [6]. In surgical studies, the control group usually receives the "traditional" procedure. In all cases, blinding might be very challenging and even impossible on certain levels (e.g., the surgeon performing the procedure). What about acupuncture? What would you consider a good control? What about cosmetic procedures?

Using Adverse Events as the Primary Research Question

Important questions concerning adverse effects can be answered in a clinical trial. However, as the typical clinical trial is performed in a controlled setting, the information regarding adverse effects is not always generalizable to the real-world setting. Thus, the clinical translation of the results needs careful consideration when carrying out a safety-focused study. The adverse reports from phase 4 (post-marketing marketing surveillance) are considered more generalizable information in drug development, although minimum safety data from phase 1 are required to proceed to subsequent study phases.

Also, it might not be easy to formulate a specific research question regarding adverse effects, as they might not be fully known in the early stage of drug development. This will also make it difficult to power the study properly (e.g., how many patients do we need to examine to show the statistically meaningful difference?).

When the Research Question Leads to Other Research Questions

Medical history is filled with interesting stories about research questions. And sometimes, it is not the intended hypothesis to be proven that yields a big discovery. For example, Sildenafil (Viagra) was initially developed by Pfizer for the treatment of cardiovascular conditions. Although clinical trials showed Sildenafil to have only little effect on the primary outcomes, it was quickly realized that an unexpected but marked "side effect" occurred in men. Careful investigation of clinical and pharmacological data generated the new research question, "Can Sildenafil improve erectile dysfunction?" This question was then answered in clinical trials with nearly 5,000 patients, which led to Sildenafil's FDA approval in 1998 as the first oral treatment for male erectile dysfunction [7]. The investigator must be attentive to novel hypothesis that can be learned from a negative study.

CASE STUDY: FINDING THE RESEARCH QUESTION

André Brunoni and Felipe Fregni

Dr. L. Heart is a scientist working on cardiovascular diseases in a large, busy emergency room of a tertiary hospital specialized in acute coronarian syndromes. While searching PUBMED, she found an interesting article on a new drug—which animal studies have demonstrated to be a powerful anti-thrombotic agent—showing its safety in healthy volunteers. She then feels that it would be the right time to perform a phase II trial, testing this new drug in patients presenting myocardial infarction (MI). She sees this as her big career breakthrough. However, when Dr. Heart starts writing a study proposal for the internal review board (ethics committee), she asks herself, "What is my research question?"[1]

Introduction

Defining the research question is, perhaps, the most important part of the planning of a research study. That is because the wrong question will eventually lead to a poor study design and therefore all the results will be useless; on the other hand, choosing an elegant, simple question will probably lead to a good study that will be meaningful to the scientific community, even if the results are negative. In fact, the best research question is one that, regardless of the results (negative or positive), produces interesting findings. In addition, a study should be designed with only one main question in mind.

However, choosing the most appropriate question is not always easy, as such a question might not be feasible to be answered. For instance, when researching acute MI, the most important question would be whether or not a new drug decreases mortality. However, for economic and ethical reasons, such an approach can only be considered when previous studies have already *suggested* that the new drug is a potential candidate. Therefore, the investigator needs to deal with the important issue of feasibility versus clinical relevance. Dr. Heart soon realized that her task would not be an easy one, and also that this task may take some time; she kept thinking about one of the citations in an article she recently read: "One-third of a trial's time between the germ of your idea and its publication in the *New England Journal of Medicine* should be spent fighting about the research question."[2]

"So What?" Test for the Research Question

Dr. Heart knows that an important test for the research question is to ask, "So what?" In other words, does the research question address an important issue? She knows,

---

[1] Dr. André Brunoni and Professor Felipe Fregni prepared this case. Course cases are developed solely as the basis for class discussion. The situation in this case is fictional. Cases are not intended to serve as endorsements or sources of primary data. All rights reserved to the authors of this case.

[2] Riva JJ, Malik KM, Burnie SJ, Endicott AR, Busse JW. What is your research question? An introduction to the PICOT format for clinicians. *J Can Chiropr Assoc.* 2012 Sep; 56(3):167–71.

for example, that the main agency funding in the United States, the NIH (National Institutes of Health), considers significance and innovation as important factors to fund grant applications. Dr. Heart also remembers something that her mentor used to tell her at the beginning of her career: "A house built on a weak foundation will not stand." She knows that even if she has the most refined design and uses the optimal statistical tests, her research will be of very little interest or utility if it does not advance the field. But regarding this point, she is confident that her research will have a significant impact in the field.

Next Step for the Research Question: How to Measure the Efficacy of the Intervention

Dr. L. Heart is in a privileged position. She works in a busy hospital that receives a significant amount of acute cardiovascular patients. She also has received huge departmental support for her research, meaning that she can run a wide range of blood exams to measure specific biological markers related to death in myocardial infarction. Finally, she has a PhD student who is a psychologist working with quality of life post-MI. Therefore, she asks herself whether she should rely on biological markers, on the assessment of quality of life, or if she should go to a more robust outcome to prove the efficacy of the new drug. She knows that this is one of the most critical decisions she has to make. It was a Friday afternoon. She had just packed up her laptop and the articles she was reading, knowing that she will have to make a decision by the end of the weekend.

Dr. Heart is facing a common problem: What outcome should be used in a research study? This needs to be defined for the research question. She knows that there are several options. For instance, the outcome might be mortality, new MI, days admitted to the emergency room, quality of life, specific effect of disease such as angina, a laboratory measure (cholesterol levels), or the cost of the intervention. Also, she might use continuous or categorical outcomes. For instance, if she is measuring angina, she might measure the number of days with angina (continuous outcome) or dichotomize the number of angina days in two categories (less than 100 days with angina vs. more or equal to 100 days with angina). She then lays out her options:

- *Use of clinical outcomes (such as mortality or new myocardial infarction)*: She knows that by using this outcome, her results would be easily accepted by her colleagues; however, using these outcomes will increase the trial duration and costs.
- *Use of surrogates (for instance, laboratorial measurements)*: One attractive alternative for her is to use some biomarkers or radiological exams (such as a catheterism). She knows a colleague in the infectious disease field who only uses CD4 for HIV trials as the main outcome. This would increase the trial feasibility. However, she is concerned that her biomarkers might not really represent disease progression.
- *Use of quality of life scales*: This might be an intermediate solution for her. However, she is still concerned with the interpretation of the results if she decides to use quality of life scales.

More on the Response Variable: *Categorical or Continuous?*

Even before making the final decision, Dr. Heart needs to decide whether she will use a continuous or categorical variable. She wishes now that she knew the basic concepts of statistics. However, she calls a colleague, who explains to her the main issue of categorical versus continuous outcomes—in summary, the issue is the trade-off of power versus clinical significance.

A categorical outcome usually has two categories (e.g., a yes/no answer), while a continuous outcome can express any value. A categorical approach might be more robust than a continuous one, and it also has more clinical significance, but it also decreases the power of the study due to the use of less information.[3] She is now at the crossroad of feasibility versus clinical significance.

Choosing the Study Population

Now that Dr. Heart has gone through the difficult decision of finding the best outcome measure, she needs to define the target population—that is, in which patients is she going to test the new drug? Her first idea is to select only patients who have a high probability of dying—for instance, males who smoke, are older than 75 years, with insulin-dependent diabetes and hypercholesterolemia. "Then," she thinks, "it will be easier to prove that the new drug is useful regardless of the population I study. But does that really sound like a good idea?"

The next step is to define the target population. Dr. Heart is inclined to restrict the study population, as she knows that this drug might be effective to a particular population of patients and therefore this increases her chances of getting a good result. In addition, she does remember from her statistical courses that this would imply a smaller variability and therefore she would gain power (power is an important currency in research, as it makes the study more efficient, decreasing costs and time to complete the study). On the other hand, she is concerned that she might put all her efforts in one basket—this is a risky approach, as this specific population might not respond, and she knows that broadening the population also has some advantages, for instance, the results would be more generalizable and it would be easier to recruit patients. But this would also increase the costs of the study.

But How about Other Ideas?

After a weekend of reflection, Dr. Heart called the staff for a team meeting and proudly explained the scenario and stated her initial thoughts. The staff was very eager to start a new study, and they made several suggestions: "We should also use echocardiography to assess the outcome!"; "Why don't we perform a genotypic analysis on these patients?"; "We need to follow them until one year after discharge." She started to become anxious again. What should she do with these additional suggestions? They all seem to be good ideas.

---

[3] These concepts will be discussed in details in Unit II of this volume.

When designing a clinical trial, researchers expose a number of subjects to a new intervention. Therefore, they want to extract as much data as possible from studies. On the other hand, it might not be possible to ask all of the questions, since this will increase the study's duration, costs, and personnel. Also, researchers should be aware that all the other outcomes assessed will be *exploratory* (i.e., their usefulness remains in suggesting possible associations and future studies) because studies are designed to answer a primary question only—and, as a principle of statistics, there is a 5% probability of observing a positive result just by chance (if you perform 20 tests, for instance, one of them will be positive just by chance!). But Dr. Heart knows that she can test additional hypotheses as secondary questions. She knows that there is another issue to go through: the issue of primary versus secondary questions.

Defining Her Hypothesis

After going through this long process, Dr. Heart is getting close to her research question. But now she needs to define the study hypotheses. In other words, what is her educated guess regarding the study outcome?

An important step when formulating a research question is to define the hypothesis of the study. This is important in terms of designing the analysis plan, as well as estimating the study sample size. Usually, researchers come up with study hypotheses after reviewing the literature and preliminary data. Dr. Heart can choose between a simple and a complex hypothesis. In the first case, her hypothesis would only have one dependent variable (i.e., the response variable) and one independent variable (e.g., the intervention). Complex hypotheses have more than one independent and/or dependent variable and might not be easy to use in planning the data analysis.

By the end of the day, Dr. Heart was overwhelmed with the first steps to put this study together. Although she is confident that this study might be her breakthrough and she needs to get her tenure track position at the institution where she works, she also knows she has only one chance and must be very careful at this stage. After wrestling with her thoughts, she finished her espresso and walked back to her office, confident that she knew what to do.

CASE DISCUSSION

Dr. Heart is a busy and ambitious clinical scientist and wants to establish herself within the academic ranks of her hospital. She has some background in statistics but seems to be quite inexperienced in conducting clinical research. She is looking for an idea to write up a research proposal and rightly conducts a literature research in her field of expertise, cardiovascular diseases. She finds an interesting article about a compound that has been demonstrated to be effective in an animal model and safe in healthy volunteers (results of a phase I trial). She now plans to conduct a phase II trial, but struggles to come up with a study design. The most vexing problem for her is formulating the research question.

Dr. Heart then reviews and debates aspects that have to be considered when delineating a research question. The main points she ponders include the following: determining the outcome with regard to feasibility (mainly concerning the time of follow-up when using a clinical outcome) versus clinical relevance (when using a surrogate outcome) and with regard to the data type to be used for the outcome (categorical vs. continuous); the importance of the research proposal (the need for a new anticoagulant drug); whether to use a narrow versus broad study population; whether to include only a primary or also secondary questions; and whether to use a basic versus complex hypothesis. Important aspects that Dr. Heart has not considered include the following: whether to test versus a control (although not mandatory in a phase II trial, it deserves consideration since she is investigating the effects of an anticoagulant and therefore adverse events should be expected, thus justifying the inclusion of a control arm) or to test several dosages (to observe a dose-response effect); logistics; the budget; and the overall scope of her project.

All these aspects are important and need careful consideration, but you have to wonder how this will help Dr. Heart come up with a compelling research question. Rather than assessing each aspect separately and making decisions based on advantages and disadvantages, it is recommended to start from a broad research interest and then develop and further specify the idea into a specific research question.

While Dr. Heart should be applauded for her ambition, she should also try to balance the level of risk of her research given her level of experience.

Finally, we should also question Dr. Heart's motives for conducting this study. What is her agenda?

CASE QUESTIONS FOR REFLECTION

1. What are the main challenges faced by Dr. Heart?
2. Should she be really concerned with the study question?
3. Which variable response should she choose? Justify your choice to your colleagues (remember, there is no right or wrong).
4. How should she select the study population?
5. Should her study have secondary questions?
6. Finally, try to create a study question for Dr. Heart in the PICOT format, depending on your previous selections.

FURTHER READING

Text

Haynes B, et al., Clinical epidemiology: how to do clinical practice research forming research questions; part 1. *Performing clinical research*, 3rd ed. Haynes B, Sackett DL, Guyatt GH, and Tugwell P; 2006: 3–14

Portney LG, Watkins MP. *Foundations of clinical research: applications to practice*. 3rd ed. Pearson; 2008: 121–139.

Surrogate Outcomes

D'Agostino RB. Debate: The slippery slope of surrogate outcomes. *Curr Contr Trials Cardiovasc Med.* 2000; 1: 76–78.

Echt DS, Liebson PR, Mitchell LB, et.al., Mortality and morbidity in patients receiving encainide, flecainide, or placebo: The Cardiac Arrhythmia Suppression Trial. *N Eng J Med.* 1991; 324: 781–788.

Feng M, Balter JM, Normolle D, et al. Characterization of pancreatic tumor motion using Cine-MRI: surrogates for tumor position should be used with caution. *Int J Radiat Oncol Biol Phys.* 2009 July 1; 74(3): 884–891.

Katz R. Biomarkers and surrogate markers: an FDA perspective. *NeuroRx.* 2004 April; 1(2): 189–195.

Lonn E. The use of surrogate endpoints in clinical trials: focus on clinical trials in cardiovascular diseases. *Pharmacoepidemiol Drug Safety.* 2001; 10: 497–508.

Composite Endpoint

Cordoba G, Schwartz L, Woloshin S, et al. Definition, reporting, and interpretation of composite outcomes in clinical trials: systematic review. *BMJ.* 2010; 341: c3920.

Kip KE, Hollabaugh K, Marroquin OC, et al. The problem with composite end points in cardiovascular studies. The story of major adverse cardiac events and percutaneous coronary intervention. *JACC.* 2008; 51(7): 701–707.

Examples of Ancillary Studies

Krishnan JA, Bender BG, Wamboldt FS, et al. Adherence to inhaled corticosteroids: an ancillary study of the Childhood Asthma Management Program clinical trial. *J Allergy Clin Immunol.* 2012; 129 (1): 112–118.

Udelson JE, Pearte CA, Kimmelstiel CD, et al. The Occluded Artery Trial (OAT) Viability Ancillary Study (OAT-NUC): influence of infarct zone viability on left ventricular remodeling after percutaneous coronary intervention versus optimal medical therapy alone. *Am Heart J.* 2011 Mar; 161(3): 611–621.

Controls, Sham/Placebo

Finnissa DG, Kaptchukb TJ, Millerc F et.al., Placebo effects: biological, clinical and ethical advances. *Lancet.* 2010 February 20; 375(9715): 686–695.

Macklin R. The ethical problems with sham surgery in clinical research. *N Engl J Med.* 1999 Sep 23; 341(13): 992–996.

Pilot Studies

Lancaster GA, Dodd S, Williamson PR. Design and analysis of pilot studies: recommendations for good practice. *J Eval Clin Pract.* 2002; 10(2): 307–312.

REFERENCES

1. The Belmont Report. Office of the Secretary. *Ethical principles and guidelines for the protection of human subjects of research.* The National Commission for the Protection of Human Subjects of Biomedical and Behavioral Research. Washington, DC: U.S. Government Printing Office, 1979.

2. Ferguson L. External validity, generalizability, and knowledge utilization. *J of Nursing Scholarship*. 2004; 36:1, 16–22.
3. CONSORT statement, http://www.consort-statement.org/consort-statement/]
4. Echt DS, Liebson PR, Mitchell LB, et al. Mortality and morbidity in patients receiving encainide, flecainide, or placebo: The Cardiac Arrhythmia Suppression Trial. *N Engl J Med*. 1991; 324: 781–788.
5. Morgan GA, Harmon RJ. Clinician's guide to research methods and statistics: research question and hypotheses. *J Am Acad Child Adolesc Psychiatry*. 2000; 39(2): 261–263.
6. Macklin R. The ethical problems with sham surgery in clinical research. *N Engl J Med*. 1999 Sep 23; 341(13): 992–996.
7. Campbell SF. Science, art and drug discovery: a personal perspective. *Clin Sci (Lond)*. 2000 Oct; 99(4): 255–260.
8. Lonn E. The use of surrogate endpoints in clinical trials: focus on clinical trial in cardiovascular disease. *Pharmacoepidemiol Drug Safety*. 2001; 10: 497–508.
9. Kip KE, Hollabaugh K, Marroquin OC, et al. The problem with composite end points in cardiovascular studies: the story of major adverse cardiac events and percutaneous coronary intervention. *JACC*. 2008; 51(7): 701–707
10. Katz R. Biomarkers and surrogate markers: an FDA perspective. *NeuroRx*. 2004 April; 1(2): 189–195.

3

STUDY POPULATION

Authors: *Sandra Carvalho and Felipe Fregni*

Case study authors: *André Brunoni and Felipe Fregni*

Science is facts; just as houses are made of stones, so is science made of facts; but a pile of stones is not a house and a collection of facts is not necessarily science.
—Henri Poincaré (1854–1912)

INTRODUCTION

The previous chapter provided an overview of the selection of the research questions. Now that you have picked a topic and have decided *what* to study, you now have to think about *whom* you want to study in order to test your hypothesis. This chapter will begin with the general definition of *study population*, followed by an introductory session about validity (internal and external) and sampling techniques (probability and non-probability). Then you will be invited to think critically about a hypothetical case study titled "Choosing the Study Population." This chapter will conclude with some practical exercises and review questions.

The next chapter will teach you *how* to answer your research question. You will learn about basic study designs and how to choose the appropriate design for your study.

OVERVIEW OF THE STUDY POPULATION

Imagine that you want to test a new intervention for patients with chronic pain. What do you need to define?

1. The target population
2. The accessible population
3. The study population.

The design of a study often begins with the formulation of the research question, followed by the decision about whom the researcher will study: the study population.

The portion of the general population a researcher wants to draw robust conclusions or inferences about is called the *target population* or *reference population* (Figure 3.1). This population of ultimate interest is usually large and diverse (it may be from all around the world), making it impractical (or even impossible) and cost-ineffective to study it entirely.

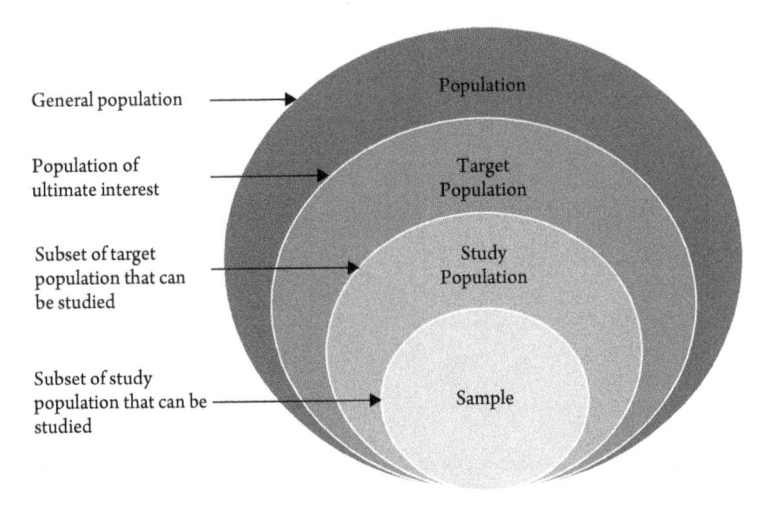

Figure 3.1. Levels of the sampling process.

The subset of the target population that is actually accessible to the researcher is called the *accessible population* (see Figure 3.1). In order for this group to be representative of the target population, it is important to clearly characterize the target population, and to define all elements within the target population that would have to be equally represented in the accessible population. In other words, the accessible population has to be (1) accessible; (2) representative of the target population; and (3) in agreement with the criteria for patient and disease characteristics, with a good ratio between risks and benefits (including both inclusion and exclusion criteria).

The group of individuals that are drawn from the accessible population and on which the research is conducted is called the *study sample* (or simply *sample*). Often only a certain number of people of the accessible population are enrolled to participate in the study (by design, but also with respect to time, budget, or logistical constraints) [1] (Figure 3.1). However, in some cases it is possible that the sample and the accessible population are exactly the same [see Sim and Wright, *Research in Health Care: Concepts, Designs and Methods*].

FIRST CHALLENGE: DEFINING THE TARGET POPULATION

The clinical investigator has usually clear in his or her mind the specific condition to be studied (i.e., patients with neuropathic pain, patients with stroke, patients with diabetes). However, the challenging task is to define among, for instance, patients with stroke, what are the characteristics of patients to be included in the study.

There are two extremes when making this decision: (1) not defining any specific characteristic (including any patients with stroke); and (2) using a very large number of characteristics to define the population to be studied (for instance, gender, age, weight, race, marital status, socioeconomic status, smoking, alcohol use, other comorbidities, specific characteristics of stroke, family history). Which extreme should we use? Probably neither one. Choosing a broad strategy of inclusion criteria (any patients with stroke) will result in a study with likely significant heterogeneity and no significant results. On the other hand, a very narrow strategy of inclusion criteria may likely not be able to find enough patients with these characteristics who are willing to be part of the study.

The strategy for choosing the study population should first take into consideration what is the study phase (early on, or phase I or II study; or a later stage, or phase III or IV) and then understanding what are the factors associated with response and safety to treatment. With these factors well established, the investigator needs then to maximize the "cost-effectiveness" of the chosen strategy. The cost would be the consequence of being too broad and increasing heterogeneity or being too strict and hurting the recruitment, and the effectiveness would be maximizing both internal and external validity.

Study Phases versus Study Population

An important consideration to determine the population of a given study is the study phase. A study can be formally classified as phase I, II, III, or IV, or simply an early development phase or later stages of a development phase.

Here we will discuss phases II and III, as phase I study is specially designed to assess safety and in most of the cases tested in healthy subjects, and phase IV studies are open-label studies usually assessing post-marketing safety.

Phase II is often the first time the efficacy (and also again safety) is tested in the population of efficacy. The goal of this phase of investigation is to detect a signal in a small population. Given the small sample size, in this phase the criteria for inclusion are more restrictive so as to increase the power of the study and detect a signal of the new intervention. See the following for a discussion of a phase II study in which criteria may not have been adequate.

Urfer et al., in a phase II study assessing a new drug for acute stroke, had the following inclusion/exclusion criteria [2]:

> The study included men or women aged ≥18 years with ischemic stroke between 48 and 72 hours before randomization confirmed by computed tomography or MRI and a National Institutes of Health Stroke Scale (NIHSS) score of ≥4 (total score) or of ≥2 on the arm or leg motor function scores of the NIHSS. Subjects had to be medically stable within the 24 hours before randomization. Excluded were subjects with a transient ischemic attack or who were unable to take medication by mouth at the time of baseline assessments. Thrombolysis during the acute phase of stroke before study enrollment was allowed.

This study included 60 subjects. Authors restricted the population by defining the time window of stroke, baseline stroke severity, and age. Likely authors hypothesized a priori that these characteristics would increase response to this new intervention in stroke. It is interesting, however, that authors concluded that

> [c]utamesine was safe and well tolerated at both dosage levels. Although no significant effects on functional end points were seen in the population as a whole, greater improvement in National Institutes of Health Stroke Scale scores among patients

with greater pretreatment deficits seen in post hoc analysis warrants further investigation. Additional studies should focus on the patient population with moderate-to-severe stroke.

Therefore the authors demonstrated that they should have in fact restricted this small study to patients with increased stroke severity.

In a phase III study, on the other hand, the goal is to be as broad as possible so as to increase the generalizability of the study, as the overall goal of phase III study is to gain knowledge for its use in the clinical practice. For example, a phase III trial in acute stroke had the following inclusion criteria that were mainly "(i) Patients presenting with acute hemispheric ischemic stroke; (ii) Age ≥18 years; (iii) National Institutes of Health Stroke Score (NIHSS) of ≥4–26 with clinical signs of hemispheric infarction." In fact, these criteria are broad and therefore increase the generalizability of this study [3].

Response to Treatment versus Study Population

In a smaller study, as well as in a larger study, the response to treatment is an important factor to consider when trying to decrease variability and therefore increase the likelihood of detecting a study signal. Investigators should be careful not to make the mistake of considering the variability of the sample with the variability of response. The investigator needs to be concerned with response to treatment variability and variability of sample characteristics. For instance, if response to treatment is not correlated to age, it does not matter that the sample has patients who are very young and very old. The challenge is to determine which factors are associated with response to treatment. The response to this question is usually in the literature or is based on clinical expertise.

For instance, Kheirkhah et al. showed that baseline sub-basal nerve fiber length (SNFL) in dry eye disease is critical in determining the response to artificial tears and loteprednol. Patients with low SFNL had no response to this treatment [4]. Thus a phase II trial in dry eye disease should include mostly patients with near to normal SFNL.

Safety versus Study Population

The final important factor to consider when selecting the study population is safety. Unless the trial is designed specifically to test whether a new intervention is safe in patients with a particular condition, clinical trials should exclude characteristics that could compromise the safety of research subjects; for instance, excluding patients with epilepsy when testing an intervention that can decrease seizure thresholds.

Validity: Internal, External, and Generalizability

In order for the sample to be valid, it must represent the main characteristics of the accessible population and by extension of the target population. Only then will results obtained from sampled individuals be generalizable to the entire target population. Ensuring representativeness is the key to be able to generalize the results.

Target population:
Patients with chronic pain

Accessible population:
Patients registered in three hospitals

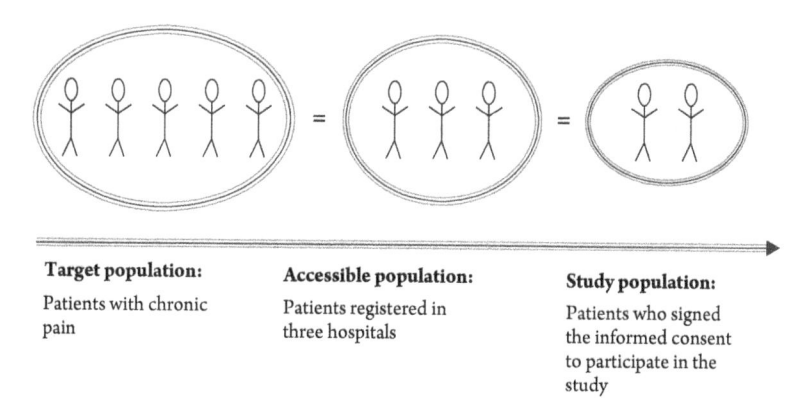

Study population:
Patients who signed the informed consent to participate in the study

Figure 3.2. Example of a simple sampling process.

Concerning validity, two important concepts must be considered: internal validity and external validity.

Internal validity refers to how accurate the outcomes and the conclusions drawn from the findings are (Figure 3.2). An experiment is considered internally valid when the measured response (outcome/dependent variable [DV]) differs only because of the manipulation introduced through the intervention (independent variable [IV]), without any other confounders. As an example, one experiment is considered internally valid if we have clear evidence that what we had manipulated during the study (e.g., the use of two different drugs to treat the same condition in similar groups) caused the difference in the outcome between groups (e.g., patients who received drug A improved 35% more than patients who received drug B).

Threats to internal validity include confounding and bias (e.g., selection bias, recall bias, detection bias, testing [sometimes testing per se influences and interferes with the results]); maturation (both physiological and psychological changes in the participant over the course of the study); instrumentation (when an effect assessed is due to a change in the measuring instrument between pre- and post-treatment, rather than due to the manipulation of the IV); and even the experimenter expectancy effect (when, for instance, the subjects responses are influenced and biased in the direction of the researcher's expectations) [5,6].

A narrow or very homogeneous sample has a good chance to demonstrate high internal validity, as it can reduce response variability and increase study power. There is, however, a trade-off with external validity and recruitment feasibility.

External validity and generalizability refer to how accurately the outcomes and conclusions drawn from the findings can be safely generalized to the target population (Figure 3.2). For example, when testing the effects of a certain drug in a group of subjects with hypertension, generalizability refers to the degree to which researchers can safely conclude that drug A is safe in this particular population (i.e., people with hypertension).

The estimates of the relationship between intervention/exposure and response/outcome may have internal validity while lacking external validity. That is, when strict inclusion/exclusion criteria yield a homogeneous sample, the observed results may be unbiased estimates of the relationship between exposure and outcome in the sample

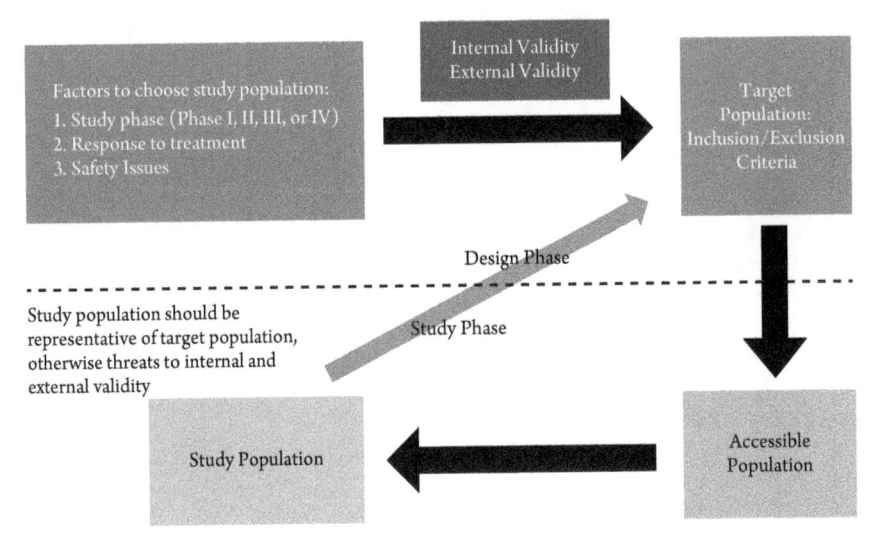

Figure 3.3. The relationship between internal and external validity and the study population.

studied. However, the sample might be too narrow to generate benefits for clinical care because the results are not generalizable or applicable to other samples or to the general population. It should be noted that an experiment that is not internally valid cannot be externally valid. If the sample is not representative of the target population, both external and construct validities of the study are at risk, so it is not possible to generalize safely. The only way to make sure that the sample is representative of the broader population is to obtain direct information from the population [7].

SECOND CHALLENGE: SAMPLING

To maximize the generalizability of your study, you must ensure representativeness. You must first clearly define the target population, carefully specify inclusion and exclusion criteria for the accessible study population, and structure the sampling method in a way that the enrollment yields a random sample of the accessible population (Figure 3.3). Remember, the more representative the sample, the more generalizable will be the study findings be to the target population.

Here the investigator should know the difference between sampling and inclusion criteria. A study can have a broad inclusion criteria; however, during the sampling process, only patients with a single characteristic enter the study, therefore affecting the generalizability of the findings (see also Chapter 7 in this volume).

Why Do We Use Sampling?

It is the best method to get information from the population with

- Low costs
- Simplicity
- Reduced field time
- Increased accuracy
- Possible generalizability.

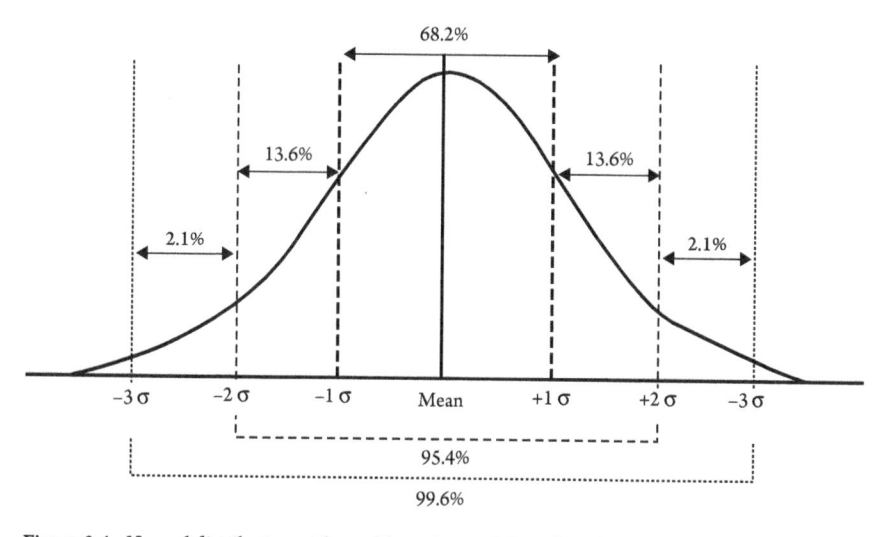

Figure 3.4. Normal distribution with confidence intervals based on the standard deviation.

After defining the study population, researchers need to select the method of sampling (i.e., the method to select individuals). *Sampling* refers to the process by which researchers select a representative subset of individuals from the accessible population to become part of the study sample under consideration to recruit a sufficient size to warrant statistical power (e.g., 3, 4) (see Chapter 11 for more information on sample size calculation). Increases in the heterogeneity of the target population (greater variability) require an increase in the sample size, thus guaranteeing that individuals are homogenous on the variables under study (see Figure 3.4 later in this chapter for representation of normal distribution).

What can we do in order to select a study population that is representative of the accessible population and, by extension, of the target population? One way to proceed is to define clearly the eligibility criteria for the accessible population.

Sampling Bias

As stated before, a sample has to be representative to ensure generalizability from the sample to the population. A sample is considered representative of a given population when it represents, at least, a similar heterogeneity for the relevant characteristics. This means that the variations found in the sample reflect to a high degree those from the broader target population. However, the process of collecting the sample is open to systematic errors that can lead to non-random, biased sample—this is called the *sampling bias* (also known as *ascertainment bias* or *systematic bias*).

A sampling method is considered biased when the subjects who were recruited from the accessible population favor certain characteristics or attributes over others compared to the target population. This imbalance of characteristics or attributes influences the outcome of the study—either because they are overrepresented or underrepresented relative to others in the population [8,9]. Sampling bias is a threat to *external* validity (generalizability) and cannot be accounted for by simply increasing the sample size. In order to minimize the degree of bias when collecting the sample, special sampling techniques should be employed (see discussion later in this chapter).

It is important to distinguish sampling bias from *selection bias*. While sampling bias creates a difference between the target population and the accessible population, selection bias causes a difference between study groups. Selection bias occurs when there is a failure to implement successfully random allocation and concealment of allocation. Selection bias can be intentional or unintentional. Intentional selection bias occurs when, for instance, researchers consciously select into the interventional study group subjects with some specific characteristics that will make it more likely for the study phenomenon to be demonstrated (e.g., researchers choose only patients with a low level of disease severity to demonstrate the efficacy of a certain treatment because they think that they are more likely to respond to it). Unintentional sampling bias occurs when subjects were supposed to be enrolled "randomly," but the researchers were unaware that they were selecting only subjects with certain characteristics (e.g., subjects who were more motivated to participate, or were more accessible). This is clearly an example of unintentional selection bias. Selection bias is a threat to *internal validity* [10].

Some authors [e.g., 9] even defend that sampling bias is inevitable. Therefore it is important to recognize and report all the exceptions during enrollment, maintaining accurate reports about the selection process.

But in practice, what are the most common sources of bias? One type of bias occurs when only volunteers participate in the study because this type of sample usually includes people who are highly motivated and/or people who don't care about the study ("professional volunteers") [11]. This is called a *voluntary response sample*. Convenience samples, in which researchers use only subjects who are easily accessible, are also a potential source of bias, as only a subset of people of the target population is assessed. Lack of blinding, for example in open-label studies (for more details, see Chapter 4), is also a great source of bias. Poor allocation concealment will compromise the balance of groups in the sample, as researchers may assign participants differentially to the different groups (e.g., placebo and treatment group) or may even exclude those who may compromise the expected results.

In summary, sampling bias occurs when the sample is not randomly selected, and limits generalizability, hence making it difficult to draw valid inferences from the sample toward the target population.

Sampling Error(s)

Sampling error or *estimation error* (or precision) refers to the standard error that gives us the *precision* of our statistical estimate [12]. In this case, the degree from which an observation differs from the expected value is called an error.

So, sampling error is a statistical error that is obtained from sample data, which differs to a certain degree from the data that would be obtained if the entire population were used [6]. Low sampling error means less variability in the sample distribution, based on the standard deviation. A simple rule of thumb is that standard deviation and sampling error will increase in the same fashion.

The sampling error depends on the sample size and the sampling distribution (Figure 3.4), based on the characteristics of interest. Unlike sampling bias, sampling error can be predicted and calculated by the researcher taking into account the following measures: standard error, coefficient of variance, confidence intervals, and P values.

When simple random sample of size "n" is selected from population of size N, standard error (s) for population mean or proportion is

$$\frac{\sigma}{\sqrt{n}} \text{ or } \sqrt{\frac{p(1-p)}{n}}$$

Used to calculate, 95% confidence intervals (see also Chapter 14 for these calculations):

$$\overline{X} \pm 2 \times S_{\overline{x}}$$

Sampling Techniques

There are two broad types of sampling designs in quantitative research: *probability sampling* and *non-probability sampling* (Figure 3.5). With probability sampling techniques, every subject has, in theory, equal chances of being selected for the sample. On the contrary, with non-probability sampling techniques, the chance of every subject being selected is unknown [13,14].

Probability sampling methods are based on random selection. This means that every person in the target population has an equal and independent chance of being selected as a subject for the study [15]. This procedure decreases the probability of bias, even when using a small sample size, because bias depends more on the selection procedure than on the size of the sample. So, the main advantage of this method is that the selection process is randomized, therefore minimizing bias (reducing sampling bias) and thus increasing confidence in the representativeness of the sample [15]. Other advantages of the probability sampling methods are objectiveness, requiring little information from the population, and increasing accuracy of the statistical methods after the study [e.g., 16]. On the other hand, the main disadvantages of these methods are that the process is expensive and time-consuming, and a complete list of the entire population is needed [7,16]. There are different types of probability sampling

Internal validity
- Refers to the extent to which we can accurately state that the independent variables (IVs) produced the observed effect.
Internal validity is achieved when the effect on dependent variable is only due to variation in the IVs.
- Threats to internal validity: Confounding and bias.

External validity or generalizability
- Refers to the extent to which we can generalize our findings to or across target population which happens when study participants (sample from the accessible population) are representative of the target population.
- The resulting outcomes and conclusions are unbiased estimations.

Figure 3.5. Internal and external validity or generality [based on 12].

Probability Sampling	Non-Probability Sampling
Simple Random Sampling	Convenience Sampling
Systematic Sampling	Consecutive Sampling
Stratified Sampling	Quota Sampling
Cluster Sampling	Judgmental Sampling
Disproportional Sampling	Snowball Sampling

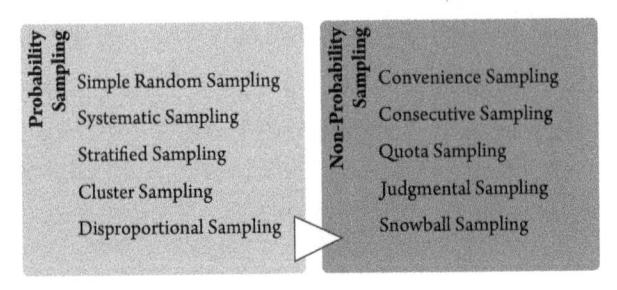

Figure 3.6. Probability sampling and non-probability sampling techniques.

methods: simple random, systematic, stratified, cluster, and disproportional sampling (Figure 3.5).

Simple Random Sampling

Definition and Method

Probably the most simplistic and basic form of sampling is simple random sampling. It uses a random number generator as the sampling frame (such as a random number table, a telephone directory, or a computer program) to select and numerate a subset of people from the population. Using this method, each individual of the population has equal, independent chances of being selected and participating in the study, without selection bias from the researcher [17].

Advantages

It is an easy method of sampling.
It can be done manually.
This method is ideal for statistical proposes because confidence interval around the sample can be defined using statistical analyses.

Potential Problems

This method requires complete lists of the population, which may be very unpractical and costly when individuals are scattered in a vast geographic area.
Difficulties completing the list of the entire population may systematically exclude important cases in the population.

Example
Suppose you want to study the entire population with Parkinson's disease who received deep brain stimulation (DBS) in all hospitals in the United States.
   First, you will need a list (organized by letters or numbers) of all Parkinson's patients who received DBS for each hospital in the United States that performs these invasive procedures. These lists are named the *sampling frame*. After that, you need to choose a process to select numbers randomly in each list, in a way that every patient has the same chance of being selected.

Systematic Sampling

Definition and Method

In systematic sampling, a set of study participants is systematically and randomly selected from a complete and seriated list of people (N = Population). Then a sampling interval is obtained by dividing the accessible population by the desired sample size. So, suppose that each individual in the accessible population is organized by alphabetical order. The researcher establishes a sampling interval (SI) to select subjects, which is the distance between the selected elements. For instance, we can specify taking every third name or every tenth name.

Advantages

It is an easy method of sampling,
It can be done manually, especially if lists are already organized into sections.
It is ideal for large target populations, where simple random sampling would be difficult to perform.
It ensures that the selected individuals are from the entire range of the population.

Potential Problems

This method can be expensive and time-consuming if the sample is not conveniently located.
The selection method chosen could introduce bias when systematically some members of the target population are excluded. So, it is inadequate when there is periodicity in the population.

Example
Suppose that the population size is N = 5,000 and the desired sample size is n = 100. The first step would be to organize the population by alphabetical order and then divide: k: 5,000/100 = 50.
This means that every 50th person listed will be selected to integrate in the sample.
In summary, *first you need to create a sampling frame* (e.g., list of people), then choose randomly a starting point on the sampling frame, and finally pick a participant at constant and regular intervals in order to select sets of participants.

Stratified Sampling

Definition and Method

With stratified sampling, the accessible population is first divided into two or more strata or homogenous subgroups to which each individual is randomly assigned, according to specific characteristics relevant for the study purpose. The groups to which individuals are allocated must not overlap. This method uses simple random or systematic sampling within defined strata in order to enhance the representativeness of the sample [18]. Stratification is based on attributes that often are of relevance for the study purpose, such as age, gender, race, diagnostic, duration of disease, geographic localization, socioeconomic status, education, and so on. With this method, each element has an equal chance to be assigned to a specific subgroup, and thus an equal chance of being represented.

Advantages

This method increases the representativeness in the target population by ensuring that individuals from each strata are included.

It is ideal when subgroups within the target population need to be analyzed separately and/or compared (subgroup statistical analyses).

It is less expensive—great precision is obtained even with smaller samples.

Potential Problems

The process of selecting the sample is more complex and requires more information about the population in order to classify and organize elements from the target population. Sometimes, difficulties in identifying the main characteristics of the target population may require some adjustments during the study. There is also another problem, if the proportions in the target population are not reflected in the strata. For instance, if one stratum has two times more representatives in a target population than another stratum, then the sample size of each stratum should reflect this. This process is called *proportional stratified sample*, where the sample size in each stratum aims to reflect the proportion of those individuals in the target population. Please note that this should only be used when the proportions in the target population are different, but they are not very disproportionate. If they are disproportionate (for instance, group A, $N = 100$; group B, $N = 2,000$), disproportional sampling should be considered instead.

> **Example**
> Suppose you want to study the incidence and prevalence of disease A by gender. After selecting the accessible population, you need to randomize each individual within each stratum (stratum 1: female; stratum 2: male). Sample would have 50% of individuals in each gender group.
>
> In summary, first you need to divide the target population into characteristics of interest—named stratification factors—(gender, age, level of education, etc.), and then the sample is selected randomly within each group.

Cluster or Multistage Sampling

Definition and Method

Cluster sampling, or multistage sampling, involves the successive selection of random samples from "natural" or "meaningful" units (clusters; e.g., cities, schools). In a one-stage cluster sample, a random sample of clusters is selected, and all individuals from that cluster are included in the study. A second stage can be added if not all, but only a fixed number of individuals will be randomly selected from a particular cluster to be studied. The clusters that provide the sample should be representative of (or similar to) the target population. Clusters may be geographic, racial, and so on.

The difference between cluster sampling and stratified sampling is that in stratified sampling, the entire study population is divided into strata based on a certain characteristic (covariate) and all strata are sampled. In cluster sampling, only a selected number of clusters are included for sampling. Also, clusters are defined by geographical aspects, and the individuals within a cluster do not necessarily have a common biological characteristic (covariate).

Advantages

This method is ideal for large and disperse target populations.
There is reduced cost and it is less time-consuming (e.g., sampling all students in a few schools vs. some students from all schools).
There is reduced variability.
Sampling frame is not required.

Potential Problems

The main problem of cluster sampling is a loss in precision. This can lead to biased samples when clusters were chosen based on biased assumptions about the population, for instance, when the clusters are very similar and therefore less likely to represent the whole population. Or, if clusters differ substantially from one another, sampling will lose efficiency.

> **Example**
> Suppose you want to study medical students; you may select randomly five universities in the state of Massachusetts and then select randomly 500 students in each university.
>
> *In summary, first you need to identify the study units (clusters), and then you recruit a fixed number of participants within each if they meet the criteria for the study.*

In *non-probability sampling methods*, subjects are selected from the accessible population by non-random selection. This is the most common method used in human trials. But often it is difficult to assume that they produce accurate and representative samples of the population, and therefore generalizability to the target population is limited. This method is often used in preliminary and exploratory studies, and in studies in which it is difficult to access or identify all members of the population. So, this method is used only when it is not possible (or not necessary) to use probability sampling methods. The disadvantage of this technique is that it is less likely to produce representative samples, which affects generalizability to the target population [7,16]. There are different types of non-probability sampling methods: convenience, consecutive, quota, judgmental, and snowball sampling.

Convenience Sampling

Definition and Method

In convenience sampling, participants are selected because they are easily accessible, and the researcher is not concerned about the representativeness of the sample in the population. This sample could also be random, but usually it is biased.

Advantages

It can be used when other sampling methods are not possible. In some cases, it may be the only choice.
It is practical.

Potential Problems

There is usually sampling bias.
The sample is not representative of the population (low external validity, or none).
It is impossible to assess the degree of sampling bias.

> **Example**
> Probably one of the most common situations where convenience sampling occurs is when university students or volunteers are recruited through advertisement, an easy form of recruitment.
> Another example would be to study all patients who present to a clinic within a specific time frame.

Consecutive Sampling

Definition and Method

Consecutive sampling is very similar to convenience sampling. However, in this case, researchers include all accessible subjects from the accessible population, who met the eligibility criteria over a specific time or for a specified sample size.

Advantages

Compared with convenience sampling, the sample better represents the population.

Potential Problems

There is poor representativeness of the entire population, with little potential to generalize.
The sample is not based on random selection.
It is impossible to assess the degree of sampling bias.

> **Example**
> Suppose you want to study all patients who received treatment A during the first 6 months of use, so all the patients are eligible and are consecutively assigned to form the sample.

Snowball Sampling (Network or Chain Sampling)

Definition and Method

In snowball sampling, researchers ask the first participants of the study to identify and try to enroll in the study other potential participants who will possibly meet the study criteria. This technique is usually used when the size of the available population is very small, and thus has the disadvantage of low representativeness.

Advantages

It is ideal for very small population sizes.
It is ideal when participants are very difficult to locate or contact.
It is easy to implement.
In some cases it is the best sampling method to implement (e.g., when there are no records of the population).

Potential Problems

The generalizability of the results is questionable.
It is impossible to assess the degree of sampling bias.

> **Example**
> Suppose you want to study the prevalence of a certain disease in homeless people or in a rare ethnic group. Asking the first subjects assigned to the study could be the best or even the only option that the researcher has to identify and access other subjects.

HOW SHOULD THE RESEARCHER SELECT THE APPROPRIATE SAMPLING METHOD?

Please also note that the choice of sampling method (see Scheme 3.1) will affect the results. Therefore, it is necessary to carefully plan the sampling method, to base it on the study objectives, and to consider what the accessible part of the target population is. There are also factors that should be taken into consideration, such as enrollment time, budget, and the sample size required to reach a certain power and significance level when performing such study (see also Chapter 11).

The following case study will help to further address these critical issues.

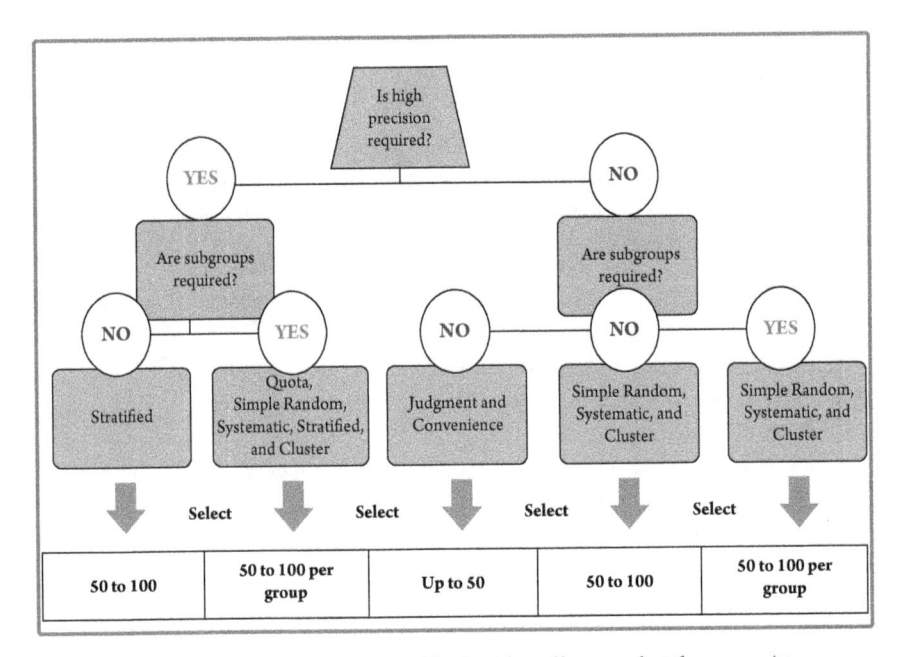

Scheme 3.1. This scheme represents one possible algorithm of how to select the appropriate sampling method [adapted from 2].

CASE STUDY 3: CHOOSING THE STUDY POPULATION

André Brunoni and Felipe Fregni

Professor Anderson is a renowned researcher in the field of rheumatology. He has published many articles on several rheumatologic diseases, which have become references in the field. He has been recently promoted to full professor and now works at Brigham and Women's Hospital in Boston. His team, composed of basic and clinical researchers, has been developing a new drug for rheumatoid arthritis (RA)—the drug "RA-007"—for many years. Animal studies as well as phase I and phase II studies showed promising results. Now Prof. Anderson is preparing himself for a huge step— to be the PI (principal investigator) of a large phase III trial to prove the efficacy of RA-007. He has just hung up a telephone call with the program director of NIH (National Institutes of Health—the main funding agency for biomedical research in the United States) confirming that he will receive the funds for the study he is proposing. Because he has been planning this study for several months, he has designed it very carefully, but one issue still bothers him: the study population.[1]

Introduction

For logical reasons, it is impossible to conduct a trial on the entire population. Therefore, when designing a clinical trial, it is necessary to choose who is going to be studied. Although it may be a trivial task in the trial, choosing the study population— or sample—correctly might be the difference between success and failure, and will also influence how other researchers and clinicians see your trial.

There are important points that the researcher needs to consider when choosing the right population. First, it is interesting to exclude conditions that might mimic the disease under study but that do not respond to the therapeutic intervention or that need to be treated differently. For instance, a clinical trial testing a new antibiotic for bacterial pneumonia should not include patients with viral pneumonia, as these patients will have a lower response rate or even no response to the new antibiotic. Second, there is the issue of competing risk, for instance, patients with other comorbidities who might worsen because of these conditions and, therefore, confound the clinical trials results.

Although it is appropriate to select very carefully and to dedicate some time to choosing the study population, over-choosing by adding more *inclusion* or *exclusion* criteria items might also be dangerous, as it would *restrict* the generalizability or external validity of the study—especially because the study population will usually be different from the "real world" population or the population that will be seen in the clinical practice, which might not represent the studied population.

---

[1] Dr. André Brunoni and Professor Felipe Fregni prepared this case. Course cases are developed solely as the basis for class discussion. The situation in this case is fictional. Cases are not intended to serve as endorsements or sources of primary data. All rights reserved to the authors of this case.

There are other issues that need to be addressed when choosing the study population—one of them is the feasibility of recruitment—*would it be feasible to recruit patients, or would the trial need to be interrupted for lack of subjects?*

Another important point to consider is ensuring that the research team is able to apply the diagnostic criteria you have developed—for instance, a study might determine that a brain biopsy is necessary to diagnose a brain tumor. This would highly limit the ability of investigators to enroll patients and might indeed exclude patients with a diagnosis of a brain tumor. The researcher needs to be extremely attentive to situations in which a sample bias might occur (sample bias occurs when the study population differs from the target population).

Choosing the Target Population

Prof. Anderson is really confident that RA-007 might finally represent a good treatment for RA. Because he is one of the leading names in the treatment of RA, he has seen hundreds of patients with RA and knows how devastating this disease can be to his patients. Phase II studies showed that this new drug is 50% better than placebo in terms of quality of life and progression of disease. However, these phase II studies used the principle of "decrease the noise to amplify the signal" (i.e., these studies used a very homogeneous population to decrease the variability of the sample and thereby to amplify the signal—the efficacy of RA-007). But although the data from phase II studies—some collected in his laboratory at Longwood Medical Area (Boston, United States)—showed impressive results, as also confirmed by a recent meta-analysis that his group has conducted, this drug is not yet approved for use in humans. Therefore, he needs to be very precise in choosing the population for his study so as to maintain the internal validity of his trial, but also to show some external generalizability.

Although Prof. Anderson has already determined the study population for this study as laid out in his grant application, Prof. Anderson and his team are reviewing the eligibility criteria of his target population—that is, the inclusion and exclusion criteria—and thus are repeating the mental process of choosing the study population to determine whether the study will need to be amended. So they need to review some important questions. Everyone on his team is aware that the fate of this study, and consequently the investment from the government/US taxpayers (the NIH has awarded Prof. Anderson a grant of $4 million to run this study), is highly dependent on how they choose the study population:

1. *The trade-off of internal versus external validity*: Prof. Anderson can choose anything from enrolling all patients with RA to including only patients with severe, advanced RA. However, if he chooses the first option the sample will be too heterogeneous—for instance, there will be patients with mild RA that would get better even with a simple analgesic (he is planning to compare RA-007 against a control group)—and then the results would tend to go toward the null hypothesis. On the other hand, targeting a strict population might be good to prove the efficacy of an intervention, as patients with more severe disease are more likely to respond, but not to increase the external validity of the study—therefore, this drug would only be approved by the regulatory agencies or by the insurance companies for specific situations,

preventing the use of RA-007 in other subgroups of patients. In addition, there is the issue of *regression to the mean* effect when targeting patients with very severe disease—that is, since RA is a chronic, relapsing disorder, it is possible that a patient is recruited in the most severe phase of the disease to get better a few weeks later—not because of RA-007, but for the natural history of the disease/regression to the mean and, since patients of the control group will also present this effect, the clinical difference between groups will decrease. Also, patients with severe disease will likely be having other treatments that may confound the results of this trial. This is an issue that needs to be carefully considered during this phase. Prof. Anderson and his team need to weigh these factors very carefully.

2. *The issue of RA diagnosis*: The next important issue to review is to define the specific criteria for diagnosis of RA—in other words, how the study investigators will determine whether or not a patient has RA. Prof. Anderson knows that this is not an easy task. Being too simplistic (such as clinical diagnosis only) might select wrong cases or may miss correct cases. However, being too complex (for instance, with imaging and even anatomo-pathological exams) will increase the costs of the study and also exclude patients with RA who do not have these exams as; this will influence the external validity of the study. In addition, he needs to find criteria that will produce consistent results across different research investigators to increase inter-rater reliability.

Recruiting the Subjects

It is a cold fall morning in Boston, and during the drive from his home to his office, Prof. Anderson now realizes that he needs to address another important issue: recruitment. On that morning, Prof. Anderson is starting a meeting with his recruitment team. He sighs quietly, as he knows it will be a long day. "Recruiting is a very hard task," he thinks, while hearing the suggestions of his staff. The sample size estimation they calculated is 1,800 subjects. His thoughts start wandering... "I could advertise in the newspaper... or maybe on the Internet..."... "No, I think it's best to talk with my colleagues and ask their patients..."... "I could use the patients from my ambulatory of severe RA..."... "Or maybe patients from my office...." And he knows that he will have to deal with the annual reports that he will need to submit to NIH describing the status of his study and recruitment.

Prof. Anderson is aware that there is no perfect recruitment strategy. In addition, the recruitment strategy will have an important influence on the study population. The issues of generalizability and target population apply, in fact, at this point. If he chooses to recruit patients from his ambulatory or from his colleagues, his recruitment yield will probably be higher—as these patients are very severe and, therefore, are willing to try a new treatment. Advertisement will probably reach more patients, but it's expensive and also will bring a large number of patients who are not eligible for the study—therefore increasing the study costs.

Also there is the issue of probability versus non-probability samples. The methods mentioned would select non-probability samples—for example, only patients who frequent Brigham and Women's hospital, or only patients with RA who read newspapers, or only those who access the web will be selected—therefore not representing a random sample of the entire RA population with the characteristics defined by the study criteria.

In fact, in clinical research, it is often impossible to obtain a true random population—that is, all subjects of the target population should have the same probability of being chosen. Although using non-probability samples is more convenient (easier, faster, and more affordable) and sometimes the only possible method, such an approach brings important consequences to the phase III trial of Prof. Anderson: generalization with a non-probability sample needs to be made with extreme prudence as the methods of statistical inference are usually violated with this approach. As Prof. Anderson wants to generalize the results of his study to clinical practice, he knows that this will be an important challenge. In a conversation earlier with a colleague from the social sciences department about results of the polls from the last presidential election, this issue has arisen. His colleague commented on the issue that election polls showed very different results in the last election. Prof. Anderson then commented, "Well my friend, I have the same problem in clinical research. If in an election poll, you select most of the respondents in wealthy neighborhoods in the South, then you may get more conservative votes; similarly, if I select my patients for a study from an alternative medicine clinic, then the placebo response might be higher, for instance. However, unlike conducting election polls, selecting a random population of patients to participate in a study is not an easy task."

Final Considerations: The Challenges Are Not Finished

Prof. Anderson is at Logan Airport waiting for his flight to Seattle—for the American College of Rheumatology's 2008 Annual Meeting. While seated in the boarding area, he goes over his plan for the study population and although he is quite satisfied now, he still has some issues to consider, such as adherence and future difficulties in recruitment.

Adherence is an important issue that might also affect the study population significantly. Patients might leave a study for several reasons. First, patients might present adverse effects of the active drug and/or the absence of any effect of the placebo group (if a placebo is used). The attrition can significantly bias the results of a given study. One option to decrease the dropout rate is to have a run-in phase (i.e., giving placebo or another active drug to all patients at the beginning of the study, usually for one or two weeks) so as to select patients who will adhere to the study treatment—the idea is that patients with poor adherence will drop out, and the study starts with a more "dedicated" sample. But that might bias the study population even more, as it essentially re-selects patients one more time; and it also poses ethical problems (e.g., how to state in the informed consent a placebo run-in phase?). His flight has just started boarding; he closes his study notebook and while he waits to board he knows he needs to reassess his study population criteria and make the necessary amendments in the protocol before the study starts, and also ask for approval from the NIH. He wishes he had done this before he submitted the grant.

CASE QUESTIONS FOR REFLECTION

Now that you have had a chance to familiarize yourself with the case, we will consider some of the questions that the case raises. After each question there is a summary of the main topics that can help you to reflect on them.

1. What are the challenges for Professor Anderson? Why are these challenges so important?

Professor Anderson's concerns are related to the study population for a phase III clinical trial to test the efficacy of drug RA-007. He is so concerned with choosing the study population because he is aware of the implications that a low representativeness of his sample may have, especially with running a phase III study. So, let's summarize the main challenges: (1) Should he exclude medical conditions that mimic the disease in study? What are the main risks if he enrolls subjects with conditions with similar clinical manifestations to the ones that are the objective of the study? (2) Should he exclude competing risk factors? Why would it be so important to exclude such risk factors? (3) Should he restrict the inclusion criteria in order to have a more homogenous sample? Or should he broaden the focus, accepting, for instance, patients in different stages of the disease? (4) What would be the strategy used to diagnose subjects? (5) How should the recruitment be done? (6) How can he increase or guarantee adherence?

These questions that Prof. Anderson stated have importance because, depending on the choices he makes, they will impact the feasibility and validity of the study, and ultimately its generalizability. These questions include the target population and how to define it, then how to define further what population will be studied by using inclusion and exclusion criteria, and finally, the trade-off between internal and external validity.

2. Considering the trade-off between internal and external validity, do you think that Prof. Anderson should consider enrolling a broader sample (for a more heterogeneous sample), or should he restrict the eligibility criteria (for a more homogeneous sample)?

Prof. Anderson needs to find a balance between how restrictive the eligibility criteria are and how much he wants to compromise the generalizability of his study. Please remember what impacts the degree to which results are generalizable from the sample to the target population. In general, all experiments have some degree of artificiality to them and it is not possible to create a "perfect" sample. Increasing homogeneity of the sample may help to understand better a phenomenon in a specific group—however, at the cost of being able to make reliable inferences about the more heterogenic target population. In contrast, increasing heterogeneity, by having less restrictive eligibility criteria, may approximate the sample's characteristics with those of the target population, with the trade-off of increasing the variability of results, introducing more chances of bias and ultimately risking to obtain results that are more difficult to interpret. What is the best trade-off, and how can this be included in the study design?

3. What type of recruitment strategies should Prof. Anderson choose in this case?

Prof. Anderson considers several recruitment strategies: recruiting his own patients, recruiting patients from referral from other professionals, or advertising the study in several media (e.g., journals, Internet, radio). The appropriate strategy needs to be selected in order to increase the efficiency of enrollment, by increasing the probability of accessing correctly diagnosed patients and thus saving time by screening primarily individuals that meet the inclusion criteria.

4. What type of sampling method do you think is more suitable in this case? Can you provide reasons?

Prof. Anderson wants to ensure internal validity (controlling for confounders and bias, like selection bias, recall bias, detection bias). And simultaneously he wants to increase generalizability by ensuring the representativeness of the recruited sample. So, probability-sampling techniques may be a more appropriate choice. Within probability-sampling techniques, Prof. Anderson then may choose simple random, systematic, stratified, cluster, or disproportional sampling. Concerning the objective, and each method's advantages and disadvantages, what would be the more most suitable method in this case? And, what about non-probability sampling techniques? What are the main issues and advantages of choosing theses sampling procedures in this specific case? Please remember that there is no universally applicable sampling technique. Choosing the ideal sampling technique depends always on several factors, such as the study objective, the budget available, time, and the accessibility of the population, among others.

OTHER QUESTIONS FOR FURTHER REFLECTION

1. What challenges does Prof. Anderson face?
2. What is at stake in this case?
3. Is there a right answer?
4. Should he consider recruitment as an important factor to decide the inclusion/exclusion criteria for his population study?

FURTHER READING

Sim J, Wright C. *Research in health care: concepts, designs and methods*. Cheltenham: Nelson Thornes; 2000.

REFERENCES

1. Gay LR, Mills GE, Airasian PW. *Educational research: competencies for analysis and applications*. 9th ed. New York: Pearson; 2008.
2. Urfer R, et al. Phase II Trial of the Sigma-1 Receptor Agonist Cutamesine (SA4503) for recovery enhancement after acute ischemic stroke. *Stroke*. 2014; 45: 3304–3310.
3. Ma H, et al. A multicentre, randomized, double-blinded, placebo-controlled Phase III study to investigate Extending the time for Thrombolysis in Emergency Neurological Deficits (EXTEND). *Int J Stroke*. 2012; 7(1): 74–80.
4. Kheirkhah A, et al. Effects of corneal nerve density on the response to treatment in dry eye disease. *Ophthalmology*. 2015 Apr; 122(4): 662–668.
5. Cook TD, Campbell DT, Day A. *Quasi-experimentation: design and analysis issues for field settings*. Boston: Houghton Mifflin; 1979.

6. Finger MS, Rand KL. Addressing validity concerns in clinical psychology research. In: Roberts MC, Ilardi SS, eds. *Handbook of research methods in clinical psychology*. 2. Malden, MA: Blackwell; 2003: 13–30.
7. Nieswiadomy RM. *Foundations of nursing research*. 6th ed. New York: Pearson; 2011.
8. Weisberg HI. *Bias and causation: models and judgment for valid comparisons*. New York: Wiley; 2010.
9. Heckman JJ. Sample selection bias as a specification error. *Econometrica*. 1979; 47(1): 153–161.
10. Gaertner SL, Dovidio JF. *Reducing intergroup bias: the common ingroup identity model*. Psychology Press; 2014 Apr 4.
11. Wallin P. Volunteer subjects as a source of sampling bias. *Am J Sociol*. 1949; 54(6): 539–44.
12. Särndal CE, Swensson B, Wretman J. *Model assisted survey sampling*. Berlin: Springer Verlag; 2003.
13. Ary D, Jacobs LC, Sorensen C, Razavieh A. *Introduction to research in education*. 8th ed. Belmont, CA: Wadsworth; 2009.
14. Parahoo K. *Nursing research: principles, process and issues*. Basingstoke, UK: Palgrave Macmillan; 2006.
15. Polit DF, Beck CT. *Nursing research: generating and assessing evidence for nursing practice*. 8th ed. Philadelphia: Lippincott, Williams, & Wilkins; 2008.
16. Bryman A, Bell E. *Business research methods*. 3rd ed. New York: Oxford University Press; 2011.
17. Moore DS. *The basic practice of statistics*. 5th ed. New York: W. H. Freeman; 2009.
18. National Audit Office. *A practical guide to sampling*. London: National Audit Office; 2001.

4

BASIC STUDY DESIGNS

Authors: *Alexandra Gomez-Arteaga, Felipe Fregni, and Vera Novak*

Case study authors: *André Brunoni and Felipe Fregni*

Study lends a kind of enchantment to all our surroundings.
—Honore de Balzac (Novelist, 1799–1850)

INTRODUCTION

This chapter provides an overview of basic study designs for interventional studies and introduces important concepts for the design of clinical trials. Later, in Unit III of this volume, you will learn about types of observational studies and the main differences between an observational study and a clinical trial. More complex research designs, such as adaptive designs, will also be covered in Unit III.

STUDY DESIGN

The study design delineates the methodology of how to obtain the answer to the research questions. As Sackett et al. (1997) stated, the question being asked determines the appropriate research architecture, strategy, and tactics to be used—not tradition, authority, experts, paradigms, or schools of thought [1,2]. Knowing the advantages and limitations of each design will play an important role, but the decision of which one to choose is going to be based on which design can answer the defined research question with the most compelling evidence—but at the same time, in the most straightforward and fundamental way.

In the most basic form, the type of study can be described either as experimental or randomized. The most important characteristic of an experimental study is the manipulation of the treatment variable (independent variable) using randomization to control for confounding. The experimental studies look for a *cause–effect relationship* where the investigator is systematically introducing a specific change (intervention) and controls for everything else to remain the same. Experimental studies and quasi-experimental studies are interventional studies that differ in the concept of randomization. Even though randomized clinical trials are the source of the strongest evidence for evidence-based medicine, it is by no means the only or even the most appropriate approach for all of the clinical research questions [3]. On the other hand, in observational studies the independent variable (most commonly referred to as *exposure*) is not controlled by the investigator; thus its relationship with the outcome (also referred to as *disease*) is usually confounded by other variables (see Chapter 16 for more

details). (See Figure 4.1 for a depiction of the main types of study design and their relationship with manipulation of intervention).
The study design is the methodology used in order to

- Eliminate systematic error (bias)
- Minimize random error (chance, variability)
- Increase precision
- Ensure the generalizability of study findings [1].

Experimental studies test the efficacy of a new intervention that can be either therapeutic (e.g., drugs, devices, surgery) or preventive (e.g., vaccine, diet, behavioral modification). In order to ensure the validity of a study, an attempt must be made to optimize the design. Therefore, the intervention is usually tested against placebo or a standard intervention. Another very important concept of an experimental study is that the patients are allocated at *random* to each treatment group, including the control arm. In fact, administration of the intervention (independent variable of the study) but not the allocation needs to be manipulated by the experimenter (for instance, the patients receive a given intervention not because of clinical reasons but because of study assignment). Randomization is a sine qua non characteristic of an experimental study because it is the best method to guarantee that all variables will be equally distributed between groups, except, naturally, the intervention (see Chapter 5 for Randomization). Therefore, if at the end of the study there is a difference between

Experimental Variable/Intervention

Full Manipulation   **No Manipulation**

EXPERIMENTAL DESIGNS:	QUASI-EXPERIMENTS:	OBSERVATIONAL STUDIES
– Intervention is manipulated – Assignment is random	– Intervention is manipulated – Assignment is NOT random	– Intervention is NOT manipulated – Assignment is NOT random

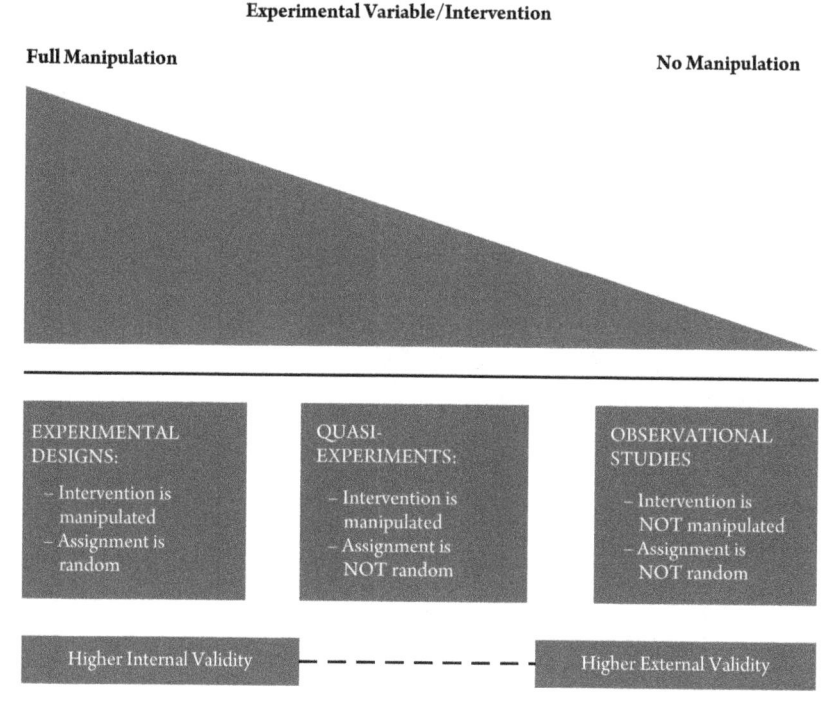

Higher Internal Validity – – – – – – – Higher External Validity

Figure 4.1. Main types of study design and their relationship with manipulation of intervention.

groups, it shall be concluded that such difference occurred due to the intervention. Other interventional studies not using randomization are considered quasi-experimental studies (*quasi*: Latin for "almost"). In this type of study, allocation is made using non-random methods such as allocation by the medical record number, date of birth, or sequential inclusion. In some cases, however, the researcher can control study allocation, thus introducing intrinsic bias to the study.

Note: The study design will pre-define what statistical methods you will use to analyze the study data (see Unit II).

STUDY DESIGN CLASSIFICATIONS FOR INTERVENTIONAL STUDIES

Figure 4.2 shows the most commonly used designs in interventional studies. There are many more complex designs (e.g., mixed designs, adaptive designs) that are not included.

Experimental Designs

Parallel Group Designs

This design is the most common type in experimental studies. It compares two or more groups that are established by random assignment. Subjects are randomized to

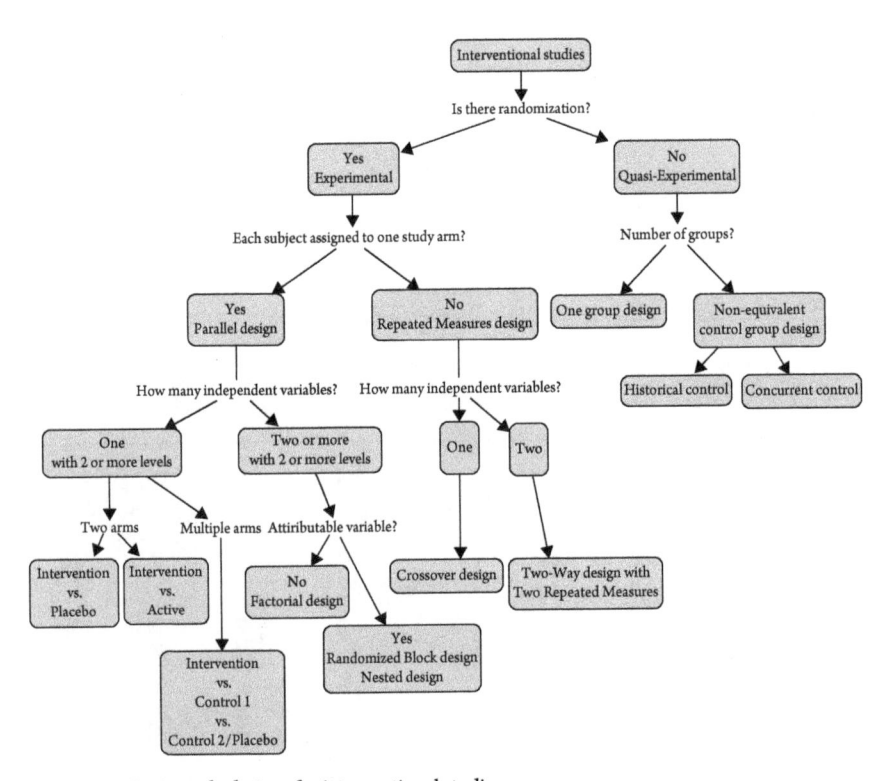

Figure 4.2. Basic study designs for interventional studies.

> **Box 4.1** Advantages and disadvantages of parallel group designs
>
> The major advantages in general for a parallel design are:
> - Simplicity.
> - Universal acceptance in the academic world
> - Applicability to acute settings
> - Facility for analysis and results interpretation
> - There are well-established and accepted methods to compare their findings and use them in a meta-analysis
> - There is no concern for carryover effect
> - It can be used in a trial of superiority, non-inferiority, or equivalence
> - Is optimal for any phase of research
> - Allows for different number of subjects in each arm
>
> Its disadvantages are:
> - It is not so powerful to account for within-patient variability
> - Confounding
> - Expensive
> - Longitudinal, long follow-up period
> - Requires larger samples
> - Dropouts
> - Very controlled conditions different to medical practice

different treatment arms that can either be the experimental intervention or the control group—which can be another intervention or placebo, or a combination of both. The groups are compared based on the measurement of the endpoint of the intervention; it can be pre-test–post-test control group design, where the outcome is measured at baseline and after the intervention in each group (e.g., visual analogue scale before and after the intervention to assess pain), or post-test control group, where the outcome is measured only after the intervention and is compared with the control (e.g., time [in days] of hospitalization after surgery). See Box 4.1 for the advantages and disadvantages of parallel group designs.

One Independent Variable

The first type consists of one independent variable with different levels, or one treatment in different formats (for instance, active drug and placebo drug).

Intervention against placebo This is used to detect a difference between the intervention versus no intervention (i.e., placebo or sham surgery). An important disadvantage of this design may be the ethical concerns of using placebo, since it may be unethical to receive the placebo intervention when an available standard treatment already exits. Another potential limitation of this design is the delay in recruitment, as not all the subjects will agree to participate in a trial where there is a chance of receiving placebo.

Table 4.1 Biostatistical Plan for Analysis of Parallel Group Designs

Number of Groups	Parametric Data	Non-Parametric Data
2	Unpaired t-test	Mann-Whitney U-test
≥ 3	One-way analysis of variance (ANOVA), regression model and analysis of covariance*	Kruskal-Walllis analysis of variance by ranks

*When there is an extra variable that is assumed to influence the dependent variable.

Intervention against active agent This type is also known as a Standard of Care Concurrent Control Trial, where both groups are receiving standard care and in one group we are adding the investigational intervention. This design is adequate to detect the difference against standard of care, but does not show us that it is better than no intervention. These trials can use the double-dummy design for blinding (which will be discussed more in Chapter 5). The main disadvantage of this design is that it cannot investigate the pure effects of the intervention, and any potential interaction between the standard intervention and the experimental intervention will either increase or decrease the therapeutic effects.

Multigroup design The three-arm design is very common and is used to compare a new intervention with two controls (one can be placebo). This design can also be used in a specific subtype of trials where different dosages or timing of a new intervention are tested.

An analysis of parallel group designs with one independent variable with different levels is shown in Table 4.1 (this topic will be further discussed in other chapters).

For two groups, the unpaired t-test for parametric data or Mann-Whitney U-test for non-parametric data can be performed depending on the data distribution. For three or more groups, a one-way analysis of variance (ANOVA) for parametric or Kruskal-Walllis analysis of variance by ranks for non-parametric data may be performed. An analysis of covariance can also be used when there is an extra variable that is assumed to influence the dependent variable. Regression model is also applicable [3].

Two or More Independent Variables with Different Levels or Two Treatments in Different Formats

For this category, the investigator is interested in manipulating two treatments simultaneously.

Factorial design This is considered a parallel design that includes two or more independent variables. In this design, a subject is randomly assigned to different combinations of levels of the two independent variables. Usually, the most used are two-factor or three-factor designs. From Figure 4.3 we can conclude that this design allows us to answer three questions [3]:

1. Is there a differential effect between intervention A and control?
2. Is there a difference between intervention B and control?
3. Is there an interaction between intervention A and intervention B?

	Levels	Intervention A		Mean	Difference
		Placebo	Active		
Intervention B	Placebo	I Placebo	II Intervention A	(I + II)/2	I–II
	Active	III Intervention B	IV Intervention A & B	(III + IV)/2	III–IV
Mean		(I + III)/2	(II + IV)/2		
Difference		I–III	II–IV		

Figure 4.3. Factorial design: Two factors with each two levels = 2 x 2 factorial design. To get the main effect of A, we compare the mean of the active intervention A to the mean of the control. We use the same reasoning for the main effect of B, but here we compare the means of the row's total. On the other hand, to get the interaction, we focus on the differences within each of the columns and within each of the rows. If the differences are different, then there is an interaction effect.

The first two questions are to answer the *main effect*, as in the previous designs with only one independent variable. The third question is something unique to this type of study; it allows us to determine if the use of one intervention affects the other (*interaction effect*); that is, the effect of intervention A varies across the levels of the intervention B.

Factorial designs can be very helpful as they can be used to gain efficiency when studying two different treatments, or they can be used to study the interaction between two treatments. However, one very important concept here is that it cannot be used for both goals simultaneously. If there is a positive interaction, the main effect varies according to the value of the other variable; therefore the main effect of each variable can only be assessed when they are being tested alone. Many factorial trials are not powered to detect this interaction, and false negative results for the interaction may be concluded [4]. The most common use of factorial design is to test for the main effect and not for interaction.

In factorial design, the options for the biostatistical plan include a two-way or three-way analysis of variance, or multivariable regression modeling [3].

Example 1: Physicians' Health Study (PHS) I. This study began in 1982 with two objectives: to test whether aspirin prevented myocardial infarction and other cardiovascular events and to examine whether beta-carotene prevented cancer.

Trial design was a 2 x 2 factorial design. Arms: active aspirin and active beta-carotene, active aspirin and beta-carotene placebo, aspirin placebo and active beta-carotene, or aspirin placebo and beta-carotene placebo.

The efficiency is gained by testing two interventions (two main effect questions) on the same trial, saving resources by using the same pool of participants and methodology.

Main conclusions of PHS I:

1. Aspirin reduced the risk of first myocardial infarction by 44% ($P < 0.00001$) [5].
2. 12 years of supplementation with beta-carotene produced neither benefit nor harm in terms of the incidence of malignant neoplasms, cardiovascular disease, or death from all causes [6].

> Some of the disadvantages of using this design to gain efficiency were the following:
> - It needed many more participants for the study to be powered enough to detect both main effect questions.
> - The assumption of no interaction needed to be met. The main effects would not have been concluded if the protective effect of aspirin was modified by the amount of beta-carotene. There is a formal statistical test to assess interaction, but this test is not very powerful.

Non-parallel Design

Repeated measures design is a specific type of design where one group of subjects is tested at baseline and then at repeated time points during/after intervention. These studies are often referred to as *longitudinal studies*. Two main types of this design can be used: the *between-subjects design*, in which subjects received only one intervention but are tested several times, or the *within-subjects design*, where the subjects receive all the interventions in the same study—also called cross-over design. However, the investigator should be careful, as these designs usually (and should whenever possible) involve randomization.

Cross-over Design

It is the simplest form of this design, where a subject is assigned to one intervention, followed by measurement of the outcome variable, and then is assigned to the second intervention, followed by the measurement of the outcome variable. The order is systematically varied among the participants: we randomize participants to define which intervention they receive first (this is what makes it a randomized trial). The greatest advantages of this design are that it reduces the individual variance among participants and it increases power, as each participant serves as its own control, decreasing the number of subjects needed to test an intervention.

The main weaknesses that are important to consider and address in cross-over trials are the following:

- *Carry-over effect*: Subjects can have residual effects of the first intervention as they undergo the second intervention. Usually this requires a wash-out period, a time where participants do not receive any intervention, for them to come to the same baseline before starting the new intervention.
- *Practice (learning) effect*: Subjects repeat the same measurement method over and over.
- *Order effect*: Depending on which intervention is being tested first, subjects may respond differently to the second.

In cross-over design, the efficacy of the intervention over the control is assessed on the basis of the within-subject difference between the two treatments with regard to the outcome variable [7]. It can be analyzed by a paired t-test, or a two-way analysis of variance with two repeated measures if it uses parametric data. Non-parametric data are analyzed by a Wilcoxon signed-rank test. The analysis should include a preliminary testing to assess that the wash-out period was long enough and that there was no carry-over effect influencing the results.

Multifactor Design with Two Repeated Measures

As in factorial design, participants can be assigned to two or more interventions (independent variables). Here all participants are sequentially assigned to the four conditions.

Quasi-Experimental Designs

Designs where group assignment is not randomized, or if there is no control group at all, are considered quasi-experimental designs. The research designs are very similar to experimental designs, but we will describe specifically two types: *the one-group design* and the *non-equivalent control group design*.

One-Group Design

In one-group design, one set of repeated measures is taken before and after treatment on one group of subjects. Here the outcome variable is compared within the two points of assessment (pre-test and post-test). It resembles a repeated measure design, but there is no randomization of order to any control as all subjects are receiving the intervention [3].

Non-equivalent Control Group Design

The comparison group is "external" to the trial; that is, patients are not prospectively enrolled, treated, and assessed within the study protocol [8]. These types of trials tend to overestimate the effect.

There are two types:

- Historical control trial: it can be from a previous trial or clinical database.
- Concurrent control trial: patients in the same period but in a different, uncontrolled setting.

Designs with Non-random Allocation

There are other methods to define allocation of subjects in different interventions that are not random. For instance, subjects who come to appointments on Tuesdays receive treatment A and patients who come to appointments on Wednesdays receive treatment B.

Other Designs

N-of-1

The common definition of N-of-1 trial is a single or multiple cross-over study performed in a single individual. According to a systematic review [9] the N-of-1 trials serve three purposes:

1. They bridge the gap between the broad probabilities established in large parallel trials and treatments that work in an individual patient.
2. Second, the individual treatment effects estimated from a series of N-of-1 trials can be combined across patients to provide an estimate for the average treatment effect, averaged across patients participating in these trials. Therefore, N-of-1 trials can supplement or substitute for traditional parallel-group randomized controlled trials (RCTs) as a way to estimate the average treatment effect.
3. They provide an estimate of heterogeneity of treatment effects across patients.

Types of Trials: Quick Introduction

Superiority: whether the investigational intervention has superior clinical benefit relative to a placebo or a comparative active therapy.

Equivalence: whether the investigational intervention has comparable efficacy to an approved intervention.

Non-inferiority: whether the investigational intervention is not worse than a comparative intervention by a certain margin.

SPECIAL CONSIDERATIONS

Designs for Rare Diseases: Are They Different?

One difficult challenge in clinical research is the study design for rare diseases (diseases with low prevalence). The problem is not trivial; according to Ravani et al. [10], there are approximately 6,000 rare diseases identified in the United States. In 1983 the US Congress passed the "Orphan Drug Act" [11]. This landmark act instructs the US Food and Drug Administration to label a disease as "rare" if it has a prevalence of <200,000 persons in the United States. In the most recent years, the revolution of the Internet and the ability to congregate patients with rare disorders in centers and groups have provided new opportunities for their study.

Although RCTs are the gold standard, sometimes it is not possible to get the number of patients to run an RCT for a condition that is rare. What should you do in this situation? In fact, Ravani et al. list some of the situations in which RCT might not be used (for instance, large treatment effect, lack of equipoise, rare outcome) and also gives some alternative designs. Box 4.2 summarizes the challenges and potential study designs for rare diseases.

Example 2: Effect of enzyme therapy in juvenile patients with Pompe disease: a three-year open-label study [12].

"Pompe disease is a rare neuromuscular disorder caused by deficiency of acid α- glucosidase. Treatment with recombinant human α-glucosidase recently received marketing approval based on prolonged survival of affected infants. The current open-label study was performed to evaluate the response in older children (age 5.9–15.2 years). The *five patients* that we studied had limb-girdle muscle weakness and three of them also had decreased pulmonary function in upright and supine position. They received 20-mg/kg recombinant human α-glucosidase every two weeks over a 3-year period. No infusion-associated reactions were observed. Pulmonary function remained stable ($n = 4$) or improved slightly ($n = 1$). Muscle strength increased. Only one patient approached the normal range. Patients obtained higher scores on the Quick Motor Function Test. None of the patients deteriorated. Follow-up data of two unmatched historical cohorts of adults and children with Pompe disease were used for comparison. They showed an average decline in pulmonary function of 1.6% and 5% per year. Data on muscle strength and function of untreated children were not available. Further studies are required."

Box 4.2 Challenges and potential study designs for rare diseases

Main challenges with studying Rare Diseases:
- Limited target; therefore limited accessible population
- Incomplete understanding of the pathophysiology involve
- Endpoints and surrogate outcomes for their study may not be optimal
- Ethical concerns for control with Placebo
- Lack of controls
- Underpowered results.

Some of the research design options include:
1. Two-Group crossover study: As discussed, patients serve as their own controls, requiring a smaller sample size. However, assumptions about period effects, carryover effects, and drop-outs should be consider carefully.
2. Use of external historical controls: Use registry data and perform Quasi-experimental studies.
3. Use of observational studies: case reports, case series, etc. Main problem: How to reduce selection bias for choosing controls?
4. Factorial design: use of the available sample to answer two questions on the same trial.
5. Adaptive design: Use some of the new strategies such as "Play the winner" (Discussed in Chapter 17).
6. N-of-1 design: Here the aim is to estimate individual treatment effects from the available patients and then build an average of the treatment effect.
7. Use of multicenter trials
8. Open-label studies.

Designs According to the Study Phase Development

One interesting part of the article by Freudenheim (13) is the discussion of study phases (I, II, III, and IV) and different study designs. This is important in clinical research—for instance, it is OK to conduct an open-label study in phase I, but not appropriate for a phase III trial. Even though it is true that some study designs fit certain study phases better, it does not mean that it is an attribute of that phase and that it cannot be used for others. Box 4.3 provides some examples of designs according to the study phase from www.clinicaltrials.gov.

Box 4.3 Study design according to the study phase

Phase I
- Open-label parallel design: Phase I, Multicenter, Open-label, Dose-escalating, Clinical and Phamiacolcinetic Study of PM01183 in Patients With Advanced Solid Tumors. NCT00877474 (19).
- Double-blind randomized parallels design: A Phase Ib Double-blind Randomized Placebo Controlled Age-deescalating Trial of Two Virosome Formulated Anti-malaria Vaccine Components (PEV 301 and PEV 302) Administered in Combination to Healthy Semi-immune Tanzanian Volunteers. NC T00513669 (20).
- Crossover: A Phase I, A Single-Centre, Double-Blind, Randomized, Placebo-Controlled, Three-Period, Three-Way Crossover Study Of The Hemodynamic frier:actions Of Avanafil And Akohol In Healthy Male Subjects.NCT01054859 (21).
- Factorial: A Phase I lead-in to a 2x2x2 Factorial Trial of Dose Dense Temozolomide, Memantine, Mefloquine, and Metfomtin As Post-Radiation Adjutant Therapy of Glioblastoma Mukiforme.NCT01430351 (22).
- Historical controls: Phase I/II Multicenter Trial of Intra-Arterial Carboplatin and Oral Temozolomide for the Treatment of Recurrent and Symptomatic Residual Brain Metastases. NCT00362817 (23).

Phase II
- Open-label: An Open-label, Phase II Trial of ZD1839 (IRESSA) in Patients With Malignant Mesothelioma.NCT00787410 (24).
- Parallel: Active control - A Randomised, Double-blind, Parallel Group, Multi-centre, Phase II Study to Assess the Efficacy and Safety of Best Support Care (BSC) Plus ZD6474(Vandetanib) 300 mg, BSC Plus ZD6474(Vandetanib) 100 mg, and BSC Plus Placebo in Patients With Inoperable Hepatoceliular Carcinoma (HCC). NCT00508001 (25).
- Crossover. A Phase 2, Dose-finding, Cross-over Study to Evaluate the Effect of a NES/E2 Transdemial Gel Delivery on Ovulation Suppression in Normal Ovulating Women. NCT00796133 (26).
- Factorial: A Randomized, Double-Blind, Placebo-Controlled, 3/6 Factorial Design, Phase II Study to Evaluate the Antihypertensive Efficacy and Safety of Combination of Fimasartan and Amlo dipine in Patients With Essential Hypertension.NCT01518998.(27)
- N-of-1: N-of-1: Serial Controlled N-of-1 Trials of Topical Vitamin E as Prophylaxis for Chemotherapy-InducedOral Mucositis in Pediatric Patients.NCT00311116(28)

Phase III
- Parallel, Crossover and Factorial designs are common.
- Historical controls and Open label: Open Label, Phase III Study of NABI-IGIV 10% [Immune Globulin Intravenous(Human), 10%] In Subjects With Primary Immune Deficiency Disorders (PIDD) NCT00538915 (29). Primary Outcome Measures: To Assess the Efficacy of Nabi-IGIV 10% in Preventing Serious Bacterial Infections (SBIs) Compared to Historical Control Data.

Phase IV
- Again Parallel, Crossover and factorial can be common
- Open-label: An Open Label, Multi Centre Phase IV Study of Adefovir Dipivoxil in Korean Patients With Chronic Hepatitis B (CHB). NC T01205165.(30)

These examples illustrate how we can find different types of designs in all study phases. However, you should know when it is common and scientifically acceptable to use certain designs. Again, the option depends on what you are asking and in what population; as such, you can still have a Phase III open-label trial if the disease is rare, life threatening, or there are no available controls, among other reasons.

Large Simple Trials for Drug and Vaccine Safety Research

Large simple trials (LSTs) are randomized interventional studies that test the worth of interventions in large populations without the extensive data collection and other infrastructure needed for intensive clinical trials [14]. The goal is to obtain reliable and unbiased results similar to those from a well-performed randomized clinical trial. The advantages include more generalizability, more heterogeneity in the studied population, and more convincing interpretation of effects in "real-life" situations. A recent review of the published literature identified 13 ongoing or completed safety LSTs [15].

The characteristics of LSTs include the following [16]:

- Large sample sizes, often in the thousands
- Broad entry criteria consistent with the approved medication label
- Randomization based on equipoise
- Minimal, streamlined data-collection requirements
- Objectively measured endpoints (e.g., death, hospitalization)
- Follow-up that minimizes interventions or interference with normal clinical practice
- Considered to be less expensive than more complex trials
- Results that are relevant for clinical practice

Why do we need them?

- To reduce, as much as possible, random error
- To have the power to assess moderate effects
- To have the power to assess effects on rare conditions
- To have the power to assess effects in clinically important subgroups
- To have the power to demonstrate clinical equivalence
- To make it possible to do cluster randomization studies
- So that results are applicable to a wide range of people and settings

The main limitations include the following:

- How much can the definition of treatment be relaxed?
- How heterogeneous can the study sample be?
- Objectively measured endpoints such as death may be more costly at the end.
- Operational: How to define study protocol? How to account for deviations in protocol, measure compliance, account for drop outs?
- How to plan for the biostastistical analysis?

CASE STUDY: CHALLENGES FOR A STUDY DESIGN IN DERMATOLOGY

André Brunoni and Felipe Fregni

Dr. Garden, a dermatologist from California, sat at the coffee shop at Stanford University with his two work colleagues. They are clinicians and researchers with a very special interest in psoriasis, a severe dermatological disease characterized by erythematous plaques, which has no satisfactory treatment. They talked about a phone call Dr. Garden received last year from a big pharmaceutical company interested in testing a new topical therapy for psoriasis. In this phone call, they initially agreed to wait until the conclusion of phase I studies and, indeed, the studies showed that this new topical treatment (drug "P-SOLVE") is safe. They also agreed on some ethical aspects, including that the results would be published regardless of the results. Although Dr. Garden is very excited about this potential study (he is receiving a fairly good grant to lead a phase II study with 80 patients with severe psoriasis who will be recruited by the pharmaceutical company), he is also aware of the challenges of running this study. In fact, Dr. Garden knows that in a matter of days, he and his team need to make a series of decisions that will have a significant impact on the results of this study and his academic career. Now, it is his responsibility to design the most optimal randomized clinical trial to test the hypothesis that P-SOLVE is an effective therapy for severe psoriasis.[1]

Introduction

Experimental studies are designed to test the efficacy of a new intervention against placebo or a standard intervention. The most important aspect of an experimental study is that the patients are allocated at random to each treatment group. In fact, the independent variable of the study (for instance, the intervention) needs to be manipulated by the experimenter (for instance, the patients receive a given intervention not because of clinical reasons but because of study assignment) and, in addition, a control or comparison group is necessary. Randomization is a *sine qua non* characteristic of an experimental study because it is the best method to guarantee that all variables will be fairly distributed between groups, except, naturally, the intervention—therefore, if, at the end of the study, there is a difference between groups, it shall be concluded that such difference occurred due to the intervention. In fact, in experimental designs, the goal is to reduce random variation and systematic error, and to increase precision. Other interventional studies not using randomization are considered *quasi-experimental* studies.

There are several variations of RCTs, though the most frequently used is the design in which patients are allocated into two parallel groups and their endpoint scores are compared between groups. There are other designs that can bring some benefits

---

[1] Dr. André Brunoni and Professor Felipe Fregni prepared this case. Course cases are developed solely as the basis for class discussion. The situation in this case is fictional.

according to the study design (such as a cross-over design)—in fact, the researcher needs to consider the advantages and disadvantages of each design before deciding the final study design.

Dr. Garden can be considered a successful clinician and researcher. With almost 40 articles published in journals of relatively high impact, he has acquired a satisfactory experience in running clinical trials. Although he has run studies in a variety of dermatologic diseases, his great passion is psoriasis—that was the reason he chose dermatology as a specialty. Dr. Garden sent an email scheduling a meeting with his three postdoctoral fellows at his office to discuss the project. They arrived at the conference room and could notice that Dr. Garden wrote on the white board the potential study designs with large capital letters. They realized that this would be a long meeting.

Massimo Rossini, a postdoctoral fellow from Italy, begins, "Well . . . I would go for a classic RCT to compare P-SOLVE against placebo (we use an inert skin cream). We don't have many patients and we might not achieve a significant effect size with two active drugs. Besides, severe psoriasis is a disease with no satisfactory treatment . . . so my idea is P-SOLVE versus placebo—this would be a cleaner and better strategy!

Two-Arm Design: New Drug versus Placebo

Massimo suggested a very common, simple, and applied RCT design that is used in many different situations (e.g., for small and large samples, for pharmacological and non-pharmacological treatments, for phase II and III studies). It has several advantages, as it allows the use of several powerful and statistical methods, and it also provides an easier interpretation of the results. In addition, such a design can be pooled together with similar studies in meta-analysis. Finally, that might be a good design to assess the adverse effects of drugs.

However, such a design also has some drawbacks: first, there might be ethical concerns on using placebo when there is a standard treatment that is available. Even if the trial is short, this would go against the Helsinki Declaration, which says that a new therapeutic method should be tested against the best current therapeutic method. Massimo, aware of this important ethical concern, suggests that patients with a severe disease should be excluded and that the trial should have a short duration. However, Dr. Garden immediately replied that the drug could have the best benefits for patients with a severe disease. Another concern is that offering placebo in a trial would decrease the recruitment rate. Finally, using only placebo might lead to more dropouts in this group, which can under-power the study.

Catherine Hill, a postdoctoral fellow from Canada, quickly replied, "I'm sorry, Massimo—I have a different opinion," and after a pause, she continued, "We should not use placebo since there are effective treatments for psoriasis and some patients do respond . . . . Therefore, a future clinician might want to combine P-SOLVE with the other treatments. So, I suggest using a potent systemic drug, such as methotrexate [a drug used for chemotherapy and also for severe psoriasis] in all patients (we would select severe disease), in addition to P-SOLVE or placebo. So, my suggestion is methotrexate + P-SOLVE versus methotrexate + placebo!"

Two-Arm Design: Standard Drug + New Drug versus Standard Drug + Placebo

This approach is an adjustment of the "classic" RCT in which the standard drug will be used (open label or blinded) in all patients. This design might be the only option in certain fields in which using placebo would be unethical—for example, a new drug for AIDS. Also, the dropouts would be lower and, in addition, blinding might be more robust—since both groups will have side effects—that is, patients and physicians would not easily guess the allocated group. Although this design would satisfy potential ethical concerns, a negative result might be difficult to interpret, since the absence of difference between groups can be related to the large effect size in the standard drug group or to a negative interaction between both; in fact, even a positive result might underestimate the effect of the new drug, therefore leading to a larger sample size requirement. Finally, with this design, it would be difficult to analyze the adverse effects of P-SOLVE.

"It's my turn to disagree, Catherine," replies Edward Williams, a postdoctoral fellow from Colorado who has just started his fellowship with Dr. Garden. Suppose that, by using your idea, we came to negative findings—in this case, you can't conclude that P- SOLVE is ineffective, as you should consider that both methotrexate and P-SOLVE might act in the same pathways of the disease; therefore, methotrexate might be as effective as P-SOLVE, but with P-SOLVE having fewer side effects, as it is a topical treatment. So, I think we should keep placebo, to compare the new drug against it, but also methotrexate, to compare it against P-SOLVE and placebo. Therefore, I suggest a three-arm design: P- SOLVE versus placebo versus methotrexate."

Three-Arm Design: Standard Drug versus New Drug versus Placebo

A three-arm design is also a possible option in RCTs. The new drug is compared against the standard treatment and also against placebo—in this case, the use of placebo needs to be considered—that is, a delay in treatment would not significantly harm the patients given that there is an available effective drug. There are some advantages to this approach: first, this design can simultaneously prove whether the new drug is more effective than placebo and at least as effective as the standard drug—although this option seems attractive as it resolves some of the issues, such as giving information as to whether the drug is effective and comparable to the standard treatment, this design nevertheless has some drawbacks.

The most important drawback is that it requires more power as more comparisons will be performed—therefore the sample size will be larger than two-arm studies. In addition, lack of differences between standard versus new drug might be a type II error (the error of failing to observe a difference between groups when, in fact, there is a difference).

There are also some blinding issues here. Because the new drug is a topical agent and the standard drug is an oral (or IV) agent, this adds a complication to blinding. One alternative here would be the use of a double-dummy design in which one group receives a placebo pill and active topical medication, the other an active pill and placebo topical medication, and the third a placebo pill and topical medication—which, although feasible, adds complication to the trial. Also, if the standard drug requires flexible dosages to reach efficacy (e.g., lithium for bipolar disorder, which should be adjusted accordingly to the serum levels), then blinding might be an issue (although it is possible to have blinded strategy for dose adjustment, this adds complication to the trial design). Another threat to blinding is that physicians would easily "guess" patients on the standard treatment. Finally, the target population should exclude patients who have already used the standard treatment; otherwise this design would favor the new treatment (since the standard treatment would be used in patients in which such treatment was already proven ineffective).

Dr. Garden is writing frenetically on the whiteboard. The postdoctoral fellows are anxious, thinking about the pros and cons of their ideas. Suddenly, Dr. Garden stops writing, walks to the window, and asks without turning his eyes away from the beautiful garden in front of his office: "Although I liked your suggestions, let us explore all the options. I would also like to hear your ideas on cross-over studies."

Massimo immediately says, "Well, a cross-over might increase the efficiency of our study as the within-subject variability is smaller than between-subject variability. But there is the issue of carry-over effects and therefore data analysis should be planned carefully."

Crossover Design: New Drug → Placebo versus Placebo → New Drug

In a cross-over study, subjects receive both treatments at different times of the study: those who start using the new drug will change to placebo for the second half of the study, and vice versa. The advantage of this approach is to maximize the number of subjects in each group, as all patients will take placebo and the new drug. Also, it is possible to perform within comparisons, that is, to compare the effect of the new drug versus placebo in the same patient, therefore increasing the study power. Finally, this design might help recruitment, as patients know they will receive the active treatment at one point during the study.

On the other hand, this design is logistically more complicated, as the treatment should be changed without harming blinding. Another important issue is the carryover effect, that is, the effect of one treatment that will be carried on when the treatment is switched. In fact, there are several issues here: (1) persistent physiological effects of drugs (e.g., drugs with large half-lives might take weeks to be washed out from the body); (2) the first treatment might cure or permanently change the disease; (3) a treatment by period interaction. Therefore, the carry-over effect can bring serious concerns to the study's validity. Finally, the issue of placebo still needs to be addressed in this design.

After hearing Massimo, Dr. Garden turns to his staff. "Thanks, Massimo, I appreciate your comments." Dr. Garden remains quiet for a moment and starts walking through the room. His team knows that his attitude is demonstrating that he is thinking about something else. He then stops, goes back to his whiteboard and says, "Now, Edward and Catherine, I liked your suggestions about using methotrexate. Can you imagine a design in which we can put your ideas together?"

Catherine was faster this time, "A factorial design! We can compare both treatments against each other separately and also against placebo." Catherine continued, "OK, but you are decreasing even more the number of subjects in each group! This decreases power and we might not prove efficacy due to a type II error."

Factorial (2 x 2) Design: New Drug + Standard Drug versus New Drug versus Standard Drug versus Placebo

A factorial design randomizes patients into four groups to simultaneously test, usually, two interventions. A factorial design is used for two reasons: (1) to test two independent interventions using only one sample—therefore to increase efficiency (testing two treatments with one sample size)—for example, the famous Physician's Health Study trial that tested aspirin and beta-carotene for prevention of cardiovascular disease and cancer,[2] respectively; or (2) to test the interaction effects between two independent interventions—the plan in this case. Note that, despite having two interventions, there is still one dependent variable (outcome).

Factorial design can then be used to increase efficiency or to test the interaction effect (i.e., the synergistic or antagonistic effect occurring between two interventions). In this case, for instance, it would be interesting to test if P-SOLVE and methotrexate ameliorates psoriasis better than each drug separately or, alternatively, that using both drugs does not increase the overall effect.

The main disadvantage of this design is that the interaction effect should be estimated carefully, otherwise no group difference will be observed due to lack of power—for instance, if the combined intervention is expected to be just slightly more effective than each intervention separately, then this would require a larger sample in order to detect an effect size.

Dr. Garden looks at his watch and sees that his weekly outpatient clinic is about to start in 15 minutes. He then wraps up the meeting, "Thank you everyone. Let us all think on all these ideas and try to choose the best design—it will not be easy. Also, one additional question to Catherine: should we have a factorial design but the two factors being phototherapy and P-SOLVE, as we are also interested in this new phototherapy treatment?" He then heads to his clinic, knowing that it would be a busy afternoon. By the end of the day, he finds himself preoccupied. He knows that in two days he will have a meeting with the CMO (chief medical officer) and some vice presidents of the pharmaceutical company and he will need to present the study design to them. He refuses dinner and also the baseball game and goes directly to his home office to work on this study.

Authors' note: In this chapter we did not consider non-inferiority studies, in which a new drug is compared directly against a standard drug. We will review this topic further in the course.

CASE DISCUSSION

In order to select the best approach, it is important to put the disease into context. Some of the main points Dr. Garden should consider are the following:

1. He is studying severe psoriasis. Current guidelines for severe psoriasis recommend phototherapy or systemic therapies such as retinoids, methotrexate, cyclosporine, or biologic immune-modifying agents. Sometimes it requires upfront combination therapy. Improvement usually occurs within weeks [13,14]. *Is placebo an option?*
2. It is a grant for a phase II trial with 80 patients. Depending on the complexity of the comparison, the sample size will have to be bigger in order to have enough

---

[2] To learn more about this famous factorial study go to http://phs.bwh.harvard.edu/phs1.htm.

power to detect a difference. *Will the number of patients limit his availability of designs?*
3. What has been done for this disease? Examples of previous trials:
   a. "Efficacy and safety results from the randomized controlled comparative study of adalimumab vs. methotrexate vs. placebo in patients with psoriasis (CHAMPION)" [15].
   b. "Phase 3: A randomized, double-blind, double-dummy, placebo controlled, multicenter study of subcutaneous Secukinumab to demonstrate efficacy after twelve weeks of treatment, compared to placebo and Etanercept, and to assess the safety, tolerability and long-term efficacy up to one year in subjects with moderate to severe chronic plaque psoriasis. (ClinicalTrials.gov Identifier: NCT01358578)" [16].

The advantages and disadvantages are of each study design for Dr. Garden trial are summarized in Table 4.1.

Conclusions: Based on our discussion, since it is a phase II trial, where the main objective is to assess efficacy and safety and where there is a limitation of the number of patients available, the simplest design would be to select a randomized, double-dummy design of P-SOLVE versus placebo. Placebo would be an acceptable option since the outcomes of the intervention would be tested fairly quickly and participants would then receive additional interventions. If the phase II is positive, a phase III trial design would be done to test P-SOLVE against other interventions available (parallel design or factorial design). Theoretically, cross-over is an appealing option; however, the carry-over and order effect might be important cofounders in a disease with rapid improvement to interventions.

CASE QUESTIONS FOR REFLECTION

1. What challenges does Dr. Garden face in choosing the study design?
2. What are his main concerns?
3. What should he consider in making his decision?

REFERENCES

1. Wypij D, ed. Clinical trials: basic study design. Class Lecture. *Principles and practice of clinical research*. Boston, MA. May, 2012.
2. Sackett DL, Wennberg JE. Choosing the best research design for each question. *BMJ*. 1997 Dec 20–27; 315(7123): 1636. PubMed PMID: 9448521. Pubmed Central PMCID: 2128012.
3. Portney L, Watkins M. *Foundations of clinical research: applications to practice*, 3rd ed. Upper Saddle River, NJ: Pearson Prentice Hall; 2009.
4. Green S, Liu PY, O'Sullivan J. Factorial design considerations. *J Clin Oncol*. 2002 Aug 15; 20(16): 3424–3430. PubMed PMID: 12177102.
5. Group* SCotPHSR. Final Report on the Aspirin Component of the Ongoing Physicians' Health Study. *N Engl J Med*. 1989; 321(3): 129–135. PubMed PMID: 2664509.
6. Hennekens CH, Buring JE, Manson JE, Stampfer M, Rosner B, Cook NR, et al. Lack of effect of long-term supplementation with beta carotene on the incidence of malignant

neoplasms and cardiovascular disease. *N Engl J Med.* 1996 May 2; 334(18): 1145–1149. PubMed PMID: 8602179.

7. Wellek S, Blettner M. On the proper use of the crossover design in clinical trials: part 18 of a series on evaluation of scientific publications. *Dtsch Arztebl Int.* 2012 Apr; 109(15): 276–281. PubMed PMID: 22567063. Pubmed Central PMCID: 3345345.

8. Fawcett JW, Curt A, Steeves JD, Coleman WP, Tuszynski MH, Lammertse D, et al. Guidelines for the conduct of clinical trials for spinal cord injury as developed by the ICCP panel: spontaneous recovery after spinal cord injury and statistical power needed for therapeutic clinical trials. *Spinal Cord.* 2007 Mar; 45(3): 190–205. PubMed PMID: 17179973. Epub 2006/12/21. eng.

9. Gabler NB, Duan N, Vohra S, Kravitz RL. N-of-1 trials in the medical literature: a systematic review. *Med Care.* 2011 Aug; 49(8):761–8. PubMed PMID: 21478771.

10. Wühl E, van Stralen KJ, Wanner C, Ariceta G, Heaf JG, Bjerre AK, Palsson R, Duneau G, Hoitsma AJ, Ravani P, Schaefer F. Renal replacement therapy for rare diseases affecting the kidney: an analysis of the ERA–EDTA Registry. *Nephrology Dialysis Transplantation.* 2014 Sep 1; 29(suppl 4): iv1–8.

11. Public Law 97–414.

12. Van Capelle CI, van der Beek NA, Hagemans ML, Arts WF, Hop WC, Lee P, Jaeken J, Frohn-Mulder IM, Merkus PJ, Corzo D, Puga AC. Effect of enzyme therapy in juvenile patients with Pompe disease: a three-year open-label study. *Neuromuscular Disorders.* 2010 Dec 31; 20(12): 775–782.

13. Freudenheim JL. A review of study designs and methods of dietary assessment in nutritional epidemiology of chronic disease. *J Nutrition.* 1993 Feb; 123(2 Suppl): 401–405.

14. Schön MP, Boehncke W-H. Psoriasis. *N Engl J Med.* 2005; 352(18): 1899–1912. PubMed PMID: 15872205.

15. Saurat JH, Stingl G, Dubertret L, Papp K, Langley RG, Ortonne JP, et al. Efficacy and safety results from the randomized controlled comparative study of adalimumab vs. methotrexate vs. placebo in patients with psoriasis (CHAMPION). *Br J Dermatol.* 2008 Mar; 158(3): 558–566. PubMed PMID: 18047523.

16. Novartis-Pharmaceuticals. A randomized, double-blind, double-dummy, placebo controlled, multicenter study of subcutaneous secukinumab to demonstrate efficacy after twelve weeks of treatment, compared to placebo and etanercept, and to assess the safety, tolerability and long-term efficacy up to one year in subjects with moderate to severe chronic plaque-type psoriasis (FIXTURE). In: ClinicalTrialsgov [Internet] NLM Identifier: NCT01358578 [Internet]. 2012.

5

RANDOMIZATION

Authors: *Juliana C. Ferreira, Ben M. W. Illigens, and Felipe Fregni*

Case study author: *Felipe Fregni*

Chance favors only the prepared mind.
—Louis Pasteur (French scientist, 1822–1895)

INTRODUCTION

Randomization is a key feature of randomized controlled trials (RCT), which are considered the gold standard in evaluating the efficacy of new interventions. In this chapter, we will discuss what randomization is, why it is important, methods of randomization, and their advantages and disadvantages. We will also discuss a case that illustrates the options faced by researchers when designing a RCT and choosing the randomization method.

WHAT IS RANDOMIZATION?

Randomization is the process of allocating study participants to one of the study groups, in which each participant has an equal chance of being allocated to the treatment or control group [1]. When randomization is properly conducted, neither the investigator nor the participants can foresee the group to which the participant will be assigned, nor can they interfere with allocation. Randomization ensures that treatment groups in a clinical trial are comparable in terms of known and unknown risk factors, since participants with a given set of risk factors have equal chances of being allocated to the control or the intervention (treatment) group [2].

In clinical practice, and in observational studies, treatment is determined by the patient's clinician, and/or the patient's preferences. As a result, it is common that patients with more severe disease are treated with more aggressive strategy than asymptomatic patients [1]. For example, in an observational study of the use of inhaled corticosteroids for asthma and the risk of asthma exacerbation, we could expect participants with moderate asthma to be more likely to be using daily inhaled corticosteroids than asymptomatic participants. So, if the study showed that the use of daily corticosteroids was associated with a greater risk of exacerbation, this finding could be erroneously attributed to the medication use rather than the baseline disease severity (as sicker patients were given the medication). For non-randomized studies evaluating invasive procedures, for example surgery, participants with better overall health (such as younger participants with no comorbidities) might be more likely treated with surgery, while older, sicker participants might be treated with a less invasive strategy. In these two examples, the two groups are not comparable at the beginning of the trial, and treatment group allocation is influenced by baseline characteristics.

CONSEQUENCES FOR LACK OF RANDOMIZATION OR FAILURE IN RANDOMIZATION: SELECTION BIAS

The aim of randomization is to avoid selection bias and produce treatments groups that are truly comparable. Selection bias is defined as a systematic error that results from participants being allocated one of the study groups based on their baseline characteristics (i.e., participants are *selected* to receive one type of treatment). When selection bias occurs, the two groups in a clinical trial may differ considerably regarding known and unknown covariates at baseline, before treatment starts. Therefore, differences in outcomes between the two groups observed at the end of the trial could be a result of the intervention that is being evaluated, or a result of the baseline differences [3].

When treatment allocation is randomized, and each participant has an equal chance of being allocated to treatment or control, the two groups will be balanced for known and unknown baseline characteristics. Also, only when treatment allocation is randomized can we say that the two groups came from the same source population—an important assumption for most statistical tests.

Although selection bias is very likely in non-randomized trials, it can also occur in randomized trials, when randomization fails. An example of that is when the randomization method is proper but the list of randomization order is disclosed to investigators recruiting participants—also called *failure of allocation concealment* (see the following section).

SELECTION BIAS IN RANDOMIZED TRIALS: POOR ALLOCATION CONCEALMENT

For randomization to work, and in fact produce comparable groups, two points are essential:

- The researcher and the participant must be unable to predict their allocation group—what we call *allocation concealment*.
- The researcher must be unable to change a participant's allocation, once he or she has been randomized.

You may be thinking that if allocation is randomized, there is no way to predict the next participant's allocation. However, in order to use randomization in practice, a randomization list must be generated, which contains the sequence of allocation for all trial participants. As we will see when we discuss methods of randomization, this list cannot be available to the researchers who are recruiting and registering participants for the trial. It may be known only by a pharmacist who delivers medication, or it can be used by someone not involved in participant recruitment to prepare numbered, opaque sealed envelopes, or it can be created by a computerized system of registration and randomization of participants. In any case, if the researcher can guess the allocation group for the next participant, he or she might be able to select participants. For example, suppose that a researcher is conducting a trial to test a new rehabilitation program for patients with traumatic brain injury, and preliminary data on a small series of patients led her to believe that the new treatment works. Now suppose she has access to the randomization list and knows that the next participant will be allocated to the control arm. If the next eligible participant is a young patient with a severe disability, whom she feels would benefit from the new treatment, she might not discuss the trial with this patient until other participants were registered, and the next participant's group was known to be active treatment.

Therefore, for randomization to truly prevent selection bias, there needs to be *allocation concealment*: allocation group of the next participant must be unknown to investigator and participants [4]. Moreover, once the participant is randomized to one of the study groups, allocation cannot be changed by the investigator. For example, suppose that randomization was being done by the researcher flipping a coin every time a new participant was to be randomized to treatment or control. If the researcher from the rehabilitation trial flipped the coin, and it ended in tails (control), she might flip the coin again and again until it landed in heads (treatment). That is why the randomization procedure should be implemented in a way that this type of manipulation is not possible. We will discuss methods for implementing randomization later in this chapter.

METHODS OF RANDOMIZATION

There are many methods of randomization, each with its advantages and disadvantages. In this chapter, we will discuss simple randomization, blocked randomization, stratified randomization, and adaptive randomization.

Simple randomization is one of the most commonly used methods of randomization, because it is easily implemented and inexpensive. In simple randomization, a random digit table, usually generated by a computer, is used to generate the randomization list. Several computer programs, including Stata, can generate a random digit table. The number of digits in the table is set as the number of participants to be enrolled in the trial. The table contains digits from 0 to 9, and the sequence of the digits is random. Each set of digits will be paired with a study group. For example, suppose you determine that 0 to 4 corresponds to treatment (T) and 5 to 9 correspond to control (C). Figure 5.1, panel 1A, depicts the random digit table generated for a trial with 24 participants, and the randomization list resulting from it.

The advantages of simple randomization are that it is inexpensive, easy to be implemented, and the fact that allocation concealment is a natural feature of simple randomization, since every participant has an equal chance of being randomized to treatment or control group. The major disadvantage of simple randomization is that, for small sample sizes (<100), there is a considerable chance of imbalances in the number of participants randomized for each group [1]. For trials of 20 participants, for example, the chance of an imbalance of having 6 participants or less in one of the groups is approximately 11%. Simple randomization can also lead to imbalances in terms of important baseline covariates between groups, since it does not take any baseline characteristic into account when randomizing participants. For example, in a trial of a new drug to treat congestive heart failure (CHF) planning to include

1A

Random numbers	8	8	4	8	3	0	5	4	8	1	3	6	3	7	6	2	5	9	8	2	9	5	6	7
Ramdomization list	C	C	T	C	T	T	C	T	C	T	T	C	T	C	C	T	C	C	T	C	C	C	C	C
Subject ID	1	2	3	4	5	6	7	8	9	10	11	12	13	14	15	16	17	18	19	20	21	22	23	24

Control arm: n=15
Treatment arm: n=9

1B

Random numbers: 3 | 6 | 5 | 2 | 5 | 3

Ramdomization list	C	T	T	C	T	C	C	T	C	T	C	C	T	C	T	T	C	T	C	T	C	C	T	T	C
Subject ID	1	2	3	4	5	6	7	8	9	10	11	12	13	14	15	16	17	18	19	20	21	22	23	24

Control arm: n=12
Treatment arm: n=12

1C

Random numbers: 7 | 3 | 17 | 1 | 6

Ramdomization list	C	C	C	T	T	T	C	T	T	C	T	C	C	C	T	C	C	T	T	C	T	T	C	C	T
Subject ID	1	2	3	4	5	6	7	8	9	10	11	12	13	14	15	16	17	18	19	20	21	22	23	24

Control arm: n=12
Treatment arm: n=12

1D

Stage: moderate

Random numbers: 4 | 2 | 6

Ramdomization list	T	T	C	C	C	T	C	T	T	C	C	T
Subject ID	1	2	4	6	7	10	12	15	16	18	19	21

Stage: severe

Random numbers: 5 | 3 | 1

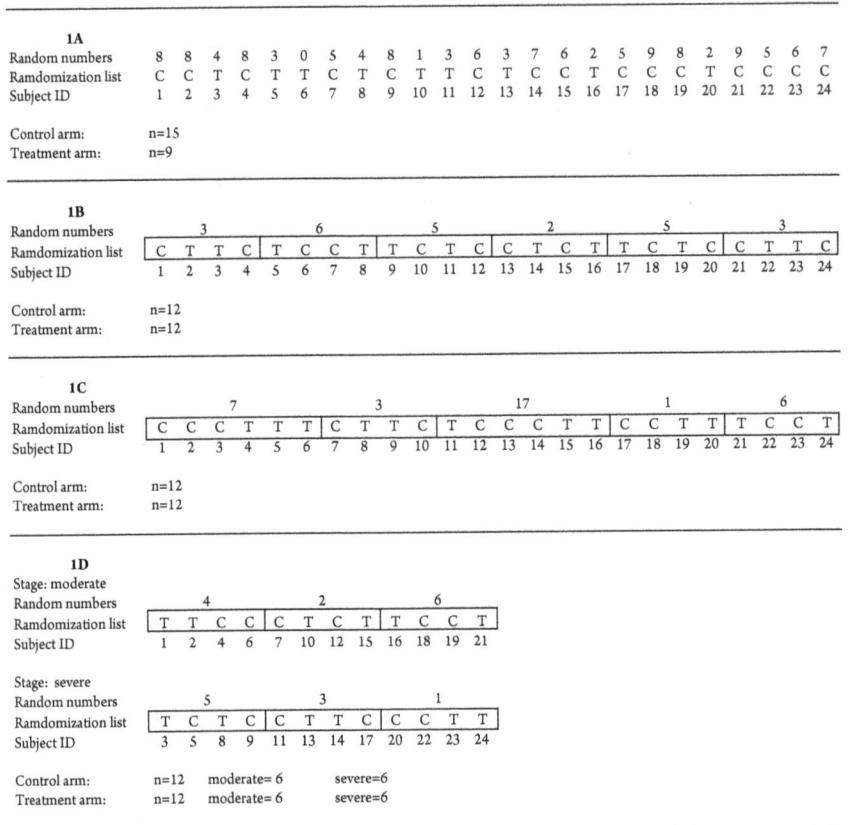

Ramdomization list	T	C	T	C	C	T	T	C	C	C	T	T
Subject ID	3	5	8	9	11	13	14	17	20	22	23	24

Control arm: n=12, moderate=6, severe=6
Treatment arm: n=12, moderate=6, severe=6

Figure 5.1. Methods of randomization for a two-arm trial comparing treatment (T) and control (C). A) Simple randomization: A computer generates a sequence of 24 random numbers from 0 to 9. The investigator pre-determines that 0 to 4 will correspond to treatment (T) and 5 to 9 will correspond to control (C). This random sequence results in 15 subjects being assigned to the control arm and 9 to the treatment arm;
B) Blocked randomization: Blocks have a size of 4. There are 6 possible combinations of the order of randomization for these 4 patients: 1) CCTT; 2) CTCT; 3) CTTC; 4) TTCC; 5) TCTC; and 6) TCCT. A computer generates list of 6 random numbers, from 1 to 6, which corresponding to one of the 6 possible blocks of 4 participants. This random sequence results in 12 subjects being assigned to the control arm and 12 to the treatment arm;
C) Blocked randomization with variable block sizes: Blocks have a size of 4 or 6. There are 26 possible combinations for blocks of 4 or 6 participants: 1) CCTT; 2) CTCT; 3) CTTC; 4) TTCC; 5) TCTC; 6) TCCT; 7) CCCTTT; 8) CCTCTT; 9) CCTTCT; 10) CCTTTC; 11) CTCCTT; 12) CTCTCT; 13) CTCTTC; 14) CTTCCT; 15) CTTCTC; 16) CTTTCC; 17) TCCCTT; 18) TCCTCT; 19) TCCTTC; 20) TCTCCT; 21) TCTCTC; 22) TCTTCC; 23) TTCCCT; 24) TTCCTC; 25) TTCTCC; 26) TTTCCC. A computer generates list of 6 random numbers, from 1 to 26, which correspond to one of the 26 possible blocks of 4 or 6 participants. This random sequence results in 12 subjects being assigned to the control arm and 12 to the treatment arm, and allocation concealment is preserved.
D) Stratified randomization with blocks: Eligible patients are first separated into two strata according to stage of disease. Each stratum has a separate randomization list. For each stratum, the computer generates a list of 3 random numbers, from 1 to 6, which correspond to one of the 6 possible blocks of 4 participants. This random sequence results in 12 subjects being assigned to the control arm and 12 to the treatment arm. There is balance in sample size between groups, and balance for the stage of disease between treatment groups.

40 participants, simple randomization might result in more participants with severe CFH in the treatment group than in the control group just by chance. As a result, outcomes might be worse for the treatment group than the control group even if the intervention (the new drug) was effective, because participants in the treatment group were sicker than those in the control group. Therefore, simple randomization is not a good option for trials with small sample sizes, or when balance for key covariates is desired.

Blocked randomization is a randomization method that randomizes participants within blocks, instead of randomizing each participant individually. The blocks have a predetermined size, for example blocks of 4 or 6 participants, and within each block, there is balance in terms of number of participants in each group. For example, suppose that we use blocked randomization with block sizes of 4 for our trial of 24 participants. Each block will have 4 participants—2 must be allocated to the treatment group and 2 to the control group. There are six possible combinations of the order of randomization for these 4 participants: CCTT, CTCT, CTTC, TTCC, TCTC, and TCCT. To generate a randomization list, the randomization program will randomly select one of the six combinations for each block of 4 participants. Therefore, the randomization list is a random sequence of these 6 possible blocks. For a trial with 24 participants, the program will randomly select of one the combinations six times. Figure 5.1, panel 1B, depicts the random blocks generated for a trial with 24 participants, and the randomization list resulting from it.

The major advantage of blocked randomization is that it will result in balanced groups in terms of number of participants per group. If the trial is terminated before the completion of a block, an imbalance may occur, but will be small. For our 24 participants' trial, for example, the worst case scenario if the last block was interrupted with 2 participants would be 10 participants in one group versus 12 participants in the other group.

Blocked randomization can have a disadvantage: if the trial is not blinded, and researchers know the assignment of previous participants and the block size, they might be able to predict the allocation of the next participant, compromising allocation concealment and allowing for selection bias [2]. For example, suppose that in a trial comparing surgery with medical treatment, the researcher knows that the block size is four and first three participants were randomized to surgery, control, control. He will then deduce that the next participant is going to be randomized to surgery, since blocks are balanced (two treatments and two controls). To overcome this problem, the block size should be variable within the trial (i.e., blocks can have random sizes of 4 or 6, for example). Figure 5.1, panel 1C, depicts the random blocks with variable block sizes generated for a trial with 24 participants, and the randomization list resulting from it.

Blocked randomization will lead to balance in sample size between groups; however, it may still result in imbalances for important covariates between the groups, since baseline characteristic are not taken into account in the randomization process.

Stratified randomization is an alternative method when baseline covariates have a strong impact on the study outcome, and balance for these covariates between the groups is important. In stratified randomization, eligible participants are first separated into strata according to baseline characteristic, for example, gender, or stage of disease. Each strata has a separate randomization list, and after being categorized into one of the strata, the participant is randomized to control or treatment arm. With this method, each participant in each strata has an equal chance of being allocated to control or treatment group, and if the sample size is big enough, there will be balance in terms of the number of subjects allocated to control or treatment within each strata.

Stratification is commonly associated with blocked randomization, so that participants are first categorized into one of the strata, then randomized in blocks within that stratum [5]. In this method, we can achieve balance in sample size between groups with the block, and balance for the covariate with the stratification. Figure 5.1, panel 1D, depicts stratified, blocked randomization generated for a trial with 24 participants, and the randomization list resulting from it. The block has a size of four, and stratification is for stage of disease.

Stratification and blocks will result in balanced groups as long as there are not too many strata, so that each stratum has a minimum number of subjects. Otherwise, it can actually lead to imbalances. For example, for our trial of 24 participants, if we decided to stratify by disease severity, gender, and age (greater or less than 65), there would be six strata. But since there are probably fewer severe than moderate patients in our accessible population, we might have only two older females with severe disease. If the first block randomly chosen for this stratum was TTCC, it would be imbalanced, with the two participants allocated to the treatment group [5].

Therefore, stratification should be done with few strata, only the most relevant ones, preferably using dichotomous variables, instead of choosing an arbitrary cut-off for continuous variables. Balance is expected to begin to fail with stratified blocked randomization when the number of strata approaches one-half of the sample size. Keeping the number of strata to a minimum is also important for the sample size calculation, because covariates used for stratification must be entered into the multivariate analysis, if it is planned, and approximately 10 outcomes are needed for each variable entered in the multivariate analysis model [6]. Variables typically used for stratified randomization include site center in multicentric studies, and disease severity.

Adaptive randomization is a generic name for randomization methods that use algorithms which include baseline covariates and the allocation of previous participants into consideration to allocate the next participants [7,8]. We will discuss the most popular of the adaptive methods, minimization.

The minimization method uses a computerized algorithm that lists the baseline covariates of interest for the participant, evaluates the balance (or imbalance) of these covariates among the participants already included in each of the study groups, and then allocates the participant to the control or the treatment arm in order to minimize the imbalances [7].

Let's suppose for a hypothetical trial—with two covariates, gender and disease severity—that there are 11 participants already included in the trial and the next participant to be randomized is a male with severe disease (see Table 5.1). The minimization algorithm will take into account the total number of participants in each group, as well as their distribution across the covariates, to assign this next participant to the control or treatment group. In total, there are 6 participants in the treatment group and 5 participants in the control group, so if balance in terms of number of participants in each group was the only important factor, this participant should be randomized to the control group. However, there are two severe patients in the control group and only one severe patient in the treatment group, so to obtain balance in the number of

Table 5.1 Randomization with the Minimization algorithm

Disease Severity	Female	Male	Marginal Total
Mild and moderate	2C 3T	1C 2T	3C 5T
Severe	1C 1T	1C 0T	2C 1T
Marginal total	3C 4T	2C 2T	5C 6T

Adaptive randomization—minimization: a trial of 24 participants with two important baseline covariates, gender and disease severity. There are 11 participants already registered in the trial and the next participant to be randomized is a male with severe disease. A computerized algorithm categorizes participants into strata, and evaluates the number of patients in the control and the treatment arm in terms of all the covariates and allocates the participant in order to minimize imbalances.

severe patients in each group the participant should be randomized to the treatment group. The algorithm takes into account the imbalances for each covariate and assigns the participant to one of the groups in order to minimize imbalances. Some algorithms assign scores for each covariate and add up the total score for each group in order to make the decision; others use other strategies. For all the algorithms, the rationale is to weigh in all the covariates and try to balance the groups as the trial progresses.

The minimization method allows for more covariates to be taken into account to influence randomization than traditional stratification, and usually generates balanced groups in terms of most of the covariates.

A disadvantage of minimization technique is that it requires the implementation of the algorithm using a computerized system for randomization. The randomization list cannot be generated in advance and used to prepare sealed envelopes, since the allocation of previous participants is used to determine the allocation of the next one. As a result, the computerized system must be available at the moment when the participant is considered eligible for the study and needs to be randomized. If the trial is multicentric, the system must be web-based, online, and accessible to all centers at all times. Another potential disadvantage for non-blinded trials is that investigators may be able to predict the allocation of the next participant, leading to selection bias. To overcome this problem, the algorithm may be programmed to use a "biased coin" strategy: it determines the group allocation that would minimize imbalances, and then randomizes the participant with a 70% or 60% chance of being allocated to that group, but with 30% or 40% chance of being allocated to the other group. This strategy protects allocation concealment, but may lead to small imbalances for trials with small sample sizes.

WHAT IS THEN THE BEST TYPE OF RANDOMIZATION? THE CHALLENGE FOR SMALL TRIALS

The response to this question in a few words would be: for large trials, any method would work well—in fact, in most of the cases a simple randomization method is adequate, and for small trials, none of the methods is fully adequate.

In summary, simple randomization is easy to implement and inexpensive, but can lead to considerable group imbalances in trials with small sample sizes. Blocked randomization produces balance in terms of number of participants in each group, but not in terms of baseline covariates. Stratification is usually combined with blocked randomization to provide balance between groups in the number of participants and important covariates. However, depending on the number of covariates used for stratification and the sample size, this method could lead to imbalances, going back to the problem of simple randomization method. Adaptive randomization methods, especially minimization, allow for more baseline covariates to be taken into account and produce balanced groups in terms of both the number of participants and covariates, but are more complex and should be implemented with statisticians and information

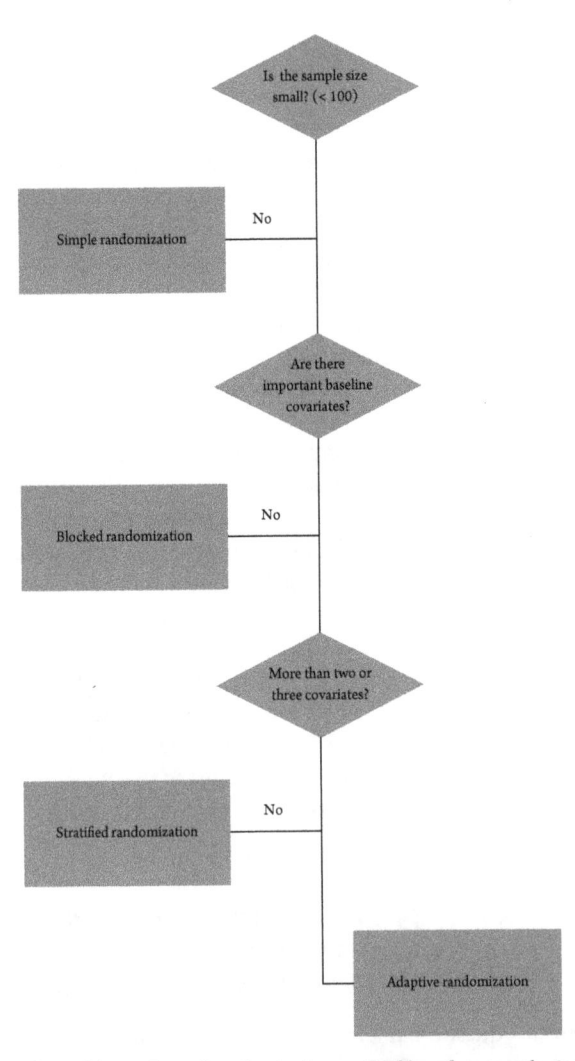

Figure 5.2. Flow chart of the options of randomization method based on sample size and number important baseline covariates to be balanced among the treatment arms.

technology (IT) support. Figure 5.2 shows a flow chart of the many options of randomization methods and potential limitations, especially in small sample size trials.

CHECKING WHETHER THE RANDOMIZATION METHOD WAS ADEQUATE

Given the importance of randomization, one important issue is to check whether the randomization method was properly chosen and implemented. There are no formal methods to check that, but investigators and clinicians assessing a randomized trial should look at some studies' characteristics to decide whether or not randomization was proper and therefore the results are valid.

First, clinicians should look at the methods of the study and then, based on the sample size and study characteristics, assess if theoretically the choices for the randomization and allocation concealment methods were adequate, as discussed earlier. Second, they should look at the paper's Table 1. Table 1 in articles reporting the results of clinical trials usually describes the demographic and clinical characteristics of each group according to the randomized group. This table is essential and can provide valuable information for the clinician to assess whether randomization was adequate. This table has the number of subjects per group, and thus it indicates whether the groups are balanced. Next, the randomization should have resulted in balanced groups regarding the covariates. Here one challenge is to define what is acceptable as balanced, and how to assess that factor. Usually, investigators compare baseline characteristics between groups using statistical tests and conclude that if there are no significant differences, then groups are likely balanced. However, this conclusion is not proper, as the trial was not designed to test for the hypothesis that there are differences in baseline characteristics between groups. In other words, there is not enough statistical power for that testing; thus a non-significant test does not indicate balanced groups. The investigator should look at the absolute values. Are they too different? If they are, then there may be an indication that an imbalance may have occurred, and this may explain the different results. (The next chapters of this text will discuss how to address these differences.) A final important concept is that there may be variables (unknown confounders) that are not shown in Table 1 and thus even if the randomization method used was adequate and no obvious imbalances are seen across the measured covariates, there may still be differences between groups.

IMPLEMENTING THE RANDOMIZATION METHOD: ENSURING ADEQUATE ALLOCATION CONCEALMENT

After choosing the best randomization method for a particular study, investigators need to plan how to implement it. For example, if sealed envelopes will be used, who will be responsible for preparing the envelopes? If a telephone-based randomization service is chosen, how it will be put into practice? In this section, we discuss some practical issues related to randomization.

Envelope systems are widely used because this system can be developed locally, with little cost. To put such a system into practice, the investigators should follow these steps:

1. Determine the randomization method (simple, blocked, stratified).
2. Create a randomization list. This can be done using statistical packages or websites (see a list later in this chapter). If the method chosen is stratified randomization, separate lists should be generated for each strata. This should ideally be done by someone outside the trial, for example a statistician, or a colleague not involved in the trial. If this is not possible, the person generating the list should at least not be responsible for recruiting and enrolling participants for the trial.
3. Prepare numbered, opaque, inviolable envelopes according to the list, with the randomization code inside. It is safer to prepare more envelopes than the number of participants planned to be enrolled in the trial, in case of dropouts or eligibility errors.
4. Envelopes should be opened only after eligible participants have been registered into the trial. Write the date and participant trial number on the outside of the envelope, and sign. Keep the opened envelopes as a record.

In some cases, a randomization list, without envelopes, can be available for a pharmacist, for example. If that is the case, make sure that investigators have no access to the list and that the person who has access to it understands the need for allocation concealment.

Telephone systems and web-based randomization systems are usually done by companies that offer their services for a fee. Computerized systems can also be created by the trial staff, of course, as long as members of the team are experts in computer programming and web design; they will have to work together with the trial statistician.

CASE STUDY: RANDOMIZATION: THE DILEMMA OF SIMPLICITY VERSUS IMBALANCES IN SMALL STUDIES

Felipe Fregni

Professor Luigi Lombardi is sitting in his office after a full day of work. He is trying to finish his grant proposal, but he is having trouble writing the randomization method section. He had an unpleasant experience in the past when he submitted a paper from one of his studies and his method of randomization was highly criticized by one of the reviewers. He did not want to repeat the same mistake this time. He is therefore taking extra time to write this section. He is staring at his computer screen and going over all his options. It is almost 11 p.m. and the last train to his house is about to leave. He packs his notes and starts walking to the train station, but his thoughts are focused on how to resolve this issue.

Introduction

In clinical research, one of the goals is to compare two (or more) different groups of subjects that have been exposed to different interventions or have different risk factors. In clinical trials, these groups might receive two different interventions (e.g., drug A vs. drug B, or a placebo vs. experimental treatment). If there are two groups, it becomes critical to define how subjects are allocated to such groups. If the treating physician or the researcher interacting with the subjects is allowed to decide allocation, then bias will probably occur as sicker patients (or the patients with an increased likelihood of response) might be randomized to the active, experimental treatment. This effect can typically be observed in observational studies, where usually the treating physician decides the treatment based on clinical characteristics and personal preferences, and is called *selection bias*.

For instance, in a previous observational study comparing three antipsychotic drugs (risperidone, olanzapine, and clozapine) for the management of chronic schizophrenia, physicians chose the drug that participants were to receive. In fact, significant changes across the three treatment groups were seen for illness duration and number of hospitalizations: Participants taking clozapine had longer illness duration and higher number of hospitalizations compared to those taking olanzapine.[1]

Therefore, unbiased methods of allocating participants are necessary to produce comparable groups of intervention. In addition, most of the statistical tests are based on the notion that groups are comparable; therefore randomization becomes a critical issue to increase the internal validity.

However, randomization comes with a price: research subjects (and investigators) need to accept the fact that they may not be aware of the treatment group until the trial

---

[1] Strous RD, Kupchik M, Roitman S, Schwartz S, Gonen N, Mester R, Weizman A, Spivak B. Comparison between risperidone, olanzapine, and clozapine in the management of chronic schizophrenia: A naturalistic prospective 12-week observational study. *Human Psychopharmacology: Clinical and Experimental*. 2006 Jun 1; 21(4): 235–243.

is over (if it is a blinded trial), and their treatment will be determined by randomization, not personal choice. In addition, randomization is not always easy to implement and can also add bias to a study.

There are several methods of randomization. They can be divided into two main categories: fixed allocation randomization and adaptive randomization. In the fixed allocation randomization, subjects are allocated with a fixed probability to the study groups, and this probability does not change throughout the study. Examples of fixed allocation randomization are simple, blocked, and stratified randomization. For the adaptive randomization, however, the allocation probability changes as the study progresses and can be based on the group characteristics (baseline adaptive randomization) or response to the treatment (response adaptive procedure).

Is the Randomized Design Always Necessary?

Randomized clinical trial (RCT) is the gold standard of clinical research for comparison of two interventions. This method is considered the gold standard, as it is the only method that has the potential to avoid systematic error due to imbalance of unmeasured or unknown factors. However, is it always possible and worthwhile to perform such trials? In some situations, such as for trials with a very small sample size, randomization might produce critical imbalances between groups that might invalidate the results. Although some methods might be used to prevent potential imbalances, such as the method of minimization, these methods are not free of bias. In fact, alternative solutions, such as cross-over trials, might be considered for such small trials.

Professor Lombardi's Randomization Dilemma: Simplicity versus Imbalances in Small Studies

Prof. Luigi Lombardi is a clinical pulmonary physician dividing his time between clinical research and clinical work. He works in the large Policlinico Universitario Hospital in Rome and is the chief of the Pulmonary Physiology Department of this hospital, and he holds an academic appointment of associate professor. His research is focused on the clinical development of new pharmacological interventions for asthma. In fact, he also has a personal interest in this condition as his younger daughter has frequent asthma attacks, most of them triggered by exercise. He has recently discovered a new compound (QB0024) that he believes will be effective for the treatment of asthma—especially in cases where the main component is exercise-induced asthma. The preliminary animal, toxicologic, and phase I studies have shown that this compound is safe.

He then sees an opportunity to conduct the first phase II trial in this area. His plan is to compare this new drug against placebo as an add-on treatment (all participants would receive standard treatment) for exercise-induced asthma. He then starts writing the grant to get funds for this study. In fact, he could not ask for better conditions, as the number of participants with asthma in his outpatient service has increased significantly in the last two years, and three senior pulmonary fellows have approached him recently expressing interest in participating in his research team.

Although everything seems to be in place, he is having trouble finishing the grant application as he cannot decide on the randomization strategy. He has several options, such as simple randomization, blocked randomization, stratified randomization, and the methods of adaptive randomization. He knows that there is no gold standard method and that each of the methods has its advantages and disadvantages. As he is applying for a pilot grant, he will have limited funds to run this study—that will add some challenges to his randomization strategy.

In his grant application, he planned a small phase II study with 60 participants that, according to his sample size calculation, will be enough to show significant differences between the placebo and experimental drug groups. Although he prefers simpler methods of randomization due to his limited resources, he is concerned that these methods might add some biases to his study. What randomization method should Prof. Lombardi use in his study?

Main Issues Associated with Randomization

After a long week of little progress with the grant, Luigi hopes that he will be able to make a decision over the weekend. After waking up early Saturday morning, he now sits at his table in the garden with a bunch of notes and his computer. He first reviews the main issues associated with randomization for this study.

Challenges for Small Clinical Trials: The Risk of Imbalance

Although randomization is a method to reduce bias in clinical trials, it is also associated with an undesirable effect: generating imbalanced groups (by chance). This effect is more likely to occur in small samples. Suppose that a fair coin is tossed twice: what is the chance that heads will come up twice? This will be 1 in 4 (25%). However, if you toss the coin 10 times, the chance that heads will come up 10 times is 1 in 1,024 (approximately 0.1%). Suppose now that you are randomizing a small group of 20 subjects (16 men and 4 women) into two groups of 10 subjects. Using simple randomization, it is possible that one of the groups will have only men (instead of 8 men and 2 women per group). If men respond better to a given treatment, then this imbalanced sample will bias the results.

Examples of imbalance in small studies are commonly found in the literature. In a study with 40 subjects with cerebral palsy, the two groups (placebo and botulinum toxin A) showed important differences regarding the demographic data: for instance, while the gender ratio (female:male) was 12:10 for the botulinum group, it was 5:13 for the placebo group. In addition, participants in the placebo group had more severe disease (according to the functional scale GMFM).

For Prof. Lombardi, this potential bias is critical, as he knows that some factors, such as disease severity and level of physical activity, are extremely important as they are associated with the response level of QB0024. If the group receiving the experimental treatment has a higher proportion of participants with high level of physical activity or less severe disease, then the results might be biased toward QB0024. He therefore is concerned with this randomization strategy as he wants to make sure that groups are balanced regarding these two important factors. Besides this issue of imbalance for simple randomization method, the other methods also present some challenging issues, such as unblinding, difficulty in implementation, and validity.

Additionally, Luigi has to consider ethical and power issues. For instance, he was recently considering using a 1:3 strategy of randomizing participants to placebo and active treatment. He decides then to review each strategy separately.

Simple Randomization: Simplicity versus Imbalanced Groups

The first option Luigi considers is the simple randomization strategy, in which every participant has a 50% chance of receiving either active or placebo treatment. This option seems interesting to him in regard to feasibility, given his lack of staff and limited budget. This strategy is in fact commonly used in clinical trials and would not compromise the statistical inference of the study. In addition, because the chances that the next participant will be randomized to either placebo or treatment is not affected by the allocation of previous participants, unblinding due to this randomization strategy is not a concern.

However, despite the potential advantages, Prof. Lombardi is afraid that, due to the small sample size, the risk of imbalanced groups is elevated.

Blocked Randomization: A Method Trying to Reduce Imbalance Between Groups

Next, Luigi considers using the method of blocked randomization. In this method, participants are randomized in blocks of a fixed number, being, for instance, half randomized to active treatment and half to placebo in each block. Block sizes can be defined by the principal investigator. This method has the potential advantage of decreasing the likelihood that at the end of the study there will be differences in the number of subjects across groups of treatment (unless the study is interrupted in the middle of a block, then small imbalances are possible). Although Luigi is attracted to this option, he understands that this would not eliminate the possibility that the groups would be imbalanced regarding other factors, such as level of physical activity and severity of disease.

In addition, another potential issue of this design is that investigators might guess the treatment at the end of the block. For instance, in a study using a block size of 4 and a randomization ratio of 1:1 (two participants randomized to active treatment and two randomized to placebo in each block), an investigator could guess that in one block two participants have already been randomized to receive active treatment and one to receive placebo (for instance, based on efficacy or adverse effects) and therefore the next participant would be randomized to placebo to complete the block; in this case, he or she might consider not randomizing the next patient if he or she wants to give the active treatment to this patient.

Luigi stops for a couple of minutes and then has the idea of using random block sizes—for instance, block sizes can randomly vary between four and six participants. With this method, the possibility of unblinding during allocation of participants is smaller. He is initially satisfied with this option, but he is still concerned with the possibility of imbalances regarding other important covariates.

Stratified Randomization: Controlling Imbalances for Important Covariates

As Luigi considers the importance of ensuring that both covariates (physical activity and disease severity) are distributed proportionally in the two groups of intervention, he decides to explore the method of stratified randomization. In this method, participants are initially separated into strata of really important covariates that might affect results significantly, and then randomized within that stratum. It is recommended to minimize the influence of important baseline covariates at the level of trial design or randomization, instead of using post-adjustment during data analysis. In Prof. Luigi Lombardi's study, there are two factors, with two levels each. Luigi would need to create four strata: high physical activity level and severe disease, high physical activity level and moderate to mild disease, low physical activity level and severe disease, and low physical activity level and moderate to mild disease. After a given participant is assigned to each stratum, then he or she is randomized into active treatment or placebo. This option is attractive to Luigi, and he also thinks that this will be easily accepted by his colleagues; however, he knows that this option has some shortcomings.

A potential drawback of this strategy is that if randomization is conducted using the method of simple randomization in each stratum, the risk of imbalances is actually increased as the total sample size of 60 participants is divided into four smaller strata and, in fact, one of the strata might contain only three or four participants. Therefore, the initial concern of having imbalanced groups is again a problematic issue, but now with the addition of using a more complicated method. Something that worries Prof. Lombardi is that the research staff for this study still needs to receive appropriate training in clinical research.

He then considers one option: to use blocked randomization in each stratum. This seems at first glance to be a solution that may address most of the issues he has been dealing with; however, he goes back to the potential problem of unblinding subjects at the end of blocks. In addition, Luigi is not quite satisfied with two levels for each factor; he actually would like to have four levels of physical activity (no physical activity, low physical activity, moderate physical activity, and high physical activity). But then he would need to create eight strata, and he quickly realizes that this method might fail due to the low number of subjects in each stratum. He decides to take a break for lunch to explore the more sophisticated approaches: the methods of adaptive randomization.

Methods of Adaptive Randomization

After lunch, Luigi returns to his quiet spot in his garden and explores the methods of adaptive randomization. For this method, the randomization of subjects changes as the trial progresses. The main disadvantage of this method is that it is complicated to run and also adds complication during the statistical analysis as statistical inference may be guaranteed using simple methods of statistical analysis. Luigi decides to explore two methods: minimization technique and randomization adaptive response.

Minimization Technique: Randomizing Participants According to an Algorithm

The first method Luigi decides to explore is the minimization technique, in which participants are randomized according to the covariates important for the study (in this case, physical activity and severity of disease) using an algorithm that changes the likelihood that a given participant will receive active treatment or placebo according to his or her baseline characteristics. For instance, if an eligible patient has high physical activity level and severe disease and if in this category all the previous subjects received active treatment, the computer/algorithm might give this participant a 75% chance of receiving placebo as to try to balance groups. This method has the advantage of addressing some of the issues with a large number of strata in a small study and also the issue of unblinding. But the two main issues are the challenges to run this method and the modifications that are necessary to be made in the statistical analysis.

Adaptive Randomization According to the Response: Playing the Winner Strategy

Although Luigi is satisfied with his strategy, he saw an old note entitled "playing the winner strategy." Although he will not likely use this method, he reviews it quickly. In this method, every new participant is randomized according to the response of the previous participant. For instance, participant 1 is randomized to active treatment, if he responds to the treatment, then participant 2 also receives active treatment until a participant does not respond, then there is a switch to the other treatment. Although this is an interesting method, it has several issues associated with it, such as choosing the appropriate method of statistical analysis and other biases that can be introduced.

He then quickly reviews his notes and makes a preliminary decision. He types the method of randomization in his computer and writes three paragraphs justifying the method. He is quite confident with the chosen method.

CASE DISCUSSION

Randomization

Prof. Lombardi is writing a grant proposal to get funding for a small phase II placebo-controlled, randomized trial to test a new drug for exercise-induced asthma attacks. He thinks the drug is promising and is eager to start the trial. He has a large clinic where he can recruit participants, and a small team to help him conduct this trial. However, he wants to make sure the randomization method is the best for his study design and characteristics.

This case is a classic example of the challenges inherent to choosing a randomization method for a small sample size trial. Here the investigators need to weigh the pros and cons of each possibility. Ultimately, investigators need to decide how important covariates are for the study and whether it is necessary to have a stratified randomization method.

Another important factor that needs to be considered in this study is the allocation concealment (i.e., making sure that investigators and participants cannot anticipate to which study arm participants will be randomized, in order to avoid selection bias). As we discussed earlier, certain randomization methods may compromise allocation concealment, such as blocked randomization with fixed block sizes, or some minimization algorithms. Moreover, the procedure used with randomization to effectively reveal the allocation once participants have been randomized, such as sealed envelopes, or computerized or telephone-based systems, need to be implemented in a way to avoid manipulation of the allocation.

- One of the most frequently used approaches is the envelope randomization method, where numbered envelopes that contain a treatment allocation are opened sequentially as participants are entered into the study. However, investigators can abuse and, for instance, open several envelopes at the same time and choose the most desirable treatment for a given participant.
- Another method is the use of a central randomization service with a dedicated telephone randomization (this is useful especially for multicenter trials). But this is an expensive method, especially if it depends on 24-hour coverage. One alternative is web-based randomization—this would eliminate some of the problems mentioned earlier, but technical support is needed. Based on these initial suggestions, which method would you choose? Why? Why is the allocation so important, and sometimes all the effort made to decide and implement a randomization strategy is lost if allocation concealment is not adequate? Is there any difference between allocation concealment and blinding?

CASE QUESTIONS FOR REFLECTION

1. What challenges does Prof. Lombardi face in choosing the randomization strategy?
2. What are his main concerns?
3. What should he consider in making his decision?

WEB RESOURCES

- http://www.randomization.com/
- http://www-users.york.ac.uk/~mb55/guide/randsery.htm

REFERENCES

1. Kang M, Ragan BG, Park JH. Issues in outcomes research: an overview of randomization techniques for clinical trials. *J Athletic Training.* 2008; 43: 215–221.
2. Bridgman S, Dainty K, Kirkley A, Maffulli N. Practical aspects of randomization and blinding in randomized clinical trials. *Arthroscopy.* 2003; 19: 1000–1006.
3. Schulz KF, Grimes DA. Generation of allocation sequences in randomised trials: chance, not choice. *Lancet.* 2002; 359: 515–519.
4. Vickers AJ. How to randomize. *J Soc Integr Oncol.* 2006; 4: 194–198.

5. Randelli P, Arrigoni P, Lubowitz JH, Cabitza P, Denti, M. Randomization procedures in orthopaedic trials. *Arthroscopy*. 2008; 24: 834–838.
6. Thall PF, Wathen JK. Practical Bayesian adaptive randomization in clinical trials. *Eur J Cancer*. 2007; 43: 859–866.
7. Taves DR. The use of minimization in clinical trials. *Contemp Clin Trials*. 2010: 31: 180–4
8. Harrell FE Jr, Lee KL, Mark DB. multivariable prognostic models: issues in developing models, evaluating assumptions and adequacy, and measuring and reducing errors. *Statistics Med*. 1996; 15: 361–387.

6

BLINDING

Authors: *Rita Tomás and Joseph Massaro*

Case study authors: *Rui Imamura and Felipe Fregni*

The only way to get rid of a temptation is to yield to it.
—Oscar Wilde, *The Picture of Dorian Gray* (1891)

INTRODUCTION

One of the most important strategies in conducting a research study is to minimize bias. A randomized controlled trial (RCT) using blinding (or masking) of patients and study personnel to the study treatment the patient is receiving, along with randomization, is now considered the gold standard in clinical research. Randomization is done to greatly increase the likelihood that study groups are balanced at baseline (avoiding selection bias, confounding). Blinding, on the other hand, encompasses the methods and strategies used to keep study participants and key research personnel unaware of treatment assignment status throughout the duration of the trial, as well as after completion of the trial during data analysis. Blinding can be achieved in the absence of randomization, but they are usually used together.

The knowledge about treatment allocation can compromise the quality of the study, hindering internal validity by increasing the risk of bias. Lack of blinding of health-care providers, study staff, and subjects (patients) can alter expectations, change behaviors toward the intervention (compliance, dropouts), and influence side-effect report as well as the reporting and assessment of efficacy outcome variables.

Despite investing extensive efforts, some interventions make it very difficult, or nearly impossible, to achieve or maintain blinding of patients and providers (e.g., clinical trials of surgery, psychotherapy, rehabilitation). Nonetheless, investigators should counter this aspect, by blinding at least some important research personnel, such as outcome assessors (raters) or endpoint adjudicators.

Despite being extensively recommended by expert panels and advisory agencies, blinding status is often not reported by authors. If mentioned at all, commonly not enough information is provided about who exactly was blinded, by what means blinding was accomplished, and how successful it was. It is then important that the investigator really understands not only how to design studies with effective blinding, but also the potential limitations when blinding is not possible or has some inherent limitations.

HISTORY

Blinding and blinding assessment in the medical field have more than two centuries of history. Blinding was initially used to expose fraud when the healing properties of magnetism, perkinism, and homeopathy were tested [1,2]. One of the first studies using a sham intervention in a blinded manner was published by Austin Flint in 1863 [3].

At the beginning of the twentieth century, concerns were raised that bias could be introduced through "patient's expectations" and "physician's personality." This initiated the use of blinding in the fields of physiology and pharmacology. In addition, blinded trials promoted recruitment and decreased attrition in the comparison group; instead of being offered "no treatment," patients received a placebo/sham intervention in a blinded manner [2].

A *double-blind* randomized clinical trial is sometimes defined as a study where neither the treating physician nor the subject knows the randomized treatment the subject is receiving (this definition will be discussed later in the chapter). In Michigan, from 1926 to 1931 [4], sanocrysin was tested against distilled water to treat tuberculosis. One of the authors was unaware of group allocation and presumably so were the patients. This trial is considered to be the first study incorporating a double-blind approach [2].

DEFINITION

Blinding or masking is the methodological principle of concealing group allocation (intervention or control/placebo/sham) from subjects and study staff *after* randomization [5]. This concept should not be confused with allocation concealment, which refers to hiding group allocation *during* the randomization process, preventing selection bias [6]. Allocation concealment and blinding maintain "unawareness" of group status at different points in time and guarantee the methodological soundness of clinical trials. Allocation concealment protects the allocation sequence before and until assignment, and blinding protects the sequence from then on (Figure 6.1). It can be achieved in all clinical trials, in contrast with blinding, which sometimes can be *unfeasible to achieve or to maintain*.

WHO CAN BE BLINDED

Many groups of individuals can and should be blinded as much as possible to the treatment received by the patient while the study is ongoing [5,8,9]:

1. Participant/subject/patient/volunteer: receives the trial intervention (one of them)
2. Health-care provider/clinician/attending physician: provides the intervention
3. Outcome assessor/data collector/rater/evaluator/observer: provides outcome data
4. Outcome adjudicator/endpoint committee member/judicial assessor: ensures that outcome data adhere as defined a priori
5. Data handlers/data entry clerk: enters data from patient file to trial database
6. Data analyst/statistician: conducts data analysis
7. Manuscript writer: writes a paper with trial results.

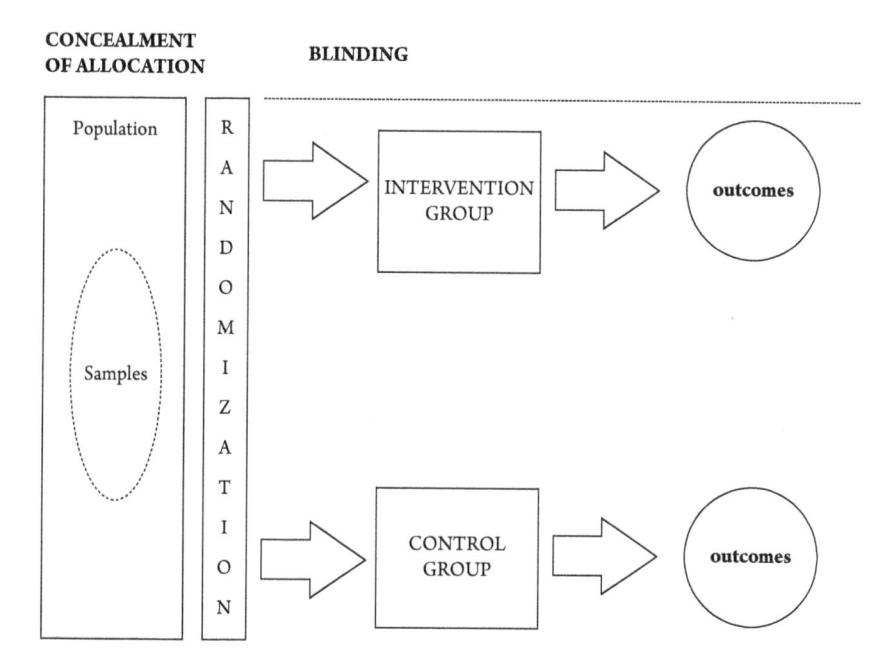

Figure 6.1. Allocation concealment and blinding.
Adapted from Viera and Bangdiwala [7].

Some groups may be unblinded due to the nature of their role in the study, such as treatment manufacturer, pharmacist, and medical monitor. The medical monitor deals with patient safety issues and often has access to the randomization schedule containing the record of the randomized treatment each patient receives (this access is needed in case an individual patient's randomized treatment needs to be made known in the event the patient experiences a serious adverse event), as do members of the data safety monitoring board (DSMB).

BLINDING TERMINOLOGY

Blinding terminology can be confusing and ambiguous [1,5,10]. Many terms often used in papers and study protocols are not universal and may not mean the same to all members of the clinical research community. A study encountered 17 unique interpretations of the meaning of "double-blinding." When surveying textbooks, nine different combinations of blinded groups were found. For the majority, "double-blinded" meant that both participants and health-care providers were unaware of group allocation, but double-blinded has been interpreted in many different ways, by various groups such as data collectors, data analysts, and judicial assessors [10].

Instead of describing a trial vaguely as "blinded," researchers are now encouraged to describe the blinding status of all personnel involved in the trial, complying with the CONSORT recommendations [11].

Nevertheless, some authors have proposed the adoption of standardized terminology [12]. A tentative flowchart is described in Figure 6.2.

```
┌─────────────────────────┐
│ Were subjects blinded to│  ──NO──▶  NOT BLINDED
│ treatment assignment?   │
└───────────┬─────────────┘
            │ YES
            ▼
┌─────────────────────────┐
│ Were those who administered│         SINGLE BLIND STUDY
│ the treatment and outcome  │──NO──▶  List or groups that were
│ assessors blinded to       │         blinded, if applicable.
│ treatment assignment?      │
└───────────┬─────────────┘
            │ YES
            ▼
┌─────────────────────────┐
│ Were data managers and  │         DOUBLE BLIND STUDY
│ biostatisticians blinded│──NO──▶  List or groups that were
│ to treatment assignment?│         blinded, if applicable.
└───────────┬─────────────┘
            │ YES
            ▼
┌─────────────────────────┐
│     TRIPLE BLIND STUDY  │
│ List other groups that  │
│ were blinded,           │
│ if applicable.          │
└─────────────────────────┘
```

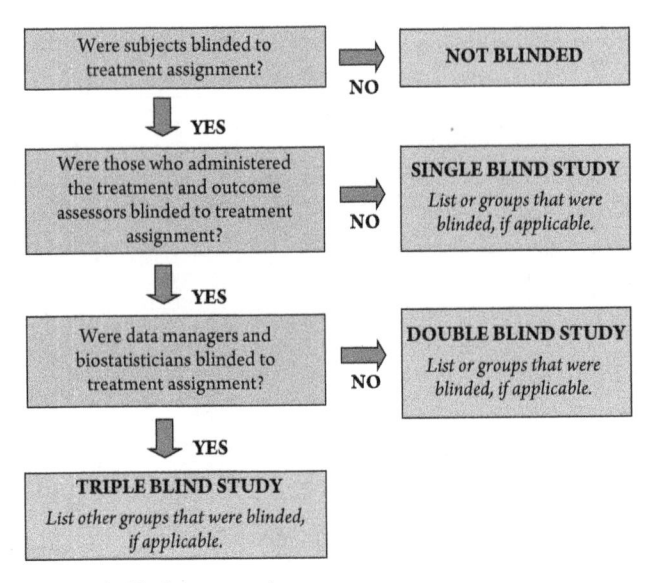

Figure 6.2. Flowchart for blinding terminology. Adapted from Miller and Stewart [12].

As can be seen in Figure 6.2, a definition of a triple-blind study is that patients, treating and evaluating personnel, and data managers and biostatisticians be blinded to treatment assignment. This definition is not consistently used. Overall, as many personnel as possible should remain blinded to study treatment allocation as much as possible, even in a single-blind and open-label trial.

The terms "blinding" and "masking" may be used interchangeably, although "masking" may be preferred when blindness is an outcome of interest [1]. The term "masking" started to be used as an euphemism for "blinding," which was thought to be offensive to some trial participants [13].

Depending on the context, the words "blinding" and "masking" may also have different meanings: a placebo can be used to mask (or conceal) an intervention, and assessments can be performed in a blinded fashion to prevent unblinding.

An *open-label trial* is when participants and treating physicians are always aware of group assignment. Even in this setting, care should be taken that all other individuals involved in the trial be as blinded as possible (for instance, an evaluator). "Open-label" methodology can also be used after a well-conducted randomized controlled blinded trial, when an *open-label extension* period may follow. This extension may allow for further detection of adverse effects and can monitor efficacy during more prolonged use. In addition, this extension period may allow the control group to switch to the active drug. Despite the interest of gathering further data, there is increased risk for bias intrinsically bonded with open-label trials [14].

An alternative trial, derived from this design, is an *open trial with blinded endpoints* (sometimes called PROBE—prospective randomized open-label blinded endpoint). This design could be described as a single-blind study, where only endpoint assessors are blinded. Still, there are plenty of opportunities for bias to occur, as referrals to adjudication are often done by unblinded study personnel [15].

A *single-blind trial* is when one group of interest in the study is unaware of group allocation. This is usually interpreted as subjects being blinded to the treatment assignment [10]. When only one group is blinded and the participants group is unblinded, a more descriptive approach should be used, rather the designation of "single-blind" [12].

A *double-blind trial* is usually understood as participants and investigators being unaware of group assignment [12]. The term "investigator" is intentionally imprecise, as it can mean either the health-care provider or the outcome assessor. Interpretation of this term can lead to many different definitions, but the most common definition found in textbooks includes patients and evaluators [10]. In some studies, it is used to describe all three categories (patients, providers, and evaluators [1].

In a *triple-blind trial*, three different groups are unaware of the treatment allocation, but there is no consensus regarding which three. Usually, blinded groups are all those involved in a double-blind trial plus the data managers and/or biostatisticians [1,12]. If health-care provider and the evaluator are not the same person, this term can comprise these two staff members in addition to the participant [1].

Quadruple-blind trial is a term rarely used by authors. It can be applied when four different groups were blinded to treatment assignment: participant, health-care provider, evaluator, and data analyst [1].

When stating blinding methodology, a more qualitative approach is recommended [11]. Researchers should clearly state which groups were blinded (rather than just mentioning how many) and how that was accomplished.

BLINDING IN CLINICAL RESEARCH

Blinding is of one the hallmarks of methodological quality. Nevertheless, not all authors report blinding status in their papers, leaving the reader with an unanswered question: "Did the author indeed blind key players within the study and forget to report it, or is this an unblended, less "sound" trial?" It is usually assumed that if blinding is not reported, it probably was not performed (properly).

In 2000, an analysis of the top five medical journals found an explicit report of blinding status in less than 25% of articles [16]. From a random sample of 200 papers of blinded clinical trials, 78% were described as being double-blind, but only 44% reported explicitly the blinding status of each trial group. When authors were contacted, in almost a fifth of the studies neither patients, providers, nor evaluators were blinded. This resulted in 15 different definitions of a double-blind trial [17]. Despite the unquestioned importance of blinding, results from non-blinded studies should not automatically be invalidated [18,19].

In a 2010 survey of all controlled trials registered in the ClinicalTrials.gov database as of September 2010, 60% were open trials and allocation status was missing in almost a fourth of studies. When comparing just the last decade with the last three years (2000–2010 and 2007–2010), the percentage of missing information decreased substantially, from 9% to 3%, respectively. The percentage of open-label remained stable [20]. Reports about gynecology and obstetrics and orthopedics trials have shown that in many open-label studies, blinding could have been accomplished easily [21,22].

A recent survey from the field of rehabilitation also found a significantly increased percentage of papers reporting blinding status in the last 10 years from 56% to 85% [18]. This may represent the call of action for researchers and journal editors for better quality when reporting results, summarized in the CONSORT statement since 1996 [23].

CONSEQUENCES OF UNBLINDING

Lack of blinding increases the risk of bias, which can be a threat to the internal validity of a clinical trial. A subject or an investigator who is aware of group allocation may consciously or unconsciously change his or her attitude, beliefs, or behavior regarding the study.

The main types of bias associated with unblinding are *performance, detection/observer,* and *attrition bias* [5,8,24,25].

> *Performance bias*: unequal provision of care from study staff, independent of study protocol (e.g., when adjusting a dose or referral for adjudication);
> *Detection/observer bias*: partiality in evaluation of outcome of interest (especially subjective variables), usually favoring the experimental group;
> *Attrition bias*: increased dropout rate from subjects who know that they are in the control group.

Other phenomena that could be also linked with unblinding include the following:

> *Loss of placebo effect*: effect of the treatment ritual and patient–health-care provider interaction is lost if control group allocation is known;
> *Response/self-report bias*: tendency for subjects to report (or not) efficacy/side effects according to what the investigator expects or to "please" him or her;
> *Non-compliance*: subjects may have a tendency not to follow the protocol (e.g., trial regimen) if they are in the control group;
> *Co-intervention*: subjects may have tendency to seek adjunct treatment (if they are in the control group) and/or systematic differences in basic care from study personnel among study groups; also can be called *contamination*.

BLINDING VERSUS BIAS

The need for adequate blinding is essential to avoid bias. Importantly, it is not only adding a blinding that will prevent bias, but how the blinding was implemented. The goal of the researcher is to understand potential flaws in the blinding method, and that of the reader is to assess whether the blinding method was adequate.

We discussed in the previous section the types of biases that can be found when blinding is not implemented or is flawed. Bias is defined as a "systematic error, or deviation from the truth, in results or inferences" [26]. The main problem with bias is that it cannot be estimated or corrected. In fact, bias can go in both directions. A study that has results biased will likely have little or no value. Figure 6.3 summarizes the types of biases according to each component of a randomized clinical trial.

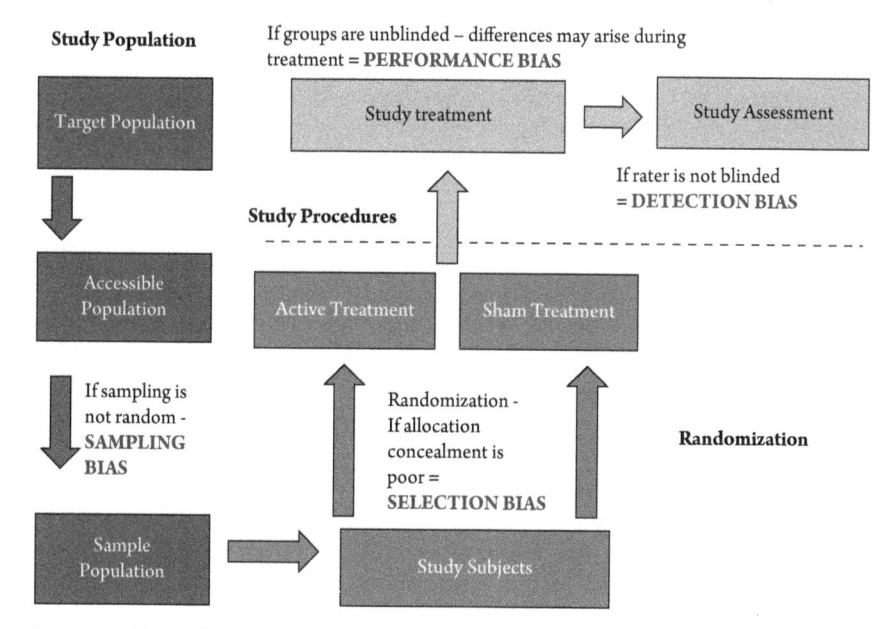

Figure 6.3. Types of bias associated with unblinding.

THE IMPACT OF BLINDING

Some researchers have questioned the importance of blinding. The risks of non-blinded outcome assessors was clearly shown in trial by Noseworthy and colleagues [27]. In this study, the effect of weekly plasma exchange in multiple sclerosis patients was only significant when assessed by non-blinded neurologists. Neurologists who were unaware of group allocation did not find any benefit of adding plasma exchange to the treatment regimen. This novel paired-evaluator design, back in 1994, clearly showed the importance of physician blinding to prevent "erroneous conclusion about treatment (false positive, type 1 error)" [26].

A systematic review of 250 randomized controlled trials from 33 meta-analyses concluded that trials that were not double-blind had larger estimates of effects, with odds ratios being exaggerated by 17%. Trials that were inadequately concealed also overestimated treatment effect by 30% [28]. Allocation concealment appears to have a stronger effect in bias reduction when compared to blinding [6,8,27,28]. Other studies confirmed this trend, with lower methodological (e.g., open-label) quality being associated with larger treatment effects [19,24,29,30].

The effect of blinding on bias might also be related to the outcome of interest. More subjective outcomes might be more vulnerable to bias when subjects and evaluators are unblinded. Pain scores, depressive symptoms, patient's function, and quality of life are examples of subjective ("soft") outcomes. Mortality from all causes could be considered a hard, objective outcome, and might make it unnecessary to have blinded evaluators [6,8]. On the other hand, an outcome such as mortality from a certain cause (e.g., cardiovascular) might add a certain degree of subjectivity and therefore the adjudicators should be blinded.

Other examples of robust outcomes are biochemical markers (e.g., glycosylated hemoglobin level) assessed by calibrated machines [6]. If these continuous variables are transformed into dichotomous outcomes, such as "disease" or "disease-free," discretion is advised when determining the cut-off point. This decision needs to be made a priori or by a blinded data analyst [9]. There are many opportunities for bias to occur, even when the primary variable is thought to be relatively immune to subjectivity.

Wood and collaborators reviewed 146 meta-analyses and found that effect estimates were exaggerated by 25% in studies with subjective outcomes and lacked blinding. Open-label trials with objective outcomes were not associated with overvalued effect sizes [31]. This accentuates the need for objective outcomes or the use of more than one subjective variable to evaluate the same outcome (e.g., self-reported variable) to allow for reliability testing [6].

A recent survey of 25 studies that used both blinded and non-blinded assessment of the same binary outcome concluded that the odds ratios were overestimated by 36% (ratio of odds ratio of 0.64) when performed by unblinded evaluators. In general, non-blinded assessments were more optimistic for both groups, with less 26% failure events (e.g., wound or fracture healing). In addition, misclassification was characterized by "intervention preoccupation," with discordant (more positive) evaluations in 35% of the intervention group and only 18% in the control group [32].

HOW TO ACCOMPLISH BLINDING

To blind both patients and caregivers, ideally both interventions (treatment and control) should "look the same." This could be easily done if a placebo intervention can be used as control. A placebo is considered a "pharmacologic inactive agent" [8].

If the treatment being tested is a new drug delivered in the form of a tablet, the placebo tablet should be identical in appearance (size, color, weight, odor, and touch). De Craen and collaborators have shown that certain colors are associated with specific effects: red, yellow, and orange were associated with a stimulant effect, and blue and green were related to a tranquilizing effect [33]. The distinct taste of ascorbic acid and zinc gluconate led to unblinding in trials evaluating the efficacy of these drugs treating the common cold [34,35]. Unblinded patients reported additional benefit, but not the patients who remained blinded [36]. The route of administration should also be the same (oral administration, subcutaneous, intravenous, etc.). Another work by De Craen and colleagues demonstrated that a subcutaneous placebo showed enhanced relief in acute treatment of migraine when compared to an oral placebo (32% vs. 26%) [37].

Ideally, the placebo should also mimic the side effects associated with the drug being tested (e.g., anti-muscarinic effects of the tricyclic antidepressants like dry mouth and constipation). This is called an *active placebo* [8]. Having a matching placebo can be useless when testing drugs with extreme side effects, like chemotherapy agents [6].

When a new drug is being tested against another active treatment (standard treatment) a double-dummy design can be used. This means having placebo formulation of both drugs. All patients are given two different formulations: (1) one active new drug and a placebo standard treatment; or (2) placebo new drug and active standard treatment (Figure 6.4). This adds an additional challenge in terms of compliance because patients have to take more than one tablet/capsule.

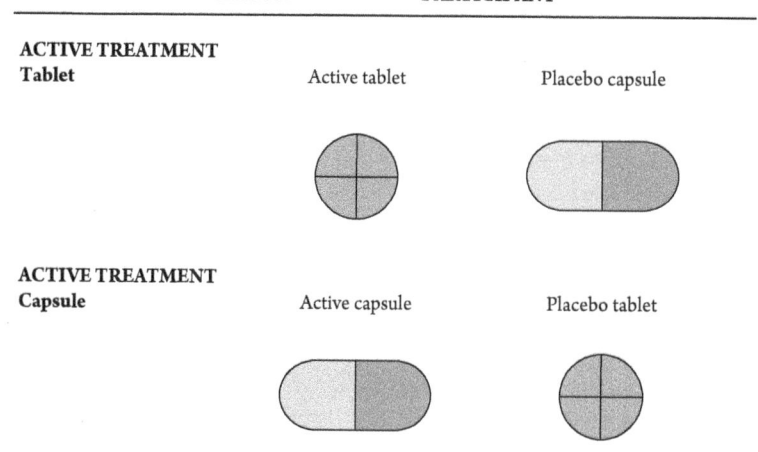

RANDOMIZED ALLOCATION	PARTICIPANT	
ACTIVE TREATMENT **Tablet**	Active tablet	Placebo capsule
ACTIVE TREATMENT **Capsule**	Active capsule	Placebo tablet

Figure 6.4. An example of how blinding is accomplished in a double-dummy design trial. Adapted from Forder, Gebski, and Keeck [6].

Blinding procedures in a double-dummy setting can be burdensome, especially when drugs have different prescription schemes (b.i.d. vs t.i.d.) or one needs frequent dose adjustments (e.g. warfarin vs ximelgatran [38]). Table 6.1 illustrates the complexity of dose titration in a double-dummy design of drugs with different administration schemes: for example, gabapentin was administered two to three times a day and amitriptyline only once a day.

Boutron and collaborators reviewed the methods of blinding of pharmacological treatment trials published in 2004 in high-impact factor journals. Only 41% of the trials properly described the strategies deployed to blind patients and health-care providers. Several methods were used: similar capsules/tablets, embedded treatment

Table 6.1 An example of dose titration in a double-dummy design

Dose level	9 AM dosage	3 PM dosage	9 PM dosage	Total daily dosage
Initiation phase day 1	Placebo Placebo	Placebo Placebo	12.5mg AMT or 300 mg GBP	12.5mg AMT or 300 mg GBP
Initiation phase day 2	Placebo or 300mg GBP	Placebo Placebo	25mg AMT or 300mg GBP	25mg AMT or 600mg GBP
Level 1	Placebo or 300mg GBP	Placebo or 300mg GBP	25mg AMT or 300mg GBP	25mg AMT or 900mg GBP
Level 2	Placebo or 300mg GBP	Placebo or 300mg GBP	2x 25mg AMT or 2x 300mg GBP	50mg AMT or 1200mg GBP
Level 3	2x Placebo or 2x 300mg GBP	Placebo or 300mg GBP	3x 25mg AMT or 3x 300mg GBP	75mg AMT or 1800mg GBP

AMT—amitriptyline; GBP—gabapentin

Adapted from Morello et al. [39].

in hard gelatin capsules, similar syringes or bottles, peppermint flavor or sugar to coat treatment (mask taste of active substance), and opaque coverage of intravenous treatment [40].

Non-pharmacologic treatments pose an even greater challenge. Interventions that involve medical devices, rehabilitation, surgical procedures, education, and psychotherapy are difficult to blind from patients and providers [41,42]. This can translate into lower methodological quality, as shown in a survey of clinical trials evaluating non-pharmacological and pharmacological treatments of hip and knee osteoarthritis. Non-pharmacological interventions were less likely to be compared to placebo/sham, and blinding of patients and assessors was reported less often [43].

In surgical or technical interventions, some options include concealing incisions and scars from assessors, use of a sham dressing, altering digital radiographs or images, and providing video/audiotape/photography for assessment [41,44].

When the treatment is an intervention requiring the participation of a subject/patient, such as physical therapy or educational sessions, the control group could have sham intervention (without therapeutics effect) or an attention-control intervention [41].

If a medical device is being tested (e.g., transcutaneous electrical nerve stimulation), a sham apparatus should be used. The sensorial experience induced by the sham treatment should be similar to the active device: same lights, noise, or sensation. If this is too complex to be accomplished, patients can be told that they may or may not feel something on the treatment site and that this fact is unrelated to the efficacy of the treatment. Sham devices have greater effect than placebo tablets, so testing placebo pills against an active device is not advisable, and may inflate the treatment effect [45]. If neither option is available, it is always possible to blind patients and evaluators to study purpose or hypotheses, ask patients not to tell assessors their group allocation, or not have surgeon or providers involved in outcome evaluations [41].

If the device delivers a treatment that is not "felt" by the patients (e.g., ultrasound treatment), the same treatment procedures should be repeated for both groups (e.g., switching "on" and "off" the device, session duration, patients positioning, etc.), but the sham device has been tampered and does not operate. The use of curtains or boxes to blind a device can also be useful [41].

ASSESSMENT OF BLINDING SUCCESS

Some researchers argue that "to be blinded and "were blinded" are not to same thing, so trialists should evaluate blinding efficacy systematically at the end of the trial [46]. This can be achieved by thoroughly evaluating the appearance of the active treatment and the control prior to the trial, by running a pilot study searching for flaws and threats to blinding, or by asking key study persons about their guesses with regard to randomized treatment allocation.

The absolute need to measure this is still controversial, as a new therapy that is highly effective or has an adverse event profile will necessarily unblind patients. Success of blinding "[...] is that there should be unblinding through efficacy" [47]. In addition, frequently asking subjects about their hunch concerning their group allocation might trigger their curiosity and encourage unblinding actions [48]. Those who correctly decipher their assignment may disguise it and not answer truthfully [49].

The most recent update of the CONSORT statements does not recommend that this assessment be done routinely [11,49].

Surveys found that only 2%–7% of all trials reported tests for the success of blinding [40,51]. One of the reasons for this low reporting is the lack of a standard method to accomplish this. Some questions remain without a definite answer: Which timing is the best to survey subjects and study personnel? Should "do not know" be offered as an category? Should success be a binary or a scale variable? Which is the cut-off value for successful blinding? What statistical analysis should be done? [49,50].

In these surveys, three or five responses categories can be used:

- "active," "control," "do not know"
- "strongly believe active," "somewhat believe active," "somewhat believe control," "strongly believe control," "do not know."

Data can be structured in a 2-by-3 or 2-by-5 contingency table (Figure 6.5).

Instead of a simple chi-square, comparing the number of correct and incorrect answers, more elaborated statistical approaches have been tried. James and colleagues have proposed a disagreement measure, a modified version of the kappa coefficient known as James's blinding index (BI) [51]. The index varies between 0 and 1: BI = 0, or "total lack of blinding"; BI = 0.5, or 50% of correct and incorrect guesses (random guesses); and BI = 1, or "complete blinding" [51]. It puts a great weight on the "do not know" answers, which means that there is a true uncertainty about group status. This index aggregates data from both the active and control group, not allowing detection of differences in unblinding between groups [51]. There is another statistical method, the Bang's BI, that allows a separate analysis of all treatment arms, which can be useful when groups behave differently in terms of unblinding. An index ranging from −1 to 1 is given to each group. When blinding was successful, BI = 0. When BI >0 there was a failure in blinding above random chance and patients guessed their treatment allocation correctly (e.g., BI = 0.21 means that 21% of the participants guessed their treatment allocation beyond chance). If BI <0 there was a failure in blinding above random chance and patients mistakenly guessed their treatment allocation. Bang's BI

	Response		
Assignment	Active	Control	Do not know
Active			
Control			

Figure 6.5. An example of a 2-by-3 contingency table.

advantages are the ability to detect not only the magnitude but also the direction of unblinding for each group [51].

BLINDING GUIDELINES

American and European advisory agencies recommend that studies should be blinded, including the subject, investigator, sponsor staff involved in treatment, and clinical evaluations. Ideally, all study personnel should be blinded, but if "practically or ethically possible," single-blind and open-label are also option. In this case, emphasis should be placed on random allocation, and when possible, assessment should be done by a blind evaluator [53,54]. Also, in single-blind and open-label, it is our opinion that as many study personnel as possible should remain unblinded if at all possible.

The CONSORT expert panel, originally gathered in mid-1990, issued a statement that recommended that researchers elaborate on blinding methodology when reporting their findings:

> Describe mechanism (e.g. capsules, tablets); similarity of treatment characteristics (e.g. appearance, taste); allocation schedule control (location of code during trial and when broken); and evidence for successful blinding among participants, person doing intervention, outcome assessors, and data analysts. [23]

In 2001, the statement was updated to include a checklist of 22 items to mention when reporting a clinical trial. This list included an item regarding blinding (#11):

> Whether or not participants, those administering the interventions, and those assessing the outcomes were blinded to group assignment. If done, how the success of blinding was evaluated. [55]

In the most recent statement, from 2010, the panel goes into detail and recommends that more information about blinding be given, namely how similar the intervention were (#11a, #11b):

> 11a If done, who was blinded after assignment to interventions (for example, participants, care providers, those assessing outcomes) and how; 11b If relevant, description of the similarity of interventions. [11]

The evaluation of the success of blinding, once included in the 2001 statement, was dropped due to its controversial aspect [5,56].

Blinding Data Analysis

Data analysts can be blinded in any trial, but this is only rarely reported [16]. Though data analysis is seen by many as an "objective process," analysts do make "semi-subjective" decisions during the process of analysis [9]. Therefore, all personnel performing data entry and analysis should be blinded [57]. In addition, statistical analyses should be determined a priori, to avoid "fishing expeditions."

The strategies for dealing with missing data (deletion, imputation, etc.), handling outliers, what to do with non-normal distributed data (transformation, violating test assumptions, dichotomize variables), how variables will to be analyzed (continuous or transformed in binary, which cut-off for dichotomous variable) and which subgroup analyses will be done have to be addressed before the knowledge of any preliminary results [9].

CHALLENGING DESIGNS FOR BLINDING
Blinding in Rehabilitation Trials

The physical medicine and rehabilitation field is still lacking high-quality research that recognizes the benefit of some of its treatments. There has been a trend for improvement in the last decade, but it is still suboptimal [18]. It is particularly difficult to blind certain rehabilitation treatments that involve a high interaction between patient and therapist, and often clinical endpoints are subjective, such as pain, quality of life, or function [42]. Many times, treatments are delivered in the form of medical devices, and developing a sham device is far more complicated than manufacturing a placebo pill. Nevertheless, it is always feasible to blind data collectors, outcome assessors, and data analysts and to use more "hard" outcomes or surrogate variables [18]. Recruiting naïve patients, without previous experience with treatment being studied, is preferable. Interaction between patient and provider should be standardized among groups to limit the placebo effect in both groups [42]. When possible, more objective outcomes should be used, such as isokinetic dynamometry to assess strength, the H-reflex to assess spasticity, imaging, urodynamic testing, nerve conduction studies, or electromyography.

Blinding in Chronic Obstructive Pulmonary Disease Trials

Some drugs used in the treatment of chronic obstructive pulmonary disease (COPD) are delivered by different kinds of inhalers. It can be challenging to prevent unblinding of the patient with certain drugs that have certain characteristics, like a distinct taste. Tiotropium is one good example: it cannot be removed from the capsules displaying the manufacturer's logo, as the drug is very unstable. As the logo is visible from the inhaler, unblinding occurs automatically. Researchers in this field have found strategies to minimize the bias that arises from an open-label trial, including the use of objective outcomes such as spirometry and cross-over designs [58].

Blinding in Acupuncture

One field where a "true" placebo use is extremely difficult is acupuncture. There is no placebo for a needle, because needling, pinching, even light touching someone's skin will always have some physiologic effect. Many approaches have been tried (e.g., blunt needle, non-penetrating needle, retractable needles, using non-standard acupuncture points, recruiting only naïve subjects, mock electro-acupuncture) [41,42,59]. Ultimately, it is impossible to blind the practitioner, so more emphasis should be put on having blinded outcome assessors [59].

CONCLUSION

Blinding, along with randomization, protects patients and researchers from contaminated findings and decreases the subjectivity of clinical trials [2,5]. One should aim to blind all key categories of personnel in a trial. If blinding of all individuals is not possible, an effort should be made to blind as many parties as possible. "Some" is better than "none." Researchers should report the blinding status of participants and all study personnel and accurately describe how that was accomplished. Despite not being unanimous, assessment of the blinding success can be done to quantify the occurrence of unblinding throughout the study. "Intentionally inducing a state of ignorance" will minimize the risk of bias and therefore increase the internal validity of the study [5].

CASE STUDY: STUDY BLINDING: HOW FAR SHOULD RESEARCHERS GO TO DECREASE THE RISK OF CONSCIOUS OR UNCONSCIOUS BIAS?

Rui Imamura and Felipe Fregni

It is springtime in the beautiful city of Paris. One of the main teaching hospitals has just launched a large clinical research center, and the director of this newly formed center expects to have several clinical trials conducted there. Dr. Bejout, an ENT (ear, nose, and throat) specialist with a special interest in allergic rhinitis, plays an important role in this center. He works in the large and busy ENT department and is the coordinator of a postgraduate program in the field, with several PhD students working with him. He has participated in several clinical trials and feels prepared to assume a leadership role in this clinical research center; he therefore starts shifting his effort from clinical work to research. In addition, with the globalization of clinical research, the competition has increased, therefore adding an additional level of pressure.[1]

Besides the current challenges, he just received news from his research assistant that his grant application to test a new topical steroid drug ("RHINO-A") for allergic rhinitis has been approved. This is the opportunity that he has been waiting for. He immediately calls his PhD student, Isabelle Giroud, to give her the good news that her PhD study will be funded. He also tells her that now important decisions on the study need to be made. After hanging up the call, he looks at his calendar on his desk: he has only 10 days to finish the last details of this study before leaving for summer vacation with his family. Although the study is designed, one point concerns him: study blinding.

Introduction

Current Development of RHINO-A

After promising results in pre-clinical and phase I trials, Dr. Bejout feels it is the proper time to run a phase II trial. In fact, Isabelle has been working on this project for several months and she is anxious to move on to the next step. The plan for this study is to perform a randomized parallel phase II trial testing RHINO-A versus placebo (and an option that was not ruled out yet was to include a third group of oral antihistamine) for four weeks in perennial allergic rhinitis patients. Ethical issues regarding placebo use in this setting were extensively discussed with the IRB (institutional review board) and resulted in the conclusion that it was acceptable due to the nature of the disease and short duration of the trial.

The main goal of the study is to assess initial efficacy, as measured by decrease in total nasal sign and symptom scale (TNSSS)—the main outcome, a composite scale that consists of grading symptoms and signs of allergic rhinitis. Symptoms include congestion, runny nose, sneezing/itchy nose and postnasal drip and are self-rated by

---

[1] Dr. Rui Imamura and Professor Felipe Fregni prepared this case. Course cases are developed solely as the basis for class discussion. The situation in this case is fictional.

the patients. Signs are assessed by an ENT specialist on physical examination: color and edema of the nasal mucosa, presence of nasal secretion, and posterior pharyngeal wall abnormalities. Evaluation of symptoms and signs are planned at baseline and at study completion, after the four-week treatment period. Secondary endpoints will focus on safety (adverse reactions questionnaire).

One of the main challenges for Dr. Bejout and Isabelle is that the main outcome variable (TNSSS), being a clinical scale, is subject to bias, due to subjectivity in symptoms assessment. Knowledge of treatment allocation by the patient, the evaluating physician or both may lead to a biased result and threaten the validity of the study. So, they believe blinding will be a critical consideration for the success of the trial. On the other hand, blinding will increase the study costs and also will make the assessment of adverse effects difficult—especially potential systemic effects of corticosteroids.

Main Issues Associated with Blinding

The expectations of patients and investigators may influence the findings of a trial, especially when the outcome measure is not so robust, i.e., there is some subjectivity in its assessment. It has been shown that lack of blinding in clinical trials has little or no effect on objective outcomes (such as death), but usually yield exaggerated treatment effect estimates for subjective (soft) outcomes (such as pain levels). When blinded studies on the same subject are performed, these effect estimates tend to decrease or disappear. This effect was demonstrated by an elegant trial from Noseworthy et al. (1994)[2] in which cyclophosphamide and plasma exchange were compared to placebo for multiple sclerosis treatment. Interestingly enough, neither one of the active treatment regimens was effective when compared to placebo when assessed by the blinded neurologists. On the other hand, the results from the unblinded neurologists showed a treatment benefit at 6, 12, and 24 months when compared to placebo.

In fact, observer (or detection) bias is an example of deviated research outcomes in unblinded studies and might be associated with the issue of human behavior being influenced by what we believe. It does not mean that investigators or participants in clinical trials are necessarily untrustworthy. Bias associated with knowing the treatment allocation is often unconscious. In addition, when patients know their group of treatment, they may also look for alternative forms of treatment outside the study protocol (co-interventions), or may change their behavior just because they are participating in a study—this is called the *Hawthorne effect*, influencing efficacy results. On the other hand, if a patient knows that he or she is in the experimental arm, adverse events may be over-reported. In a similar way, if the evaluating physician knows that the patient received the experimental treatment, then he or she may be more probing when evaluating adverse events. Finally, blinding is necessary when a researcher wants to assess the effects of a given treatment beyond the placebo effects. In other words, blinding is also useful to prevent other biases associated with the placebo effect. One

---

[2] Noseworthy JH, et al. The impact of blinding on the results of a randomized, placebo-controlled multiple sclerosis clinical trial. *Neurology.* 1994; 44(1): 16–20.

important issue that researchers should be aware of is the perceived bias. In other words, even if an unblinded study finds the true effect estimate of a given treatment, it is not possible to prove that the result is not biased due to unblinding.

Although blinding should be used whenever possible as it reduces the chance of intentional or unintentional bias being introduced into the study, there are some issues associated with blinding, such as an increase in study costs, feasibility, adherence, and adverse effects monitoring.

As Dr. Bejout will be leaving soon for his long overdue family vacation, he knows that he and Isabelle need to finalize the study plan in the next few days, and the last outstanding issue is study blinding. He was able to cancel his morning administrative meetings and calls Isabelle for a long meeting. He places a bunch of paper and a pencil on his table and asks his secretary to redirect his clinical calls to the on-call ENT physician. He then starts the meeting with Isabelle, "Let us review all the potential options so that we can choose the best one."

The Simplest Blinding Option: A Single-Blind Study

Isabelle and Dr. Bejout started with the simplest blinding option: a single blind study. Although it can refer to a study in which either the investigator or the study subject is unaware of the treatment, a single-blind study usually blinds the patients to treatment allocation, and the investigators remain unblinded.

"This method definitely has advantages," ponders Dr. Bejout. He then continues, "It is simpler and it will also allow for better monitoring of adverse effects, as treating physicians/investigators would be more attentive to possible adverse reactions in the experimental drug group. Something that concerns me is that steroids, even when topically administered, may cause local and systemic adverse effects." He speculates that, with this approach, referring physicians may also feel safer in sending their patients to join the trial, making the recruitment process easier as it increases physicians' adherence. Finally, this would also reduce the study costs as it would reduce staff work to make the investigators blinded.

Isabelle then quickly replies, "On the other hand, single-blind studies have several disadvantages that might decrease the internal validity of our study. For instance, if the treating or evaluating physician is not blinded, there is a risk of biased results. Although the part of the main outcome (TNSSS) that is dependent on patients (the symptoms) would be less affected, there is still the investigator-dependent component on TNSSS."

There is also a risk that treating physicians may consciously or unconsciously influence the behavior of the subject when rating the patient's symptoms. That is called experimenter (psychology) bias. Furthermore, non-blinded evaluating physicians (raters) may be prone to observer bias (i.e., their preconceptions may influence observer judgment of the study endpoint). Another important aspect of unblinded studies is that physicians may influence or choose patients who might respond better to a given treatment. As noted earlier in the chapter, this is called selection bias. For example, if a physician wants the experimental treatment to be successful, he or she may consciously or subconsciously select patients with a better prognosis for improvement in the experimental arm.

The Traditional Option: A Double-Blind Study

Dr. Bejout then moves to the next option and lays out his thoughts, "Well, Isabelle, there is the option of a double-blind study where both the subject and the investigator are blinded to treatment allocation. This design would be easily accepted by our colleagues as the best approach to achieve a higher standard of scientific rigor, as it minimizes/eliminates different types of bias. However, I am still concerned with adverse effects monitoring and physicians' adherence."

In some double-blind studies there is concern over the extent to which the investigator remains blinded. Coding and matching the drug is of utmost importance to maintain the blinding. Even managing all the details to ensure study blinding, in some cases a fully double-blind study might not be possible. Investigators may become unblinded during the study period by a differential treatment efficacy, especially if placebo is used as the control. In some cases, the side-effects profile of the experimental drug may unblind investigators, as well. Similar effects might be observed with study subjects. To limit this possibility, active and placebo treatment must be identical in odor, appearance, and taste (and induce similar sensory experience if an external device is used).

A Compromise Solution: A Single-Blind Study with a Third Blinded Rater

Now it is Isabelle's turn: "Well, another possibility is a single-blind study with an external blinded rater. That would be a compromise between the two options we discussed before." Then she continues, "Although the unblinded investigator can still influence patients and therefore add bias to the study, and this would increase the costs of the study."

This method requires two investigators to be in contact with the patients: the treating investigator/physician, who knows treatment allocation (and may assess adverse effects), and the blinded evaluating investigator (rater), who is responsible for assessing the efficacy outcome of the study. So, the study becomes more complex and costly. Also, it increases patients' visit duration and therefore might decrease adherence. Finally, it does not eliminate the possibility of the unblinded physician/rater unintentionally influencing patients' behavior.

Adding Another Control Group: Double-Dummy Design

Although Dr. Bejout and Isabelle decided to have only two groups (placebo vs. RHINO-A), there is still the possibility of adding a third group to compare the effects of this new intervention with the oral standard drug. Isabelle then asks, "Dr. Bejout, if we add the third group that will be a control group testing the oral drug, how are we going to blind patients if they will quickly be able to identify the treatments as they are different (topical vs. oral medication)?" Dr. Bejout quickly responds to this question, "In this case, we would need to use the double-dummy design in which patients receive two interventions, the topical and oral drug; however, only one of them is active, or both are placebo (for the placebo group)." He then stops for a couple of minutes to answer an urgent call from a patient in need of a prescription. When he comes back to the discussion, he concludes, "But Isabelle, we will not have funds to run three groups of patients, so let us focus on the other options for this study and use this for perhaps a follow-up study."

The Safest Option: A Triple-Blind Study

Dr. Bejout looks at his watch as it is almost noon and he knows that he does not have much time left before his afternoon clinic. He wants then to move to the last option: a triple-blind study. "Isabelle, how about if we add another level of blinding, having the statistician or the investigator responsible for data analysis blinded?"

There is no rule of thumb for the additional blinding level in triple-blind studies. Besides the treating/evaluating investigator/physician, the sponsor or investigator responsible for data analysis may be blinded—or, according to Forder et al.,[3] "[t]hose who adjudicate the study outcomes (the outcomes assessment committee) or those who monitor the study safety (the safety and data monitoring committee)." It has advantages, as blinding data analysis. For example, it may prevent errors due to biased handling of data, such as choice of analytical strategies or methods. However, it also adds costs and complications to the study protocol, and in addition, when the database is locked at the end of the study, the need to blind the statistician becomes less important.

Final Issues: Blinding Assessment

After a four-hour discussion, Dr. Bejout and Isabelle felt ready to decide how to proceed regarding the study blinding. But Isabelle then realizes that they did not decide whether they are using blinding evaluation. This has been a recent concern in well-designed clinical trials, and she believes they should consider it in their study.

It has been suggested that the success of blinding should be assessed systematically in clinical trials. Blinding can be evaluated using an informal assessment of the reported blinding practices, but this approach is subjective. The alternative is to assess the success of blinding with a formal test. However, there is still no consensus on the appropriate methodology. One method consists of asking participants and investigators to guess treatment assignment and compare the answers with the actual treatment. Results may be flawed, as there is a tendency that patients feeling better will tend to guess they are in the experimental arm rather than in the control. Consequently, if the experimental treatment is really effective, blinding reliability may be questioned, although the method of blinding was adequate. With this method, blinding is more likely to be considered successful when a treatment is ineffective. An alternative is to compare patient- versus investigator-based questionnaires.

Dr. Bejout's secretary enters the room and mentions that he is running late for his outpatient clinic service. He quickly gets his white coat and tells Isabelle that they

---

[3] Forder PM, Gebski VJ, Keech AC, Allocation concealment and blinding: when ignorance is bliss, *Med J Aust.* 2005 Jan 17; 182(2): 87–89

should meet the next day at 7 a.m. to make this decision and submit the final version of the study. Isabelle leaves the office feeling energized and glad that she will finally be able to start working on her PhD project.

CASE DISCUSSION

After a successful pre-clinical and phase I trial, Dr. Bejout is developing a project to run a phase II trial for a new topical steroid drug for allergic rhinitis. The trial will last four weeks, and because of its short duration and the nature of the disease being studied, the IRB has agreed to the use of a placebo. His main outcome is going to be the Total Nasal Symptoms Score Scale (TNSSS), a score given by reported symptoms (by patient) and signs assessed by an ENT physician. Symptoms and signs will be evaluated at baseline and after study completion. Side effects also will be evaluated with a questionnaire, as a secondary endpoint. Like any scale of signs and symptoms, TNSSS is subjective and more prone to bias than "hard," objective outcomes. Knowledge of group allocation may involuntarily influence signs and symptoms reports by the patients and physician, leading to biased results. Dr. Bejout's challenge is to choose a blinding procedure that will ensure a high-quality trial but also feasibility and cost control. On the other hand, Dr. Bejout is worried about adverse effects of the steroid, and thinks than the attending physician might underreport side effects if unaware of group allocation. Indeed, this trial illustrates the challenge of making the trial feasible versus preventing bias.

As in any trial, five main groups of individuals can be blinded according to the CONSORT statement: patients, health-care provider, data collectors, outcome adjudicator, and data analysts. One must remember that the variable of interest is a subjective, "soft" outcome and depends on the report of symptoms by the patient and an evaluation of signs from the assessors.

Several options were discussed: single-blind, double-blind, single blind with a third blind rater.

In a single-blind study, the patient would be blinded, but the physician would still know group allocation. This option has advantages, as it is relatively simple and keeps the placebo effect, but still leaves the physician vulnerable to observer/detection bias and differential treatment among patients from the two groups (performance bias).

A double-blind (both patient and physician) is a well-balanced solution, but other issues such as adherence and adverse-event reporting may come to play. In other to keep both parties blinded, a placebo has to be developed. It should be identical in shape, color, size, and taste to the active drug. This adds cost to the study and sometimes is hard or nearly impossible to achieve. Unblinding may still occur, if the active drug is highly effective in comparison to the placebo, and physicians and patients become aware who is in the active drug group. Attending physicians might be less motivated to recruit their patients to a study where they are kept "blind" to study allocation and underreport side effects while monitoring for adverse events.

A compromise solution is blinding the patient and having an external, blinded, assessor. This would keep the attending physician aware of group allocation, therefore maintaining the possibility of physician unintentionally influencing the patient behavior and thus performance bias.

In addition to the patients, health-care provider, and evaluators, data analysts/ statisticians could also be blinded. If this would be too complex, statistical analyses should be determined a priori, guaranteeing unbiased analysis.

If Dr. Bejout wishes to test his RHINO-A against a standard oral treatment, then a double-dummy design should be considered, but this will add an extra burden in terms of logistics and cost. There would be three different groups of subjects: (1) topical RHINO-A plus placebo tablet; (2) topical placebo plus active tablet; (3) topical placebo plus placebo tablet. Furthermore, this could be troublesome in terms of compliance, as patients would have to take not one, but two medications. In terms of data analysis, having three groups may decrease power to detect differences among the groups, if sample size is not increased.

Dr. Bejout also has to decide if he wishes to assess for blinding success. This adds extra work to his project as well as challenges in terms of interpretation of results. Asking investigators and patients to guess group allocation might raise their interest in this topic and incentivize unblinding efforts. If the treatment is truly effective, then "unblinding through efficacy" may occur, which is not necessarily bad. Blinding is more likely considered "successful" when the new treatment is not effective, as both control and intervention group will "feel the same." Using blinding assessment is therefore highly debatable.

Blinding groups of interest in a study adds complexity and cost to the study. With limited funding, the investigator has to compromise and determine what is the most important. Blinding increases the methodological soundness of the study, but it is not the only aspect that has to be addressed. As "some is better than none," Dr. Bejout must decide how far can he go in terms of blinding to go improve the internal validity of his trial. Any weaknesses concerning this aspect should be commented in the project/paper, and strategies to overcome potential study limitations should be mentioned. There are no "right" or "wrong" answers in this case. The pros and cons of each design should be weighed by the investigator, and a compromise must be achieved. Limitations and weaknesses of the study (concerning blinding) should be acknowledged and addressed as best as possible.

CASE QUESTIONS FOR REFLECTION

1. What are the challenges faced by Dr. Bejout and Isabelle in choosing the study design?
2. What are their main concerns?
3. What should they consider in making their decision?

FURTHER READING

In these references you will find an inventory of blinding methods in pharmacological and non-pharmacological trials:

Boutron I, et al. Methods of blinding in reports of randomized controlled trials assessing pharmacologic treatments: a systematic review. *PLoS Med.* 2006; 3(10): e425.

Boutron I, et al. Reporting methods of blinding in randomized trials assessing nonpharmacological treatments. *PLoS Med.* 2007; 4(2): e61.

This paper summarizes the rationale for blinding and bias mechanisms:

Hrobjartsson A, Boutron I. Blinding in randomized clinical trials: imposed impartiality. *Clin Pharmacol Ther.* 2011; 90(5): 732–736.

REFERENCES

1. Schulz KF, Chalmers I, and Altman DG. The landscape and lexicon of blinding in randomized trials. *Ann Intern Med.* 2002 136(3): 254–259.
2. Kaptchuk TJ. Intentional ignorance: a history of blind assessment and placebo controls in medicine. *Bull Hist Med* 1998; 72(3): 389–433.
3. Flint A. Contribution toward the natural history of articular rheumatism; consisting of a report of thirteen cases treated solely with palliative measures. *Amer J Med Sci.* 1863; 46: 17–36.
4. Amberson JB, McMahon BT, Pinner M. A clinical trial of sanocrysin in pulmonary tuberculosis. *Amer Rev Tuberc.* 1931; 24: 401–435.
5. Hrobjartsson A, Boutron I. Blinding in randomized clinical trials: imposed impartiality. *Clin Pharmacol Ther.* 2011; 90(5): 732–736.
6. Forder PM, Gebski VJ, Keech AC. Allocation concealment and blinding: when ignorance is bliss. *Med J Aust.* 2005; 182(2): 87–89.
7. Viera AJ, Bangdiwala SI. Eliminating bias in randomized controlled trials: importance of allocation concealment and masking. *Fam Med.* 2007; 39(2): 132–137.
8. Schulz KF, Grimes DA. Blinding in randomised trials: hiding who got what. *Lancet.* 2002; 359(9307): 696–700.
9. Polit DF. Blinding during the analysis of research data. *Int J Nurs Stud.* 2011; 48(5): 636–641.
10. Devereaux PJ, et al. Physician interpretations and textbook definitions of blinding terminology in randomized controlled trials. *JAMA.* 2001; 285(15): 2000–2003.
11. Moher D, et al. CONSORT 2010 explanation and elaboration: Updated guidelines for reporting parallel group randomised trials. *J Clin Epidemiol.* 2010; 63(8): e1–37.
12. Miller LE, Stewart ME. The blind leading the blind: use and misuse of blinding in randomized controlled trials. *Contemp Clin Trials.* 2011; 32(2): 240–243.
13. Lang, T., Masking or blinding? An unscientific survey of mostly medical journal editors on the great debate. MedGenMed, 2000. 2(1): p. E25.
14. Taylor, W.J. and M. Weatherall, What are open-label extension studies for? J Rheumatol, 2006. 33(4): p. 642–3.
15. Psaty, B.M. and R.L. Prentice, Minimizing bias in randomized trials: the importance of blinding. JAMA, 2010. 304(7): p. 793–4.
16. Montori VM, et al. In the dark: the reporting of blinding status in randomized controlled trials. *J Clin Epidemiol.* 2002; 55(8): 787–790.
17. Haahr MT, Hrobjartsson A. Who is blinded in randomized clinical trials? A study of 200 trials and a survey of authors. *Clin Trials.* 2006; 3(4): 360–365.
18. Villamar MF, et al. The reporting of blinding in physical medicine and rehabilitation randomized controlled trials: a systematic review. *J Rehabil Med.* 2012; 45(1): 6–13.
19. Balk EM, et al. Correlation of quality measures with estimates of treatment effect in meta-analyses of randomized controlled trials. *JAMA.* 2002; 287(22): 2973–2982.
20. Califf RM, et al. Characteristics of clinical trials registered in ClinicalTrials.gov, 2007–2010. *JAMA.* 2012; 307(17): 1838–1847.

21. Schulz KF, et al. Blinding and exclusions after allocation in randomised controlled trials: survey of published parallel group trials in obstetrics and gynaecology. *BMJ*. 1996; 312(7033): 742–744.
22. Karanicolas PJ, et al. Blinding of outcomes in trials of orthopaedic trauma: an opportunity to enhance the validity of clinical trials. *J Bone Joint Surg Am*. 2008; 90(5): 1026–1033.
23. Begg C, et al. Improving the quality of reporting of randomized controlled trials. The CONSORT statement. *JAMA*. 1996; 276(8): 637–639.
24. Juni P, Altman DG, Egger M. Systematic reviews in health care: Assessing the quality of controlled clinical trials. *BMJ*. 2001; 323(7303): 42–46.
25. Higgins JPT, Green S. *Cochrane handbook for systematic review of interventions*. London: John Wiley & Sons; 2008.
26. http://bmg.cochrane.org/assessing-risk-bias-included-studies
27. Noseworthy JH, et al. The impact of blinding on the results of a randomized, placebo-controlled multiple sclerosis clinical trial. *Neurology*. 1994; 44(1): 16–20.
28. Schulz KF, et al. Empirical evidence of bias: dimensions of methodological quality associated with estimates of treatment effects in controlled trials. *JAMA*. 1995; 273(5): 408–412.
29. Moher D, et al. Does quality of reports of randomised trials affect estimates of intervention efficacy reported in meta-analyses? *Lancet*. 1998; 352(9128): 609–613.
30. Pildal J, et al. Impact of allocation concealment on conclusions drawn from meta-analyses of randomized trials. *Int J Epidemiol*. 2007; 36(4): 847–857.
31. Wood L, et al. Empirical evidence of bias in treatment effect estimates in controlled trials with different interventions and outcomes: meta-epidemiological study. *BMJ*. 2008; 336(7644): 601–605.
32. Hrobjartsson A, et al. Observer bias in randomised clinical trials with binary outcomes: systematic review of trials with both blinded and non-blinded outcome assessors. *BMJ*. 2012; 344: e1119.
33. de Craen AJ, et al. Effect of colour of drugs: systematic review of perceived effect of drugs and of their effectiveness. *BMJ*. 1996; 313(7072): 1624–1626.
34. Desbiens NA. Lessons learned from attempts to establish the blind in placebo-controlled trials of zinc for the common cold. *Ann Intern Med*. 2000; 133(4): 302–303.
35. Hemila H. Vitamin C, the placebo effect, and the common cold: a case study of how preconceptions influence the analysis of results. *J Clin Epidemiol*. 1996; 49(10): 1079–1084; discussion 1085, 1087.
36. Karlowski TR, et al. Ascorbic acid for the common cold. A prophylactic and therapeutic trial. *JAMA*. 1975; 231(10): 1038–1042.
37. de Craen AJ, et al. Placebo effect in the acute treatment of migraine: subcutaneous placebos are better than oral placebos. *J Neurol*. 2000; 247(3): 183–188.
38. Francis CW, et al. Comparison of ximelagatran with warfarin for the prevention of venous thromboembolism after total knee replacement. *N Engl J Med*. 2003. 349(18): 1703–1712.
39. Morello CM, et al. Randomized double-blind study comparing the efficacy of gabapentin with amitriptyline on diabetic peripheral neuropathy pain. *Arch Intern Med*. 1999. 159(16): 1931–1937.
40. Boutron I, et al. Methods of blinding in reports of randomized controlled trials assessing pharmacologic treatments: a systematic review. *PLoS Med*. 2006; 3(10): e425.
41. Boutron I, et al. Reporting methods of blinding in randomized trials assessing nonpharmacological treatments. *PLoS Med*. 2007; 4(2): e61.

42. Fregni F, et al. Challenges and recommendations for placebo controls in randomized trials in physical and rehabilitation medicine: a report of the international placebo symposium working group. *Am J Phys Med Rehabil.* 2010; 89(2): 160–172.
43. Boutron I, et al. Methodological differences in clinical trials evaluating nonpharmacological and pharmacological treatments of hip and knee osteoarthritis. *JAMA.* 2003; 290(8): 1062–1070.
44. Kaptchuk TJ, et al. Sham device v inert pill: randomised controlled trial of two placebo treatments. *BMJ.* 2006; 332(7538): 391–397.
45. Bang H, Park JJ. Blinding in clinical trials: a practical approach. *J Altern Complement Med.* 2012; 19(4): 367–9.
46. Senn SJ. Turning a blind eye: authors have blinkered view of blinding. *BMJ.* 2004; 328(7448): 1135–1136; author reply 1136.
47. Park J, Bang H, Canette I. Blinding in clinical trials, time to do it better. *Complement Ther Med.* 2008; 16(3): 121–123.
48. Altman DG, Schulz KF, Moher D. Turning a blind eye: testing the success of blinding and the CONSORT statement. *BMJ.* 2004; 328(7448): 1135; author reply 1136.
49. Fergusson D, et al. Turning a blind eye: the success of blinding reported in a random sample of randomised, placebo controlled trials. *BMJ.* 2004; 328(7437): 432.
50. Hrobjartsson A, et al. Blinded trials taken to the test: an analysis of randomized clinical trials that report tests for the success of blinding. *Int J Epidemiol.* 2007; 36(3): 654–63.
51. James KE, et al. An index for assessing blindness in a multi-centre clinical trial: disulfiram for alcohol cessation: a VA cooperative study. *Stat Med.* 1996; 15(13): 1421–1434.
52. Bang H, Ni L, Davis CE. Assessment of blinding in clinical trials. *Control Clin Trials.* 2004; 25(2): 143–156.
53. US Food and Drug Administration. Guidance for Industry E9 Statistical Principles for Clinical Trials. 1998 [cited 2012]; Available from: http://www.fda.gov/downloads/Drugs/GuidanceComplianceRegulatoryInformation/Guidances/ucm073137.pdf.
54. European Medicines Agency. ICH Topic E 9 Statistical Principles for Clinical Trials. 2006 [cited 2012]; Available from: http://www.ema.europa.eu/docs/en_GB/document_library/Scientific_guideline/2009/09/WC500002928.pdf.
55. Moher D, Schulz KF, Altman DG. The CONSORT statement: revised recommendations for improving the quality of reports of parallel group randomized trials. *BMC Med Res Methodol.* 2001; 1: 2.
56. Sackett DL. Commentary: measuring the success of blinding in RCTs: don't, must, can't or needn't? *Int J Epidemiol.* 2007; 36(3): 664–665.
57. Gotzsche PC. Blinding during data analysis and writing of manuscripts. *Control Clin Trials.* 1996; 17(4): 285–290; discussion 290–293.
58. Beeh KM, Beier J, Donohue JF. Clinical trial design in chronic obstructive pulmonary disease: current perspectives and considerations with regard to blinding of tiotropium. *Respir Res.* 2012; 13: 52.
59. White A, Cummings M, Filshie J. *An introduction to Western medical acupuncture.* 1st ed. Edinburgh: Churchill Livingstone Elsevier; 2008.

7

RECRUITMENT AND ADHERENCE

Authors: *Timo Siepmann, Ana Isabel Penzlin, and Felipe Fregni*

Case study authors: *Rui Imamura and Felipe Fregni*

Drugs don't work in patients who don't take them.
—C. Everett Koop. Improving medication compliance: proceedings of a symposium. Reston: National Pharmaceutical Council; 1985.

INTRODUCTION

This is the final chapter of Unit I, Basics of Clinical Research. In this unit, you have already learned how to select your research question (Chapter 2) and how to choose the study population (Chapter 3) in which you will test your hypothesis. But how do you identify and reach these potential study subjects? And how do you ensure that they adhere to the protocol? In this chapter we present the role of recruitment and adherence of study participants in clinical trials. The term *recruitment* refers to the identification and enrollment of study participants, including operational aspects such as advertising, overcoming recruitment barriers, and management of financial, logistic, and time-related aspects throughout the process of enrollment. The term *adherence* refers to the compliance of study participants to act in accordance with the study protocol and to remain in the study. *Retention* is often used synonymously with adherence, but rather refers to actions aimed at keeping patients in the study so that they are available at follow-up (alive and not lost to dropout or withdrawal). *Attrition* is defined as loss of subjects during the course of the study, which can be due to death, stopping of the assigned intervention, dropout, or intentional withdrawal. In this chapter we describe the methodological principles of achieving effective recruitment, adherence, and retention in clinical research.

RECRUITMENT

It frequently happens that during the study design phase, only limited thought is given to recruitment strategies. In reality, though, one of the most difficult parts of a study is the recruitment process, and it is this factor that often decides whether a study will fail or succeed [1,2].

The two main objectives of the recruitment process are the following:

1. To recruit a study sample that is representative of the target population (see Chapter 3);

2. To recruit a sample that is large enough to fulfill the requirements of the sample size and power calculations (see Chapter 11) [3].

RECRUITMENT: STUDY SAMPLE, DEFINITION, AND SIZE

Before enrolling individuals from your target population in your trial, you have to consider the first important step in the process of participant recruitment: defining the target population (see Chapter 3 for more details). The target population will be determined based on the research question and the hypothesis to be tested. It is important to define the target population by specifying clear inclusion/exclusion criteria. These criteria will be used to screen subjects/patients for enrollment and to determine who will be entered in the study. Once the screening criteria are defined, you will have to decide how many subjects you want to recruit. The sample size depends not only on the desired power and the effect size, but also on budgetary and logistic considerations. This decision is based on several factors, and it is not always easy to find the right balance between them (see Chapter 11 for more details). The main concern is that if the sample size is too small, the study result might be negative due to insufficient power, resulting in a type II error; on the other hand, if the sample size is too large, unethical issues become a concern, in addition to the unnecessary expenditure of time, resources, and labor.

It is important to consider that sample size goals are affected before the start of a study by the recruitment response rate (with the potential of introducing non-response bias) and during the study by the attrition rate. The *response rate* is the number of screened subjects who ultimately agree to enroll in a study. During the screening process, the pool of potential study subjects shrinks substantially from initially 100% to 10%–15% eligible and finally as low as 1% enrolled [4]. This phenomenon is mainly due to the fact that the number of subjects who are available and willing to enroll is overestimated; this is referred to as the funnel effect, or Lasagna's Law (see Figure 7.1) [5,6]. But even from that small part of enrolled subjects, not

THE FUNNEL EFFECT

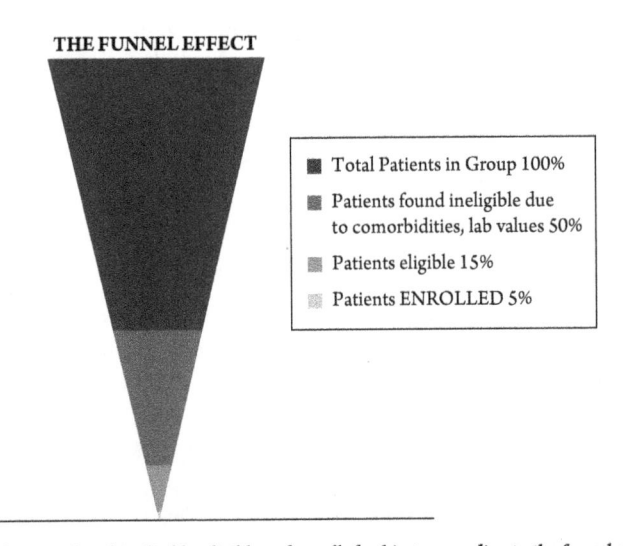

- Total Patients in Group 100%
- Patients found ineligible due to comorbidities, lab values 50%
- Patients eligible 15%
- Patients ENROLLED 5%

Figure 7.1. The distribution of total, ineligible, eligible and enrolled subjects according to the funnel effect.

all can be randomized. Many reasons can be attributed to a low response rate, such as patients' lack of motivation, as well as practical issues such as travel expenses. The funnel effect demonstrates that, at the end, only a small portion of all identified potential study patients or subjects will be enrolled in the study.

The candidate's decision of whether or not to participate in a research study is usually based on the participant's perception of risks/costs and benefits in enrolling in a clinical trial. The investigator should therefore be aware of potential risks/costs and benefits that are associated with the investigation.

Participants' Decision-Making Process

In order to estimate and improve recruitment rates, it is important to consider the factors that patients weigh when deciding whether or not to participate in a research study. The challenge is to understand the weight of these factors in the decision-making process. The main factors are the following:

Benefits and motivation:

- Medical: Access to cutting-edge treatment that would not be available in a non-research setting
- Financial: Access to novel treatments at no cost or reduced cost
- To advance science
- To earn extra money
- Altruism: To improve public health.

Risks and concerns:

- Medical: Side effects, assignment to placebo, lack of efficacy
- Continued access to study drug/intervention
- Logistical: Trade-off with other time commitments, medical or opportunity costs.

Identification of Participants, Recruitment Methods, and Obstacles

When we conduct a clinical trial, how do we reach the target population? How do we use our financial resources efficiently to advertise our study? How do we design our advertising in order to draw the attention of as many potentially eligible participants as possible without introducing bias? What are the appropriate means to distribute the advertising material? There are several ways to identify potential participants for a research study:

- Medical records review
- Clinic log
- External referrals: primary care, specialists (collaborations)
- Clinical research centers
- Specialized clinics and general hospitals
- Registries
- Recruitment/call center

- Patient support groups
- Patients' community websites
- Clinical trial registration sites
- Government
  - clinicaltrials.gov
  - clinicaltrialsregister.eu
- Patient advocacy groups
  - ciscrp.org (international)
- Institutional Resources
  - rsvpforhealth.org (local)
- http://searchclinicaltrials.org/
- Databases: AWARE for All, RSVP for Health
- Advertising: paper flyers, radio, newspapers, web.

After the target population has been chosen and defined by inclusion/exclusion criteria, the next step of the study recruitment plan is to determine the best medium of advertising to reach potential study candidates. Easy and effective ways to reach a specific group of patients are *health-care-provider-based strategies* (also referred to as targeted strategies), such as clinician invitation letters (invitation letters to physicians treating patients who are potentially eligible for study participation, or the distribution of leaflets and promotional posters in hospitals). However, these strategies may only be sufficient when a highly specific group of patients affected by the same (or similar) disease constitute the target population and require the collaboration of clinicians to refer patients to the study. But if we identify an appropriate way to address the potential participants through *community-based strategies* (also referred to as broad-based strategies), such as advertising through television or the Internet, how do we know that this specific medium doesn't exclude a group within this population that does not have access to this medium? For example, what if we choose to perform a study in patients with type II diabetes and decide to advertise our study through Internet advertisement on webpages of diabetes support groups? As older people commonly have less access to the Internet, online advertising would be more likely to reach younger type I diabetes patients than older type II diabetes patients.

Besides the age-dependent behavior, there are other important factors that should be considered when choosing the form of advertising. These influencing factors include the following:

- Access to the medium of advertising
- Complexity of language and information
- Number of media selected for advertising
- Time and budgetary limitations.

In the process of determining the adequate medium of advertising, we need to balance both the available time and monetary resources of the study and the efficiency of the advertising. Common media of advertising include the following:

- Leaflets
- Promotional posters

- Television
- Newspapers
- Internet (i.e., social or professional networks)
- Mails
- Emails.

Both leaflets and promotional posters are useful to reach local target groups with low costs, but may fail to reach larger populations that exceed regional borders.

While television can reach broad target groups in a short time, it is costly and therefore usually requires industrial financial support. Regional newspaper advertisement can be useful to reach high numbers of individuals within the scope of the newspaper's circulation, but might exclude subjects who are using the Internet or television to get access to news. Internet ads are useful to reach a broad number of subjects or patients, but also to address specific groups. However, as Internet usage in most countries correlates with demographic factors such as age and income, the exclusive use of the Internet for advertising might bias the selection of study participants. Advertising by regular mail is time-intensive but may help to reach a very specific population. Advertising by email has several advantages over regular mail, but low perception might be a problem, and an email might never even reach the attention of an individual by being filtered out (spam/advertisement filters). Additionally, both mail and email require access to contact information (street addresses or email addresses, respectively). Due to data protection regulations, mail and email lists can be preserved. Therefore advertising by mailing or emailing in a community-based setting may be restricted to subjects or patients whose addresses are included in those address lists that are openly available. Alternatively, public *awareness campaigns* through specialized medical societies can be an effective tool to raise awareness of the study among physicians and patients, thus facilitating health-care-provider-based recruitment.

> *Health-care-provider-based recruitment strategies* (e.g., clinician invitation letters) are sufficient to reach specific groups of patients but require the collaboration of colleagues to refer patients to the study. Public awareness campaigns can facilitate health-care-provider-based recruitment.
>
> *Community-based recruitment strategies* (such as newspaper or Internet advertisement) must be planned in consideration of the individual conditions of the research study, including financial resources, specific properties of the target population, and access of the target population to different media forms.

Sometimes it might be useful to combine different forms of advertisement to increase the efficiency of reaching potential study participants. For example, it can be useful to increase visual *exposure to the advertisement* through the *combined use* of leaflets and promotional posters when addressing healthy subjects in a certain buildings, for example in a university. The combination of different media might be also useful when subgroups within the target population have different access to different media forms (e.g., young subjects preferring Internet, older subjects preferring newspaper).

In addition to choosing the appropriate form of advertisement, attention also has to be paid to the contents. On one hand, complex information (i.e., the pharmacokinetic adverse effects of a certain investigational new drug in a newspaper ad) might be

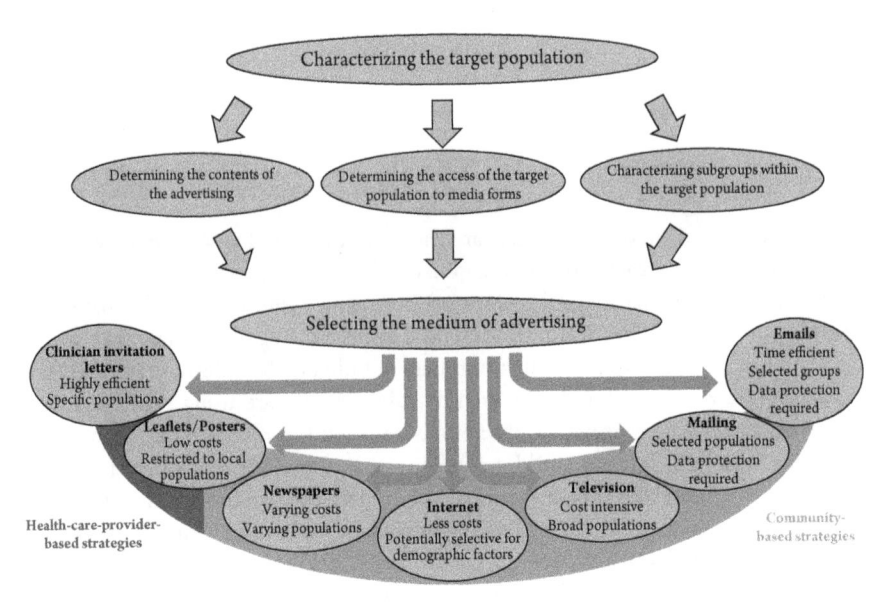

Figure 7.2. The consecutive steps in planning the study advertisement in consideration of the individual properties of different media.

difficult to understand. On the other hand, not naming significant potential adverse effects of the study intervention in an advertisement might raise a feeling of being deceitfully "concealed" when learning about this effect during the informed consent stage and might further decrease the recruitment response rate.

In conclusion, before starting the recruitment of study participants, it is crucial to carefully design a *detailed recruitment strategy plan (including an advertisement plan)*, considering both the properties of the medium of advertising and the feasibility of conducting the advertisement, the latter mostly being restricted by financial resources. The process of planning the study advertising plan is also illustrated in Figure 7.2.

THE EFFECTIVENESS OF RECRUITMENT STRATEGIES

Which single or combined strategy is most effective depends on several factors, such as the study design, the target population, and the intervention. A recent paper asserted that "physician referrals and flyers were the most effective recruitment method" in their trial [7]. The use of combined (multi-tiered) recruitment strategies was found to be beneficial in enrolling those subjects who had been previously indecisive or doubtful [8].

Human Factors

Once a potential candidate shows interest in participating in the advertised research study, the individual skills and behavior of the research staff gain upmost importance in the process of recruiting. In order to successfully enroll a participant, it is crucial for the study staff to show empathy and professionalism, beginning with the first contact and the initially provided information. Gorkin et al. demonstrated that successful enrollment is higher for those patients who read and understood the informed consent than in those patients who did not fully read and understood it [9]. An empathic way of explaining the study to the potential participant is important in order to achieve a high degree of understanding. Therefore, both *empathy* and *sufficient clarification* are important contributors to successful recruitment.

From Screening to Enrollment

After potential candidates are identified and contacted, the next step in recruitment is the screening process: Based on inclusion and exclusion criteria, subjects are screened for eligibility. Those who are selected and are able to accommodate the study protocol schedule will be asked to sign the *informed consent*. The informed consent is a document that describes the study to the study subject in lay terms and explains risks and benefits. The most important points are to ensure that obtaining the informed consent and participation in the study are voluntary and that the study subject is being protected (i.e., confidentiality, adverse events). An informed consent has to be approved by the institutional review board (IRB).

After informed consent is obtained, subjects are enrolled in the study and are assigned to a treatment arm with or without randomization (for more details about randomization, see Chapter 5). The process of enrolling subjects in a trial is also referred to as *accrual*. After enrollment is completed, it is very important to ensure the adherence and retention of study subjects, which we discuss in the next section.

ADHERENCE

Adherence in Clinical Practice

The WHO defined *adherence* in June 2001 as "the extent to which the patient follows medical instructions" [10]. However, this definition is somewhat limited, since "medical" is too narrow a description; not including other forms of care and "instructions" implies that the patient is a passive, obedient recipient, rather than an active participant. In 2003 the definition of adherence was therefore modified as "the extent to which a person's behavior—taking medication, following a diet, and/or executing lifestyle changes, *corresponds with agreed recommendation from a health care provider.*"

Another definition of adherence is the "active, voluntary, and collaborative involvement of the patient in a mutually acceptable course of behavior to produce a therapeutic result" [11,12]. Although synonymous, the term adherence is preferred over *compliance*, since the latter suggests that the patient is a passive, acquiescent receiver of a treatment protocol.

Adherence in Clinical Research Studies: Definition

In the context of clinical research, the term *adherence* refers to the degree to which study participants act in concordance with the study protocol or the instructions or advice of the research physician. Two primary types of adherence have been described previously: The term *follow-up adherence* refers to the degree to which the participant undergoes the scheduled sequence of research measurements (i.e., keeping follow-up appointments or undergoing repeated blood tests) until reaching the endpoint [13]. The term *regimen adherence* refers to pursuing the study protocol (or regimen) consistently (i.e., being on schedule in taking medication at the specified dose).

Retention and Attrition

Whereas *retention* describes the degree to which study participants stay in the trial, the term *attrition* refers to the loss of subjects during the course of the investigation. Both retention and attrition affect the final adherence rate.

There is no general consensus on what rate of adherence is considered acceptable. The actual rate of adherence in clinical trials varies substantially, depending on several factors, but rates of 51%–79% are not uncommon [14]. In general, studies of chronic conditions usually report lower rates of 43%–78% [15–17].

Barriers to Adherence and Consequences of Low Adherence

Adherence is influenced by various factors. Osterberg and Blaschke identified major *predictors of poor adherence* that include "presence of psychological problems, particularly depression, presence of cognitive impairment, treatment of asymptomatic disease, inadequate follow-up or discharge planning, side effects of medication, patient's lack of belief in benefit of treatment, patient's lack of insight into the illness, poor provider-patient relationship, presence of barriers to care or medications, missed appointments, complexity of treatment, cost of medication, copayment, or both" [18]. Also, adherence is affected by the degree of severity and chronicity of a disease, or by treatment side effects. Examples of populations that display more difficulties to adhere to treatments include the following:

- HIV patients (side effects of drugs, multiple drugs, and food intolerance)
- Patients with arterial hypertension (asymptomatic condition)
- Patients with psychiatric conditions (behavioral difficulties)
- Pediatric populations (non-compliance during testing).

Problems related to regimen adherence can be classified as *omission errors* (i.e., taking a medication too late, failing to take a medication, or taking under-dosed amounts of a medication) and *commission errors* (i.e., taking an overdose of a medication, or taking a medication too frequently). Factors leading to a decreased adherence can also be classified as *random adherence problems* (i.e., unfavorable provider-participant interaction) and *non-random adherence problems* (i.e., fatigue of the patient due to the duration of the study).

Consequences of adherence problems in clinical research studies not only may put the study participant's health at risk, but also can prevent the investigator from successfully completing the trial, or can increase the duration of data acquisition that is necessary to achieve sufficient statistical power (consequently increasing costs).

Data acquired through trials with small numbers of adherent subjects can have higher statistical power than data obtained in studies with high numbers of non-adherent subjects [19]. This effect is, in large part, due to the increased amount of missing data through adherence problems (i.e., missing of follow-up visits; see also Chapter 13). The main issues of failed adherence are dropouts or premature withdrawals, which lead to several substantial problems in the conduction of a clinical trial:

- Threaten the statistical power of the trial
- Can introduce bias if dropouts are not randomly distributed across treatment groups
- Necessitate that sites access adverse effects and mortality status via alternate mechanisms where appropriate
- Threaten perception of the trial results.

Techniques of Facilitation

There are several strategies to facilitate adherence. In general, patients are acting more compliantly when they think that the clinical trial may result in a potential improvement of their health, or effective treatment of their disease, respectively. Study participants may also value the additional monitoring and care from health providers throughout the study, or may show high adherence because of altruistic reasons (i.e., improvement of medical treatment for future generations). Also, compensation and reimbursement for study-related expenses such as parking and travel expenses can contribute to the degree of adherence.

Two specific techniques to increase adherence have been described by Robiner: *pre-randomization screening* and *adherence-enhancing strategies*. [13]

In clinical research studies, *pre-randomization screening* can be used as a preventive measure to exclude subjects from participation who are at high risk of non-adherence, and lack of compliance.

The *run-in* approach includes assessment of compliance, by means of pill counts or quantitative analysis of serum concentration of the administered agent during a study pre-phase where study subjects receive a predefined prescription regimen (i.e., a certain number of placebo pills or low-dose active treatment at predefined times). This analysis is undertaken before the actual study begins and allows for the identification of patients who are likely to display insufficient compliance during the study. Furthermore, through another approach referred to as *test-dosing*, researchers can identify candidates who may drop out of the study because of dose-dependent adverse drug effects. In this pre-randomization screening method, potential study participants also receive a low dose of the experimental agent prior to the actual study. In contrast to the run-in method, test-dosing does not include assessment of compliance, but detects individual adverse effects to identify those subjects who have a high risk of dropping out due to intolerance.

Although pre-randomization screening methods are controversial because of their negative impact on sensitivity, specificity, and external validity, they can increase statistical power by 20%–41% and might pose a valid option to improve the design of potentially underpowered studies. However, as data on these techniques are limited, a consensus on their utility in clinical research has yet to be achieved [20].

Another approach to increase adherence is to perform *adherence-enhancing strategies* during the trial. These strategies aim to influence the subject to be compliant with the research protocol and instructions of the research staff. Adherence-enhancing strategies include those listed in Table 7.1.

Table 7.1 Adherence-enhancing strategies

Recruitment strategies	Giving detailed information on the trial, spending appropriate time with the subject to achieve understanding of the protocol
Social strategies	Involving family members to promote study participation or providing social support
Health-care strategies	Providing health-related information or involving other health-care providers in promoting study participation
Protocol strategies	Minimizing frequency of medication intake or quantity of follow-up visits
Logistical support	Providing child care and free parking during the study visits
Staff strategies	Training the research personnel in adherence-enhancing behavior
Adherence monitoring	Obtaining feedback on the degree of adherence during the study from the subjects, questionnaires, counting pills, using logs, using of tracer substances, electronic monitoring

Adherence monitoring can be useful as a direct adherence-enhancing strategy, but also helps to identify and evaluate the impact of possible protocol-related causes of adherence problems. This knowledge on the causality of problematic adherence can be used to prevent adherence problems in future studies with a similar design. Methods of how to adjust for problems with adherence at the data analysis stage will be discussed in Chapter 13.

Figure 7.3 summarizes the important points of recruitment and adherence that need to be taken into account when designing a trial.

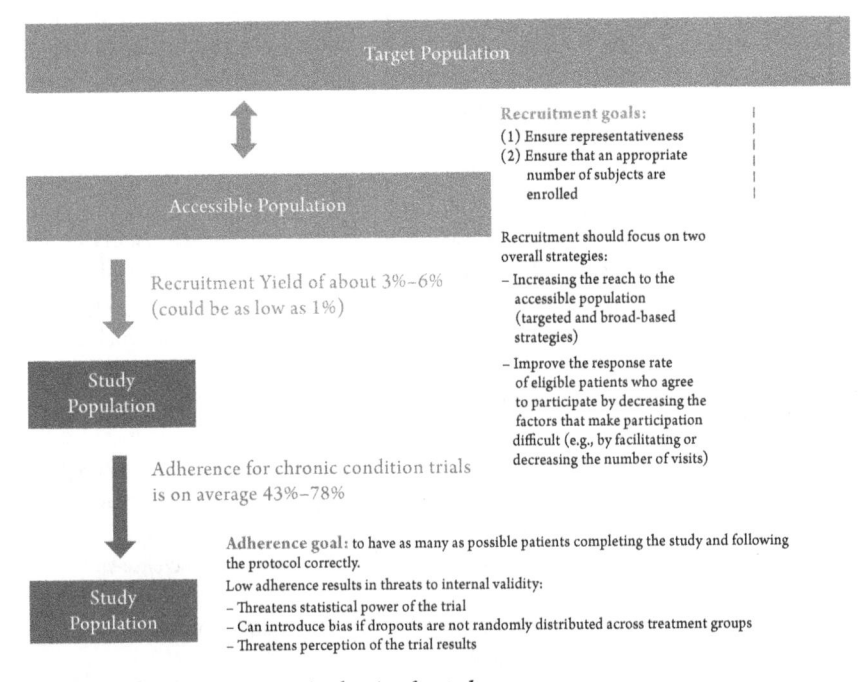

Target Population

Recruitment goals:
(1) Ensure representativeness
(2) Ensure that an appropriate number of subjects are enrolled

Accessible Population

Recruitment Yield of about 3%–6% (could be as low as 1%)

Recruitment should focus on two overall strategies:
- Increasing the reach to the accessible population (targeted and broad-based strategies)
- Improve the response rate of eligible patients who agree to participate by decreasing the factors that make participation difficult (e.g., by facilitating or decreasing the number of visits)

Study Population

Adherence for chronic condition trials is on average 43%–78%

Adherence goal: to have as many as possible patients completing the study and following the protocol correctly.
Low adherence results in threats to internal validity:
- Threatens statistical power of the trial
- Can introduce bias if dropouts are not randomly distributed across treatment groups
- Threatens perception of the trial results

Study Population

Figure 7.3. The consecutive steps in planning the study.

CHALLENGES FOR RECRUITMENT

Recruitment and Retention in Alzheimer's Disease Trials

Currently there are no effective treatments or preventive strategies available for Alzheimer's disease. This might be one of the main reasons why it is extremely difficult to recruit and retain patients for research studies. The recruitment of 400 subjects requires participation of more than 200 international centers to compensate for the low number of recruited patients and the high number of dropouts per center [21]

Issues that may affect recruitment and retention:

- Strict inclusion criteria (e.g., acetylcholinesterase inhibitor–treated patients only)
- Requirement of lumbar punctures and imaging studies
- Frailty of the patients
- Caregivers' additional burden provided by additional visits to the research center other than medical appointments
- Patients' stress imposed by repeated cognitive testing.
- Patients' comorbidities leading to hospitalizations for other reasons than the studied conditions, resulting in loss of follow-up.

The problem of a multicenter setup is that the unit "center" adds another level of variance and therefore makes results even more difficult to interpret. Despite the availability of several promising drug candidates, the methodological issue of recruitment and retention is currently the major roadblock to finding successful treatment options in Alzheimer's disease.

Recruitment of Children in Clinical Research

As much as for adults, there is a need to test new therapeutic options in the pediatric population. In this population, consent for the participation in the research study is given by the guardian. As the consent is thus not given by the individuals who suffer the possible risks of the investigational intervention, clinical research in minors is ethically problematic. Addressing this ethical conflict, Caldwell provided recommendations for research practice with minors [22]:

- Researchers should obtain the subject's assent to participate in the investigation if possible. However, a child's initial expression of dissent may be recognized as a usual rejection of medical procedures and need not necessarily lead to automatic exclusion from the study.
- Pre-selection of eligible subjects (i.e., based on the researcher's evaluation of the assumed degree of compliance) should not be performed in order to avoid low recruitment rates.
- Children and guardians should be informed in an age-appropriate, brief, and clear way.
- The financial compensation to the guardians must not influence their decision regarding the participation of their child. An IRB must therefore evaluate the appropriateness of incentives given to the guardians.
- If a child's clinician also acts as an investigator in a study that includes an investigational intervention performed on the child, the clear differentiation of the roles of "physician" and "research investigator" must be ensured.

Recruitment in Psychiatric Research

In order to address some challenges in the enrollment of potential candidates for psychiatric clinical studies, the patient's perspective should be considered. Candidates usually appraise costs and benefits when deciding whether or not to join the proposed study [8]. In addition, the study design can influence the decision of the candidates. For example, the required commitment to a long-term follow-up or the risk to be randomly assigned to the placebo group may negatively affect the candidate's decision to join the study. Furthermore, the possible adverse effects of an investigational new psychopharmacological treatment may scare eligible subjects. Also, the necessity of discontinuation of an ongoing psychopharmacological treatment may negatively affect the candidate's decision. Subjects' enlistment and adherence can also be compromised by long, boring, and repetitive psychometric examinations and procedures.

In order to balance these disadvantages of enrollment, the investigator can emphasize the benefits of participating in the investigation. For example, altruistic intent can attract individuals to clinical psychiatric research. In addition, the accessibility and affordability of a new psychopharmacological therapy may be decisive for some patients. Another beneficial aspect of the participation in a clinical study can be the increased amount of contact with health-care providers. Also, reimbursement of travel expenses, small financial incentives to compensate for patients' time, or alternative incentives such as movie or theater tickets, may influence the candidate's decision positively. Additionally, flexibility of schedules can be decisive, in particular for employed candidates.

CASE STUDY 18: RECRUITMENT OF STUDY PARTICIPANTS

Rui Imamura and Felipe Fregni

Dr. Angela Nasser was returning from a long period of traveling in Brazil, during which time she went to Rio de Janeiro, Sao Paulo, and Belo Horizonte to give talks. She also took advantage of this trip to talk to some colleagues regarding her phase III study testing a new intervention (ImmuneD) for the treatment of type I diabetes mellitus in youth. She was both thrilled and exhausted as she was getting close to her home of Florianopolis—the capital of Santa Catarina State in southern Brazil. Although she enjoyed seeing her colleagues, she now needed to make an important decision: choose the strategy of recruitment so as to decide if it would be feasible to run this study.[1]

Due to poor weather, Dr. Nasser's return flight had to land in Curitiba, a city 200 miles away from Florianopolis. Since she was eager to get home, she decided to get a taxi. Those few hours in the cab would be a good opportunity to review the meeting notes she took during her trip regarding the study recruitment.

While she was waiting for the cab, she quickly looked at the front page of the newspaper, which was announcing that the Ministry of Health had recognized the importance of special programs for health assistance and research for children in Brazil. In fact, she received a large grant from the federal government to continue her research on new treatments for juvenile diabetes.

Introduction: Diabetes Type I in Youth

As a pediatric endocrinologist, one of Dr. Nasser's passions includes juvenile diabetes. Although its clinical importance is unquestionable, juvenile diabetes (type I diabetes) in youth is not a very common disease. So, she was mainly concerned with the recruitment process, especially for the large study she was planning.

Dr. Nasser's clinical trial was based on the idea that short-term treatment with immune therapy in patients with type I diabetes at the beginning of the disease can induce long-term remission and therefore decrease the need for insulin. Because this effect seems to be more pronounced in patients younger than 20 years and concerns with adverse effects in the youth population are critical, Dr. Nasser planned this study for patients younger than 20 years only. The phase I and II trials showed that patients treated with immunotherapy (ImmuneD) had better beta-cell function after one year and lower insulin dosage needs. In fact, Dr. Nasser's group was involved in one of the previous phase II trials.

The planned design involves direct tests with ImmuneD versus placebo in the context of standard therapy in patients younger than 20 years recently diagnosed with diabetes. The outcome variable would be daily insulin doses. The sample size estimation using data obtained from the phase II study was 500 patients. This is

---

[1] Dr. Rui Imamura and Professor Felipe Fregni prepared this case.

wherein the problem lies: according to some studies, approximately 10,000 youth are diagnosed with diabetes in Brazil each year. Given the size of Florianopolis (a city with approximately 1 million inhabitants), Dr. Nasser's estimate was that approximately 50 children are diagnosed yearly with diabetes in her city, and therefore would qualify for the study. Although she was the director of the largest diabetes center in Florianopolis, it would take several decades to complete this study.

Recruitment: A Fundamental but Often Neglected Step in Clinical Trials

Recruitment of study participants is a fundamental and often neglected step in study planning and grant proposal projects. A proper recruitment strategy ensures that eligible patients, representative of the target population, will be correctly selected. Trial recruitment that is slower than expected can result in prolonged trial duration, increased costs, limited statistical power, and even early termination of the study. In fact, researchers often overestimate recruitment rates. A previous study reported that cancer trials usually have patient accrual at a slower rate than planned.[2] Problems with recruitment and the methods used to solve them may influence the study design and interpretation of the results. The CONSORT statement on recruitment requires that the period of recruitment is clearly defined.

Dr. Nasser interrupted her thoughts on the study and looked at the beautiful scenery outside—the cab driver chose to go along the coast to avoid traffic and they were now passing through a series of beautiful beaches. But she quickly resumed her thoughts on the study, reviewing the discussion she had with her colleagues. Dr. Nasser was very systematic and took notes of everything. She hoped to review her notes again before arriving to Florianopolis in order to have a good idea of the recruitment plan for this study.

First Stop—Rio de Janeiro: Discussion of Broad-Based Recruitment

Dr. Nasser had begun her trip in Rio de Janeiro—where she had to give a lecture at the Brazilian Society of Endocrinology meeting. But she also had scheduled a meeting with her colleague—Dr. Marcio Correa—one of the most important researchers in this area in Brazil. After explaining the study to Dr. Correa, they began the discussion.

Dr. Correa started, *"Well, you should first consider the eligibility criteria of the study population and define your target and accessible population. As you know, juvenile diabetes is not a prevalent disease, so the size of the target population is somewhat restricted—especially given the fact that you need newly diagnosed patients at the beginning of the disease. On the other hand, as ImmuneD does seem to apply to the entire population of newly diagnosed type I diabetes patients (younger than 20 years), I suppose eligibility criteria can be quite unrestricted. That would be aligned to the objectives of a phase III study, allowing for generalizability of study findings. Uncomplicated entry criteria will also*

---

[2] Pocock SJ, Size of cancer clinical trials and stopping rules. *Br J Cancer.* 1978 Dec;38(6): 757–766.

facilitate recruitment in different centers if you wish to do so. So, what would be our accessible population?"

Dr. Nasser quickly responded that she wanted to enroll patients with newly diagnosed type I diabetes aged 20 years or younger. She then asked him, *"What would be your ideas for broad-based strategies?"*

"With a broad-based strategy, you could use advertisements in the media (TV, radio, printed, and Internet) and deliver brochures in heavily concentrated areas, such as malls, parks, and cultural events to reach a broader accessible population," Dr. Correa responded, and continued, *"which would mean broader geographic diversity and larger absolute recruitment yield. In addition, sometimes it is easier to recruit patients by attracting their attention rather than trying to get referrals from our colleagues."*

"The only issue with this strategy," Dr. Correa pondered, *"is that you will get a large population of non-eligible patients. And you know, it is not easy to deal with them! Furthermore, the screening process will be time-consuming and very expensive. Cost-benefit analysis should be taken into account, as it is not uncommon to have yields lower than 10% of screened patients with this strategy."*[3]

Dr. Nasser thought about these issues for a couple of minutes and then commented on generalizability, *"Another advantage with this strategy is that we would get a sample with patients from both outpatient and inpatient facilities and primary to tertiary hospitals that we would not easily get using patient referral or examining medical records. In addition, in Brazil, prompt access to medical care is not universal and many patients with initial phases of the disease may not be accessible using other methods of recruitment."*

Dr. Correa's secretary interrupted their conversation, as he had to run to another meeting. This meeting was very productive to Dr. Nasser's study. While she waited for a cab in Ipanema Beach outside Dr. Correa's office, she made the final notes in her precious research notebook before the next stop of this trip, Sao Paulo.

Second Stop: Sao Paulo: Discussion of Targeted Enrollment Strategies

The second stop on Dr. Nasser's trip was Sao Paulo—the largest city in Brazil. She needed to give a lecture in the morning and had two meetings in the afternoon—one of them with the director of the pediatric endocrinology center at the University of Sao Paulo—Dr. Paulo Costa. She arrived on a rainy day, which made her life more difficult as she needed to beat the already difficult traffic in Sao Paulo. But she made it to her meeting with Dr. Costa.

After Dr. Nasser explained the study in detail, including the fact that she will need to expand the study to the population of the entire state of Santa Catarina or perhaps to the neighbor states, she asked his thoughts on recruitment methods.

Dr. Costa then started, *"As juvenile diabetes is a relatively severe condition, most diagnosed patients are linked to some hospital or outpatient clinic. So, asking these*

---

[3] Friedman L, Furberg C, DeMets D, *Fundamentals of clinical trials*, 3rd ed. New York: Springer; 1998.

health facilities for patient lists and also sending invitation letters to physicians may yield a reliable accessible population. In addition, because in your trial, the intervention (ImmuneD) consists of only one application of the intervention and the outcomes can be measured in other centers, there is no problem if patients are in other cities. The advantage of this method is that it has a lower cost (emails or invitation letters) and it provides a more reliable population (decreasing costs of screening), therefore increasing recruitment yield. This would be the simplest and cheapest solution."

In addition, Dr. Costa continued, *"As the study involves direct tests in the context of standard therapy, physicians who are concerned with the integrity of their patients may find the study ethical which would also facilitate referral as it increases the buy-in for this study—in fact, if a patient is recruited through the Internet, the physician might advise the patient not to participate in the study."*

However, Dr. Costa pointed out, *"Even though this seems like a good strategy, you need to be prepared for a low number of referrals by colleagues, as their perception of the importance of the trial (having a busy agenda as the background) might be low. This would be the main problem for you."*

Dr. Nasser reviewed the main points raised in this meeting, adding everything in her notebook. It was almost 9 p.m. and she was going to the hotel—at least the traffic was better and she only needed to worry about getting to the airport on time the next day.

Third Stop: Belo Horizonte—Discussion of Public Awareness Campaigns as a Recruitment Strategy

Although Dr. Nasser was tired of this long trip, she was looking forward to getting to Belo Horizonte as she had some family there and really enjoys the city, food, and people there. For this stop, she had a meeting with the director of the local society of juvenile diabetes—Dr. Marcia Motta.

Dr. Marcia Motta is an endocrinologist with a passion for diabetes, who has dedicated all her time to the local population of juvenile diabetes in order to improve medical access for these patients. Dr. Motta, after hearing the study Dr. Nasser was planning and her challenges for recruitment, gave her some advice: *"As you know, Angela, a practical way to reach physicians would be to contact the related medical local societies (pediatrics and endocrinologists), such as ours in your state, and ask for their approval and support to raise awareness of the study among physicians and even patients, through their websites or small public campaigns. Besides being relatively easy to perform and having low costs, you would get more reliable patients than media advertisement. I believe that the clinical relevance of the study (a new promising treatment for pediatric diabetes) where medical needs are relatively unmet should facilitate referral and also get their support. Also, as the study involves direct tests in the context of standard therapy, physicians concerned with the integrity of their patients may find the study ethical, which would also facilitate referral."*

Dr. Nasser, as usual, took note of everything and considered that she had at that point some material to decide the method of recruitment in her study.

Back in Florianopolis, Dr. Nasser entered the city and was looking forward to arriving home. After reviewing her notes, she had an initial plan to discuss with her research team. She felt thrilled with the prospect of completing this study.

CASE DISCUSSION

Dr. Angela Nasser intends to test a novel pharmacological add-on medication for the treatment of patients with type I diabetes, which may help to reduce the necessary daily dosages of insulin in these patients. As type I diabetes is not as highly prevalent as type II diabetes, Dr. Nasser has to carefully consider her options of patient recruitment in order to enroll a sufficient number of study participants. The first mandatory step in this process is to define the target population and the accessible population in consideration of the eligibility criteria defined.

In this case, the target population can be easily identified as newly diagnosed type I diabetes patients of a certain age, whereas the population accessible to Dr. Nasser's recruitment efforts depends in large part on the advertisement strategy chosen by her. The scope of advertising and consequently the size of the population she can reach are restricted by both the financial resources available and the accessibility of disease-specific medical institutions, such as clinical type I diabetes centers or type I diabetes support groups. Accordingly, Dr. Nasser is facing the challenge of choosing a recruitment strategy that allows for both enrolling a sufficient number of eligible study participants and keeping a balance between internal validity and external generalizability. For example, the restriction of patients recruitment to a dedicated clinical type I diabetes centers would be time and cost efficient and would result in high internal validity, but could fail to produce data that can be extrapolated to a larger population. Furthermore, the generalizability of Dr. Nasser's study findings is influenced by the chosen eligibility criteria. Selecting only few or very broad inclusion criteria will make it is easier to enroll subjects and results will have a higher degree of generalizability; however, the sample will be more heterogeneous, which will affect sample size/power calculations and will require adjustments in the statistical analysis such as covariate adjustments [23]. On the other hand, too many or too restrictive eligibility criteria make it difficult to enroll patients and may lead to a narrow study population with low generalizability.

In addition to the considerations regarding the study population, Dr. Nasser needs to select a strategy to advertise the trial among this population. Therefore, she must select between various possible recruitment methods, all of them presenting with different advantages, disadvantages, and outcomes: community-based strategies (broad-based) ensure both fast progress in recruitment and a high degree of diversity of patients, but might attract many non-eligible subjects, whereas health-care-provider-based strategies (targeted) provide a more reliable population but highly depend on the degree to which the health-care provider collaborates by referring patients to the study. Consequently, the decision of using either a broad-based or targeted recruitment strategy may influence the demographic constitution of the study population. While referrals from private practice may include more patients with higher education and social status, some community-based strategies such as advertisement in newspapers or on Internet platforms such as "craigslist" may address more patients with low income and lower education. In order to increase the heterogeneity of the study population, Dr. Nasser might also consider a combination of broad-based and targeted strategies.

Although there is no ultimate rule for the selection of the best technique to recruit participants in a clinical research study, it remains crucial for the success of

Dr. Nasser's promising project to carefully consider the available options of recruitment strategies and to weigh their impact on the outcome of her study and the interpretation of its results.

CASE QUESTIONS FOR REFLECTION

1. What are the issues involved in this case that resulted in the disagreement?
2. What are the author's concerns? And the institution's?
3. What should the author consider to make the decision?
4. Have you experienced a similar situation?

FURTHER READING

Recruitment

Campbell MK, Snowdon C, Francis D, Elbourne D, McDonald AM, Knight R, et al. Recruitment to randomised trials: strategies for trial enrollment and participation study. The STEPS study. *Health Technol Assess.* 2007; 11: ix–105.

Daley AJ, Crank H, Mutrie N, Saxton JM, Coleman R. Patient recruitment into a randomised controlled trial of supervised exercise therapy in sedentary women treated for breast cancer. *Contemp Clin Trials.* 2007; 28(5): 603–613.

Gillan MG, Ross S, Gilbert FJ, Grant AM, O'Dwyer PJ. Recruitment to multicentre trials: the impact of external influences. *Health Bull (Edinb)* 2000; 58: 229–234.

Gorkin L, Schron EB, Handshaw K, Shea S, Kinney MR, Branyon M, et al. Clinical trial enrollers vs. nonenrollers: the Cardiac Arrhythmia Suppression Trial (CAST) Recruitment and Enrollment Assessment in Clinical Trials (REACT) project. *Control Clin Trials.* 1996; 17(1): 46–59.

Grunfeld E, Zitzelsberger L, Coristine M, Aspelund F. Barriers and facilitators to enrollment in cancer clinical trials: qualitative study of the perspectives of clinicalresearch associates. *Cancer.* 2002; 95(7): 1577–1583.

Johnson MO, Remien RH. Adherence to research protocols in a clinical context: challenges and recommendations from behavioral intervention trials. *Am J Psychother.* 2003; 57: 348–360.

Ngune I, Jiwa M, Dadich A, Lotriet J, Sriram D Qual. Effective recruitment strategies in primary care research: a systematic review. *Prim Care.* 2012; 20: 115–123.

Peto V, Coulter A, Bond A. Factors affecting general practitioner's recruitment of patients into a prospective study. *Fam Pract.* 1993; 10(2): 207–211.

Rengerink O, Opmeer BC, Loqtenberg SL, Hooft L, Bloemenkamp KW, Haak MC, et al. Improving participation of patients in clinical trials—rationale and design of IMPACT. *BMC Med Res Methodol.* 2010; 10: 85.

Spilker B, Cramer JA. *Patient recruitment in clinical trials.* New York: Raven Press; 1992.

Adherence

Connolly NB, Schneider D, Hill AM. Improving enrollment in cancer clinical trials. *Oncol Nurs Forum.* 2004 May; 31(3): 610–614.

Ickovics JR, Meisler AW. Adherence in AIDS clinical trials: a framework for clinical research and clinical care. *J Clin Epidemiol*. 1997; 50(4): 385–391.

Osterberg L, Blaschke T. Adherence to medication. *N Engl J Med*. 2005; 353(5): 487–497.

REFERENCES

1. Ashery RS, McAuliffe WE. Implementation issues and techniques in randomised trials of outpatient psychosocial treatments for drug abusers: recruitment of subjects. *Am J Drug Alcohol Abuse*. 1992; 18(3): 305–329.
2. Spilker B, Cramer JA (eds.). *Patient recruitment in clinical trials*. New York: Raven Press; 1992.
3. Hulley SB, Cimmings SR, Browner WS, et al. *Designing clinical research: an epidemiologic approach*, 2nd ed. London: Lippincott Williams and Wilkins; 2001.
4. Cooley ME, Sarna L, Brown JK, Williams RD, Chernecky C, Padilla G, et al. Challenges of recruitment and retention in multisite clinical research. *Cancer Nursing*. 2003; 26: 376–384.
5. Fedor C, Cola P, Pierre C (eds.). *Responsible research: a guide for coordinators*. London: Remedica; 2006.
6. Sinackevich N, Tassignon J-P. Speeding the critical path. *Appl Clin Trials*. 2004; 13(1): 42–48.
7. Feman SPC, Nguyen LT, Quilty MT, Kerr CE, Nam BH, Conboy LA, et al. Effectiveness of recruitment in clinical trials: an analysis of methods used in a trial for irritable bowel syndrome patients. *Contemp Clin Trials*. 2008; 29(2): 241–251.
8. Patel MX, Doku V, Tennakoon L. Challenges in recruitment of research participants. *Adv Psyichiatr Treat*. 2003; 9: 229–238.
9. Gorkin L, Schron EB, Handshaw K, Shea S, Kinney MR, Branyon M, et al. Clinical trial enrollers vs. nonenrollers: the Cardiac Arrhythmia Suppression Trial (CAST) Recruitment and Enrollment Assessment in Clinical Trials (REACT) project. *Control Clin Trials*. 1996; 17(1): 46–59.
10. Sabaté E. *WHO adherence meeting report*. Geneva: World Health Organization, 2001.
11. Delamater AM. Improving patient adherence. *Clin Diabetes*. 2006; 24: 71–77.
12. Meichenbaum D, Turk DC. *Facilitating treatment adherence: a practitioner's guidebook*. New York: Plenum Press; 1987.
13. Robiner WN. Enhancing adherence in clinical research. *Contemp Clin Trials*. 2005; 26: 59–77.
14. Claxton AJ, Cramer J, Pierce C. A systematic review of the associations between dose regimens and medication compliance. *Clin Ther*. 2001; 23(8): 1296–1310.
15. Cramer J, Rosenheck R, Kirk G, Krol W, Krystal J. Medication compliance feedback and monitoring in a clinical trial: predictors and outcomes. *Value Health*. 2003; 6: 566–573.
16. Waeber B, Leonetti G, Kolloch R, McInnes GT. Compliance with aspirin or placebo in the Hypertension Optimal Treatment (HOT) study. *J Hypertens*. 1999; 17: 1041–105.
17. Claxton AJ, Cramer J, Pierce C. A systematic review of the associations between dose regimens and medication compliance. *Clin Ther*. 2001; 23: 1296–1310.
18. Osterberg L, Blaschke T. Adherence to medication. *N Engl J Med*. 2005; 353: 487–497.
19. Hunninghake DB. The interaction of the recruitment process with adherence. In: Shumaker SA, Schron EB, Ockene JK, eds. *The handbook of health behavior change*. New York: Springer; 1990.
20. Lang JM, Buring JE, Rosner B, Cook N, Hennekens CH. Estimating the effect of the run-in on the power of the physicians' health study. *Stat Med*. 1991; 10: 1585–1593.

21. B Vellas. Recruitment, retention and other methodological issues related to clinical trials for Alzheimer's disease. *J Nutr Health Aging* 2012; 16(4): 330.
22. Duncanson K, Burrows T, Collins C. Study protocol of a parent-focused child feeding and dietary intake intervention: the feeding healthy food to kids randomized controlled trial. *BMC Public Health* 2012; 12: 564.
23. Roozenbeek B, Lingsma HF, Maas AI. New considerations in the design of clinical trials for traumatic brain injury. *Clin Investig.* 2012; 2(2): 153–162.

UNIT II
Basics of Statistics

8

BASICS OF STATISTICS

Authors: *Claudia Kimie Suemoto and Catherine Lee*

Case study author: *Felipe Fregni*

If you torture data sufficiently, it will confess to almost anything.
—Fred Menger (Chemistry professor, 1937–)

INTRODUCTION

In Unit I, you learned the basics of clinical research. You learned how to select the research question (*What* are you trying to study/prove?), define the study population (*Whom* do you want to study to test/prove your question?), design your study (*How* are you going to test/prove your question?). But what are you going to do with the data your study will generate? How will you analyze the data, and how will you interpret the results? Unit II will introduce you to statistics and will give you the knowledge and tools to formulate a data analysis plan that will help you to answer these questions.

The importance and impact of statistics in today's world is immense. In TV and other media, statistics is used all the time to support a certain message; it is used in surveys, to analyze trends and to make predictions (e.g., the odds of a team winning the next Super Bowl). It is also frequently misinterpreted (e.g., showing that coffee is linked to a lower risk of diabetes). More important, statistics plays an essential role in many decision-making processes. Statistics is widely used in many fields, including business, social science, psychology, and agriculture. When the focus is on the biological and health sciences, the term *biostatistics* is used.

Your journey into the world of statistics starts with a hypothesis: Is a new drug more effective than placebo in treating neuropsychiatric symptoms in patients with Alzheimer's disease? Is prostate-specific antigen screening efficient for early detection of prostate cancer? Can the combination of PET and CT scanning predict the risk of myocardial infarction in patients with coronary artery disease? Should a new social program be implemented to reduce poverty among the elderly? To find answers to these questions, we need to collect and analyze data from a representative sample from a larger population (for more details, see Chapter 3). Statistics provides methods of describing and summarizing the data that we have collected from a sample and allows us to extrapolate results to make inferences about the population from which the sample was drawn.

Statistics can be classified into two categories: descriptive and inferential statistics. The term *descriptive statistics* refers to measures that summarize and characterize a set of data that allow us to better understand the attributes of a group or population. As you will see, these measures can be graphical or numerical. Whereas descriptive statistics examine the sample data, *inferential statistics* and hypothesis testing aim to use sample data to learn about the population from which the sample was drawn based on probability theory. Inferential statistics will be discussed in the next chapter.

Suppose you want to answer the first question proposed in this chapter: "Is a new drug more effective than placebo in treating neuropsychiatric symptoms in patients with Alzheimer's disease?" After randomizing our patients into the placebo or new drug group and following allocation of the placebo or the treatment, we need to collect information about the frequency of neuropsychiatric symptoms in the two groups before and after intervention and compare the data. Therefore the first important point when learning and applying statistics is to understand the study variables and their characteristics. In fact, the investigator needs to know the main characteristics of the variables in order to know what to do with them [1].

This chapter will present the different types of data and the methods that can be used to organize and display each type of data. We will then introduce basic probability theory and probability distributions, with a particular emphasis on the normal distribution, which appears frequently in real life and plays a central role in many statistical tests.

TYPES OF DATA

It is important to classify the types of data that you are working with, since the data type dictates the method of data analysis that you will use. The different types of data and their general characteristics are described in Table 8.1.

Table 8.1 Types of Data, Their Characteristics, and Examples

Type	Characteristics	Examples
Nominal	Unordered categories or classes Special nomenclature: dichotomous or binary—2 distinct values	Race: White, Black, Asian, other Gender: Female and male
Ordinal	Ordered categories Magnitude is not important	New York Heart Association (NYHA) heart failure classification: I, II, III, IV
Discrete	Ordering and magnitude are importantNumbers represent measurable quantities Values differ by fixed amounts Often count data	Number of deaths in United States in 2012 by different causes of death
Continuous Interval Ratio	Measurable quantities Spacing between values meaningful Fractional and decimal values possible Arithmetic operations can be applied	Temperature, time, weight, cholesterol level

Nominal

Nominal data, also referred to as categorical data, represent unordered categories or classes. For instance, one of the possible ways to categorize race in humans is "White," "Black," and "Other races." Numbers may be used to represent categories. White can be arbitrarily coded as 0, Black as 1, and other races as 2. However, these numbers do not express order or magnitude and are not meaningful. Dichotomous or binary variables are a special type of nominal data. These two terms are exchangeable and are used when the variable has only two distinct categories. In the example provided in Table 8.1, gender and race are two examples of nominal data, but only gender is considered dichotomous or binary.

Ordinal

When a natural order among categories exists, data are referred to as ordinal. The New York Heart Association (NYHA) classification describes four categories of heart failure according to severity symptoms and degree of limitation to perform daily activities [2]:

I. No limitation on physical activity. Ordinary physical activity does not cause fatigue, palpitation, or dyspnea.
II. Slight limitation of physical activity. Comfortable at rest, but ordinary physical activity results in fatigue, palpitation, or dyspnea.
III. Marked limitation of physical activity. Comfortable at rest, but less than ordinary activity causes fatigue, palpitation, or dyspnea.
IV. Unable to carry out any physical activity without discomfort. Symptoms of cardiac insufficiency are present at rest. If any physical activity is undertaken, discomfort is increased.

Note that severity of heart failure increases from class I (no symptoms) to class IV (severe symptoms). However, the magnitude of the difference between adjacent classes is not necessarily equivalent. The difference between classes III and IV is not necessarily the same as the difference between classes I and II, even if both pairs are one unit apart. As with nominal data, ordinal variables may be coded using numbers, but these numbers are not meaningful; consequently, arithmetic operations should not be performed on ordinal data.

Discrete

Discrete data are numerical values that represent measurable quantities. Discrete data are restricted to whole values and are often referred to as count data. Examples of discrete data include the number of deaths in the United States in 2012 and the number of years a group of individuals has received formal education. Note that an ordering exists among possible values, and the difference between the values one and two is the same as the difference between the values five and six.

Arithmetic rules can be applied to discrete data; however, some arithmetic operations performed on two discrete values are not necessarily discrete. In our example, suppose one individual has 3 years of education and the other one has 4 years; the average number of years of education for the two individuals is 3.5, which is no longer an integer.

Continuous Data

Continuous data also represent measurable quantities, but are not restricted to whole values (integers) and may include fractional and decimal values. Therefore, the difference between any two values can be arbitrarily small depending on the accuracy of our measurement instrument. As with discrete data, the spacing between values is meaningful. Arithmetic procedures can be applied. Examples of continuous data include temperature, weight, and cholesterol level.

Variable Transformation (Continuous into Categorical Format)

If a less degree of detail is required, continuous data can be transformed into discrete, ordinal, or binary data format. Similarly, discrete data can be viewed as ordinal or categorical data; and ordinal data can be dichotomized.

It is important to keep in mind that continuous data provide more information about the measured variable than discrete, ordinal, or nominal data. The same holds true for discrete data in relation to ordinal and nominal data and for ordinal variables in relation to nominal data.

For example, an estimator for body fat is the body mass index (BMI), calculated by dividing the weight in kilograms by the square of the height in meters. A person with BMI of 30.2 kg/m^2 is certainly different from another individual with a BMI of 39.7 kg/m^2. The first one is very likely in better shape than the second one. However, if we follow the ordinal classification proposed by the World Health Organization (WHO), both fall under the obese category since they have a BMI >25.0 kg/m^2. The ordinal classification is not able to differentiate the two individuals.

If we perform a randomized clinical trial to test the efficacy of a new drug compared to placebo to reduce weight in obese patients, we will be able to better detect differences between the two groups if we use the continuous variable, BMI, as the outcome variable. Dichotomizing subjects as obese and not obese using the WHO's BMI cut-off of 25.0 kg/m^2 and using this binary classification as the outcome will result in loss of information and thus less power for the analysis.

The advantage of categorizing a continuous variable, on the other hand, is to provide clinical significance to study results. For instance, 0.2 kg statistically significant difference between two diet groups is not likely to be clinically relevant. But a statistical difference between obese and non-obese groups may be clinically significant.

CHOOSING A STATISTICAL TEST

The choice of outcome and the independent variables under consideration will influence the type of statistical test we can use to test the study hypothesis. You will learn in the next chapter that if we use a continuous variable (e.g., BMI), a t-test is appropriate to test for differences in mean BMI levels between two groups. If we use the binary variable for obesity status created using the WHO's obesity cut-off, a chi-square test of homogeneity is appropriate. You will learn that parametric tests like t-tests have more statistical power to detect possible differences in the outcome variable between two populations than non-parametric tests like the chi-square test.

However, if BMI is treated as continuous, small differences in BMI that are detected might have little clinical significance. To be specific, a small difference in BMI between groups that is considered a statistically significant difference in our trial might have limited impact on the patient's health and quality of life. In this case, when designing our study, we should carefully balance statistical power and a clinically meaningful difference in BMI.

Variables Format and Study Power

What is power exactly? In the next chapter, you will learn about various hypothesis tests that assume the following format. There will always be a null hypothesis that you are trying to disprove with the data that you have sampled. This null hypothesis usually represents the population status quo or the position that you would assume unless provided strong evidence to the contrary. There will also be an alternative hypothesis that you are trying to prove. In the obesity example, the null hypothesis would be that the outcome of obesity (measured by either mean BMI or by the proportion of obese individuals) is the same between treatment and placebo groups. An alternative hypothesis would be that there is a difference in the outcome of obesity between treatment and placebo groups. When we are able to disprove the null hypothesis, we say that we "reject" the null hypothesis. If the null hypothesis is not true, it makes sense that we would want to reject it. Statistical power is the ability to reject the null hypothesis when it is false.

Statistical power is the probability that the test will reject the null hypothesis when the null is false. In other words, it is the probability of not committing a false negative decision.

DESCRIPTIVE STATISTICS

The first step in data analysis is to describe or summarize the data that you have collected through tables, graphs, and/or numerical values. This is an important step, because it will allow you to assess how the data are distributed and how the data should be analyzed. When reporting the results of a study, including a description of the study population is essential so that the findings can be generalized to other comparable populations. You may also be interested in making inferences about the population that your data were sampled from; this will be discussed in more depth in subsequent chapters [3].

GRAPHICAL REPRESENTATION
Nominal and Ordinal Data

Nominal and ordinal data are summarized by the absolute and relative frequency of observations. Using the previous example of NYHA classification for heart failure, we can count the *number* of patients among each category. This is called the absolute frequency. The relative frequency will be the *proportion* of the total number of

Table 8.2 Distribution of Patients from a Hypothetical Outpatient Clinic According to NYHA Classification for Heart Failure

NYHA	Number of patients (Absolute frequency)	Relative frequency (%)	Cumulative frequency (%)
I	10	12.50	12.50
II	35	43.75	56.25
III	25	31.25	87.50
IV	10	12.50	100
Total	80	100	

observations that is present in each category. The relative frequency is calculated by dividing the number of observations in each category by the total number of observations, multiplied by 100 to get the percentage. The cumulative frequency for a given category is calculated by adding the relative proportion of that category to the relative frequencies of all preceding categories. Table 8.2 shows a hypothetical example of 80 patients from an outpatient clinic. Tables are important tools to organize and summarize data. Following common conventions, tables should be labeled and units of measurement should be indicated.

The same information can be presented using graphical figures. Although graphs are usually easier to understand than tables, they tend to provide a lesser degree of detail. Like tables, graphs should be labeled and the units of measurement should be provided. Bar charts are commonly used to display nominal or ordinal data. A vertical bar is plotted above each category, with the height of the bar representing the absolute or relative frequency of observations. Bars should be of equal width and separated from one another so as not to imply continuity. Figure 8.1 provides bar graphs representing the absolute, relative, and cumulative frequencies from our example of patients with heart failure.

The same information regarding absolute and relative frequencies can also be presented using pie charts (Figure 8.2), in which each pie slice is proportional to the

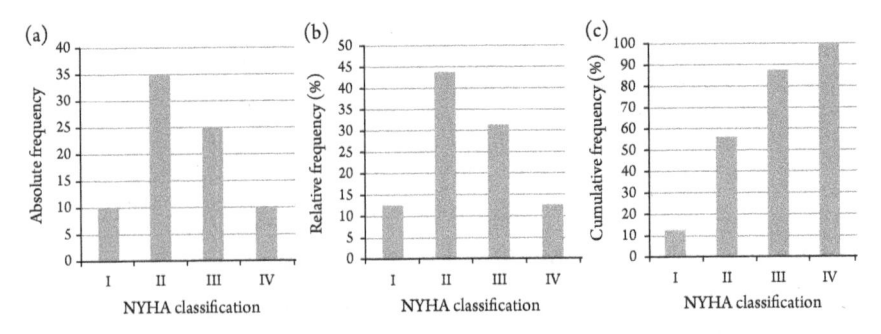

Figure 8.1. Bar chart: Distribution of patients from a hypothetical outpatient clinic according to NYHA classification for heart failure. A: absolute frequency; B: relative frequency; C: cumulative frequency.

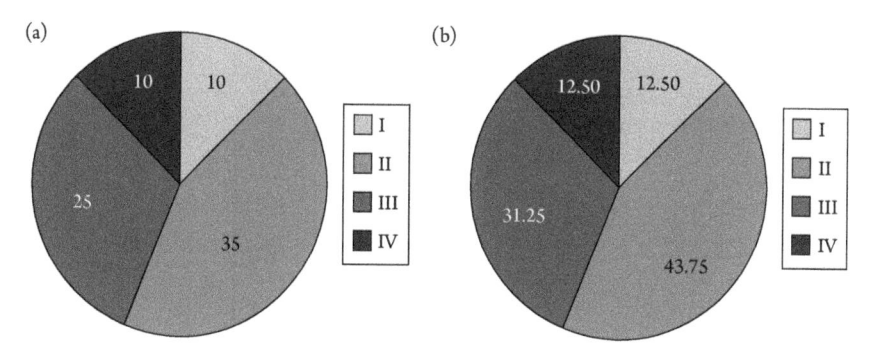

Figure 8.2. Pie chart: Distribution of patients from a hypothetical outpatient clinic according to NYHA classification for heart failure. A: absolute frequency; B: relative frequency (%).

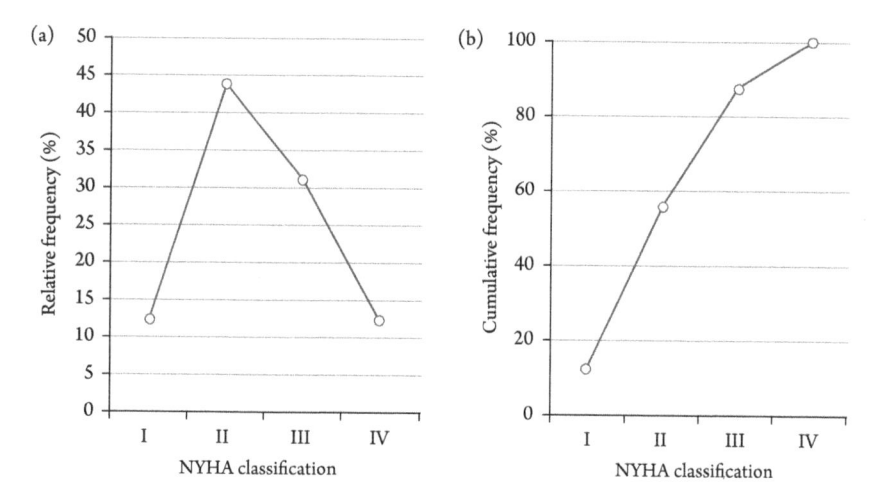

Figure 8.3. Distribution of patients from a hypothetical outpatient clinic according to NYHA classification for heart failure. A: Frequency polygon; B: Cumulative frequency polygon.

relative frequency in each category. Ordinal data can additionally be presented by relative frequency and cumulative frequency polygons, as shown in Figure 8.3.

Discrete and Continuous Data

Frequency distribution of discrete and continuous data can be represented using histograms. The first step in constructing a histogram is to order the observations from smallest to largest, and then group them into intervals, or *bins*, typically with a range that is uniform across bins; each interval will have a lower and upper value. Next, draw the axes: the horizontal axis is made up of the bins that were chosen; the vertical axis displays the absolute or relative frequency of observations within each bin. Consider the distribution of systolic blood pressure in a hypothetical group of patients depicted in Table 8.3).

Table 8.3 Absolute Frequencies of Systolic Blood Pressure in a Hypothetical Group of 117 Patients

Systolic blood pressure (mmHg)	Number of patients
100–119	15
120–139	48
140–159	36
160–179	13
180–199	5
Total	117

The histogram of these observation is shown in Figure 8.4. Note that the frequency associated with each interval in a histogram is represented by the bar's area. Therefore, a histogram with unequal interval widths should be interpreted with caution.

A histogram is a quick way to make an initial assessment of your data by showing you how the data are distributed. When studying a histogram, you might ask yourself the following: What is the shape of the distribution? (The distribution is called unimodal if it has one major peak, bimodal if it has two major peaks, and multimodal if it has more than two major peaks.) Is the histogram symmetric? (A bell-shaped distribution is symmetric, and the tapered ends of the distribution are referred to as *tails*. It is common to run into distributions that are unimodal where one tail is longer than the other; this type of distribution is called skewed.) Is there a center? How are the data points spread?

You will learn about ways to quantify the center and spread of a distribution in the next section on summary statistics.

The frequency polygon already described for ordinal data can also be used to represent discrete and continuous data. In this case, the frequency polygon uses the same

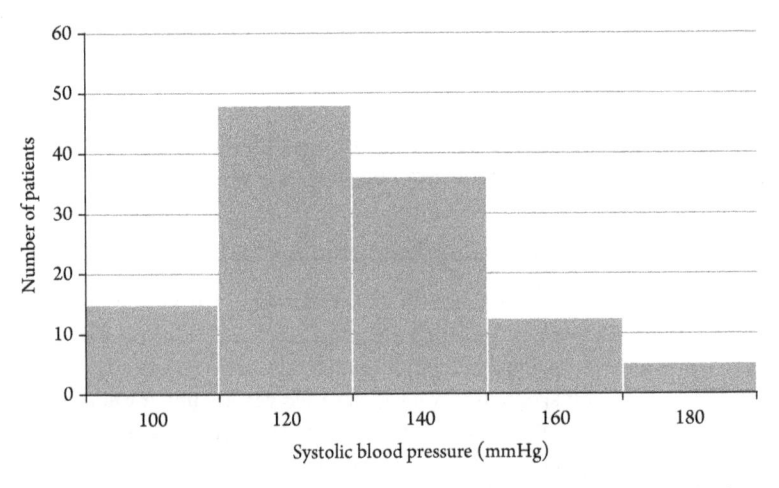

Figure 8.4. Histogram representing absolute frequencies of systolic blood pressure for the data shown in Table 8.3.

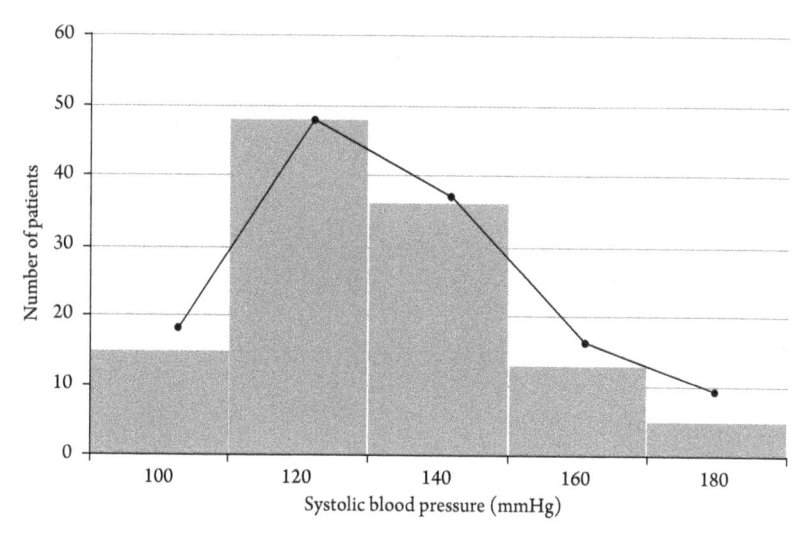

Figure 8.5. Frequency polygon: Absolute frequency of blood systolic pressure for the data show in Table 8.3.

two axes as a histogram. It is constructed by placing a point at the center of each interval and then connecting the points in adjacent bins by straight lines (Figure 8.5). The cumulative frequency polygon can also be used with discrete and continuous data, as shown in Figure 8.6.

Another way to summarize a set of discrete or continuous data graphically is the box plot, as shown in Figure 8.7, which displays a sample of 444 measures of weight in kilograms. The central box represents the interquartile range, which extends from the 25th percentile, Q1, to the 75th percentile, Q3; further explanations about percentiles will be presented in the next section. The line inside the box marks the median (50th

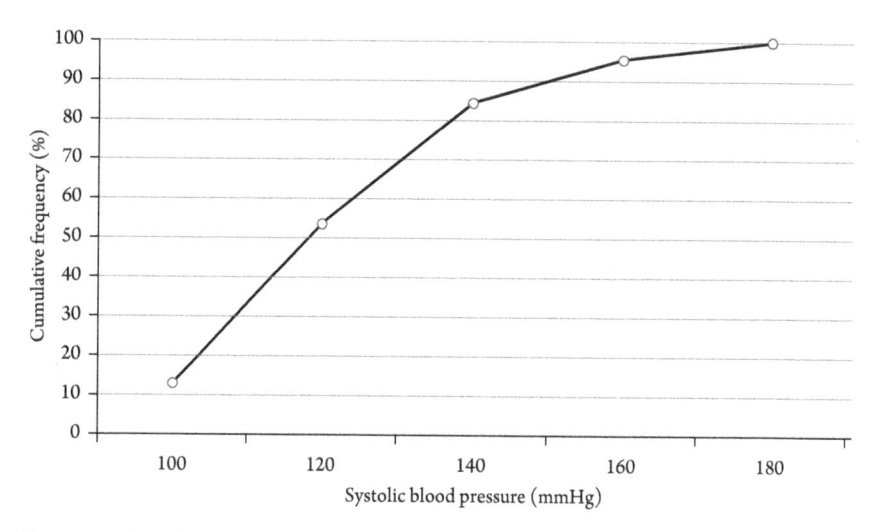

Figure 8.6. Cumulative frequency polygon: Cumulative frequencies of systolic blood pressure of data shown in Table 8.3.

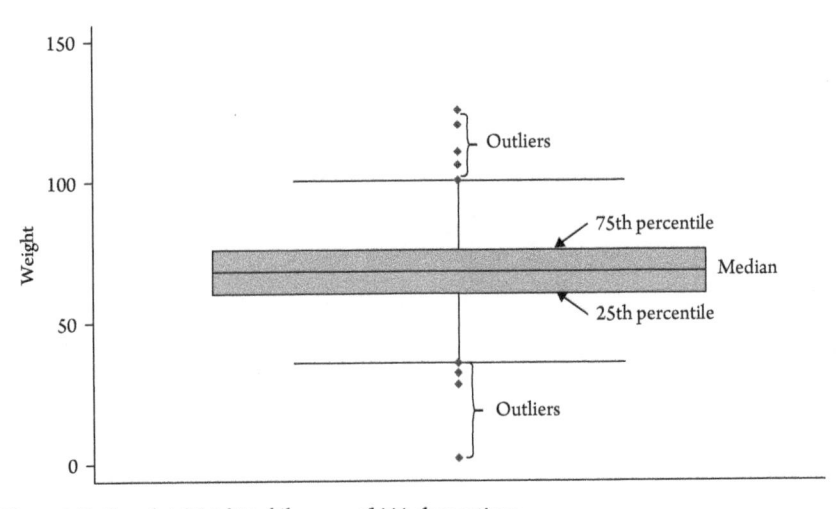

Figure 8.7. Box plot: Weight in kilograms of 444 observations.

percentile, Q2). The lines extending from the interquartile range are called *whiskers*. They extend to the most extreme observations in the data set that are within 1.5 times the interquartile range from the lower or upper quartile. To find these extreme values, find the largest data value that is smaller than Q3 + 1.5*IQR, and similarly find the smallest data value that is larger than Q1−1.5*IQR. All points outside the whiskers are considered outliers and are commonly represented by points, circles or stars.

When we are interested in showing the relationship between two different continuous variables, a two-way scatter plot can be used. Each point on the graph represents a pair of values. The scale for one measure is marked on the horizontal axis (*x* axis) and the scale for the other on the vertical axis (*y* axis).

A scatter plot gives us a good idea of the level of correlation between the two variables and also the nature of this correlation (linear, curvilinear, quadratic, etc.). Figure 8.8 shows the relationship between weight (*x* axis) and height (*y* axis) in the 444 patients shown earlier.

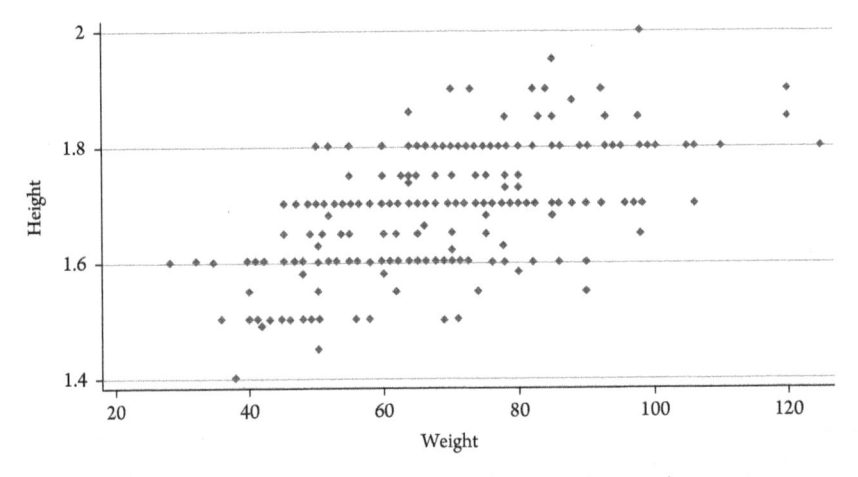

Figure 8.8. Two-way scatter plot: Weight (in kilograms) versus height (in meters) in 444 observations.

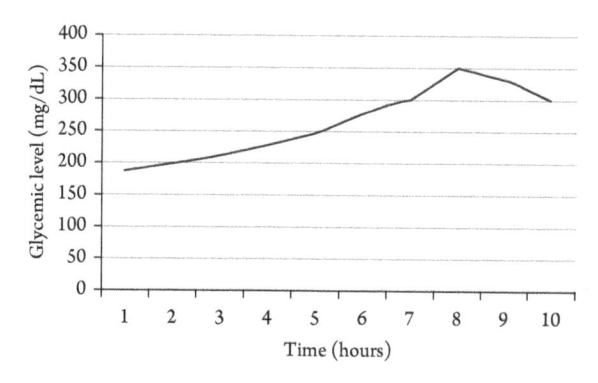

Figure 8.9. Change in glycemia over 24 hours in a hypothetical patient with diabetes.

A line graph is similar to a two-way scatter plot in that it can be used to illustrate the relationship between two discrete or continuous variables. However, in a line graph, each x value can have only a single corresponding y value. Adjacent points are connected by straight line segments. Line graphs are often used to depict the change of one variable over time. Line graph is a good resource when the goal is to show changes over time (time as represented in the x axis). Figure 8.9 shows the measures of glycemia in a hypothetical patient with diabetes.

SUMMARY STATISTICS (NUMERICAL SUMMARY MEASURES)

Graphs provide a general assessment of the data and may quickly allow you to understand how the data are distributed or find patterns and relationships between variables. Numerical summary statistics are numbers that represent the data and quantitatively summarize what might be seen through graphs. Both graphical and numerical summary measures constitute descriptive statistics. As with graphical representation, the choice of numerical representation will depend on the type of variable under consideration [4].

Dichotomous, Nominal, and Ordinal Data

As described earlier, dichotomous (binary) variables have only two categories. Dichotomous data are summarized by the proportions or frequencies of the two categories. These values are calculated by dividing the number of observations in each category by the total number of observations. For example, suppose that a sample of 450 individuals consists of 128 women and 322 men. The proportion of females is 0.284 (128/450) or 28.4%, and the proportion of males is 0.716 (322/450) or 71.6%. The sum of the proportions in both categories is equal to 1.

Similarly, nominal and ordinal variables are summarized by the proportions or frequencies of their respective categories [5].

Discrete and Continuous Data

As discussed earlier, discrete and continuous data represent measurable quantities that may take on a wide range of values. For discrete and continuous data, these representative values often address central tendency (the *location* of the center around which the observations fall) and dispersion (*variability*, or spread, of the data).

Measures of Central Tendency

Mode

The most frequent value in a particular data set is called the mode. The mode can be a useful summary statistic for categorical or ordinal data, but it is usually not informative for discrete or continuous data since unique values may occur with low frequency. In one of our previous examples of the distribution of gender in a hypothetical sample of 450 individuals, the mode is male since it is the most common of the two possible categories (male and female) with frequency 71.6%. This summary statistic is not usually used in biomedical studies.

Mean

The most common measure of central tendency for discrete and continuous data is the mean, also referred to as the average. The mean of a variable is calculated by summing all of the observations and dividing by the total number of observations. The mean is represented by $\bar{x}$ (spoken: x bar) and its mathematical notation is

$$\frac{1}{n}\sum_{i=1}^{n} x_i$$

Consider 10 measures of systolic blood samples in a hypothetical data set:

110 mmHg	134 mmHg	126 mmHg	154 mmHg	168 mmHg
128 mmHg	168 mmHg	158 mmHg	170 mmHg	188 mmHg

The mode in this example is 168 mmHg, since this value occurs twice in the data set, more than any other value. However, the mode is not really informative since it factors in only 2 observations out of 10 possible ones. The mean is more useful and is calculated as

$$\bar{x} = \frac{1}{10}\sum_{i=1}^{10} xi = \left(\frac{1}{10}\right)(110+134+126+154+168+128+168+158+170+188)$$
$$= 150.4 \text{ mmHg}.$$

It may be useful to note that the value of 1/10th is applied to every data value when calculating the mean. We can view 1/10th as the "weight" of each value, and we are essentially applying equal weight to each observation since we do not have prior knowledge about the distribution of the data.

The mean is very sensitive to extreme values. In other words, if a data set contains an outlier or an observation that has a value that is very different from the others, the mean will be highly affected by it. Suppose the last observation were wrongly recorded as 1880 mmHg. The mean in this case is

$$\bar{x} = \left(\frac{1}{10}\right)(110+134+126+154+168+128+168+158+170+1880) = 319.6 \text{ mmHg}.$$

This mean systolic blood pressure of 319.6 mmHg is more than twice that of the previously calculated mean. A systolic blood pressure value of 1880 mmHg is impossible in human beings so we should question this value and correct it. However, sometimes an error might not be so obvious, or an apparent error may not be an error at all. If we want to summarize the entire set of observations in the presence of outliers, we might prefer to use a measure that is not so sensitive to extreme observations; we will see that the median is one such measure (see later discussion in this chapter).

Sometimes we do not have access to individual measures in our data set, but only have summarized data in frequency distribution tables, as shown in Table 8.3. Data of this form are called grouped data. Because we do not have the entire data set, we cannot calculate the mean, but we can calculate the *grouped mean*, which is a different kind of average. To calculate the grouped mean, multiply the midpoint of each interval by the corresponding frequency, add these products, and divide the resulting sum by the total number of observations. The grouped mean is a weighted average of the interval midpoints, where each midpoint value is weighted by the relative frequency of the observations within each interval. (The relative frequency of an interval is the number of observations in an interval divided by the total number of observations.) The mathematical representation of the grouped mean is

$$\bar{x} = \frac{\sum_{i=1}^{K} m_i f_i}{\sum_{i=1}^{k} f_i}$$

where k is the number of intervals in the table, m_i is the midpoint of the i-th interval, and f_i is the absolute frequency of the i-th interval.

From the example shown in Table 8.3:

Systolic Blood Pressure (mmHg)	Midpoint	Number of Patients	Midpoint * # of Patients
100–119	109.5	15	1,642.5
120–139	129.5	48	
140–159	149.5	36	
160–179	169.5	13	
180–199	189.5	5	
Total		117	

$$\bar{x} = \frac{1}{117}\big[109.5(15)+129.5(48)+149.5(36)+169.5(13)+189.5(5)\big]$$
$$= \frac{16391.5}{117}$$
$$= 140.01 \text{ mmHg}$$

Median

The median is defined as the middle number in a list of values ordered from smallest to largest. (If there is no middle number, the median is the mean of the two middle values.) The median is a measure of central tendency that is not as sensitive to outliers compared to the mean. It can be used to summarize discrete or continuous data.

In the previous example, we first rank the 10 measurements of systolic blood pressure from smallest to largest:

110 mmHg	126 mmHg	128 mmHg	134 mmHg	154 mmHg
158 mmHg	168 mmHg	168 mmHg	170 mmHg	188 mmHg

Since we have 10 observations, the median is the average between the two middle values, the 5th (154 mmHg) and 6th (158 mmHg) observations; therefore, it is 156 mmHg. Observe that the median divides the data into two halves; one half is less than the median, the other half is greater than the median.

The most appropriate measure of central tendency to use depends on the distribution of the values. If the distribution of the data is symmetric and unimodal, as shown in Figure 8.10 a, the mean, median, and mode should be the same. In this scenario, the mean is commonly preferred. When the data are not symmetric, the median is the best measure of the central tendency. The data in Figure 8.10 b are skewed to the right since the right tail of the distribution is longer and fatter; similarly the data in Figure 8.10 c are skewed to the left. Since the mean is sensitive to outliers, it is pulled in the direction of the longer tail of the distribution. Therefore, in a unimodal

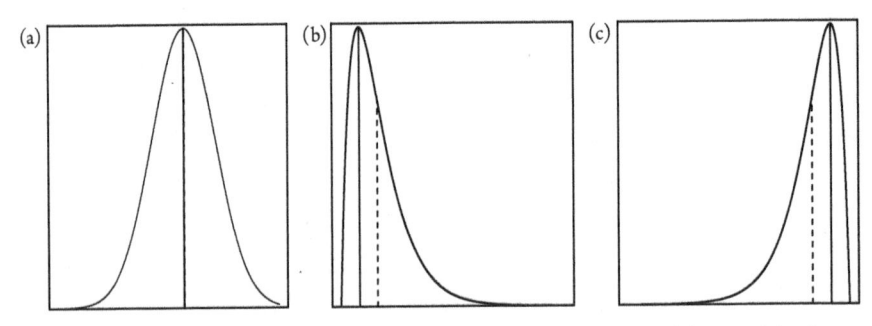

Figure 8.10. Possible distributions of the data: (a) Unimodal and symmetric; (b) unimodal and right-skewed; and (c) unimodal and left-skewed. The solid and dotted lines represent the location of the median and mean, respectively.

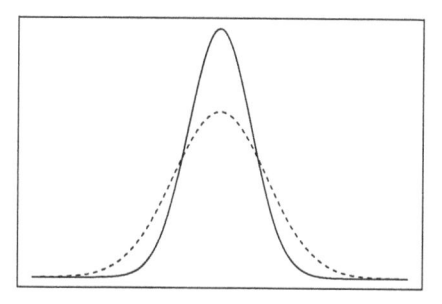

Figure 8.11. Two distributions with same mean, median, and mode, but different measures of dispersion.

distribution, when the data are skewed to the right, the mean tends to lie to the right of the median; when they are skewed to the left, the mean tends to lie to the left of the median.

Measures of Dispersion

Although two different distributions may have the same mean, median, and mode, they could be very different, as shown in Figure 8.11. Measures of dispersion are necessary to further describe the data and complement the information provided by measures of central tendency.

Range

The range of a group of observations is defined as the difference between the largest observation and the smallest. The range is easy to compute and gives us a rough idea of the spread of the data; however, the usefulness of the range is limited. The range is highly sensitive to outliers since it considers only the two most extreme values of a data set, the minimum and maximum values. In our previous example of 10 measures of systolic blood pressure, the range is 78 mmHg in the first set of observations and 1770 mmHg when the error measure of 1880 mmHg is considered!

Interquartile Range

The interquartile range (IQR) represents the middle 50% of the data. To calculate the interquartile range, you must first find the 25th and 75th percentiles. The 25th percentile, also called the first quartile and denoted Q1, is the value below which 25% of the data fall, when the data are ordered from smallest to largest. Similarly, the 75th percentile, also referred to as the third quartile and denoted Q3, is the value below which 75% of the data fall. The interquartile range is found by taking the difference between the 75th and 25th percentiles. The interquartile range is often reported with the median, as it is not affected by extreme values.

To calculate the 25th percentile of a set of measurements, first order the values from smallest to largest. Then calculate the "position" of the 25th percentile, which is equal to $n(25)/100$. In our example of 10 measures of blood pressure, the location of the 25th percentile is $10(25)/100 = 2.5$, which is not an integer. In this case, round up to the next integer. Therefore, the 25th percentile is the 2 + 1 = 3rd smallest measurement (or 3rd from the left), 128 mmHg. Similarly, the position of the 75th percentile is 10(75)/100 = 7.5, which again is not an integer; rounding up to the nearest integer, the 75th percentile is the 7 + 1 = 8th smallest measurement, 168 mmHg.

To find the kth percentile of a data set, we should begin by ranking the measurements from smallest to largest. Next, to find the position of the kth percentile, calculate $nk/100$. If $nk/100$ is an integer, the kth percentile is the average between the $(nk/100)$th smallest number and the $[(nk/100) + 1]$th smallest number. If $nk/100$ is not an integer, the kth percentile is the $(j + 1)$th smallest measurement, where j is the largest integer that is less than $nk/100$.

Variance and Standard Deviation

The most common measure of dispersion is the standard deviation. The sample variance is defined as the sample standard deviation squared. Both describe the amount of variability around the mean. The standard deviation can be viewed as the average distance of an individual observation from $\bar{x}$. A good candidate for the standard deviation might be to take the deviations of the data from the mean and average these values, as expressed in the following.

$$\frac{1}{n}\sum_{i=1}^{n}(x_i - \bar{x})$$

It turns out that this expression is equal to zero since the sum of the deviations from the mean of all observations less than $\bar{x}$ is equal to the sum of the deviations greater than $\bar{x}$, and therefore the two sums cancel each other out. To solve this problem, we might square the absolute values of the deviations from the mean and then average these values to get a single number. Note that this resulting number is a squared distance, but we are looking for a number that represents the average distance between a typical observation and the mean, so it makes sense to take the square root of the statistic. Thus a good candidate for the standard deviation is

$$\sqrt{\frac{1}{n}\sum_{i=1}^{n}(x_i - \bar{x})^2}.$$

It turns out that dividing by $n-1$ instead of n gives us a value that has better statistical properties. Thus, the standard deviation, denoted s, is given by the following equation.

$$s = \sqrt{\frac{1}{n-1}\sum_{i=1}^{n}(x_i - \bar{x})^2}$$

In summary, the standard deviation is calculated by subtracting the mean of a set of values from each of the observations squaring these deviations, adding them up, dividing the sum by the number of observations minus 1, and then taking the square

x_i	$x_i - \bar{x}$	$(x_i - \bar{x})^2$
110	−40.4	1632.16
134	−16.4	268.96
126	−24.4	595.36
154	3.6	12.96
168	17.6	309.76
128	−22.4	501.76
168	17.6	309.76
158	7.6	57.76
170	19.6	384.16
188	37.6	1413.76
	Sum	5486.40

root. For the 10 measures of systolic blood pressure, the mean is 150.4 mmHg and the variance is calculated as seen in the following:

Usually, the mean and the standard deviation are used to describe the characteristics of the entire distribution of values.

Standard Error of the Sample Mean

It is important to note that although we were able to calculate the sample mean of our collected sample, it is only an estimate of the true mean of the population that the data were sampled from, denoted μ. If we were to collect a different sample from our population, we would expect that the sample mean of the new sample might differ from the original sample mean that we calculated. There is variability between the sample means of different samples taken from our population. This variability is captured in the standard error of the sample means (SEM), which is the standard deviation of the distribution of sample means. This is not to be confused with the standard deviation (SD) of a sample, which is a measure of dispersion of just one sample. The formula to calculate the standard error of the sample mean is

$$\text{SEM} = \frac{s}{\sqrt{n}}$$

Since the SEM is equal to the SD divided by the square root of the sample size number, the SEM is always smaller than the SD.

Confidence Interval

As mentioned earlier, the mean of a sample is only an estimate of the true mean, μ, from which the data were sampled. One can conceive that there is some error involved with estimating the population by a mean of just one sample. We can create an interval around the sample mean with a margin of error that is 2 times the standard error of the mean (SEM), which is called a 95% confidence interval for the true population mean, given by the following:

$$\bar{x} \pm 2(\text{SEM}) = \bar{x} \pm 2\frac{s}{\sqrt{n}}$$

We say that "we are 95% confident that the true population mean falls in this interval." What this really means is the following: imagine that many samples of the same size are drawn from a population; then 95% of these samples will have confidence intervals that capture the true population mean.

Coefficient of Variation

It is possible to compare the variability among two or more sets of data with different units of measurement using a numerical measure known as the coefficient of variation. It relates the standard deviation of a set of observations to its mean and is a measure of relative variability. It is calculated using the following formula:

$$CV = \frac{s}{\bar{x}} \times 100\%$$

The coefficient of variation for the systolic blood pressure is

$$CV = \frac{24.69}{150.4} \times 100\%$$

$$CV = 16.42\%$$

On its own, it is difficult to assess whether this value is small or large. The usefulness of this measure is to compare two or more sets of data.

PROBABILITY

Descriptive statistics are useful to summarize and evaluate a set of data, which is the first step in statistical analysis. However, when we perform an experiment or observe a phenomenon in a particular sample, we are interested in generalizing our findings to the population from which the sample was drawn. This is achieved through statistical inference. In the next four chapters, this concept will be highly utilized to explain the basis of the statistical tests. The background necessary to understand statistical inference is probability theory. The probability of an event is commonly defined as the number of desired outcomes divided by the total number of possible outcomes. Another common definition is the proportion of times the desired event occurs in an infinitely large number of trials repeated under virtually identical conditions. Let us see how the two definitions are reasonable by considering an example, the event of getting a "head" in a fair coin toss. By the first definition, the probability of the event is 0.5, one head divided by two possible outcomes (head or tail). Now consider the latter

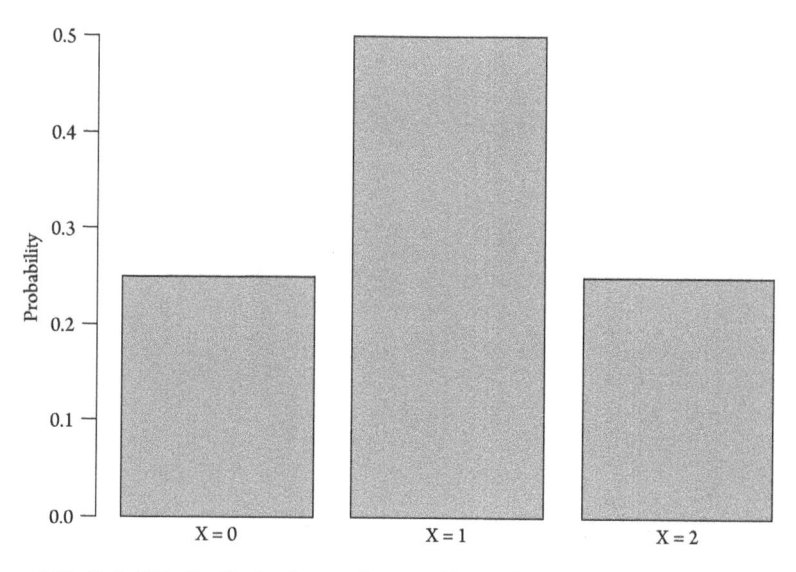

Figure 8.12. Probability distribution for a random variable, X, which is the number of heads that appear in two coin flips.

definition and imagine repeating the coin flip repeatedly. First suppose we flip the coin twice in a row; it is not guaranteed that we will only see one head due to the random nature of a coin flip. However, we will see that the proportion of heads converges to 0.5 as the number of flips becomes increasingly large. In the same way, the probability of tails will be 0.5 if the coin is tossed a large enough number of times.

A random variable is a variable that can assume different values such that any particular outcome is determined by chance. Every random variable has a corresponding probability distribution, which describes the behavior of the random variable following the theory of probability. It specifies all possible outcomes of the random variable along with the probability that each will occur. The frequency distribution displays each observed outcome and the number of times it appears in the data set. Similarly, the probability distribution represents the relative frequency of occurrence of each outcome in a large number of trials repeated under essentially identical conditions. Since all possible values of the random variable are taken into account, the outcomes are *exhaustive*, and the sum of their probabilities is equal to 1. For example, suppose we flip two fair coins and let the random variable X denote the number of heads that appear; the random variable X can take on values 0 through 2, since it is possible to observe no heads or, at the other extreme, all heads. The probability of getting no heads is ¼, the probability of getting exactly one head out of two coin flips is ½, and the probability of observing two head is ¼; the probability of all the possible outcomes of the random variable X add up to 1. The probability distribution for this random variable is displayed in Figure 8.12.

THE NORMAL DISTRIBUTION

There are many known probability distributions that correspond to different types of variables (e.g., discrete, continuous). In the context of this book, which aims to

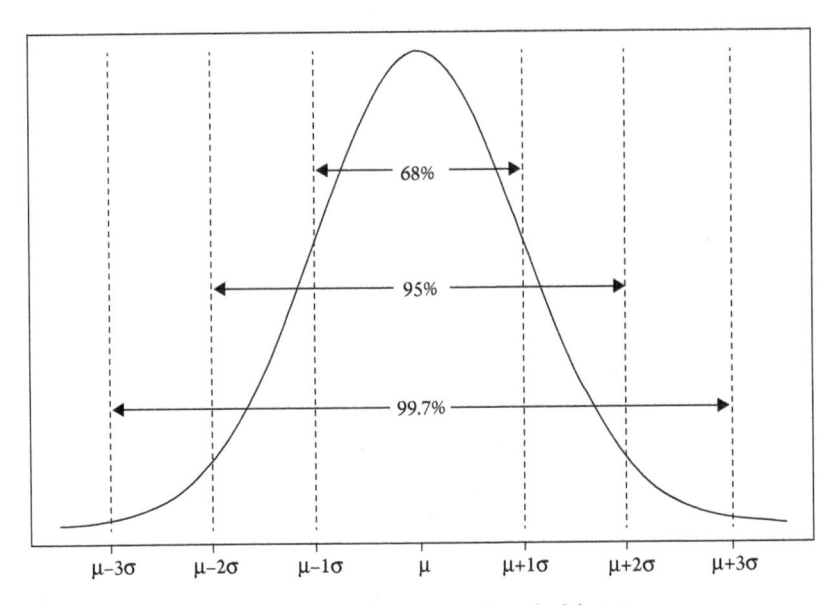

Figure 8.13. The standard normal curve with mean, μ, and standard deviation, σ.

provide the basics of statistics, we focus on the normal distribution, as it is a commonly occurring distribution for continuous variables that occur in real life and also figures prominently in several statistical tests that we will later encounter.

The normal distribution is a special unimodal and symmetric distribution. It is characterized by its mean, μ, and standard deviation, σ. Almost all of the data lie within three standard deviations of the mean; approximately 67% of the observations lie within one standard deviation around the mean, 95% lie within two standard deviations, and 99.7% lie within three standard deviations of the mean (Figure 8.13). This means that it is very unlikely that extreme values beyond three standard deviations of the mean will occur. The normal distribution is widely used because it can be used to estimate probabilities associated with many continuous variables found in biological, psychological, and social sciences, such as weight, height, blood pressure, and intelligence. You will learn that the normal distribution is used in many statistical tests [6].

A special case of the normal distribution is the standard normal distribution, where the mean μ equals 0 and the standard deviation σ is 1. In this case, approximately 68% of the data lie within the interval from −1 to 1, and 95% lie within the interval from −2 to 2. We can standardize our data by subtracting each observed value by the mean and divide the difference by the standard deviation, called a *z-score*; the resulting transformed data has mean 0 and standard deviation 1 and are on the standard normal distribution scale. We can use standardized z-scores to assess whether or not an observation is extreme (which is commonly taken to mean outside of the central 95% of the distribution) or to compare two sets of normally distributed data that are on different scales. If the underlying data are normally distributed we can use statistical tests to make statistical inferences (t-test, ANOVA, linear regression); these tests will be discussed in the next chapter.

Assessing the Distribution of a Continuous Variable

We generally do not have access to the whole target population when performing our studies. We do have access only to samples from this population, and usually the distribution of the data obtained from the sample does not exactly fit the normal curve. Therefore, an important step in descriptive statistics is to assess how the data are distributed and whether they are normally distributed or not.

Graphical assessments are the first step to assess normality. Histograms, box-plots and stem-and-leaf plots can be used for this purpose. Visual inspection of the distribution can be quite informative, although this relies on subjective assumptions.

The normal probability plot is another graphical tool to assess the normality of data. It plots the quantiles (or percentiles) of the data against the quantiles of the standard normal distribution. If the data are normally distributed, the quantiles of the data should match up with the quantiles of the standard normal distribution, and we should expect to see the plotted points fall on a straight line.

Numerical assessments can be more objective. As previously described, in a normally distributed data set, the mean and median are expected to be similar, in contrast to a skewed unimodal distribution, where one tail of the distribution is longer than the other. A measure, called *skewness*, reflects an asymmetrical departure from a normal distribution as seen in a skewed distribution. A value close to zero indicates a normal distribution. In a unimodal distribution, a positive skewness value indicates a right-skewed distribution (Figure 8.10 b); similarly, negative skewness indicates a left-skewed distribution (Figure 8.10 c). Another measure, *kurtosis*, is also helpful in assessing the normality of a distribution. Kurtosis quantifies the peakedness (width of the peak) and weight of the tails relative to a normal distribution. Values close to three are indicative of normality. In a unimodal and symmetric distribution, positive kurtosis reflects increased peakedness and heavy tails, whereas negative kurtosis suggests flatness and lighter tails. Both skewness and kurtosis are sensitive to sample size. In small samples, the values of kurtosis and/or skewness may suggest that the distribution is not normal, though the distribution in the population from which the sample was drawn may be quite normal.

Specific statistical tests, like Shapiro-Wilk and Kolmogorov-Smirnov tests, may also be used to assess the normality of a distribution; however, as with any statistical test, they are dependent on the sample size and may be poorly powered for small samples. In this case, the test statistic from the sample will preclude us from rejecting the null hypothesis of normality when, in fact, the underlying distribution may be highly non-normal.

Sampling Distribution of the Mean

If the population is small or we are dealing with census data, we are able to calculate the population mean μ and the standard deviation σ. Unfortunately, these are rarely the case in clinical research and we usually have to infer from sample data through its parameters the mean $\bar{X}$ and standard deviation s.

Suppose we select n individuals from a population and determine the mean $\overline{x1}$. Then we obtain a second sample of the same size and calculate the second mean $\overline{x2}$. Since we expect some variability in measures in our sample, it is reasonable to expect that $\overline{x1}$ and $\overline{x2}$ will be slightly different. If we continue to draw samples of size n from the population, we will end with a sample of sample means. If we draw samples of size n, the probability distribution of these sample means is known as the sampling distribution of the sample mean. This distribution has a standard deviation that is equal to $\sigma/\sqrt{n}$, where σ is the true standard deviation of the entire population, and it is referred to as the standard error of the mean. Moreover, if n is large enough, the shape of the distribution is approximately normal.

What Should Be Done When the Distribution Is Not Normal?

In reality, not all continuous variables follow a normal distribution, and if only a few observations are included in the sample it might be difficult to assess normality. While parametric tests are known to be better powered than non-parametric tests, they often assume that the data are normally distributed. If normality is not satisfied, we should decide our next steps based on four options:

1. Central limit theorem (CLT): The CLT states that if the sample size is large enough, the distribution of sample means is approximately normal. The CLT applies even if the distribution of the underlying data is not normal. However, the farther the distribution departs from being normally distributed, the larger the sample size is necessary. A sample size of at least 30 observations is usually large enough if the departure from normality is small. Therefore, if we have a sufficiently large sample size, we may use parametric tests based on CLT, even if the underlying population distribution is not normal.
2. Transformation of the data: We can modify a variable so that its distribution is more normal. Another reason for data transformation is to achieve constant variance, which is required for the use of some parametric tests. Through transformation, a new variable X' is created by changing the scale of measurement for the dependent variable X. The most commonly used transformations are the square root transformation ($X'=\sqrt{X}$), the square transformation ($X'=X^2$), the log transformation ($X'=\log X$), and the reciprocal transformation ($X'=1/X$). The most important drawbacks of data transformations are some loss of interpretability and failure to smooth the data. Regarding interpretability, if we choose, for example, to log transform our dependent variable X, all further results will be presented and interpreted in a logarithmic scale and could be difficult to interpret for the readers.
3. Use of non-parametric tests: Another possible approach for non-normally distributed data is the use of non-parametric tests, which will be presented in Chapter 10. These tests do not require any assumptions about the underlying distribution of the data; however, they often have less power to detect true differences among the compared groups, and the chance of false negative associations is higher compared to when parametric tests are used. Therefore, usually a larger sample size is required when we use non-parametric tests compared to parametric ones.
4. Categorization of the data: Another possibility is to transform continuous data that are not normally distributed into nominal or ordinal variables. A continuous variable that is recoded as categorical may be more clinically relevant, but the loss of power is very significant as discussed before in this chapter.

CASE STUDY: A LONG CANADIAN WINTER: THE DILEMMA OF CATEGORIZING THE DATA AND CHOOSING PARAMETRIC VERSUS NON-PARAMETRIC TESTS

Felipe Fregni

It is one of those harsh winters in Montreal. This year, the first snowstorm was in October and Professor Jean Rosseau knows that from now until probably April of next year, he will need to live with the white scenery. He just returned to Canada after living 15 years in North Carolina, in the United States. Being a French Canadian, he missed Canada, especially the French area, and besides, he received a proposal from University of Montreal that could not be refused: a tenure track position of full professor and research chair in the department of neurology in addition to a very large start-up package (5 M) to start his own laboratory there.

He now needs to show that he is being productive, and the first study he is planning to run is a study to assess a cholinesterase inhibitor for the treatment of behavioral symptoms in Alzheimer's disease. He has the funds for this study. He is planning to use part of his start-up package (although he needs to be conservative in his spending, as a good part of this money will be used to buy equipment for his laboratory and to pay salary for his research team and staff until he gets his Canadian grants). He has carefully planned this study, but some issues are still unresolved: whether to categorize the data as parametric versus non-parametric data. He has one week to make the decision before presenting the study to the departmental meeting. This will be the first departmental meeting, and he wants to make a good impression at this meeting.

Defining Your Variables Has Significant Implications for Data Analysis

Even before planning data analysis and sample size calculation, the investigator needs to decide whether the outcome of his or her study will be measured as continuous (and whether it is normally distributed or not), discrete (counts), or categorical. Data classification can be confusing initially, as there are different types of classification and slight variations in the terms authors prefer to use. A simple method to classify data is the following:

- Interval or ratio data (continuous variable): For both types of variables, the difference between an interval (e.g., 1°C difference in temperature) has the same meaning if comparing 35°C versus 36°C, or 40°C versus 41°C. For the case of ratio data, there is the concept of an absolute zero; for instance, a height of zero means no height. Other examples include weight, temperature in Kelvin, time since randomization. In this case, the ratio of two values has meaning.
- Ordinal variable: also referred as expressing ranks (the concept of rank will be important for non-parametric tests). In this type of data, order is important, but the differences between adjacent ranks have no meaning. For instance, the difference between "much improved" to "improved" may not be equal to the difference

between "much worsened" to "worsened" in a ordinal scale in which patients have to say: "much improved"; "improved"; "no change"; "worsened"; or "much worsened." Note that order here is important. You can say that in terms of clinical improvement "much improved" > "improved" > "no change" > "worsened" > "much worsened." On the other hand, if your variable is profession—there is no order for classifying type of profession: "occupational therapist"; "firefighter"; "psychologist"; "biologist"—this is the next type of data (categorical).
- Categorical variable (called binary or dichotomous when there are only two possibilities and nominal when there are more than two possibilities): When data can fit into categories, we call this categorical data. Examples include death (yes/no) or cardiovascular event (three categories: no cardiovascular event, unstable angina, myocardial infarction).

The investigator should know which type of data he or she is dealing with in order to define the most appropriate and valid statistical test. In addition, the type of data (e.g., continuous vs. categorical) will have a significant impact on the study power.

Another important concept here is that, in some cases, data are originally nominal or ordinal—for instance, a researcher might be measuring death (yes/no), and in this case the plan has to be to use categorical data. However, if the data are continuous, then one option is categorize it—for instance, suppose an investigator is collecting data on blood pressure (that is continuous), he or she may want to categorize it into low blood pressure and high blood pressure (after defining a cutoff). The main advantage of this approach is that a significant difference between high and low blood pressure will have a significant clinical meaning; however, the cost is a loss in efficiency and therefore a decrease in power. There are also critical considerations and limitations when using this approach (of categorizing continuous data) [7].

Another important point for continuous data is whether the data are normally distributed. This will have important implications for the choice of the statistical tests. Statistical tests for normal distribution (e.g., ANOVA and t-test—or parametric tests) usually have more efficiency than the respective options for data that are not normally distributed (or non-parametric tests).

Finding a Drug to Treat Agitation in Alzheimer's Disease

Being a neurologist who specialized in cognitive dysfunction, Prof. Rosseau was particularly interested in Alzheimer's disease and new treatments for it. In fact, that was one of the reasons he moved back to Canada—as the behavioral neurology department at the University of Montreal was particularly strong.

Alzheimer's disease causes a progressive impairment in cognitive function—loss of memory is usually one of the first evident symptoms. One of the main issues for these patients and their caregivers is behavioral and psychological symptoms (BPS). Among BPS, agitation is one of the most prevalent symptoms, observed in 24% of patients. There are only a few treatments for this condition (mainly neuroleptics), and those induce modest gains and serious side effects.

An option for agitation is the use of colinestherase inhibitors, which have shown initial positive effects in preliminary studies, but uncertainty remains as to whether they are effective when behavioral disturbance is severe. Prof. Rosseau is planning to conduct a clinical trial to test (CHOLIN001) for the treatment of agitation in patients who have not responded to psychosocial treatment.

The Trial

The study Prof. Rosseau is planning is a single-center (there was a large dementia center in the behavioral neurology unit), double-blinded, randomized, parallel group trial in which patients would be assigned to receive placebo or CHOLIN001 for 12 weeks, after four weeks of failed psychosocial treatment. The main challenge in this trial is to define the main variable in order to decide the statistical plan and sample size calculation. The main outcome for this study is Cohen–Mansfield Agitation Inventory (CMAI) scores at 12 weeks. The CMAI evaluates 29 different agitated behaviors in patients with cognitive impairment and is carried out by caregivers. The frequency of each symptom is rated on a seven-point ordinal scale (1–7), ranging from "never" to "several times an hour." A total score is obtained by summing the 29 individual scores, yielding a total score from 29 to 203.

It is Monday afternoon and the weather forecast shows five inches of snow during the evening and early morning; Prof. Rosseau knows that the traffic through old Montreal will not be easy. He goes home to prepare for the first meeting with his research team. In this meeting, there will be four of his research fellows: Catherine Moreau—a neuropsychologist from Quebec city who just finished her PhD; Scott Neil—a senior neurology resident from Toronto in his last year of residency; Hugo Frances—a PhD student in cognitive neuroscience from Montreal; and Munir Dinesh—a postdoctoral fellow from India who has recently arrived to work with Professor Rosseau. The agenda for the morning meeting was to decide how to use the variable CMAI in the study. Prof. Rosseau sends the following email to the team:

Dear Team,
The agenda for tomorrow's meeting will be the discussion to decide how to use the CMAI variable in our study. I would like each one of you to come prepared according to the following instructions:

Catherine – your task is to investigate if it is appropriate to use CMAI as a variable with parametric tests.

Scott – as I suspect that CMAI will not be normally distributed, please investigate the use of data transformation (log transformation) or use of central limit theorem.
Hugo – please investigate the use of non-parametric approaches.
Munir – please investigate the categorization of data.
We will meet tomorrow at 8 a.m. in the conference room.

Looking forward
JR

Challenges and Issues for Use of Rating Scales with Parametric Tests

The heavy snowfall has stopped and by the time Prof. Rosseau was leaving home, the snow was light and the snow-plowing trucks had cleaned most of the streets. Prof. Rosseau decided to leave earlier to avoid surprises, and this would also give him additional time to go over the options to decide the best approach to handle with the main variable.

Everyone arrives with coffee and they are all excited to start working together. After introductions and a brief summary of the study design, Prof. Rosseau asks Catherine, "So Catherine, can we use CMAI as a continuous variable—I mean to use parametric tests?"

Catherine had spent almost all night working on this topic, and she was proud of the results. She then begins, "The main challenge we have here is the use of a rating scale. In fact, rating scales are increasingly selected as primary or secondary outcome measures in clinical trials. They are used especially for health outcomes where you cannot measure directly (such as disability, mood, cognitive function, and quality of life). The main issue is that rating scales generate ordinal scores—therefore one option would be categorizing it—as Munir will discuss with us. But the main question is: can we use parametric tests (the same that is used for continuous and normally distributed data) for rating scales? If it were blood pressure, this would be easier."

After a pause, Catherine continues, "It seems that the use of parametric statistics (for instance, t-test and ANOVA) with multiple-item rating scale data is controversial and has been intensively debated. The ones against this use say that rating scales are ordinal scales and therefore must be analyzed with non-parametric statistics. This would be certainly the safer solution—no one would criticize that. However, the supporters of this use argue that when the items of these scales are summed, this creates interval levels that are satisfactory enough (similar to continuous data) to allow the use of parametric statistics (she then shows two articles that support the use of parametric statistics in this situation). In addition," she completes, "some parametric statistics (e.g., t-tests) are robust enough to handle with the weaknesses of ordinal measurements. In fact, you can see in the literature that most rating scale data are analyzed using parametric statistics. Although using parametric statistical tests will give us more power, we have to consider that this is controversial—and it is only accepted by some statisticians."

Prof. Rosseau, after a brief pause, gives his feedback, "That is very good research, Catherine. Thank you for bringing this to the group. This was very helpful. It seems that we have some basis to use parametric tests. However, the issue to use parametric tests does not depend only on making sure that an ordinal scale can be used here; it also depends on the data being normally distributed. Because I believe that most patients would have a CMAI score near the cut-off point—to define severe agitation—then the data would probably be somewhat skewed. We should then analyze two methods in order to use parametric statistics: log transformation and use of central limit theorem. Scott, it is your turn now!"

Use of Central Limit Theorem to Justify the Use of Parametric Statistics in Date That Is Not Normally Distributed

Scott Neil, a senior resident, has a special interest in clinical research. He wants to become a clinician and also a researcher. In his own words, "I think that doing clinical work only would make me crazy. I need additional intellectual stimulation." He sees this opportunity to work with Prof. Rosseau as the chance to get the necessary training to become a future clinical researcher. He wants to impress the team in their first meeting. He then starts, "I agree with Prof. Rosseau that data might not be normally distributed. The first step is to look at the sample size. Given the sample size calculation in which we want to detect an average difference of a 6 point (SD 6) change in agitation inventory score from baseline to 12 weeks between active treatment and placebo with a power of 90% at the 5% (two sided) level of significance, we would need a sample size of 22 in each group (total of 44 patients). These parameters are based on the results of similar studies." He then continues, "This number of patients is not enough for the use of central limit theorem. The idea of central limit theorem is that even for large data sets that are not normally distributed, the use of parametric tests is OK. The main idea here is that parametric tests are robust to deviations from normal distributions, as long as the samples are large. The only issue is to define what "large" is. Large in this case depends also on the nature of the particular non-normal distribution. Although this is controversial, most statisticians are comfortable to use the central limit theorem with 70–100 data points." He then pauses and goes to the whiteboard.

"Because our distribution does not deviate excessively from normality, if we double the sample, we would be able to rely on this method and use parametric tests (given the issue of the scale that was discussed before by Catherine)." Prof. Rosseau then interrupts him, "This is excellent, Scott. Great job. Although increasing the sample size would increase our costs and duration of this trial, I want to try to use parametric tests in order to use some advanced modeling with the data that requires normal distribution. In addition, increasing the sample size would increase the power of our study, especially if we underestimated the sample size; however, we need to have a strong justification to do so. But let us hear the next option: use of log transformation."

Use of Log Transformation to Create a Normal Distribution

Scott was glad that the first part had gone well and he was able to explain what took a while for him to understand. He was proud of himself. Now the second part was easier. He then begins with the explanation for the group:

> Another option is the use of log transformation of the data. Let me explain better: because we expect that most of the data would be concentrated near the cut-off point and there might be some outliers, then our data will not be normally distributed. In fact, let us assume that we will get the following CMAI scores: 50, 51, 52, 55, 56, 57, 66, 80, 82, 90. These data are not normally distributed. But if we log transform these data, we would have: 1.70, 1.71, 1.72, 1.74, 1.75, 1.76, 1.82, 1.90, 1.91, 1.95. In fact, the Shapiro-Wilk test (a test to detect whether the data are normally distributed) shows that the first original set is not normally distributed while the second (logged transformed) is normally distributed.

Prof. Rosseau is impressed with Scott. He quickly comments, "Thank you again, Scott. This is very helpful. This seems an interesting strategy as it would not be necessary to increase the sample size of our study and we would be able to use parametric tests. However, the disadvantage here would be the interpretation of the data. At the end of the study, if we find significant results, we would have to say that CHOLIN001 induces a significant decrease in the logged transformed CMAI scores as compared to placebo. Well, this is certainly an option, depending again on the nature of the data, but let us go to Hugo and the use of non-parametric tests.

Use of Non-Parametric Tests: A Potentially Safe Solution

Hugo is an outstanding PhD student. He is one of the best students in the PhD program; his CV has impressed Prof. Rosseau, and that is one of the reasons he was chosen to work with him. He has been eager to speak, and now it is his turn. He does not waste one minute and begins:

> I will try to convince you all that the approach of using non-parametric tests—tests that need much less assumptions for the data—does not require that data are normally distributed and also is OK for ordinal data—an example is Wilcoxon test—might be the best one. If we go with the non-parametric approach, we would not need to be concerned with the issues raised by Cathy and we would not need to increase the sample size or use logged transformed data.

Prof. Rosseau then continues, "Thank you, Hugo. I agree with you, you laid out all the advantages; however, if we use a non-parametric approach we would not be able to use some advanced models that require normally distributed data and also using non-parametric data, we would lose some power and would need to increase the sample size between 5% and 10%. But again, this is a good option. Let us hear Munir for the last option: categorizing the data."

Using the Data as a Categorical Outcome: Increasing the Clinical Significance

Munir is the last to speak. He arrived in Montreal three weeks ago and considers this postdoctoral fellowship extremely important for his career. He was lucky to be considered to join Prof. Rosseau's team, and the main reason was because of the contact between Prof. Rosseau and his former mentor. He was a bit nervous for this first meeting. He stuttered at the beginning but soon gained confidence:

> One option is if we categorize CMAI. I would say that a reduction of 30% or greater in CMAI can be considered clinically important. We can therefore classify patients as responders (30% reduction in CMAI scores) and non-responders and then compare the rate of responders between placebo and CHOLIN001. This approach would increase the clinical significance and also would eliminate the issue of parametric tests as we would analyze the data using tests to compare proportions such as Chi-square or Fisher's exact test.

He looks at his notes and continues, "The disadvantage of this method is that we would lose some power. I therefore calculated the new sample size. Given that the rate of response to placebo would be 30% and the rate of response to CHOLIN001 would be 55%, and assuming 90% power at the 5% level of significance, we would need 81 participants in each group (total of 162 participants)."

After this detailed explanation, Prof. Rosseau thanks Munir and gives the final words, "Well, we have four different methods, each one with advantages and disadvantages. I now want you to think carefully about all of them and come tomorrow to the meeting with an opinion about the best approach."

Prof. Rosseau looks through his window. The snowfall has finally stopped and it is possible to see some sun. He knows it will be a long winter, but his excitement about this new study makes him forget about the next six months of cold weather, short days, and longer nights.

CASE DISCUSSION

This case illustrates the importance of understanding the study variables well. The first important point is to identify the variable type (i.e., nominal, ordinal, or continuous). For most of the cases, this determination is fairly easy; however, in some cases, as in this case study, there is some room for debate. It has been discussed that the "total score" variable is built on ordinal items. Potential methods of variable transformation also have been discussed. The investigator needs to first make careful assessments and then evaluate if some of the transformation tools are advantageous, and to determine the advantages and disadvantages of these methods. Finally, the overall impact on the study needs to be carefully considered.

CASE QUESTIONS FOR REFLECTION

What challenges does Prof. Rosseau face in choosing how the variable is treated?

1. What are his main concerns?
2. What should he consider to make the decision?
3. What type of variable should he use?
4. What are the pros and cons of using the variable you have chosen?

FURTHER READING

Papers

- Grimes, DA, Schulz, KF. Descriptive studies: what they can and cannot do. *Lancet.* 2002; 359(9301): 145–149.
- Neely, JG, Stewart, MG, Hartman, JM, Forsen, JW Jr, Wallace, MS. Tutorials in clinical research part VI: descriptive statistics. *Laryngoscope.* 2002; 112(7 Pt. 1): 1249–1255.
- Sonnad, S. Describing data: statistical and graphical methods. *Radiology.* 2002; 225(3): 622–8.

Online Stata Computing Resource

Resources to help you learn and use Stata. UCLA: Statistical Consulting Group.

http://www.ats.ucla.edu/stat/stata/

Books

- Pagano M, Gauvreau K. *Principles of biostatistics*, 2nd ed. Pacific Grove, CA: Cengage Learning; 2000.
- Portney LG, Watkins MP. *Foundations of clinical research: applications to practice*, 3rd ed. Upper Saddle River, NJ: Pearson Prentice Hall; 2009.

REFERENCES

1. Cummings JL, Mega M, Gray K, Rosenbergthompson S, Carusi DA, Gornbein J. The neuropsychiatric inventory:comprehensive assessment of psychopathology in dementia. *Neurology*. 1994; 44: 2308–2314.
2. New York Heart Association. *Diseases of the heart and blood vessels: nomenclature and criteria for diagnosis*. Little, Brown and Company; 1964.
3. Hobart JC, Cano SJ, Zajicek JP, Thompson AJ. Rating scales as outcome measures for clinical trials in neurology: problems, solutions, and recommendations. *Lancet Neurology*. 2007; 6: 1094–1105.
4. Kirkwood BR. *Essentials of medical statistics*. Malden, MA: Blackwell Scientific Publications; 1988.
5. Miller RG Jr. *Beyond ANOVA: basics of applied statistics*. CRC Press; 1997.
6. Dalgaard P. *Introductory statistics with R*. New York: Springer Science & Business Media; 2008.
7. Kirsch I, Moncrieff J. Clinical trials and the response rate illusion. *Contemp Clin Trials*. 2007; 28: 348–351.

9

PARAMETRIC STATISTICAL TESTS

Authors: *Ben M. W. Illigens, Fernanda Lopes, and Felipe Fregni*

Case study authors: *André Brunoni and Felipe Fregni*

A man gets drunk on Monday on whisky and sodawater; he gets drunk on Tuesday on brandy and sodawater, and on Wednesday on gin and sodawater. What causes his drunkenness? Obviously, the common factor, the sodawater.
—Anthony Standen, *Science Is a Sacred Cow*

INTRODUCTION

This chapter begins with the fundamentals of statistical testing, followed by an introduction to the most common parametric tests. The next chapter will describe non-parametric tests and will compare them to their parametric counterparts.

The previous chapter gave you an overview over different types of data, descriptive methods, and sample distributions. You also learned the basics of probability, which leads us to what is most commonly done in applied medical statistics: hypothesis testing.

HYPOTHESIS TESTING

When we conduct an experiment, how do we know if the data from our sample group are different compared to the normal population or compared to another group? What would we use to compare both groups, how could we describe the differences of the groups? We have already learned the methods of descriptive statistics in Chapter 8, which helped us to characterize our sample. Therefore, we could, for example look at a measure of central tendency: We could select a summary statistic for our sample (commonly the sample mean) and then compare it to the reference group data [1]. But if we indeed find a difference between the groups, how do we know that this is a true difference? We have to consider that it could be due to the following reasons:

- Actual effect (there is a real difference between the groups)
- Chance
- Bias
- Confounding.

> **Difference between bias and confounder**
>
> *Bias* is a systematic error that leads to a false measurement of the dependent variable and therefore to a wrong conclusion.
>
> A *confounder* is a variable that relates to the dependent and independent variable, doesn't lie on the causal pathway (which would be called an intermediary variable), and leads to the assumption of a causal relationship between the dependent and independent variable, which, however, is either overestimated or misleading.

Statistical tests are generally designed to determine if the observed difference between the groups is likely due to chance (and therefore not meaningful). This is based on the initial assumption that groups in most of the cases are not different—unless under the "rare" circumstance that there is a real effect (due to the intervention or, more generally, due to the study design). This initial belief is called the null hypothesis (H_0: group 1 = group 2, stated as no difference between groups). In fact, remember that when you are running a study, you are doing so to add a new knowledge (this is your alternative hypothesis). You start from current knowledge (this is your null hypothesis; for instance, currently there is no evidence to support a difference between a new intervention and a placebo (even though based on other studies you have hypothesized that this is not the case, but need to run the study to confirm) [2].

Therefore, the null hypothesis is set up so that we can reject the null hypothesis if there is a real difference between the groups. If the null hypothesis can be rejected, the alternative hypothesis is true (H_A: group 1 ≠ group 2).

Importantly, statistical tests cannot account for bias or, in most cases, for confounding. The best strategy to exclude or limit those effects as much as possible is through a proper study design (see Chapter 4). An example would be comparing two groups of treatment (drug A vs. placebo), but during the trial there was no appropriate blinding (leading to detection bias). Because of this, even if the statistical test shows a difference between drug A versus placebo, this result is likely due to bias and is not valid.

The statistical test calculates the probability of the observed event to happen. If the probability of the observed result is small enough, the investigator concludes that the difference is likely not due to chance and can reject the null hypothesis.

The *p* value provides an estimate of the probability of the event, and if it is small enough, the result is called *statistically significant* [3].

The key question is, what is considered small enough? Usually the threshold is set between what is considered likely due to chance and actual effect. This threshold is called alpha (α), the level of significance. It is widely accepted to consider a *p*-value of equal or less than an α of 0.05 small enough (which corresponds to a chance of 1 out of 20). This value, though, is arbitrary. An interesting exercise can help you to understand that 0.05 is extreme enough to consider that is beyond chance: suppose someone tosses a coin and tells you "it is heads" (1st trial), and then again, "it is heads

> *P-value* definition: The probability of the observed result or something more extreme under the null hypothesis.

again" (2nd trial), then again, "it is heads again" (3rd trial), then one more time "oh, again, it is heads!" (4th trial)—at this point you become suspicious that the coin is biased and has only heads, but your colleague again tosses the coin and again it is heads (5th trial)! At this point you believe that the chance of 5 heads in a roll is so extreme that the coin is likely biased. The probability of having 5 heads consecutively is 0.032 (close to 0.05); thus you can understand that 0.05 is a reasonable threshold.

Statistical Errors

When conducting a statistical test, there are four possible outcomes:

	Fail to Reject H_0	Reject H_0
H_0 is true	Correct	Type I error
H_0 is false	Type II error	Correct (power)

We already discussed two outcomes:

1. Scenario 1 = the H_0 is true (suppose it is possible to know this). You run the experiment and indeed find a p-value greater than 0.05, thus failing to reject the H_0. Therefore the result of the experiment matches the truth (again, if it was possible to know the truth).
2. Scenario 1 = the H_0 is false (again, suppose it is possible to know this). You run the experiment and indeed find a p-value smaller than 0.05, thus rejecting the H_0. Therefore the result of the experiment matches the truth (again, if it was possible to know the truth).

In these two scenarios the experiment matches the truth. But what if it does not?
The preceding table shows that also two types of errors can occur when performing a statistical test:

1. Type I error (false positive): Rejecting the null hypothesis even though the null is true (in other words, claiming a significant difference when in fact there is no difference. Using the example of the coin, it is possible to get a normal coin and toss it 5 times and get heads in all the times).
- Level of significance = α—probability of committing a type I error.

Most studies set an alpha of 0.05. An α of 0.05 means that you are accepting a 5% maximum chance of incorrectly rejecting the null hypothesis (H_0). The lower α is, the lower this "permitted" chance will be.

2. Type II error (false negative): Failure to reject the null hypothesis when the null is false (in other words, claiming that there is no significant difference when in fact there is a difference; this happens when the experiment is underpowered).= β— probability of committing a type II error= Directly related to power (Power = 1-β, see Chapter 11).

Most studies set a β of 0.2. This means that your power will be 0.8 (80%), and that you are accepting a 20% chance of failing to reject the null hypothesis (H_0) when it is actually false.

How Does One Conduct Hypothesis Testing?

Now that you understand the idea of hypothesis testing and the concept of *p*-value, the next step is to understand how to conduct a statistical test appropriately. For the beginners in statistics, it is easier to break the process into smaller steps and to use a framework as shown here:

First step: understand the variables;
First important step: classify the study variables.

The investigator needs to determine the dependent (or the outcome) and independent variables. This has been discussed in the previous chapter (please go back to this chapter if this concept is not clear). The next step is then to classify this variable into continuous, ordinal, or categorical variable (this has been explained in detail in the previous chapter). Finally, if the variable is continuous, then the investigator needs to determine whether the distribution is normal (refer to Chapter 8 for a detailed discussion).

For those who are beginning in statistics, it may then help to visualize all the options to choosing a statistical test (see Table 9.1). If given these initial steps (variable determination and normality), the investigator finds out that one of the parametric statistical tests can be used (t-test, ANOVA, or linear regression), then the investigator needs to check whether the other assumptions for using these tests are met (as discussed in the second step in the following).

Table 9.1 Summary of Statistical Tests Based on Variable Classification

Independent Variable(s)	Continuous Data (Outcome)		Categorical / Binary Outcome
	Normal distribution	Non-normal	
Compare two groups (independent variable; binary)	Unpaired and paired t-test	Mann-Whitney Wilcoxon	Chi-square Fisher's exact
Compare three or more groups (independent variable; categorical)	ANOVA (one or n-way ANOVA)	Kruskal-Wallis or Friedman test	Chi-square Fisher's exact
Association between two variables (independent variable; continuous)	Pearson correlation	Spearman correlation	
Association between three or more variables (independent variable; continuous)	Multiple linear regression		Multiple logistic regression

Second step: check other assumptions for the use of parametric tests.

It is important also to check if other factors are met when using parametric tests (see the list of assumptions in the following). The other important assumption is whether the variance of groups is roughly equal. Although t-test and ANOVA are robust for some level of imbalance in variances across groups, it is recommended to check.

There are still other assumptions, such as that data are randomly selected and the observations are independent. These assumptions are not exclusive of parametric tests. They are important also for other statistical tests, and in fact the investigator should make all possible efforts to meet these assumptions. Nevertheless, it is known that most of the sampling method is actually non-random (see Chapter 6 for further discussion).

In summary, parametric tests rely on certain assumptions. These assumptions are

— Normal distribution of the underlying data (step 1)
— Data are measured on the interval or ratio scales (step 1)
— Random sampling from a defined population (step 2)
— Variances in the samples being compared are roughly equal (tests for homogeneity of variance) (step 2)

Understanding How Statistical Significance Is Calculated

Although the software can run the statistical test, it is important to understand how statistical significance is calculated. In order to determine whether the difference between groups is statistically significant, it is important to know the variability of the data in addition to the compared difference between groups [4]. Are the two groups different relative to the variability in the data?

The basic form of a statistical test is the ratio between signal and noise multiplied by the square root of the sample size.

$$t = \frac{signal}{noise} \times \sqrt{sample\ size}$$

This formula gives you a value that tells you how confident you can be about your data. The higher the signal is, the more confident you can be in the difference, while an increase in noise reduces the impact of the signal (sample size and power will be discussed in Chapter 11).

This concept is also demonstrated in Figure 9.1.

Mean

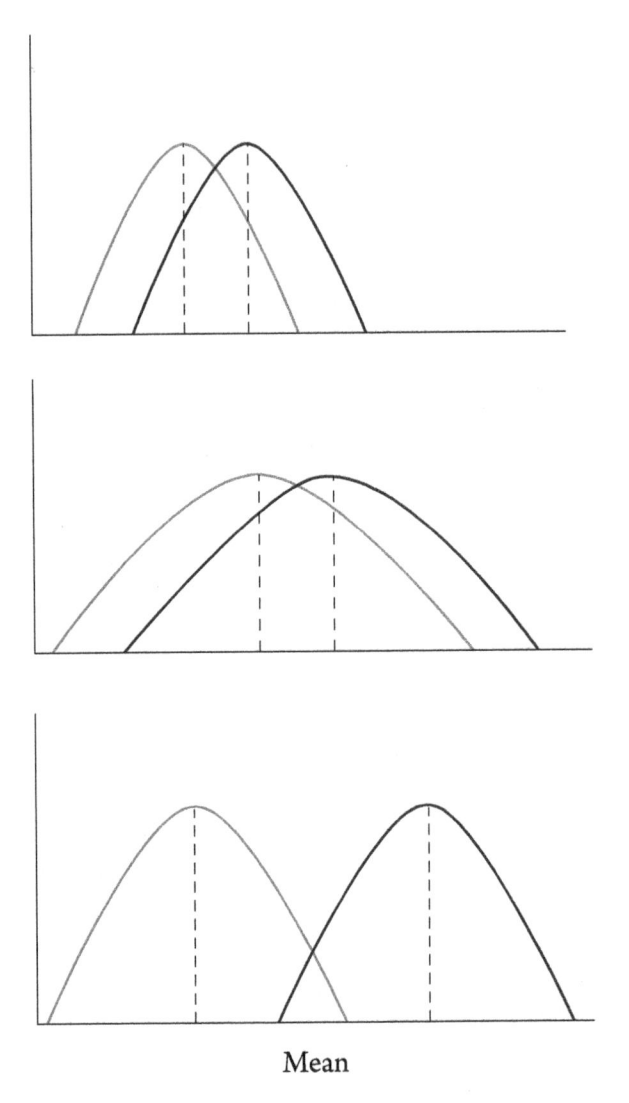

Figure 9.1. This figure shows that two parameters are important: differences between the means (difference between dashed lines) and variability (how wide is the spread of the data).

Comparing Two Means: T-Test

This is one of the most commonly used statistical tests. Why is it so common? Because it is a simple test that compares results from two groups that were assessed in a continuous outcome (for instance, blood pressure, cholesterol levels) and a good number of assessments in medicine are based on a continuous scale. It is also a relatively simple test to use and to understand its main results. Although this may be considered too simplistic a test, as it only uses one independent variable, it can answer most of the questions from a well-designed randomized clinical trial in which groups are well balanced. In addition, this test is robust to small violations in the normality assumption.

Classic examples in literature include randomized clinical trials that compare different interventions while using biological continuous measurements as outcomes. In the study performed by Salvi et al. [1], patients with asthma were randomized to receive either Ciclesonide (inhaled corticosteroid) alone or combined with Formoterol (long-acting beta-agonist) [5]. The main outcome, forced expiratory volume (continuous outcome), was compared using a t-test for independent samples.

Summary of how to use the test (see later in the chapter for statistical software use):

Independent variable (explanatory variable, X): binary—two groups
Dependent variable (outcome, Y): Continuous, normally distributed
For independent samples: unpaired t-test
For dependent samples (e.g., pre- and post-intervention comparison): paired t-test.

Comparing More Than Two Means: Analysis of Variance (ANOVA)

The next option when handling an outcome that is measured in a continuous scale and is normally distributed is the analysis of variance (ANOVA). When should this test be used instead of a t-test? ANOVA should be used when there is more than one independent categorical variable. The main independent variable in a test is the group of intervention (e.g., real drug vs. placebo). However, there are two situations in which you need to use ANOVA instead: (1) your main independent variable has more than two levels (for instance, drug A, drug B and placebo); or (2) you also want to add another variable, for instance, time of assessment (baseline and after treatment) or you want to add a variable to adjust the results, for instance for an important variable (e.g., gender). ANOVA is also a robust test in which it is relatively easy to understand the output. However, it is not a full multivariate test, as you can only add categorical variables as the independent variables. For a complete multivariate test, you need to use a regression analysis (discussed next).

Summary of how to use the test:

Independent variable (explanatory variable, X): categorical—more than two groups
Dependent variable (outcome, Y): Continuous, normally distributed.

The ANOVA tests the H_0 that all means are equal. The H_0 can be rejected when at least two means are not equal, but the ANOVA does not reveal between which groups the difference is significant. In order to determine where the difference lies, post hoc multiple comparison tests such as Bonferroni or Tukey's can be used.

Linear Regression

The final example here is the linear regression, which uses the same type of outcome (measured in a continuous scale and normally distributed) but differently from t-test (and similar to ANOVA), accepts more than one independent variable. The difference between ANOVA and linear regression is that the independent variable can be either a categorical variable or a continuous variable. Linear regression is useful in RCTs when there are covariates to adjust—in other words, variables that are related to the outcomes/response to treatment—that are continuous (e.g., baseline age) or in observational trials to adjust for variables that are confounders.

Linear regression can also be used to build prediction models (or equations that predict the outcome based on a set of independent variables). Prediction in medicine is very valuable—in fact, the linear regression model is a powerful tool to establish predictive relationship between factors and a continuous outcome, for example, predictive factors for the risk of dying from breast cancer.

Summary of how to use the test:

Independent variable (explanatory variable, X): continuous or categorical
Dependent variable (outcome, Y): continuous, normally distributed.

It is beyond the scope of this chapter to explain how to select variables appropriately to be added in the linear regression (also called *model selection*).

Parametric versus Non-Parametric Tests

In Chapter 10 we will discuss non-parametric tests that are used when not all assumptions necessary for the application of parametric tests are met.

The challenge of selecting the right statistical test is not just to understand the difference between each test, but also, what endpoint will be assessed. This case will give an example of how the process of selecting the study design, study endpoint, and the statistical test are intertwined.

How Should One Interpret Results from Statistical Software?

After reading these initial sections, the investigator needs to know then when to use these tests appropriately. (If there are still some problems in understanding dependent versus independent variables or normal distribution, please refer to Chapter 2.)

The next step is then organizing the spreadsheet with the data appropriately to be imported in the statistical software. The good news is that most of the statistical softwares accept direct import from Excel spreadsheet. It is important to organize the variables in the column. For instance, each variable should have only one column. However, it becomes a bit more complicated when it is repeated measures, meaning the same variable is collected twice at different moments from the same subject. In this case, most of the packages would still be designed to have one variable for the outcome only, and then another variable to define time of assessment. In the following we give an example for each of the three tests: t-test (unpaired and paired), ANOVA, and linear regression, using two statistical packages: STATA and SPSS.

Let's consider the following scenario: you are investigating the effect of two new antihypertensive drugs in your hospital, drugs X and Y. Your main outcome is the patient's final systolic blood pressure, measured in mmHg. Therefore, your independent (explanatory) variable is categorical, while your dependent variable (outcome) is continuous.

Comparing Two Means: TTest

Comparing two independent groups (unpaired t-test)

Entering Data

It is important to input data correctly in order to run the analysis. Each variable should have its own column. Here, the first column represents the drugs being tested (1 and 2, which represent drugs X and Y, respectively), while the second column portrays the patient's blood pressure (BP) after taking the medication.

	Drug	BP
1	1	120
2	2	110
3	1	115
4	1	140
5	1	137
6	2	112
7	1	109
8	2	133
9	2	120
10	2	125

Choosing the Analysis Test

You can perform the analysis by using the software MENU. Select the following options:

Statistics > Summaries, tables and tests > Classical tests of hypothesis > t test (mean-comparison test)

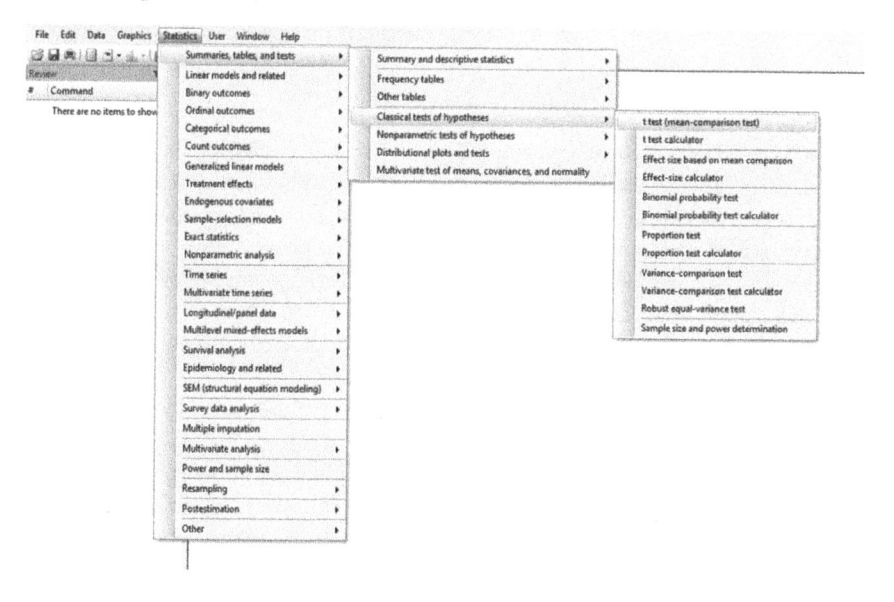

Running the Analysis

When running the analysis, the software will display some options of t-test from which to choose. Since at this moment you are comparing means of two separate, independent groups (group taking drug X and group taking drug Y), you can select the second option, *two-sample using groups*. Next, it is important to identify correctly where to place the dependent variable (outcome: BP) and the independent/explanatory variable (intervention: Drug), which can also be defined as the group variable. At last, you can choose your desired confidence interval (which generally will be 95%).

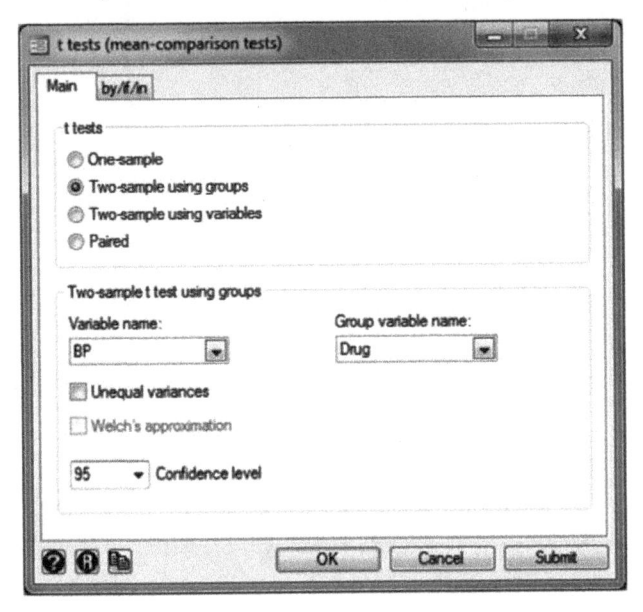

Interpreting the Output

The output shows the two-sample t test. The software will initially provide the descriptive statistics (second row), with the mean, standard error, and standard deviation for each group, as well as the 95% confidence interval. Next, the same information regarding summary statistics is provided for the entire sample, with no separation between groups (third row—*combined*) and for the difference between groups (fourth row—*diff*).

Subsequently, the *Null hypothesis is provided (Ho: dif = 0)*: There is no difference in systolic blood pressure for patients taking drugs X and Y. The t statistic (0.5651) and the number of degrees of freedom (8) are also shown.

At the bottom of the table there are three options for alternative hypotheses. The generally used alternative is located in the center (1): this is the two sided-hypothesis, in which the investigator is testing simply if the difference between groups is not equal to 0 (there is no directionality). In this case, you would fail to reject the null hypothesis, therefore concluding no difference in BP between groups ($p = 0.5875$).

In some cases, the investigator may be interested in testing a one-sided hypothesis, meaning that two different tests can be undertaken: you can test if the difference between group means is smaller than zero (left), or if the difference between groups is larger than zero (right). For both of these tests the result is also non-significant

(p = 0.7062 and 0.2938, respectively), once again concluding no difference in BP between groups.

```
. ttest BP, by(Drug)

Two-sample t test with equal variances
```

Group	Obs	Mean	Std. Err.	Std. Dev.	[95% Conf. Interval]
1	5	124.2	6.110646	13.66382	107.2341 141.1659
2	5	120	4.230839	9.460444	108.2533 131.7467
combined	10	122.1	3.572892	11.29848	114.0176 130.1824
diff		4.2	7.432362		-12.93906 21.33906

```
    diff = mean(1) - mean(2)                                      t =   0.5651
Ho: diff = 0    Null hypothesis               degrees of freedom =        8

   Ha: diff < 0                Ha: diff != 0                  Ha: diff > 0
 Pr(T < t) = 0.7062         Pr(|T| > |t|) = 0.5875          Pr(T > t) = 0.2938
```

Comparing within a Group (Paired T-Test)

Now, instead of comparing the effect of the drugs on blood pressure between two independent groups, imagine you want to evaluate the change in blood pressure before and after the treatment in the same group (for instance, patients taking drug X). In this case, the comparison happens within the group at different time points, not between two different groups.

Entering Data

In the paired comparison, data has to be organized differently in the database, since the outcome is shown in two columns, separated by time of assessment. Here, two new variables have to be inserted, representing the different time points in which data will be analyzed (BPpre and BPpost, representing the systolic blood pressure before and after taking drug X, respectively). Each horizontal line represents one patient.

BPpre	BPpost
130	120
140	115
120	110
150	140
137	137
133	112
120	112
143	106
120	120
140	115

Choosing the Analysis Test

You can perform the analysis by using the software MENU. Select the following options:
Statistics > Summaries, tables and tests > Classical tests of hypothesis > t test (mean-comparison test)

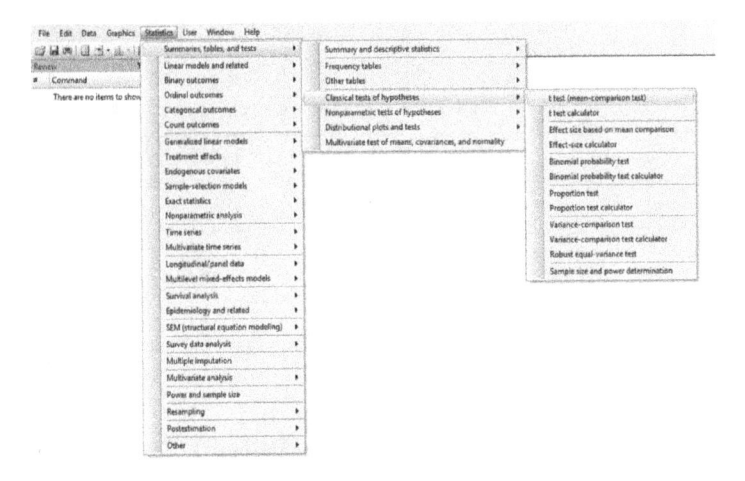

Running the Analysis

When running the analysis, the software will display some options of t-test from which to choose. Since at this moment you are comparing means within the same group (patients who are taking drug X), you can select the last option, *Paired*. Differently from what happened with the t-test for independent groups (unpaired analysis), the software will request a "first variable" and a "second variable," where blood pressure before taking the drug (BPpre) and blood pressure after taking the drug (BPpost) should be inserted (same measurement at different time points). At last, you can choose your desired confidence interval (which generally will be 95%).

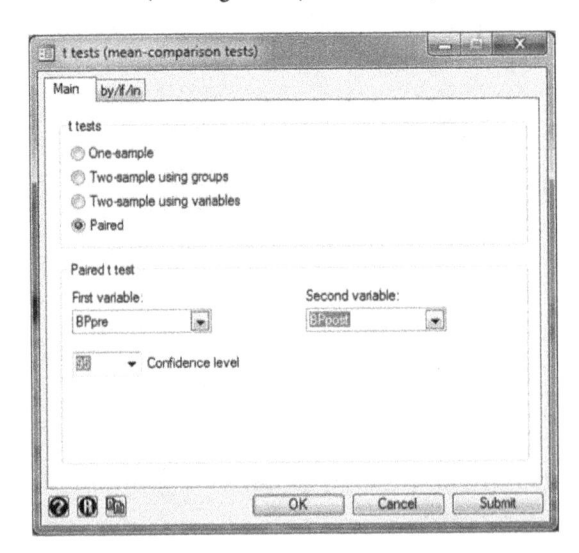

Interpreting the Output

The interpretation of the output for the paired t-test is very similar to the interpretation of the unpaired t-test, given the difference in application. The software will initially provide the descriptive statistics (second row), with the mean, standard error, and standard deviation for the two different time moments (BPpre and BPpost) as well as the 95% confidence interval. Next, the same information regarding summary statistics is provided for the difference between groups (third row—*diff*).

Subsequently, the *null hypothesis is provided* (Ho: dif = 0), stating that there is no difference in systolic blood pressure before and after taking drug X (BPpre = BPpost). The t statistic (3.8528) and the number of degrees of freedom (9) are also shown.

At the bottom of the table there are three options for alternative hypotheses. The generally used alternative is located in the center (1): this is the two sided-hypothesis, in which the investigator is testing simply if the difference between BP before and after is equal to 0 (there is no directionality). In this case, you would reject the null hypothesis, therefore concluding that drug X is able to significantly modify blood pressure ($p = 0.0039$)

In some cases, the investigator may be interested in testing one-sided hypothesis, meaning that two different tests can be undertaken: you can test if the difference in BP between the two moments is smaller than zero (left) or larger than 0 (right). In this scenario, the alternative hypothesis on the right (2) was significant, meaning that mean blood pressure before was significantly larger than blood pressure after the medication. We can therefore conclude that the drug is effective.

```
. ttest BPpre == BPpost
```

Paired t test

Variable	Obs	Mean	Std. Err.	Std. Dev.	[95% Conf. Interval]
BPpre	10	133.3	3.363365	10.63589	125.6915 140.9085
BPpost	10	118.7	3.568535	11.2847	110.6274 126.7726
diff	10	14.6	3.789459	11.98332	6.027648 23.17235

mean(diff) = mean(BPpre - BPpost)   t = 3.8528
Ho: mean(diff) = 0   Null hypothesis   degrees of freedom = 9

Ha: mean(diff) < 0	Ha: mean(diff) != 0	Ha: mean(diff) > 0
Pr(T < t) = 0.9981	Pr(|T| > |t|) = 0.0039	Pr(T > t) = 0.0019
	1	2

Comparing Three or More Means (ANOVA)

Now consider that you are also interested in the anti-hypertensive effects of a third drug that was recently launched in the market, drug Z. Since the unpaired t-test only enables comparison between two groups, a different statistical test has to be used to compare a larger amount of groups. In this case, the ANOVA test would be the most appropriate option.

Entering Data

Here, instead of analyzing solely drugs X and Y, blood pressure measurements for drug Z will also be imputed, since the purpose is to compare the differences between the three groups. The first column includes drugs X, Y, Z (1, 2, and 3, respectively), while the second column includes patients' systolic blood pressure after taking the medication.

	Drug	BP
1	1	115
2	2	90
3	2	133
4	3	95
5	1	140
6	2	125
7	3	95
8	2	112
9	1	137
10	3	100
11	3	100
12	2	120
13	1	120
14	3	102
15	1	109

Choosing the Analysis Test

You can perform the analysis by using the software MENU. Select the following options:

Statistics > Linear models and related > ANOVA/MANOVA > One-way ANOVA (note that if you want to do a two[or more]-way ANOVA, you need to select another option.

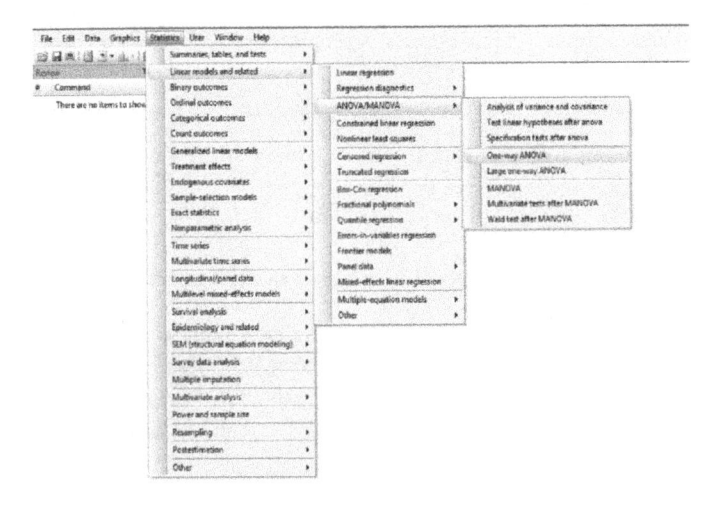

Running the Analysis

When running the analysis, the software will ask for two variables: the "response variable" and the "factor variable." The response variable can be seen as the outcome, the dependent variable that is being analyzed, while the factor variable is the independent variable. Therefore, blood pressure (BP) should be inserted in the first box, while Drug is inserted in the second box. Options for performing multiple-comparison tests are also provided.

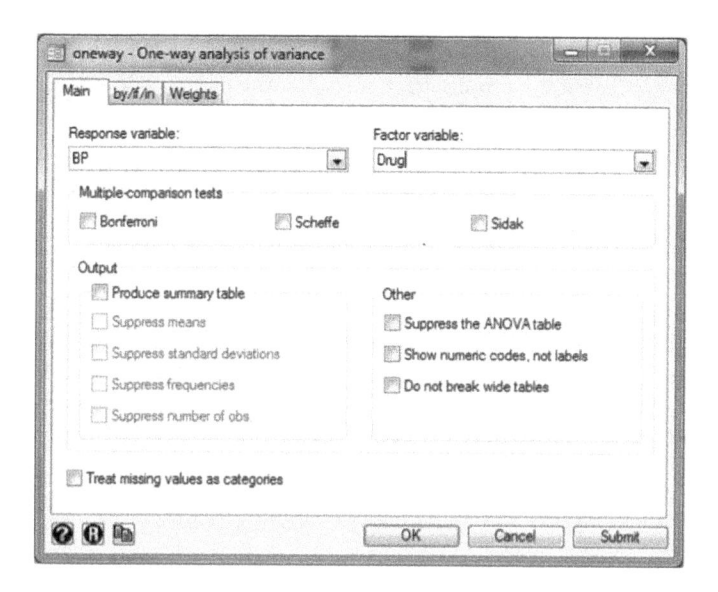

Interpreting the Output

The output for the ANOVA test is relatively simple to interpret. In this case, the null hypothesis states that blood pressure means are equal throughout the three groups.

The result indicates that there is a significant difference between at least two of the blood pressure means of the three groups (drugs X, Y, Z), with a p-value of 0.0193 (<0.05). As previously mentioned, ANOVA is not able to specify which of the group or groups were responsible for this difference, as this is a global test. Pairwise analysis in post hoc testing (e.g., Turkey's method) is therefore necessary in order to have this information (refer to software steps later in the chapter). Additionally, the software provides the sum of squares (SS), degrees of freedom (df), and the mean squares (MS), which are used to calculate the F statistic, leading ultimately to the p-value.

. oneway BP Drug

	Analysis of Variance				
Source	SS	df	MS	F	Prob > F
Between groups	1737.73333	2	868.866667	5.59	0.0193
Within groups	1866	12	155.5		
Total	3603.73333	14	257.409524		

p-value

Additionally, in case the investigator wants to pursue pairwise testing, the MENU pathway is stated here:

Statistics > Summaries, tables and tests > Summary and descriptive statistics > Pairwise comparison of means.

Linear Regression

Finally, consider that you are now interested in looking only at the effect of drug X in blood pressure levels when compared to placebo. However, at this time, you want to adjust for other covariates, such gender and age. For this purpose, linear regression is the most suitable test, since it enables adjustment for covariates. By doing so, your purpose is to obtain results that will provide an unbiased estimate of the treatment effect.

Entering Data

In order to run a linear regression, the database has to be organized with your independent variables (continuous and categorical outcomes) and dependent variable (continuous outcome). Since the software will not recognize letters (e.g., X, Y, and Z) or words (e.g., female or male), variables have to be coded in order for the analysis to be performed. In this case, drug X is coded as 1, while placebo is coded as 0. Likewise, females are coded 0, while males are coded 1. Each column represents a different variable, while each row represents an individual patient (total of 30 patients).

	Age	Sex	Drug	BP
1	56	0	1	131
2	59	1	0	135
3	34	0	1	115
4	40	1	1	130
5	58	0	1	137
6	31	1	0	146
7	4	1	1	143
8	52	1	0	112
9	35	1	1	122
10	67	0	0	127
11	45	0	1	128
12	41	1	0	122
13	57	0	1	113
14	49	1	0	151
15	40	0	1	131
16	55	0	0	115
17	51	1	1	119
18	47	0	0	129
19	53	1	1	121
20	47	0	0	120
21	56	1	1	121
22	54	0	1	123
23	53	1	1	134
24	47	1	1	131
25	45	0	0	136
26	38	1	1	113
27	59	0	0	136
28	5	1	1	125
29	39	0	0	128
30	55	1	1	117

Choosing the Analysis Test

You can perform the analysis by using the software MENU. Select the following options: Statistics > Linear models and related > Linear Regression

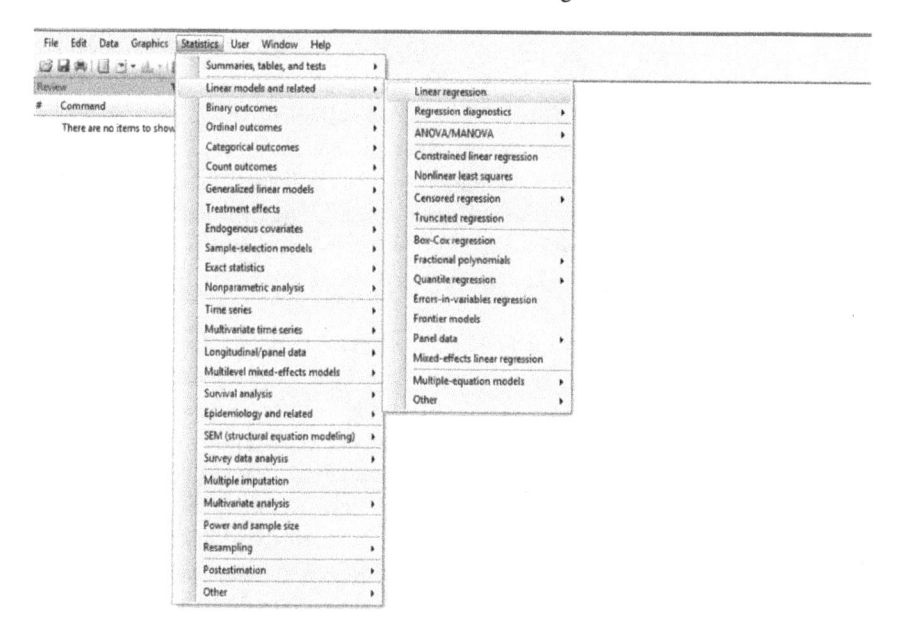

Running the Analysis

When running the analysis, the software will provide a box for the dependent variable (outcome) and the independent variables (predictors) you want to insert in your model. In this case, blood pressure (continuous outcome) is inserted as the dependent variable, while the age, sex, and the intervention drug (X or placebo) are inserted as the independent variables.

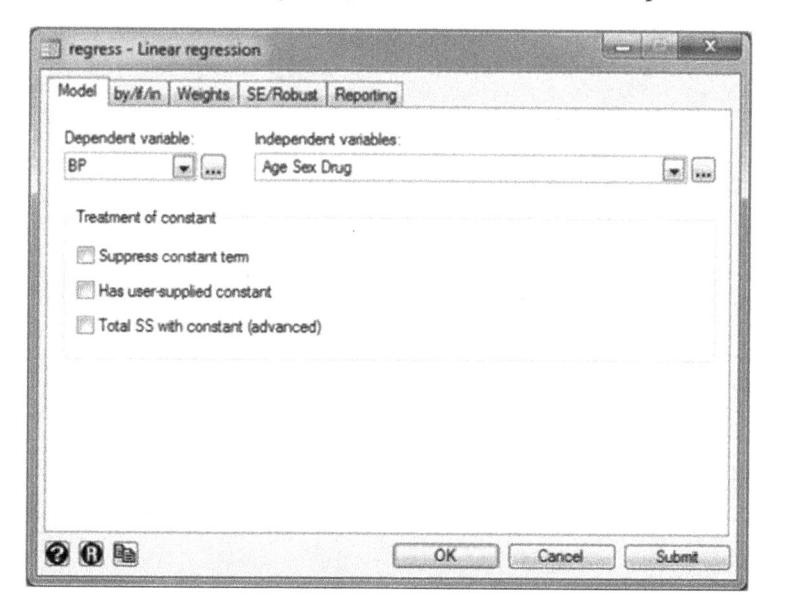

Interpreting the Output

The output for linear regression will initally provide descriptive statistics for the model, including the sum of squares (SS), degrees of freedom (df), and mean squares (MS). The number of observations (30) is stated on the right, as well as the R-squared. The R-squared represents how much of the variance of the outcome can be explained by your model (how useful the predictors are). In this case, only 10% of the variance in blood pressure can be explained by the independent variables. The adjusted R-square has the same meaning, but takes into account the number of variables that are inserted in the analysis. On the bottom of the output, the key independent variable (Drug) and all the other covariates you are interested in investigating (Age and Sex) are listed in the left column, as well as the constant for the regression equation. For each of the variables, the β coefficient, standard error, T statistic, p-value, and 95% confidence interval are provided.

The β coefficient represents the increase or decrease in the predicted value of the dependent variable (outcome) for a 1-unit increase in the explanatory variable (predictor). For instance, in case there was statistical significance for age, for every additional year, there would be a decrease of 0.15 mmHg in blood pressure, adjusted for all the other covariates. In the case of categorical variables, this interpretation changes slightly, since values are only 0 or 1. Therefore, a 1-unit increase represents switching from one group to another. The group coded 0 is considered the reference group (females), while males are coded 1. Therefore, based on the output results, if sex was statistically significant, males would be expected to have a blood pressure 1.03 mmHg higher than females, adjusted for all the other covariates.

What you are interested in here is knowing if there is evidence of a linear relationship between your explanatory variable (Drug) and the response variable (BP), while controlling for the other explanatory variables (Age and Sex). In this case, no significance was found for any of the explanatory variables.

. regress BP Age Sex Drug

Source	SS	df	MS		
Model	302.25984	3	100.75328	Number of obs =	30
Residual	2588.70683	26	99.5656472	$F(3, 26)$ =	1.01
				Prob > F =	0.4033
				R-squared =	0.1046
				Adj R-squared =	0.0012
Total	2890.96667	29	99.6885057	Root MSE =	9.9783

BP	Coef.	Std. Err.	t	P>|t|	[95% Conf. Interval]	
Age	-.1529706	.1393789	-1.10	0.282	-.439468	.1335269
Sex	1.037524	3.867191	0.27	0.791	-6.911601	8.986649
Drug	-5.626096	3.837414	-1.47	0.155	-13.51401	2.261822
_cons	136.8515	8.00353	17.10	0.000	120.4	153.303

CENTRAL LIMIT THEOREM

Checking for data normality may not always give consistent results, as it depends on some level of interpretation (looking at normality plots or performing statistical normality tests). One potential option for investigators working with large sample sizes is to use the central limit theorem to support for normal distribution.

The central limit theorem states that, when dealing with large sample sizes, the sample mean of a random, independent variable can be assumed as nearly normal. Additionally, as the sample N increases, the distribution of the sample mean will increasingly resemble a normal distribution. And what can be considered a *large* sample size? Definitions vary, but a sample size of 60–100 (or higher) can generally be considered as having a sample mean that is approximately normal.

SPSS SOFTWARE

In the SPSS software, you can use the MENU to select the three different analyses. Here we provide the sequence of commands that should be selected.

Unpaired T-Test (Independent Means)

Analyze > Compare means > 2 Independent Samples

Paired T-Test

Analyze > Compare means > Paired Sample T Test

One-Way ANOVA

Analyze > Compare means > One-Way ANOVA

Linear Regression

Analyze > Regression > Linear

CASE STUDY 9: TO T OR NOT TO T? CHOOSING THE STATISTICAL QUESTION

André Brunoni and Felipe Fregni

It is late in the evening and Dr. Maurizio Manetti is walking back home after another strenuous day of work. While he walks through the narrow sidewalks of downtown Milan, his thoughts are concentrated on an important step in his career: decreasing clinical work and dedicating more time to research. This has been his dream since he started; however, financial and family pressures have prevented him from doing so until recently. Nevertheless, he now thinks that the right moment has come, and he feels exhilarated with this feeling of change.[1]

Dr. Manetti is a senior professor and researcher at Ospedale Maggiore in Milan. In fact, Dr. Manetti started to work there as soon as he finished his orthopedic residency 35 years ago, and both his students and coworkers recognize him as a very competent and trustworthy professor. As time has passed, though, he has grown a bit tired of performing surgeries, as he feels that his body no longer has the same strength to hold up for several hours during complicated operations; his legs start to fade and his eyes start to blur. In addition, his dream when he started medical school was to become a scientist like his grandfather—a famous Italian microbiologist.

During the last five years, he has begun to finally appreciate the joy of doing clinical research. In fact, clinical research has dramatically changed since the times when Dr. Manetti was trained. For him, clinical research was done with a microscope in a laboratory, and he used to underestimate research in clinical practice ("It is not some numbers on a fancy computer program that will tell me what to do with my patients"). But now his thoughts have changed—especially since three years ago, when he took two sabbatical years to move to Boston with his family for a master's degree in clinical research, a good experience for him, where he made some good friends and established several contacts with researchers around the world.

The Trial

Dr. Manetti had decided that he wanted to spend his last years before retiring doing clinical research. He set up an orthopedic laboratory and started doing clinical research in the field of knee surgery, which used to be one of his preferred surgeries. He is especially interested in developing new treatments for alleviating postoperative pain, and particularly, a new opioid agonist (OXY004) with high affinity for opioid receptors, which seems to have a greater analgesic potency as compared with its related compound morphine. This drug is under regulatory board review, as it has been shown to be safe and efficacious for the treatment of acute pain, but has not been

---

[1] Dr. André Brunoni and Professor Felipe Fregni prepared this case. Course cases are developed solely as the basis for class discussion. The situation in this case is fictional. Cases are not intended to serve as endorsements or sources of primary data. All rights reserved to the author of this case. Reproduction and distribution without permission is not allowed.

evaluated for the treatment of postoperative pain. In addition, its immediate release form (IR) is an attractive alternative for this type of pain. Therefore, he decided to investigate the use of OXY004-IR for the treatment of postoperative pain in outpatients undergoing knee arthroscopy.

This idea has been developed together with other professors in the United Kingdom, the United States, and Brazil. Dr. Manetti decided to set up a workshop to take place in Milan and invited his colleagues. After a very warm reception and two days of intensive and productive debate, Dr. Manetti and his colleagues agreed on the terms of the trial. The initial plan was to conduct a multicenter, double-blind, randomized, placebo-controlled study in which patients are randomized to receive OXY004-IR or placebo hourly as needed for up to eight hours after the surgery to reduce pain (and in addition to standard analgesic therapy). The main outcome is the sum of pain intensity (as assessed by VAS—visual analog scale) during these initial eight hours of post-surgery. In VAS the patient quantifies the amount of pain he or she is feeling in a linear grade from 0 to 10 (a reason why VAS is considered a continuous rating scale). Regarding the ethical issues, the institutional review boards agreed with this study as placebo was offered for a short period only (8 hours), with no risk of the condition worsening due to lack of analgesic, and patients could also decide to take other medications if they wished to (but in this case they would be eliminated from the analysis). Also, patients would be prescribed standard analgesic medication.

The calculated sample size was 100 patients—25 patients for each center. This sample size would be sufficient to use parametric tests, even if data are not normally distributed due to the central limit theorem, but they are also prepared to normalize the data using logarithmic transformations if the data are excessively skewed. However, even after these two days of meetings, they are still unsure which statistical test to choose for the primary outcome.

Choosing the Statistical Test

Although the choice of statistical test depends on the research question, it is important to know the characteristics of the statistical test so as to understand the limitations and advantages of each test, and also to adjust the study design and choose the most optimal research question considering the resources and study feasibility. For instance, if the researcher wants to use linear regression, he or she needs to know the limitations of using this test, such as the assumptions associated with it (for instance, requirement of normal distribution) and also the sample size requirements. Therefore, an important step is the statistical analysis plan that needs to be done a priori (unless the investigators plan to conduct an exploratory trial). Thus, researchers need to determine the dependent and independent variables. The dependent variable is the outcome of the study (in this case, pain), and the independent variables are the factors of the study (in this case, one of the independent variables is the group—active drug or placebo). Another important characteristic is whether the data are categorical (and number of categories) or continuous. With this information, the investigator can choose the analysis plan and therefore be able to adjust his or her study design and research question.

After the two intensive days of work, the group of investigators decided to make this final decision (choosing the statistical test) at a nice dinner at an outstanding Italian restaurant near Corso Vittorio Emanuele II.

"The Antipasti"—Simple Comparison and Use of T-Test?

Dr. Manetti's colleagues are delighted with the mouthwatering meal they are about to eat. Dr. Robert Wood, a researcher from Seattle, has just chosen the *antipasti* and is now expressing his opinion, "I think our primary endpoint should be calculated by a simple comparison between the two groups eight hours after surgery—meaning that I think we should use an unpaired t-test. Our alternative hypothesis should be that active OXY004-IR would significantly reduce pain more than placebo—this is precisely what we want to prove. So we should not use complicated statistical tests—we have 100 patients and they will be randomized, which should be enough to balance them equally among the groups. And we know (from other studies) that the peak of post-surgical pain is in the first eight hours, so I think we can use the sum of pain as our endpoint. In addition, t-test is a fairly robust test that can also tolerate some degree of non-normality. Finally, I am not arguing that we should not do other statistical tests or perform other comparisons, but these should be secondary outcomes—I have a strong opinion that the primary endpoint should be as simple as it can be."

"So, the question is to t or not to t, my dear Bob," replied Professor Theodore McGrath, head of the Orthopedics Department of King's College in London and an old friend of Dr. Manetti (who deeply appreciates his British sense of humor).

"Primo Piatto": More Independent Variables and Use of ANOVA

They were now having the *primo piatto*: pasta for some, risotto for others. Professor McGrath continued, while eating his *spaghetti all'amatriciana*, "I am afraid the answer is not to t—we ought not to use t tests in our study as a primary outcome, and the reason is precisely because I think we have better options. I am particularly afraid of selecting just one time point to measure our primary outcome—sum of pain during the first eight hours might not capture the effects of this drug, as I hypothesize that in the first two or three hours after surgery, both groups would have the same results due to an initial strong placebo effect. However, during hours 3 to 8, the active group would then behave differently as the placebo effect would decrease due to lack of active drug. Therefore, I think we need to do an analysis that accounts for pain measurements after every hour (at 1h, 2h . . . 7h, and 8h)—because if we sum everything for the t-test approach, we would lose this important information in our analysis. For that, we would use a repeated- measures ANOVA model, with VAS as the dependent variable, and time and group as independent variables—'time' would have eight levels and 'group' two levels ('active' and 'placebo'). Naturally, our alternative hypothesis would be that 'the time vs. group' interaction effect is significant. Then we should use post hoc statistical tests to explore our data further and to compare the effects of active versus placebo at different time levels."

Professor McGrath stopped talking just when the secondo piatto arrived: Milan"s specialty, *cotoletta alla milanese*. They ate in silence, savoring each bite of the delicious food.

"Secondo Piatto": Controlling for Important Covariates—Use of Linear Regression

Dr. Patricia Carvalho, a Brazilian researcher with many years of expertise, decided to speak only when they all had finished eating. She said, "Theodore and Bob certainly have good arguments. I liked the simple design Bob proposed, although I have the same concerns as Theodore. However, Theodore, you must concede that your statistical model can undermine our study power, especially if we use factors with multiple levels and start performing several post-hoc comparisons between them. I am certain you remember our classes on this topic, so you know that such an approach will increase both the probabilities of type I and type II errors. Therefore, I propose that we go back to the original plan of having pain summed during these eight hours. But I am not comfortable with t-tests, as I am very concerned with some of the covariates that may confound our results—one of them is study center and the other is age. Peer reviewers and academics might question this issue, which I also think is important. Therefore, I propose using a linear regression, covarying by each center (Rio de Janeiro, Seattle, London, and Milan) and also by age. This would be similar to running an ANCOVA (analysis of covariance). I understand that this adds complications to our study design and can reduce the power of our analysis. However, if I am right, controlling for center and age would indeed decrease the variance and therefore might instead increase the power of our study. I believe this is necessary—as these two factors might be confounding variables. We could of course still use Theodore's idea and add these variables we want to control in Theodore's repeated measures model; however, as you also know, this model would not allow too many covariates due to small sample size. Therefore, using my option, we can save some statistical power to control for the variable 'study center.' Maurizio, what do you think?"

Dr. Manetti had not spoken yet. As a good host, he listened to his colleagues' ideas first and thought about each one carefully. "Well, I think you should try the tiramisu. It is easier to think with a sweet taste in your mouth. And, after that, we should have a good Italian coffee. Patricia, I believe you will prefer a lungo, as that is the way you take espressos in Brazil. Bob, you should try a lungo or an americano as well. And Theodore, they do have tea here, if you prefer."

Dr. Wood could not miss the chance, "So the question is: to tea or not to tea, Theodore?" They all laughed. Professor McGrath said, "To tea or not to tea . . . fair enough . . . I really want to make a point here, so no t test and no tea . . . I would go for a machiatto." By the time the night was over, they all felt it was a wonderful dinner and a fantastic meeting. By the next morning, their last meeting, they know they are surely going to achieve a consensus on the best statistical method for their primary outcome after a good night of sleep in gorgeous Milan.

CASE DISCUSSION

This is a classical case in which a study design may give different options of analysis. The investigator needs to be aware that the final decision of the design will impact the variables selected for their study and how they will be treated. This will also affect the power and sample size of a given study. In this example, to be didactic we consider the main options of statistical tests, but if this were a confirmatory study, the investigator would need to have its main question well defined, and that definition will indicate the direction of which test is most appropriate. This reflects, therefore, the importance of defining the research question and how that definition can affect the statistical tests to be used.

CASE QUESTIONS FOR REFLECTION

1. What challenges do Dr. Manetti and colleagues face in choosing the statistical test to be used in this trial?
2. What are their main concerns?

FURTHER READING

Papers

- Vickers AJ. Analysis of variance is easily misapplied in the analysis of randomized trials: a critique and discussion of alternative statistical approaches. *Psychosom. Med.* 2005; 67:652–655. https://insights.ovid.com/pubmed?pmid=16046383
  Online Statistical Tests

- http://statpages.org/

Books

- Feinstein AR. *Medical statistics*. Boca Raton, London, New York, Washington, DC: Chapman & Hall/CRC; 2002.
- Mc Clave JT, Sincich R. *Statistics*, 11th ed. Upper Saddle River, NJ: Pearson/Prentice Hall; 2009.
- De Veaux RD, Velleman PF, Bock DE. *Stats:data and models*, 3rd ed. Boston: Addison-Wesley/Pearson; 2009.
- Rosner. *Fundamentals of biostatistics*. Seventh Edition, Harvard University, Boston, MA: Brooks/Cole, Cengage Learning; 2010.

Webpages

http://flowingdata.com/
www.phdcomics.com/comics.php

REFERENCES

1. Page EB. Ordered hypotheses for multiple treatments: a significance test for linear ranks. JASA. 1963; 58(301): 216–230.

2. Demšar J. Statistical comparisons of classifiers over multiple data sets. *J Mach Learn Res.* 2006; 7(Jan): 1–30.
3. Salvi S, Vaidya A, Kodgule R, Gogtay J. A randomized, double-blind study comparing the efficacy and safety of a combination of formoterol and ciclesonide with ciclesonide alone in asthma subjects with moderate-to-severe airflow limitation. *Lung India* [Internet]. 2016; 33(3): 272–277. Available from: http://www.embase.com/search/results?subaction=viewrecord&from=export&id=L610379852\nhttp://dx.doi.org/10.4103/0970-2113.180803\nhttp://sfxhosted.exlibrisgroup.com/sfxtul?sid=EMBASE&issn=0974598X&id=doi:10.4103%2F0970-2113.180803&atitle=A+randomized%2C+doub
4. Carver R. The case against statistical significance testing. *Harvard Educ Rev.* 1978; 48(3): 378–399.
5. Sackett DL. Why randomized controlled trials fail but needn't: 2. Failure to employ physiological statistics, or the only formula a clinician-trialist is ever likely to need (or understand!). *CMAJ.* 2001 Oct 30; 165(9): 1226–1237. [PMID: 11706914]

10

NON-PARAMETRIC STATISTICAL TESTS

Authors: *Felipe Fregni and Fernanda Lopes*

Case study authors: *Suely R. Matsubayashi and Felipe Fregni*

INTRODUCTION

Another important class of statistical tests is *non-parametric tests*. The term *non-parametric* indicates a class of statistical tests that does not make any assumption regarding the distribution of the data. In fact, the other class of statistical tests discussed previously, parametric tests (i.e., t-test or ANOVA), requires that data are normally distributed and also that population variances are equal.

As non-parametric tests do not have any assumptions regarding distribution and variance of the data, it is indeed safer to use these tests correctly. A non-parametric test will always be valid. However, the investigator should not simply use these tests in order to select a valid test, as non-parametric tests may have less power to detect significant differences when data are normally distributed and variances are roughly equal. For instance, when using a non-parametric test, the loss of power compared to the optimal parametric test corresponds to a loss of 5% in the sample size. Thus not choosing the most effective test may indeed increase the type II error of a study.

The investigator therefore needs to choose, first, a valid statistical test and, second, the test that is also the most effective (i.e., has more power). However, this decision is not simple, as there are several situations in clinical research when it is not easy to determine what is the degree of non-normality that is accepted in order to consider that data are not normally distributed (in order to choose a non-parametric test).

Besides data that are not normally distributed, there is another situation that requires the use of non-parametrical tests: when data are classified as ordinal data rather than continuous data. *Ordinal data*, as reviewed in Chapter 8, indicates data that have order but the interval between two units has no meaning (for instance, symptom classification as poor, satisfactory, good, and outstanding). In this situation a statistical test that analyzes data as rank (or non-parametric tests) is required.

Similarly, in some situations it may not be easy to determine with certainty that a given variable cannot be classified as continuous. We will discuss some examples in the following. Here we suggest that whenever there is a situation in which there is no clear indication, the investigator needs to consider the conservative approach and choose the non-parametric option.

The final important issue is that the investigator should not choose the statistical test that provides the best result. Although the investigator needs to choose the most effective test (across the valid options), this decision needs to be made a priori, without looking at the data. If this decision comes after the investigator runs the statistical tests, then the analyses become exploratory and thus need to be acknowledged.

First we will discuss and give examples of situations in which a non-parametric test should be chosen, and then discuss each statistical test separately. The non-parametric tests that will be discussed in this initial section are Mann-Whitney (Wilcoxon Rank Sum), Wilcoxon Sign Rank, and Kruskal-Wallis. Although the names of these tests make them appear to be complicated, they are, quite the opposite, relatively simple tests to use and understand.

WHEN SHOULD NON-PARAMETRIC TESTS BE USED?

Here we will discuss when non-parametric tests should be chosen and used. We consider two conditions: (1) comparing two or more groups with continuous outcome that is not normally distributed; (2) comparing two or more groups with ordinal outcome.

Comparing Two or More Groups with Continuous Outcome That Is Not Normally Distributed

The first important category of use is when the investigator is comparing the results of two or more groups of treatments (or group of subjects) and the outcome is continuous (meaning that data is measured in a continuous scale in which the interval between units are constant and meaningful); however, the outcome is not normally distributed.

This scenario usually occurs with studies of small sample sizes in which it is not possible to determine whether data are normally distributed or not. Nevertheless, there is no fixed number to define what needs to be considered as a small sample size. For instance, groups of six or less are usually recommended to be analyzed as non-parametric data.

There are several examples in the literature.

1. For instance, Luurila et al. evaluated the effect of erythromycin on the pharmacokinetics and pharmacodynamics of diazepam. Six subjects ingested erythromycin for one week, and on day 4 they ingested a dose of diazepam. All pharmacokinetic and pharmacodynamic parameters were compared within the group using the Wilcoxon matched pairs test, not a t-test [1].
2. Bopp et al. evaluated if intubated critical care unit (CCU) patients who received twice-daily oral hygiene care with 0.12% chlorhexidine gluconate had less pneumonia incidence than those who received the standard oral care. Authors reported that the small sample size prohibited the use of parametric statistical analysis or hypothesis testing [2].
3. In a study to test the efficacy of a specific oral medication in patients with Sjögren's syndrome, Khurshudian et al. randomized patients to receive either 150 IU of interferon—(8 patients) or placebo (4 patients) for 24 weeks, with 6-week re-evaluations. Whole saliva (continuous outcome) was measured during each visit, and symptoms were assessed by questionnaires and visual analog scales. The

Wilcoxon Sign Rank test was used to detect significant changes for each of the evaluated variables [3].
4. In the study by Cruz-Correa et al. [4], five patients with familial adenomatous polyposis with prior colectomy received supplements with curcumin 480 mg and quercetin 20 mg orally 3 times a day. The number and size of polyps were assessed at baseline and after therapy. The Wilcoxon Sign Rank test was used to determine differences in the number and size of polyps.

One of the challenging issues is that when sample size is too small, non-parametric tests are also ineffective. For instance, in order to use a non-parametric test such as Kruskal-Wallis, it has been reported that no group should have fewer than five subjects in order to have an accurate estimation [5–7]. But because of the small sample, parametric tests are also not indicated. Therefore the investigator needs to consider the utility of running a small sample size given that inference statistics will likely not be valid. There are other reasons to run a small pilot study, which is beyond the scope of this chapter.

For samples that are large enough, the central limit theorem could be invoked to support the use of a normal distribution. It is also beyond the scope of this chapter to explain the theory of central limit theorem, but samples over 70 subjects (some authors say 100 or 200) usually are considered large enough to support the use of parametric tests.

For samples in the middle, or not as small and not as large, then the tests to determine normality of distribution are important to verify whether data are normally distributed or not. There are several tests to determine distribution, from statistical tests such as Wilk-Shapiro tests to graphical representation (histograms) and analysis of parameters (mean, median, kurtosis, and skewness).

As the reader will come to understand, methods to determine whether data are normally distributed or not may not be clear-cut. Again, as recommended earlier, in the case where there is not a clear-cut response, we recommend the use of non-parametric tests.

Comparing Two or More Groups with Ordinal Outcome

The other important indication for the use of non-parametric tests comes when the variable is an ordinal variable. A classical example of an ordinal variable is, for instance, classifying symptoms as "very poor," "poor," "satisfactory," "good," "very good." In this case, it is clear that there is an order, but there is no regular interval. In fact, a numerical representation of these five categories would not be appropriate. Although using tests for categorical data is an option, this option would disregard the information of the order and thus would be less effective.

In this case, the non-parametric tests discussed in this chapter are the most appropriate. Although this seems logical and the researcher would not have difficulties in understanding and applying non-parametric tests, it is not common to have these simple ordinal scales as shown here. Most of the time, these ordinal scales are part of a multi-question instrument in which each question contains an ordinal-constructed question. In these instruments (an example would be the highly used Beck Depression Inventory (BDI)), the final score is a sum of all the items. Because of this sum, most researchers consider that it has quantitative properties to be considered a continuous outcome.

There is, in fact, an intense debate regarding whether these instruments that sum up individual ordinal items can be considered a continuous outcome [8–10]. Defenders of this strategy support that when summed, this creates intervals that are similar enough to continuous data and that therefore can be analyzed with parametric tests. For instance, if BDI is considered an interval scale, then a change from 10 to 15 points on the scale would correspond to the same magnitude as a change from 20 to 25 points. On the other hand, the opposite side says that recoding the sum of ordinal items into a simple numerical value is illegitimate, since the interval between the scores cannot be considered as equivalent and it is difficult to determine constancy. This group believes that the process disrupts the relationship between the scale and the information that it portrays. Additionally, they argue that previous research has shown inconsistent results and errors when using means, Pearson's correlation r, and standard deviations with ordinal data.

Again as discussed previously, in cases where there is not a clear consensus and the investigator does not feel that he or she has all the information needed to make an appropriate decision, it may be worthwhile to be conservative and use a non-parametric test. We have cited some references that may help if this is an important issue for your field of research.

WHAT DO I NEED TO KNOW IN ORDER TO USE THESE TESTS PROPERLY?

This is an interesting question, as by definition non-parametric tests have less assumptions, and likely the investigator will be making the correct choice when using them. However, as also discussed before, it should not be the first option, as other parametric tests, if appropriate, will likely be more effective and thus hold better validity. Therefore the preceding discussion needs to be carefully considered when choosing this outcome.

Therefore, the investigator needs to use this statistical test when the outcome (or dependent variable) is (1) continuous but not normally distributed, or (2) ordinal and the independent variable needs to be categorical (i.e., groups of treatment; this is the most common scenario).

If there are two groups only, there are two options, depending whether it is two groups of treatment or two measurements in the same subjects (before vs. after). For two different groups, the correct statistical test is the Mann-Whitney (or Wilcoxon Rank Sum). For two measurements in the same subject, the Wilcoxon Sign Rank test should be used. When there are more than two groups, the investigator should use the Kruskal-Wallis.

And what should be used for situations when there are three or more groups, but the measurement was taken twice in each group? In this case, if the measurement is continuous and data are normally distributed, ANOVA would be the appropriate solution. However, if the data are ordinal or continuous and not normally distributed, then there is no solution using these non-parametric tests. In this case, the investigator can use, for instance, only one measurement and thus eliminate one of the factors (time factor), keeping only the group, and use Kruskal-Wallis, or transform the outcome into

Table 10.1 Summary Table of Non-Parametric Tests

Test	Main Outcome	Independent Variable	Analysis
Mann-Whitney	Ordinal or continuous, not normally distributed	Categorical	Compares median of two independent groups
Wilcoxon Sign Rank	Ordinal or continuous, not normally distributed	Categorical	Compares median of two dependent groups
Kruskal-Wallis	Ordinal or continuous, not normally distributed	Categorical	Compares three or more independent groups

a binary outcome and use logistic regression. The investigator needs to be cognizant of the statistical test when designing the study.

The investigator does not need to know the mathematics behind the statistical test in order to use it appropriately; however, it is useful to know that these tests compare ranks. In other words, the outcome is ranked in all the groups; therefore if one group has a much higher (or smaller) rank than the other group, then someone would expect a significant difference, depending on the sample size. By understanding this basic principle, it is therefore intuitive that it easily addresses outliers, as the important factor is not how much a data point is higher than another data point, but whether it is higher or smaller (independent of the amount).

HOW SHOULD RESULTS FROM STATISTICAL SOFTWARE BE INTERPRETED?

After reading these initial sections, the investigator needs to know when to use these tests appropriately. (If there are still some problems in understanding dependent versus independent variables or normal distribution, please refer to Chapter 8.)

The next step, then, is organizing the spreadsheet with the data appropriately to be imported into the statistical software. The good news is that most of the statistical softwares accept direct import from Excel spreadsheet. It is important to organize the variables in the column. For instance, each variable should have only one column. However, it becomes a bit more complicated when it is repeated measures, meaning that the same variable is collected twice at different moments in the same subject. In this case, most of the packages would still be designed to have one variable for the outcome only, and then another variable to define time of assessment. In the following we give an example for each of the three tests (Mann-Whitney, Wilcoxon Sign Rank, and Kruskal-Wallis) using two statistical packages: STATA 13.0 and SPSS 18.0.

Let's take a look at the following scenario: In a clinical trial, drugs A, B, and C are being tested for patients with anxiety disorder. The evaluated outcome is the patient's satisfaction level with the effect of treatment at 4 weeks post-treatment, with the scale ranging from very dissatisfied (1), dissatisfied (2), neutral (3), satisfied (4), to very satisfied (5). Thus our evaluated outcome is ordinal, while the independent variables are categorical.

Comparing Two Independent Groups

In order to initially compare patient satisfaction between drugs A and B only (two independent samples), the most appropriate statistical test is the Mann-Whitney test/Wilcoxon Rank Sum test.

- *Entering data*: It is important to input data correctly in order to run the analysis. Each variable should have its own column. Here, the first column represents the drugs being tested (1 and 2, which represent drugs A and B, respectively), while the second column portrays the level of patient satisfaction (1–5).

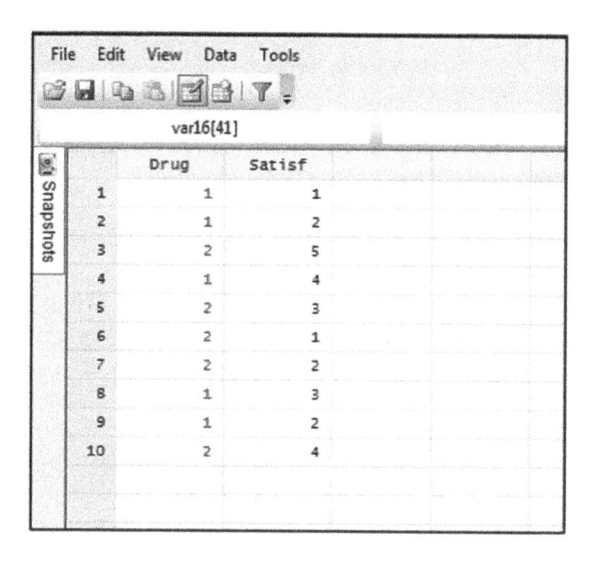

	Drug	Satisf
1	1	1
2	1	2
3	2	5
4	1	4
5	2	3
6	2	1
7	2	2
8	1	3
9	1	2
10	2	4

- *Choosing the analysis test*: You can perform the analysis by using the software MENU. Select the following options:
Statistics > Non-parametric analysis > Test of hypothesis > Wilcoxon rank-sum

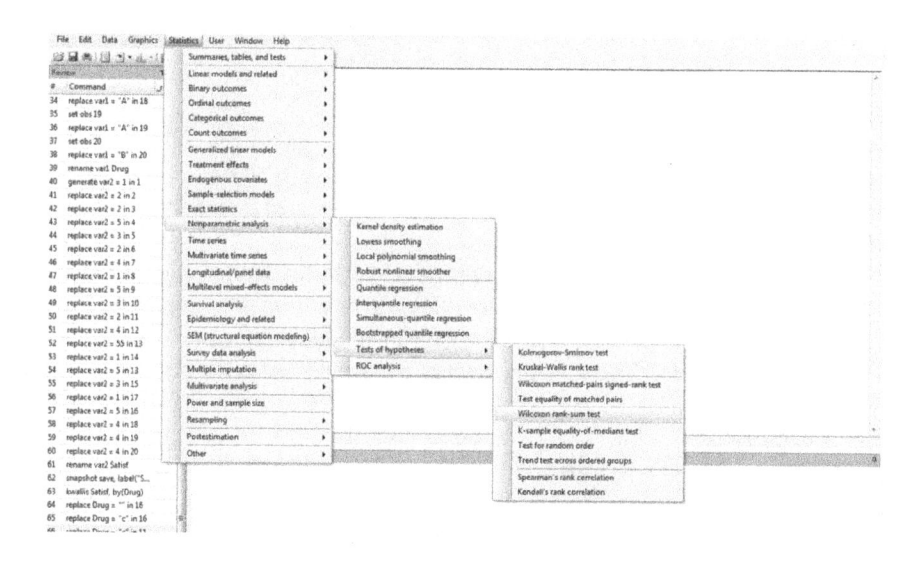

- *Running the analysis*: An important issue is to identify correctly where to place the dependent variable (outcome) and the independent variable (intervention). When running the analysis, the software will display two boxes: one for *variable* and one for *grouping variable*. The *variable* is your outcome (dependent variable), while the *grouping variable* is your intervention (independent variable). Therefore, Satisfaction with Treatment is placed in the *variable* box, and Drug being tested is placed in the *grouping variable* box.

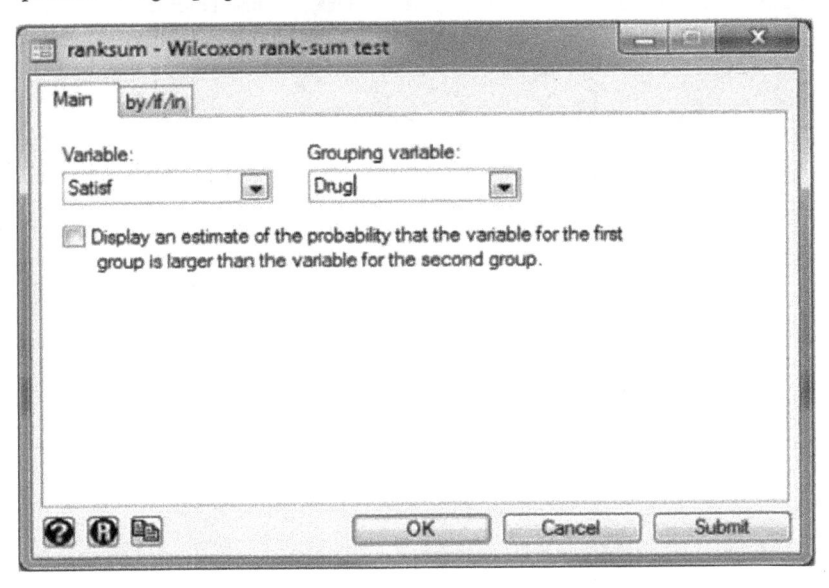

- *Interpreting the output*: The software will provide an output for the chosen test, and it is crucial not only to choose the correct test, but also to know how to interpret the given information. The table for the Mann-Whitney test provides three columns of information regarding drug A and drug B: the number of observations (number of subjects in each group), the observed rank sums values, and the expected values.

The rationale behind the Mann-Whitney/Wilcoxon Rank Sum test consists of ranking the outcomes for the given drugs (satisfaction level) and using their rank positions in the analysis, instead of their absolute values. All obtained values are ranked in order (1st, 2nd, 3rd, etc.). The ranks are then summed and compared between groups. If drug A is significantly different from drug B, then it is expected that the scores in one group will be significantly different.

Since ties may be an issue, the software provides both the *unadjusted variance* and the *adjustment for ties*. A tie occurs when a given value is in more than one sample. Next, the investigator should interpret the result of the test with the *null hypothesis*, and the *p-value*.

Null hypothesis (Ho): There is no difference in patient satisfaction between drugs A and B.

$P = 0.5219$

Conclusion: Do not reject the null hypothesis. The researcher may conclude that patient satisfaction between drugs A and B are *not* significantly different.

```
. ranksum Satisf, by(Drug)

Two-sample Wilcoxon rank-sum (Mann-Whitney) test

       Drug |      obs      rank sum      expected
    --------+--------------------------------------
          1 |       5          24.5          27.5
          2 |       5          30.5          27.5
    --------+--------------------------------------
   combined |      10            55            55

unadjusted variance        22.92
adjustment for ties        -0.97
                          ------
adjusted variance          21.94

Ho: Satisf(Drug==1) = Satisf(Drug==2)   ← null hypothesis
        z =   -0.640
    Prob > |z| =    0.5219   ⟶ p-value
```

Paired Comparison (Comparing within a Group)

If the purpose is rather to compare the patients' satisfaction with drug A at two different time points, for instance at 2 weeks post-treatment and at 4 weeks post-treatment, the chosen statistical test is the Wilcoxon Sign Rank test. In this case, the comparison is not being made between groups, but within the same group at different moments.

- *Entering data*: In the paired comparison, this may be the only case in which data are organized in a different way, since the outcome is shown in two columns separated by time of assessment. Here, two new variables have to be imputed, representing the different time points in which data will be analyzed (2 weeks and 4 weeks). Each horizontal line represents one patient. The first column represents the level of satisfaction with drug A at 2 weeks (Satisf2w) and at 4 weeks (Satisf4w) of treatment.

	Satisf2w	Satisf4w
1	1	2
2	2	3
3	5	5
4	2	3
5	4	5
6	1	4
7	3	4
8	4	5
9	5	5
10	1	3

- *Choosing the analysis test*: You can perform the analysis by using the software MENU. Select the following options:
Statistics > Non-parametric analysis > Test of hypothesis > Wilcoxon matched-pairs Sign Rank test.

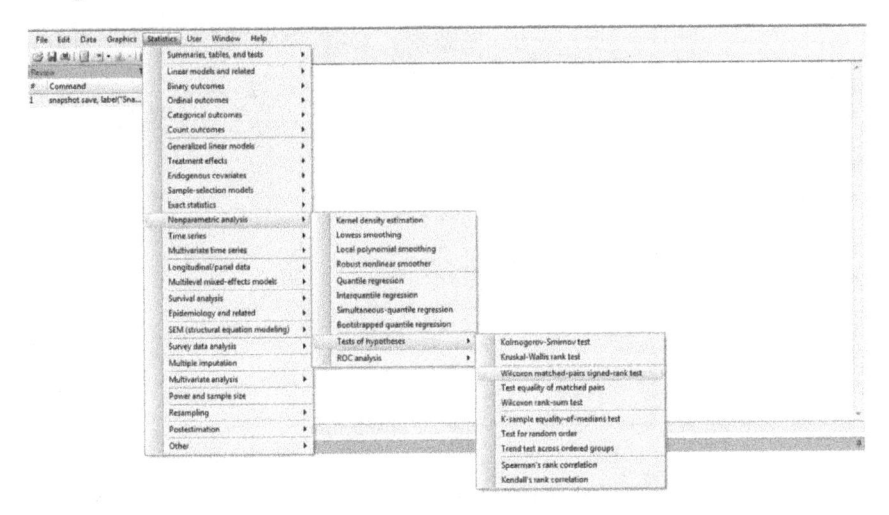

- *Running the analysis*: Sometimes, inputting data may not be the most intuitive process, as the software may provide a different framework for each test. However, it is a simple process. When running the paired analysis, the STATA software will ask for a variable and for an expression. In this case, since you are comparing the satisfaction level at 2 weeks with the satisfaction at 4 weeks, these two variables will be inserted. Satisfaction level at 2 weeks (Satisf2w) should be inserted in the *variable box*. The *expression box* enables different arithmetic calculations to be made between variables; however, in this case you should only insert Satisfaction level at 4 weeks (Satisf4w).

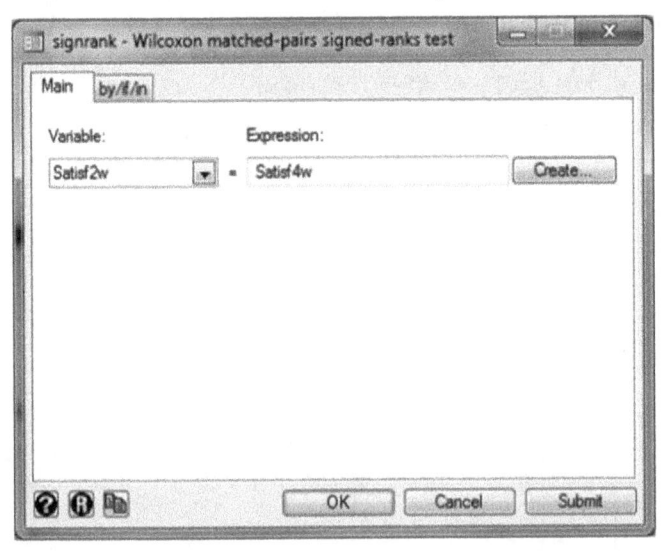

- *Interpreting the output*: The interpretation of the Wilcoxon Sign Rank test output is very similar to the Mann-Whitney test output (refer to first item). However, in this case, instead of comparing between different groups, you are comparing within the same group (Drug A).

The output table provides valuable information. In our example, we can see that 8 participants had a higher satisfaction level at 4 weeks when compared to 2 weeks, 0 patients had a lower satisfaction level with drug A at 4 weeks when compared to 2 weeks, and 2 patients did not report differences in satisfaction level between these two time points. By examining the test statistics (see later discussion), we can understand if these changes in satisfaction led to a statistically significant difference between 2 and 4 weeks post-treatment.

Null hypothesis (Ho): There is no difference in patient satisfaction between 2 and 4 weeks after taking drug A.

$P = 0.0063$

Conclusion: Reject the null hypothesis. The researcher may conclude that, for drug A, there is a significant difference in patient satisfaction between 2 and 4 weeks after taking the medication.

```
. signrank Satisf2w = Satisf4w

Wilcoxon signed-rank test

      sign |      obs      sum ranks      expected
  ---------+----------------------------------------
  positive |       0             0             26
  negative |       8            52             26
      zero |       2             3              3
  ---------+----------------------------------------
       all |      10            55             55

unadjusted variance        96.25
adjustment for ties        -4.38
adjustment for zeros       -1.25
                          ------
adjusted variance          90.63

Ho: Satisf2w = Satisf4w      ← null hypothesis
         z =   -2.731
    Prob > |z| =  0.0063     ⟶ p-value
```

Comparing Three or More Independent Groups

Finally, consider that the researcher decides to compare the effects of the three different drugs (drug A (1), drug B (2), drug C (3)) on patient satisfaction. Since now more than two groups are being compared, the most suitable test is the Kruskal-Wallis test (3 independent groups).

- *Entering data*: Here, instead of analyzing solely drugs A and B, satisfaction levels for drug C will also be imputed, since the purpose is to compare the differences between the three groups. Therefore, possible values for drug being tested are 1, 2, and 3, and for satisfaction level are 1–5.

Drug	Satisf
1	1
3	2
2	5
1	2
3	4
2	1
2	2
1	3
1	2
2	2
3	5
3	4
2	3
1	2
3	5

- *Choosing the analysis test*: You can perform the analysis by using the software MENU. Select the following options:
Statistics > Non-parametric analysis > Test of hypothesis > Kruskal-Wallis rank test.

- *Running the analysis*: Once again, the outcome variable will be the dependent variable (Level of Satisfaction), while the variable defining groups is the independent variable (Drug).

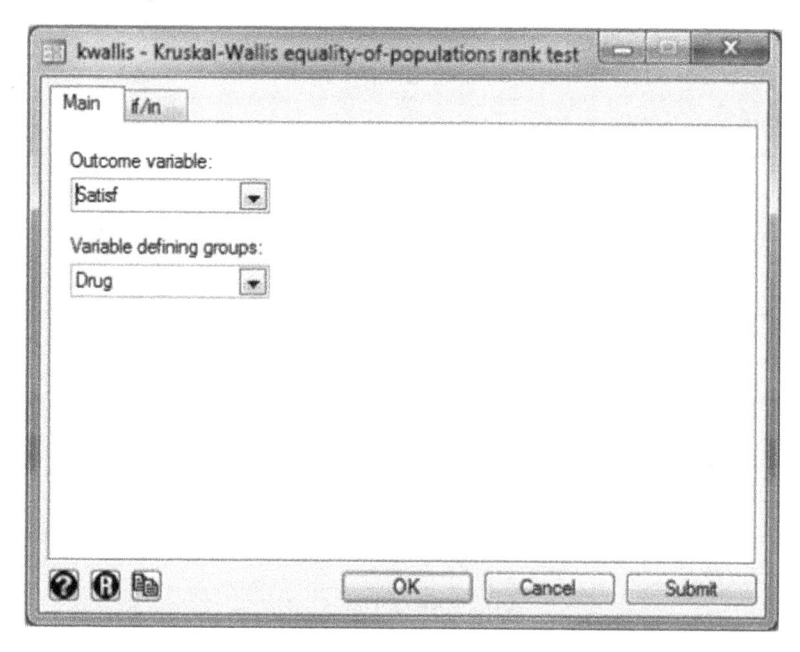

- *Interpreting the output*: The output table for the Kruskal-Wallis test provides information regarding the number of observations (obs) and the total sum of ranks for each group (Drug A, B, and C). Similarly, the software presents the unadjusted and adjusted analysis, due to the presence of ties. It is always preferable to use the adjusted analysis, as it yields estimates that are more precise.

Null hypothesis (Ho): There is no difference in patient satisfaction level between drugs A, B, and C.
$P = 0.0905$

Conclusion: Maintain the null hypothesis. The researcher may conclude that there is not a significant difference in patient satisfaction level between groups taking drug A, B, and C.

```
. kwallis Satisf, by(Drug)

Kruskal-Wallis equality-of-populations rank test

    Drug   Obs   Rank Sum
     1      5      27.50
     2      5      36.00
     3      5      56.50

chi-squared    =    4.445 with 2 d.f.
probability    =    0.1083

chi-squared with ties =   4.805 with 2 d.f.
probability    =    0.0905    ──▶ p-value
```

SPSS SOFTWARE

In the SPSS software, you can use the MENU to select the three different analyses. Here we provide the sequence of commands that should be selected.

Mann-Whitney/Wilcoxon Rank Sum

Analyze > Nonparametric Tests > Legacy Dialogs > 2 Independent Samples

Wilcoxon Sign-Rank

Analyze > Nonparametric Tests > Legacy Dialogs > 2 Related Samples

Kruskal-Wallis

Analyze > Nonparametric Tests > Legacy Dialogs > K Independent Samples

CASE STUDY 10: YIN AND YANG (阴阳) IN A CLINICAL TRIAL ON POSTPARTUM DEPRESSION: THE USE OF NON-PARAMETRIC TESTING

Suely R. Matsubayashi and Felipe Fregni

INTRODUCTION

Dr. David Wang has been anxiously waiting for this message and now it finally has arrived.

The sender was the *American Journal of Obstetrics* and the title was "Decision on manuscript 10-982." This was the email with the results of the peer review of his paper on the study that he considers to be a major contribution to the field of postpartum depression. He worked extremely hard during the past five years on this study and now the fate of his study was one click away. He had mixed feelings of anxiety and excitement.[1]

Dr. Wang is a senior psychiatrist in Beijing, China, from the Capital Medical University, and he is also an experienced investigator. He has been working intensely to publish a large clinical trial testing the efficacy of a new antidepressant for the treatment of postpartum depression. According to the World Health Organization (WHO), depression is a leading cause of disability worldwide, being the fourth in the rank of global burden of disease. In addition, women experience two or three times more depression than men, and maternal depression is directly associated with adverse child cognitive and socio-emotional development progress. It is an important issue in Western countries where the prevalence ranges from 10% to 15% of deliveries; however, this prevalence increases in developing countries such as South Africa and, in Latin America, where it nears 40%, depending on the definition evaluation criteria. Postpartum depression has great incidence in the first six months after delivery; however, it can occur until the end of the first year. These results are related to psychological, social, and economic conditions. The risk factors include depression in a previous pregnancy and/or personal or family history, single marital status (not having support from the husband or partner), low education, having experienced violence, and being unaware of pregnancy.

For Dr. Wang, postpartum depression is an extremely important issue, as he had seen in the past cases of depressed mothers hurting their babies. Another important issue is regarding breastfeeding. Because of depression, mothers stop breastfeeding their babies. The WHO recommends exclusive breastfeeding for at least the first four to six months of life and its continuation for one to two years thereafter. Because of Dr. Wang's knowledge of this specific disease, most physicians and gynecologists refer cases to him in which mothers need a drug therapy for the treatment of depression.

---

[1] Dr. Suely R. Matsubayashi and Professor Felipe Fregni prepared this case. Course cases are developed solely as the basis for class discussion. The situation in this case is fictional. Cases are not intended to serve as endorsements or sources of primary data. All rights reserved to the authors of this case.

The Trial

It was the end of the afternoon and Dr. Wang was looking through his window—his office in the Chaoyang district faced the amazing Olympic stadium that was built for the 2008 Olympic games in Beijing. Dr. Wang was particularly proud of China and in fact returned to China four years ago after a long period of research at Karolinska Institute in Sweden. His first big project after his return to his native China was to run this postpartum depression study. In fact, the view of the Olympic stadium was a constant reminder of his mission to help China gain a leading place in science.

The goal of this trial that Dr. Wang is running is to evaluate the effects of a 10-week home-based exercise program for the treatment of postpartum depression. Although the benefits of exercise for depression treatment are well documented (not only behaviorally but also via neurophysiological markers such as neurotransmitter levels), he and his team believe that they have developed a better exercise program that will have greater efficacy. Dr. Wang actually believes that his program will be a breakthrough for the treatment of postpartum depression. This treatment, besides the low cost (which would be great for his mainland China), has the important advantage of being safe and not interfering with lactation. In his trial, 50 women with postpartum depressed moods were randomly assigned to the 10-week home-based exercise program or usual care. The main outcome was the comparison of changes in the Hamilton Rating Scale for Depression (HAM-D) between baseline and immediate post-treatment when comparing exercise versus usual care. Although the sample was not large, he showed that the exercise group had significantly lower results after treatment baseline as compared with the usual care group. He expected that these findings would guide future research clinical trials and hopefully clinical practice in the future. Now, the decision was in that email.

The Email: Initial Despair—Yang (阳)

Dr. Wang then opens the email and reads it carefully:

Dear Dr. Wang,
Thank you for the submission of your manuscript to the American Journal of Obstetrics (AJO). Unfortunately, it was not accepted for publication in AJO in its current form. The manuscript was externally reviewed and was also reviewed by the Associate Editor and the Board of Editors. The overall decision is made by the Board of Editors and takes into account the Reviewers' comments, priority, relevance, and space in the journal. Substantive issues and concerns were raised that precluded assigning a high priority score to your manuscript for merit publication. However, if you can satisfactorily and completely respond to the comments of the Reviewers and the Editorial Board within three months (see the attached file), we would be willing to review a revised version of your manuscript. The revised manuscript must be submitted without exception within this timeframe. We offer no assurance that it will be accepted after resubmission. We will do our absolute best to ensure a timely re-review process so as not to cause you any delay after resubmission. We thank you again for considering AJO.

Sincerely,
Editor-in-chief, AJO

Dr. Wang then read the attachment and realized that the chief complaint from reviewers was that they used a parametric test (linear regression) to measure the main study outcome: depression as assessed by Hamilton Depression Rating Scale (HDRS) over the different time points, but the data seemed skewed, as most patients had mild to moderate depression (and few patients had severe depression). After reading the review, Dr. Wang's initial reaction was panic and despair. Several questions were going through his mind at the same time: "If I use a non-parametric approach, I am going to lose efficiency and maybe my results might not become significant? How am I going to show clinical significance with this approach? How am I going to control for age in the model using a non-parametric approach? Even if I try to transform my data to a normal distribution using mathematical transformation, this will not work as I have seen before. Can I change the method of analysis now?"

He looks again through his window and sees the Olympic stadium, and he feels inspired, as he knows that every big project has its challenges. He feels that he is extremely stressed and decides to call the day to an end and go home. He knows that after a night of sleep, the situation will be clearer.

The Light at the End of the Tunnel: Yin (阴)—Restoring the Balance

The next day, Dr. Wang feels energized again; even the traffic does not seem to bother him. He then begins to review his situation. The first issue he realized is that if he changes the analyses now, then the results of the trial would need to be considered exploratory. The next important point was the main outcome—Hamilton Depression Rating Scale—the most widely used to assess the intensity of depression symptoms. The original version contains 17 items and data can be classified as ordinal (although there is an intense debate on the appropriateness of using the sum as continuous outcome).[2,3] But if Dr. Wang decides to use data as non-parametric, then this issue would be addressed.

Another concern Dr. Wang has is the issue of not using linear regression and adjusting for continuous variables, such as age. In a survey in 1999, half of the mothers with postpartum depression were under 25 years old and the maximum age was 40 years old.[4] The proportion of adolescent to adult mothers with depression was 2:1. That ratio remains today. In addition, he believes that younger mothers might respond better to exercises and therefore confound the results. But he cannot use parametric tests to make this adjustment using common methods such as the use of ANCOVA. One of the main concerns in using non-parametric tests is the "loss of information." For instance, when dimensional data are transformed in ranks, there is a loss of

---

[2] Please see the Chapter 8 case study to read more on this issue of using ordinal scales as continuous outcome.

[3] If you want to learn more about variable classification (also discussed in Chapter 8) including a discussion of ordinal variables, go to: http://onlinestatbook.com/2/introduction/levels_of_measurement.html (this link also provides a nice exercise at the end).

[4] Cooper JP, Tomlinson M, Swartz L, et al. (1999). Post-partum depression and the mother infant relationship in a South African peri-urban settlement. *Br J Psychiatry*. 1999; 175: 554–558.

information, as two numbers will be differentiated only by which one is larger and not by the quantity of this difference; for instance 100 versus 1 would be theoretically the same as 2 versus 1 in a rank test (given there are no other numbers in between). This loss of information might then result in a loss of power/efficiency of the test and therefore might change the results. However, on the other hand, large outliers might reduce the power of a parametric approach, and this might not be a problem after all. Dr. Wang is glad he could remember his statistical courses. The other important issue is the clinical significance of the data when using a non-parametric approach, as this approach will only give a *p*-value or statistical significance, but then how does one determine whether the difference is clinically meaningful? When using continuous data, it is possible to compare two means or to calculate the effect size of the intervention; but when using ordinal data, it becomes more complicated, as median comparison might not be adequate since they might actually be quite similar or different, according to how the data were presented. One possibility here is to categorize the data—in other words, find a cut-off for the data and classify patients as responders or non-responders. In fact, it is common to define a patient as a responder if he or she has a decrease in Hamilton scores of more or equal to 50% in relation to baseline scores. Finally, it is possible to adjust for one variable using, for instance, binary (or categorical) outcomes (as discussed earlier—if we categorize the outcome in responders and non-responders). To do that, it is necessary first to create two tables according to the variable to adjust—for instance, in this case, age—and create two tables—one of adolescent pregnancy and the other of non-adolescent pregnancy. The next step is to classify the responders and non-responders in each group (exercise vs. usual care) for each table (adolescents and non-adolescents), then to use Cochran-Mantel-Haenszel (CMH) to find an adjusted odds ratio between the two groups of treatment considering these two strata.[5] The null hypothesis of this test is that the response is conditionally independent of the treatment in any given strata (in this case, adolescent and non-adolescent).

Potential Solutions: Yin and Yang (阴阳)

Dr. Wang was running to his clinics as he had a full day. He knew at that point that there would be a solution for his problem. While he was trying to get to his outpatient clinic and walking throughout the hospital, passing through hundreds of patients, he summarized in his mind his options:

- First option: Compare the improvement of depression in the exercise versus usual care group using a simple non-parametric rank test. Here there are two options: the Wilcoxon Two-Group Rank Sum Test or the Mann-Whitney Test (some authors consider these two tests as only one as they are in fact very similar—both use the principle of classifying the scores by ranks and comparing the ranks in both groups). It is a relatively simple process that can actually be done by hand if the sample is small.

---

[5] Cochran-Mantel-Haenszel Test may be a bit complicated to understand. If you want to read more, go to this link to get a more detailed explanation: http://udel.edu/~mcdonald/statcmh.html

- Second option: Categorize the data in responders and non-responders and calculate whether there is a difference in the proportion of responders using chi-square or Fisher's exact test.
- Third option: Use the same approach as the second option, but create two different tables—one for adolescents and the other for non-adolescents—then use Cochran-Mantel-Haenszel to calculate an adjusted odds ratio for these two tables and test whether there is a difference between groups.

After a full day in clinics, Dr. Wang returns to his office to get his briefcase and go home, but before leaving, he looks again at the Olympic stadium, as it is evening and the lights are on. He feels motivated and knows now he will be able to address the reviewers' concerns and have a meaningful study. He feels inspired by the chance of being able to offer something else for patients with postpartum depression and also honored for his small contribution to the scientific progress of China.

CASE DISCUSSION

This case discusses a classical example of situations in which the use of parametric tests may be criticized. In this case, the use of scale based in ordinal items may be an issue; even though the researcher is using the total sum. The investigator needs to plan well and consider the potential drawbacks of using different approaches. If the investigator is not confident, it is always best to choose a statistical test with less assumptions so as to make sure the final results are valid. The final choice should also depend on the main research question.

CASE QUESTIONS FOR REFLECTION

1. What are the challenges Dr. Wang faces when choosing the statistical test to be used in his trial?
2. What are his main concerns?
3. What should he consider when making his decision?

FURTHER READING

Callegari-Jacques SD. *Bioestatística princípios e aplicações*. Porto Alegre: Artmed; 2008: Chapter 11, pp. 94–102.

Portney LG, Watkins MP. *Foundations of clinical research applications to practice*. 3rd ed. Upper Saddle River, NJ: Pearson/Prentice Hall; 2015: Chapters 20, 22, 23, 24.

Zou KH, Tuncali K, Silverman SC. Correlation and simple linear regression. *Radiology*. 2003; 227: 617–628.

REFERENCES

1. Luurila H, Olkkola KT, Neuvonen PJ. Interaction between erythromycin and the benzodiazepines diazepam and flunitrazepam. *Pharmacol Toxicol*. 1996; 78(2): 117–122.

2. Bopp M, Darby M, Loftin KC, Broscious S. Effects of daily oral care with 0.12% chlorhexidine gluconate and a standard oral care protocol on the development of nosocomial pneumonia in intubated patients: a pilot study. *J Dent Hyg*. 2006; 80(3): 9.
3. Khurshudian AV. A pilot study to test the efficacy of oral administration of interferon-alpha lozenges to patients with Sjögren's syndrome. *Oral Surg Oral Med Oral Pathol Oral Radiol Endod* [Internet]. 2003; 95(1): 38–44. Available from: http://www.ncbi.nlm.nih.gov/pubmed/12539025
4. Cruz-Correa M, Shoskes DA, Sanchez P, Zhao R, Hylind LM, Wexner SD, et al. Combination treatment with curcumin and quercetin of adenomas in familial adenomatous polyposis. *Clin Gastroenterol Hepatol*. 2006; 4(8): 1035–1038.
5. Ofungwu J. *Statistical applications for environmental analysis and risk assessment*. New York: John Wiley & Sons; 2014.
6. Rosner B. *Fundamentals of biostatistics*. 7th ed. Boston: Cengage Learning; 2011.
7. Hothorn LA. *Statistics in toxicology using r*. Boca Raton, FL: CRC Press, Taylor and Francis Group; 2016.
8. Friedman H. *The Oxford handbook of health psychology*. Oxford: Oxford University Press; 2014.
9. Knapp TR. Treating ordinal scales as interval scales: an attempt to resolve the controversy. *Nurs Res*. 1990; Mar-Apr; 39(2): 121–123.
10. Doering TR, Hubbard R. Measurements and statistics: the ordinal-interval controversy and geography. *Area* 1979; 11(3): 237–243.

11

SAMPLE SIZE CALCULATION

Authors: *Mohammad Azfar Qureshi and Jessica K. Paulus*

Case study author: *Felipe Fregni*

Access to power must be confined to those who are not in love with it.
—Plato

INTRODUCTION

In previous chapters you were introduced to the basic concepts of study design and statistics: how to frame the right research question, how to design a study to answer this question (design, recruitment and randomization, blinding, etc.) and how to analyze the data obtained from a study (types of variables, their description, and the appropriate statistical tests). However, a crucial study design issue that has not yet been addressed is what *sample size* is required (how many study subjects or observations are needed) to have enough *power* to answer the study hypothesis with *statistical significance*.

This chapter will highlight and review the issues of type I and type II error, power, and significance level, and how these parameters are used in calculation of the sample size required to conduct a successful research study (some of these concepts have also been reviewed in Chapter 9).

The purpose of a research study is to make inferences about the target population from results obtained in a sample drawn from an accessible population. While it is important to draw a representative sample to limit systematic error (reducing or eliminating bias, confounding, etc.), it is also vitally important to select an appropriate sample size to reduce random error. Sample size calculation is an integral part of a statistical analysis plan to estimate the required number of study participants. In fact, most research funding agencies require a formal sample size calculation to demonstrate that a funded project would yield conclusive data. Similarly, International Conference on Harmonization (ICH) Good Clinical Practice (GCP) guidelines mandate outlining the details of how the number needed to conduct a trial was calculated, including the level of significance set and other parameters used [1]. Finally, most applications for human subject research at an institutional review board (IRB) require specification of a number of participants to be enrolled, with appropriate justifications. Next we will discuss the consequences of over- and underestimating the sample size.

OVERESTIMATING THE SAMPLE SIZE

There are *ethical implications* when the estimation for sample size is more than is needed, as it may add unnecessary risk for subjects in a study whose participation may not have been needed. Additionally, if the estimated sample size is very large, the researcher has to consider whether such a study is feasible (financially, logistically) and what issues arise with regard to recruitment (enrollment timeframe, recruitment strategies, available population). Studies with an overestimated sample size are a waste of resources, impose excessive strain on the research team and potentially expose an unnecessary number of study subjects to risk and discomfort.

UNDERESTIMATING THE SAMPLE SIZE

Conversely, if a sample size is underestimated, a study will be statistically underpowered to detect the pre-specified effect size, and study results might fail to reach statistical significance. Interpreting underpowered studies presents a challenge to the researcher as differences that fail to reach statistical significance could represent either a truly null effect or a false negative result. Conducting an underpowered study therefore symbolizes an impractical and unethical approach in study design, as it also wastes resources and exposes subjects to unnecessary risks, given that the results of the research will not be able to inform the study hypothesis. The problems with over- and underestimation of sample size apply not only to experimental studies, but also to many observational designs.

MIS-SPECIFYING THE SAMPLE SIZE CALCULATION

While the actual performance of a sample size calculation is relatively straightforward (especially given the proliferation of online sample size estimation tools), the estimation of the parameters and inputs required for this calculation are often challenging for the researcher. The reason for this is that a researcher must make many unverifiable assumptions in the process of pre-specifying inputs required for sample size calculations. If these assumptions do not hold true during the conduct of the research study, then the researcher will be left with an over- or underpowered study. This is the main challenge of sample size calculation: predict with accuracy some of the key inputs, such as the study effect size.

As outlined earlier, understanding the rationale behind sample size and power calculations is fundamental. The actual process of sample size calculation, on the other hand, is rather straightforward. Besides statistical software, many simple online calculators are available to perform these calculations. Tables and graphs are also available, with which the sample size can be extrapolated once the appropriate values of the relevant parameters are chosen [2].

REPORTING SAMPLE SIZE

In spite of increasing attention to the a priori specification of sample size and power by various research stakeholders, transparent reporting of sample size calculations remains inadequate. Even in randomized controlled trials, sample size calculations are still often inadequately reported, often erroneous, and based on inaccurate assumptions [3].When negative studies do not include sample size calculations, it's impossible for the reader to know whether the results were truly negative or whether the study was just underpowered. It is imperative that researchers understand the consequences of sample size and power when interpreting results and applying them to clinical practice.

PARAMETERS FOR SAMPLE SIZE CALCULATION

The specific parameters needed for a sample size calculation are driven by the choice of statistical test that is appropriate for the primary study question and outcome. However, the following parameters are commonly required for sample size calculations, and manipulation of these parameters can have a significant impact on the size of the sample needed:

1. Significance level (α)/critical p-value
2. Desired power ($1-\beta$)
3. Characteristics of the outcome: the variability in the outcome (i.e., standard deviation, σ) for continuous variables, or the frequency of the outcome for categorical outcomes
4. Anticipated treatment/exposure effect (H_a).

PROBABILITY OF ERRORS

In hypothesis testing, different types of errors were introduced (Figure 11.1).

Alpha (α): Type I error, also known as "level of significance." Type I error means rejecting the null hypothesis when it is in fact true, or a false positive. It is typically set to 0.05 or 5%. Setting alpha to 0.05 means that the investigator will accept taking 5% risk of a significant finding being attributable to chance alone. Any investigator would want to minimize this type of error as much as possible, as committing type I error can pose significant risk to the study subjects. While accepting a Type I error risk of 5%

		Truth about the population	
		H_0 true	H_a true
Decision based on sample	Reject H_0	Type I error	Correct decision
	Accept H_0	Correct decision	Type II error

Figure 11.1. Hypothesis testing and types of errors.
H_0 = null hypothesis, H_a = alternative hypothesis.

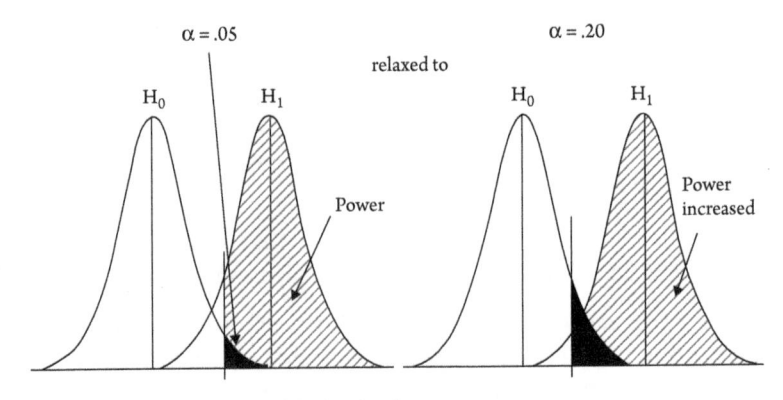

Figure 11.2. Relationship between alpha level and power.

is most common in clinical research, it is not necessarily the most appropriate value depending on the research objective and scope. In genetic and molecular studies, a large number of candidates are often compared; thus the cost of getting many false positives can be prohibitively high when screen positive hits need to be subsequently verified. For instance, if a genetic sample of 500,000 SNPs are to be scanned, then keeping alpha at 0.05 would correspond to 25,000 false positive samples that could consume extensive research resources to verify; however, setting the alpha to 0.001 would yield only 500 false positive samples. Reducing the alpha for a study will require a larger sample size.

Power (1-β): The second type of error is the Type II error (β). Type II error refers to failing to reject the null hypothesis when it is actually false (failing to detect a difference when it actually exists, or a false negative). Power is defined as 1-β, or the true positive rate. In clinical research, power is often set at 80%, meaning that the investigator will accept a risk of 20% of not detecting a difference when it truly exists.

The threshold of 80% power is an arbitrary value, much like the standard value of 0.05 for alpha. However, regarding any study with less than 80% as uninformative doesn't recognize the potential value of information gained. It may be appropriate to accept a lower degree of power for a pilot study, for example. Clinical research is often constrained by pragmatic issues regarding feasibility, and studies must be designed in accordance with sensitivity analyses that examine a meaningful array of possible findings, and follow examples set by previous analogous studies [4].

MEASURE OF VARIATION

For continuous outcome variables, there is a need to estimate the population SD (σ). How do you find this number? One option is to examine the published literature, which can be used to estimate standard deviation. In situations where no previous studies exactly matching the intervention–outcome relation are available, then studies on analogous interventions and outcomes can be used to estimate the study standard deviation. Expert opinion and subject matter expertise are needed to identify appropriate analogies in the literature. In the absence of available published estimates on the standard deviation, an investigator may conduct a pilot study to estimate the standard deviation. However, there is a risk that the pilot study may underestimate the SD for the outcome [5].

As the variability in the outcome is higher, a larger sample size will be required to detect a significant difference between study groups. To demonstrate the relationship between how variation in the sample affects the requisite sample size, consider the following example where we wish to test whether the mean weights of two populations is different. If the difference between the mean weights of the two populations is large and the within-group variability is small, then a relatively small sample would be sufficient to detect a significant difference between groups. Yet a larger sample size would be required if the within-group variability is large.

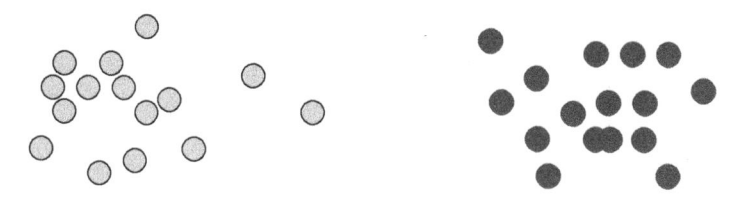

Smaller sample required—large difference in a variable that varies very little.

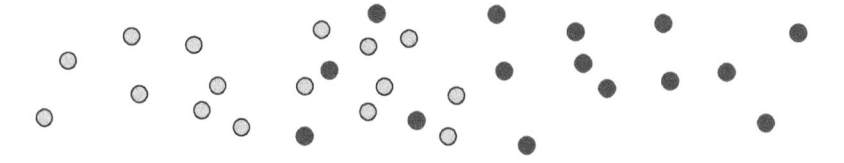

Larger sample required—small difference in a variable that varies quite a lot.

Estimates of the standard deviation may not be directly available. Sometimes the standard deviation of the outcome is not directly reported in a manuscript, but may be extrapolated from other reported statistics. Sometimes standard errors are presented; in this case, one can use the following formula to estimate the SD.

- $SE = SD/\sqrt{n}$

Similarly, 95% confidence intervals can be used to calculate the SD with the following formula.

- $95\% \ CI = 1.96 \pm SE$
- $SE = SD/\sqrt{n}$.

EFFECT ESTIMATES

The effect estimate is another important parameter for sample size calculation. The effect estimate is the actual difference expected under the alternate hypothesis, or the magnitude of treatment effect anticipated between groups. The effect estimate should reflect a clinically meaningful and feasible difference based on preliminary or published studies, and subject matter or clinical expertise.

In research, the effect estimate is measured by statistics that depend on the nature of the exposure, outcome, and research goals. Associations between the exposure and outcome be measured using a correlation coefficient (r), standardized mean difference, or relative risk, among many other options. For example, in a case-control study, the odds ratio is the most appropriate way to estimate the association between the exposure or treatment and the outcome. In summary, the nature of the exposure, outcome, and study design and research methods will determine how the effect size is calculated.

EFFECT SIZE PITFALLS

It is a relatively common mistake for an investigator to be overly ambitious about an anticipated effect size. Larger effect sizes require smaller sample sizes to detect. But overly optimistic assumptions about effect sizes can result in a study that is underpowered to detect more clinically realistic differences between study groups. Believing that a large size effect is a clinically significant result and that small size effect is clinically unimportant can be misleading [6]. Certain exposures or treatments—such as a single nutrient intervention—are physiologically likely to have a smaller magnitude effect on the outcome, though may still make a substantial clinical impact on a group of patients, and have a substantial public health impact at a population level. Finally, a large size effect does not rule out the need for replication of a study, as internal and external validity issues can account for large differences observed between treatment groups. When the investigator does not have sufficient prior evidence to justify a given effect size, they may wish to calculate the minimum effect size that could be estimated with a fixed sample size and power.

If a smaller type I error is desired (= smaller α), a larger sample size (n) will be required.
If a smaller type II error is desired (= more power), a larger sample size (n) will be required.

PROBABILITY OF THE OUTCOME

In studies where the primary outcome is a proportion, it is necessary to know the probability of the disease or the outcome itself for sample size estimation. For instance, if the outcome of the study is development of acute kidney injury in intensive care patients, the prevalence of acute kidney injury in ICU patients is needed to perform the sample size calculation.

Caveats in Sample Size Calculation

Many conditions require increase or decrease in sample size. Maximizing alpha to avoid type I error, minimizing beta to maximize power, and detecting small effect size between two groups will require large sample size and vice versa [7].

The following considerations also influence the sample size:

1. Loss to follow-up: Sample size calculation should account for dropouts that can occur during the course of a study. There is no accepted or standard figure to be

added to the calculated sample size, as the degree of drop out is highly dependent on the nature of the clinical population being studied.
2. Type of outcome variable: It is important to realize that sample size varies depending on the type of outcome variable. With all else held equal, categorical outcomes can require a larger sample size as compared to continuous outcomes. In addition, more information is lost when an outcome is set as categorical, so reconsidering the functional form of the outcome variable is a strategy if the estimated sample size turns out to be too large [8].
3. The study design is an important part of sample size estimation. Paired studies (vs. independent comparison groups) can reduce the need for larger sample sizes. Similarly, if subgroup or stratified analyses are of interest as a primary or secondary hypothesis, the study should be powered appropriately for these analyses.
4. Another issue that frequently comes up when conducting pilot studies is about the sample size of the pilot study itself. Sometimes an arbitrary number of subjects (i.e., 10 or 20 participants) are considered to be an adequate sample size for pilot studies [9]. However, there are increasing requirements to defend the pilot study sample size to justify the participation of study participants and research costs [10].

Calculating Study Power

In many research projects, your sample size may be limited due to a fixed budget, logistical or time constraints, or low rates of disease incidence, treatment, or outcome events. When the sample size is fixed due to any of these issues, an investigator should calculate the power available with the given sample size, anticipated effect size, desired alpha and other appropriate inputs.

Sensitivity Analyses

To select appropriate values for sample size calculations, it is often helpful to conduct a sensitivity analysis to evaluate how changing the alpha, power, and effect size will impact the sample size estimate. Such analysis is of great use when there are issues related to feasibility, time, and cost for a study (see Table 11.1).

Table 11.1 Sensitivity Analysis Using Different Power Values for Sample Size Calculation for an Example of a Study Looking at Proportion Rates in Two Different Groups

Sample Size (total)	Power	DM Rate in Coffee Arm	DM Rate in Control Arm
100	73%	10%	30%
200	97%	10%	30%
300	69%	10%	20%
400	81%	10%	20%
400	32%	10%	15%

Post-hoc calculation: Magnitude of Type II error can inform how you interpret null results.

Limitations in the Existing Literature Regarding Sample Size Calculation

After going through the topic and the case study, the importance of sample size calculation can be appreciated. ICH GCP guidelines, National Institutes of Health (NIH), IRBs, and (sometimes) journal reviewers require that this calculation is outlined in detail. However, it is of no surprise that on many occasions it is either not done at all, or if it is done, then there is inadequate mention of the parameters used for its calculation. A review of 70 clinical trials revealed that sample size calculations and statistical methods reported in the trial results were often explicitly discrepant with the protocol or not pre-specified [11].

Calculating Sample Size for Your Research (by Hand)

Sample size calculation is often an area of concern for researchers. Before proceeding to the calculations, the study design and its set outcome must be well defined. Once these issues have been addressed, sample size calculations can be done by the researcher or with the help of a study statistician. Depending on the study design, there are different ways of conducting a sample size calculation. We show some examples in which calculation can be done manually; however, we strongly suggest using statistical software.

Sample Size Estimation for Two Independent Means

In randomized controlled trials (RCTs) two different arms are comparing interventions to access safety and efficacy. For sample size calculation, the following information is needed:

- Alpha (level of significance set)
- Beta (power)
- Effect size
- Means of the two interventions and their standard deviations.

The formula used for calculation of sample size for comparative trials is the following [12]:

$$N = \frac{4\sigma^2 (z_{crit} + z_{pwr})^2}{D_2}$$

Sigma squared is the variance; z_{power} is the z-value for the corresponding power set, and z_{crit} is the z-value for the corresponding value of alpha set

$D = Mean_1 - Mean_2 / SD_{pooled}$

$SD_{pooled} = Sqrt(SD_1^2 + SD_2^2)/2$

Sample Size Estimation for Two Independent Proportions

When dealing with outcomes that are categorical, proportions are used to calculate the sample size. The needed information is

- Alpha
- Beta
- Effect size
- Proportions.

The formula used is the following [12]:

$$N = 2 \bullet \frac{\left[z_{crit} \sqrt{2\bar{p}(1-\bar{p})} + z_{pwr} \sqrt{p_1(1-p_1) + p_2(1-p_2)} \right]^2}{D^2}$$

p_1 is the proportion for group 1; p_2 is the proportion for group 2.

Steps for Performing Sample Size Calculation

1. Outline the specific aim of the study, with hypotheses (if appropriate), and identify the exposure/treatment and outcome, and select an appropriate study design.
2. Identify what the most appropriate statistical test is for the primary aim.
3. Gather the inputs required for a sample size or power calculation for that specific statistical test. You will likely need to specify the alpha, beta, and hypothesized effect size.
4. Consider conducting sensitivity analyses to understand how your sample size or power calculation may change depending on your assumptions (such as a condition where the hypothesized effect is slightly larger or smaller than you might expect).
5. Write up your sample size or power calculation in a short paragraph justifying your choice of inputs, and any assumptions made. Cite existing research where appropriate to defend your choice of inputs, such as the effect size or outcome variability. Be transparent about including mention of every piece of information you used to perform your calculation so that a reader could replicate it independently.

CASE STUDY 13: CALCULATING THE SAMPLE SIZE FOR A LYME DISEASE TRIAL

Felipe Fregni

It was 4 p.m. and Dr. Jennifer Hoffman was having coffee at the Massachusetts General Hospital (MGH) Cafeteria. She was thrilled that she could finally negotiate protected time for research with her department chair. It was not an easy negotiation and she was ready to move to the West Coast—UCSD—if the department did not grant her 50% of protected time to research. In fact, she initially moved to the East Coast after finishing her residency in Texas as her passion was Lyme disease—the Northeast is one of the areas with the highest prevalence of Lyme disease in the United States. However, her busy clinical practice and an increasing volume of patients prevented her from dedicating more time to research. But now she was relieved that she would have time to run the project she had been planning for several years: a clinical trial testing the treatment with antibiotic for patients with chronic Lyme disease (persistent symptoms in patients with a history of Lyme disease).[1]

Dr. Hoffman has a great deal of experience with Lyme disease, and she is one of the reference names in the state of Massachusetts for this disease. She is particularly interested in the chronic symptoms that patients develop after the acute treatment of Lyme disease. In fact, she has run a small feasibility study with 16 patients testing the use of antibiotics for this condition. Although she had just made great progress towards her career goals (getting protected time to research), now she has a very important decision to make: whether the follow-up trial testing antibiotic treatment for persistent symptoms of Lyme disease would be a small study (less than 50 patients) or a large clinical trial (around 200 patients). This decision will be mainly based on the sample size calculation and will determine whether she would be able to run this project in the near future or postpone it until she is able to secure enough funds to run a large clinical trial. She then starts to make some notes when her thoughts are interrupted by her pager: she was being called by the neurology team to see a new patient with cranial nerve paralysis, admitted with a suspected diagnosis of Lyme disease. While walking to the neurology ward, she thought about how the next weekend would be a long one: planning and working on the sample size calculation for her study.

Introduction

The size of a given study is one of the *main parameters* when designing a clinical trial and has a significant impact in the study planning and design. Calculating the sample size accurately is crucial, as an adequate number of subjects is extremely important to ensure adequate statistical inferences to the clinical results. In fact, underestimating a sample size might result in a preliminary and inadequate rejection

---

[1] Professor Felipe Fregni prepared this case. Course cases are developed solely as the basis for class discussion. The situation in this case is fictional. Cases are not intended to serve as endorsements or sources of primary data. All rights reserved to the authors of this case.

of new interventions that could be beneficial and might not be assessed again. On the other hand, overestimating a sample size might unnecessarily expose a large number of subjects to a less effective treatment (such as patients randomized to the placebo arm) and increase costs.

Besides the critical importance, sample size calculation is not easy, and the main reason is that it is often challenging to determine the parameters for sample size calculation. In other words, the investigator needs to hypothesize the difference between groups in order to calculate the sample size. But the main question is how to do it before the study is performed. There are several methods, such as using the minimal clinically significant difference, pilot studies, or previous literature. Each one has its advantages and disadvantages. Another important issue here is that clinical researchers should be comfortable in performing sample size calculations so as to better understand the methodology of their studies. In fact, sample size calculation is often not performed, and sample size ends up being determined by the duration of the trial and the ability to recruit subjects—which can lead to serious consequences for the trial.

Treatment of Persistent Symptoms of Lyme Disease with Antibiotic Treatment

Lyme disease is a widespread condition, especially in the northeast of the United States. The prevalence is around 30 cases per 100,000 in prevalent states such as Massachusetts. Although there are effective methods for the treatment of acute Lyme disease, a subset of patients who recover well from the acute phase develop persistent symptoms characterized by fatigue, myalgias, arthralgias, paresthesias, or mood and memory disturbances. There are no standard treatments for these chronic symptoms. One of the recent therapeutic approaches that has been tried is prolonged treatment with antibiotics. Although case reports and uncontrolled trials show beneficial effects of this treatment, the prolonged use of antibiotics is associated with severe adverse effects; therefore, convincing evidence is necessary to prove the effectiveness of this intervention before adopting it in clinical practice.

The Planned Trial

Dr. Hoffman was planning a randomized clinical trial in which patients with well-documented, previously treated Lyme disease—but with persistent musculoskeletal pain, neurocognitive symptoms, or dysesthesia, often associated with fatigue—would be randomized to receive either intravenous ceftriaxone for 30 days, followed by oral doxycycline for 60 days, or matching intravenous and oral placebos. Because there is no established treatment for chronic symptoms in patients with a history of Lyme disease, the use of placebo in this situation is appropriate. The primary outcome measure would be improvement on the Short-Form General Health Survey (SF-36)—a scale measuring the health-related quality of life—on day 180 of the study.

Also, in order to increase the clinical significance of the study, Dr. Hoffman decided to categorize the results of the study. She used the results of a previous study, which showed that a change of up to 7 points in SF-36 could be considered normal variation; therefore, a change higher than 7 points would be considered an improvement (responder) and if a change were less than that, it would be considered a non-responder.

Although recruitment for this study is not a problem as the infectious disease department at MGH and Dr. Hoffman are references for cases of Lyme disease in New England and she sees at least two to three new cases of suspected cases of persistent symptoms in patients with treated Lyme disease per week, it will be difficult to get funds to run a very large study. In addition, she does not want to expose an unnecessarily large number of patients to this trial. So, the calculation of an appropriate sample size is critical.

Dr. Hoffman knows that she needs to calculate the sample size very carefully. Although she has determined that the power of the study will be 90% and the alpha level will be 5% (chance that the results will be false positive), the main issue for her is how to estimate the difference between treatments. This will not be an easy task. She decides then to go to Cape Cod during the weekend where her family has a small house in the charming city of Falmouth so that she can concentrate on the task of sample size calculation for her study.

First Option: Using the Results of Her Pilot Study

The drive to Cape Cod was not easy. Although it should take only 90 minutes (from Boston) to get there, traffic during the summer is heavy and can take hours, especially on Thursday and Friday evenings. Despite the heavy traffic, she was confident that this would be a productive weekend. Moreover, besides being in a beautiful place, she would also have access to all the necessary resources, including high-speed Internet access.

Comfortable in Cape Cod, the first option she considers is to use the results of her pilot trial in order to calculate the difference between treatments. Her pilot study was a trial to assess the initial feasibility and safety of prolonged treatment with an antibiotic for persistent symptoms in Lyme disease. In this trial, 16 patients were randomized to receive active or placebo treatment (this followed the same strategy of the current trial—intravenous ceftriaxone for 30 days, followed by oral doxycycline for 60 days, or matching intravenous and oral placebos). At the end of the study, seven patients (87.5%) were considered responders in the active group and one patient (12.5%) was considered a responder in the placebo group. Therefore, if she assumes a power of 90% and alpha level of 5%, she would need a sample size of 20 patients (10 per group) to show a significant effect. She is surprised at the small sample size and repeats the calculation, but it is correct. She becomes extremely excited and sends an email to her colleague—Dr. John Davis—a clinical researcher with a lot of experience in clinical trials working at Children's Hospital. He was always a good resource for Dr. Hoffman:

> Dear John,
> Remember the chronic Lyme disease clinical trial I want to conduct? I just ran the sample size calculation using the results of my previous pilot study (with a power of 90% and alpha of 5%) and got a sample size of 20 subjects. What do you think? Although this is good, it may be too small.
>
> Jen

Dr. Hoffman was not expecting to hear from him anytime soon, but he is also working on Saturday and quickly responds to her from his Blackberry:

Dear Jen,

I do remember this study. Although this is a valid method as the methodology of your pilot study is exactly the same as your proposed study, this seems too small to me and you may be overestimating the results of your treatment. Remember the chances of overestimating are larger with small sample sizes. You might have selected a sample of patients in your pilot study that responded very well to this treatment. In addition, estimating a population's standard deviation based on small studies is known to underestimate the population's true variability. I would also suggest assessing other methods before making your final decision.

John

Dr. Hoffman decided then to go ahead and assess the other options. But before that, she stopped to have something to eat in her preferred local eatery—a small French restaurant.

Second Option: Using the Minimal Clinically Significant Difference Between Treatments

After lunch, Dr. Hoffman goes back to her work and starts assessing the use of the minimal *clinically* significant difference between treatments. The main notion for this approach is that if the difference between treatments is less than a predefined threshold, then it does not matter if the study is not powered to detect such a difference, as this difference would not be clinically relevant.

Based on her clinical experience, she then considers that a difference of 25% would be clinically relevant (anything below that would not be relevant). She also decides to assume that the placebo group might have a response as high as 35%. She then calculates the sample size using the same power and alpha parameters and comes up with the sample size of 180 (90 patients per group). That was what she feared—a large sample size if this method is used. She then decides to email John again:

John, thanks so much for your help. I recalculated the sample size using the minimal clinically significant difference and got a sample size of 180 patients. This would result in a big burden for my study budget—what should I do now?

Jen

John quickly responds:

Jen, if you use this method, your calculation will certainly be better accepted and in addition it does not hurt to have a larger sample size—it will increase the impact of your study and facilitate statistical analysis. Also remember, you are using categorical variables. However, if you are confident that the results of your pilot study are reliable, then you might be throwing away resources and exposing an unnecessary number of patients to your trial. Tough call!

John

It was getting dark and Dr. Hoffman was getting tired. She decided to call it a night and continue the next day. She then went to the porch to have a glass of wine and tried to relax so she would be sufficiently rested the next day to reach a decision.

Third Option: Using the Results from Other Trials

Dr. Hoffman wakes up and it is a beautiful day outside. It is warm and sunny and she feels energized and ready to make the final assessment: using the results of literature to calculate the sample size.

She then finds a study published four years ago in which the authors gave tetracycline to almost 300 patients with chronic Lyme disease for 1 to 11 months. Although this was a large study, it was open-label. The results of this study were remarkable: 90% of patients had a significant improvement. Using these results and given the hypothesized placebo response of 35%, the sample size would be 36 patients (18 patients per group).

She is initially surprised at the small sample size and thinks that this could be a compromise solution. However, she also considers all the issues associated with the use of results of other trials. This was an uncontrolled trial (therefore effects might be overestimated) that used another drug (tetracycline rather than ceftriaxone/doxycycline) and treatment duration was different. Also, the inclusion criteria of study participants (severity of symptoms, ages, and history of treatment) did not perfectly match those of the patients she wanted to include in her study.

Dr. Hoffman was tempted to email John again, but it was Sunday and she did not want to annoy him. But she was confident that she had enough. It was almost afternoon—she decided to pack early to return to Boston to try to beat the traffic. She was then prepared to start the next steps for this study.

CASE DISCUSSION

This case is about treatment of chronic Lyme disease and finding a way to calculate the appropriate sample size. Dr. Hoffman is an expert in the field of treating patients with Lyme disease, and although there is no standard therapy of chronic cases, she intends to test a new regimen to alleviate the symptoms of the chronic state. Chronic Lyme disease is not a common condition, and the cost of running the trial is an issue to consider as well. The main challenge is finding the best way to obtain the parameters that are needed for sample size calculation. Dr. Hoffman had conducted a pilot study on a small number of patients with promising results, and through literature search she had extracted a study in which tetracycline was used for the treatment of chronic Lyme disease. In addition, a difference of 7 points on SF-36 scale is considered to be minimally clinical significant. As this is a two-arm study with a continuous outcome, apart from the alpha, beta, and means of the two groups, standard deviations will be required to calculate the sample size.

Each of the three options mentioned can be used to estimate the standard deviation to be used for the sample size calculation. All of the options are reasonable, and all of them are used to get the standard deviations in various clinical trials. However, each of the strategies has its advantages and disadvantages. Using the parameters based on a pilot study does seem logical and relevant. The calculated sample size is also reasonable and more importantly feasible to conduct a trial for a disease that is not common. Nevertheless, there are many issues related to this strategy. First, the population of a pilot study is usually very small. Second, the pilot study population might be very homogenous and therefore results might not be applicable to a larger sample with a heterogeneous population. This frequently leads to a small sample size estimation that will render the main study underpowered. Therefore, there is a chance of increasing type II error, however, with small sample size, there is also chance of type I error. When using pilot studies which results in small sample size one has to bear in mind that the results can be overestimated.

The second option is to select the minimally clinical significant difference between the two treatments and then proceed to calculate the required sample size. It also seems like a relevant and reasonable option, but will lead to calculation of a large sample size. This can be a waste of resources, time-consuming, questionably feasible, and more important, will expose many patients to placebo, raising ethical issues and risking that the study might not achieve the grant approval. Dr. Hoffman could plan an interim analysis to assess the data and decide to stop the study if a continuation is not needed. Planning an interim analysis will be at the expense of the p-value set for the primary outcome (see Chapter 18).

The third option is to use historical values from published studies to extract the standard deviations and apply them for calculation, a strategy frequently used by researchers. It is also a cheap solution and thus helps in saving money and time. The researcher has to find a study with similar study design, outcomes, and treatment to use it as a template for obtaining the required information. This is a difficult task, and having the luxury to find a matched study is occasionally not possible, unless the study has been replicated several times in the past.

For the sheer feasibility, if literature search shows 90% improvement in tetracycline arm and taking the hypothesized 35% response to placebo, the sample size would be 36 (18 patients per arm). By doing so, Dr. Hoffman has saved time and will be able to recruit the patients needed with two to three referrals per week in 180 days. This approach helps in saving time as the calculated sample size is intermediate as compared to the ones calculated using pilot or minimal clinical difference approach. It also limits the number of patients who get unnecessarily exposed to interventions due to larger sample size if calculated using approach of minimal clinical difference.

Another option that Dr. Hoffman could apply would be simply "guesstimating" the standard deviations based on her experience in the field and do the sample size calculation. Bias can be introduced this way, and the study results could easily lose significance. This option is not recommended unless the data available are scarce.

Study design has a significant impact on the outcome and therefore the best design to conduct the study should be chosen. In case of rare diseases, one strategy is having unequal groups. Allocating more patients to the active group and then applying statistical techniques to adjust for the different ratio in group numbers and drawing conclusions is a possible strategy. This technique can also help in decreasing the number of patients who drop out, as the duration of the study is 180 days. The dropout rate is another issue that should be considered, especially in long duration clinical trials and should be accounted for in sample size calculation.

Considering dropout rate, Dr. Hoffman thinks about using the approach of unequal allocation, allowing more patients to get recruited in long-term antibiotic therapy arm. Using positive data from pilot study, this should not be against principle of equipoise. But then Dr. Hoffman thinks of using the approach of minimal clinical difference which will help in gathering clinically meaningful data with a larger sample size rather than collecting data on small number of patients using pilot or literature search data. As she decides about the way to move forward, she keeps on thinking about time, money, dropouts, etc., and says to herself that "there is much more to it rather than just plugging in values of alpha and power to calculate sample size."

CASE QUESTIONS FOR REFLECTION

Keeping all these issues in mind, the following questions are related to the case:

1. What challenges does Prof. Hoffman face in choosing the method to determine the difference between treatments?
2. What are her main concerns?
3. What should she consider in making the decision?
4. Do you have any other concerns that she should discuss for sample size (outcome variables, internal/external validity, dropping out, budget, feasibility, etc.)?

FURTHER READING

Article/Topic Review

This article discusses in detail the challenges and strategies for doing sample size calculations for different epidemiological studies:

Kasiulevičius V, Šapoka V, Filipavičiūtė R. Sample size calculation in epidemiological studies. *Gerontologija*. 2006; 7(4): 225–231. Available online at http://www.gerontologija.lt/files/edit_files/File/pdf/2006/nr_4/2006_225_231.pdf [last accessed on Jan. 16, 2013].

Grunkemeier GL, Jin R. The statistician's page: power and sample size: how many patients do I need? *Ann ThoracSurg*. 2007; 83: 1934–1939.

Review

Dattalo P. A review of software for sample size determination. *Eval Health Prof.* 2009; 32(3): 229–248. doi: 10.1177/0163278709338556.

Software Programs to Perform Sample Size and Power Calculations

You will learn in Unit III how to perform a sample size calculation in STATA, but this can be done with any statistical software package.

There are several commercially available programs:

PASS
NQuery
EAST

Many websites provide convenient sample size calculators, easing the process of calculation for researchers:

- Power/Sample size at Vanderbilt
http://biostat.mc.vanderbilt.edu/wiki/Main/PowerSampleSize
- David Schoenfeld at MGH/Harvard
http://hedwig.mgh.harvard.edu/sample_size/size.html

Books

The following reference books specifically discuss topics on sample size calculations with formulas and tables given for researchers to perform sample size calculations:

Chow S-C, Wang H, Shao J. *Sample size calculations in clinical research*, 2nd ed. Chapman & Hall/CRC Biostatistics Series; 2007.

Machin D, Campbell MJ, Tan S-B, Tan S-H. *Sample size tables for clinical studies*. 3rd Edition. Oxford, UK: Wiley-Blackwell; 2008.

REFERENCES

1. ICH Expert working group. ICH harmonised tripartite guideline: guideline for good clinical practice E6(R1). 1996. Available at: http://www.ich.org/fileadmin/Public_Web_Site/ICH_Products/Guidelines/Efficacy/E6_R1/Step4/E6_R1__Guideline.pdf [accessed on Jan. 15, 2013].
2. Machin D, Campbell MJ, Fayers PM, Pinol APY. *Sample size tables for clinical studies*, 2nd ed. Oxford, London, Berlin: Blackwell Science; 1987: 1–315.
3. Charles P, Giraudeau B, Dechartres A, Baron G, Ravaud P. Reporting of sample size calculation in randomised controlled trials: review. *BMJ.* 2009; 338: b1732.
4. Bacchetti P. Current sample size conventions: flaws, harms, and alternatives. *BMC Med.* 2010; 8(1): 17.
5. Vickers AJ. Underpowering in randomized trials reporting a sample size calculation. *J Clin Epidemiol.* 2003; 56(8): 717–720.
6. Prentice DA, Miller DT. When small effects are impressive. *Psychol Bull.* 1992; 112(1): 160–164.
7. Paulus J. Sample size calculation. Powerpoint presentation for *Principles and practice of clinical research course*. 2012. Available online from course website access http://www.ppcr.hms.harvard.edu [last accessed on Jan. 15, 2013].
8. Zhao LP, Kolonel LN. Efficiency loss from categorizing quantitative exposures into qualitative exposures in case-control studies. *Am J Epidemiol.* 1992; 136(4): 464–474.
9. Julious SA. Sample size of 12 per group rule of thumb for a pilot study. *Pharmaceut. Statist.* 2005; 4: 287–291. Available online at http://research.son.wisc.edu/rdsu/sample%20size%20pilot%20study12.pdf [last accessed on Jan. 13, 2013].

10. Johanson GA, Brooks GP. Initial scale development: sample size for pilot studies. *Educ Psychol Meas.* 2010; 70(3): 394–400.
11. Chan A-W, Hróbjartsson A, Jørgensen KJ, Gøtzsche PC, Altman DG. Discrepancies in sample size calculations and data analyses reported in randomised trials: comparison of publications with protocols. *BMJ.* 2008; 337: a2299.
12. Eng J. Sample size estimation: how many individuals should be studied? *Radiology.* 2003; 227: 309–313.

12

SURVIVAL ANALYSIS

Authors: *Jorge Leite and Sandra Carvalho*
Case study authors: *Munir Boodhwani and Felipe Fregni*

INTRODUCTION

Survival analysis denotes a specific set of standardized statistical analysis that is focused on time to event [1]—in other words, how much time elapses from exposure/intervention to the occurrence of an event. For instance, imagine that you are testing a new intervention to prevent hospitalization due to diabetic ketoacidosis (DKA). This is an acute, life-threatening condition that requires immediate medical attention, in which preventive care could have a major impact. During your trial design stage, you choose as primary outcome to measure the effectiveness of your interventions, at least one hospitalization due to DKA over a 12-month period, following the new intervention (e.g., 12 months). This metric, although suitable, can be misleading as we will see in the example that follows.

The following 2 x 2 table presents the rate of hospitalization due to DKA in the standard versus the new intervention.

	Hospitalized	Not Hospitalized
New Intervention	60	40
Standard Care	70	30

The odds ratio of being hospitalized would be 0.64 (0.36–1.16, 95% CI) or a risk ratio of 0.86 (0.70–1.05, 95% CI). Note that in both situations the 95% CI overlaps with 1, and thus there seems to be no significant difference in the number of hospitalizations due to DKA complications between the new intervention and standard of care.

A survival analysis would view this problem differently, and would focus on the time elapsed between the intervention and the outcome event (in this case, hospitalization). So instead of focusing on how many patients were hospitalized after the intervention, the main interest is how long it takes for them to develop DKA and require hospitalization.

A table for a survival analysis would be arranged differently, in order to reflect the time in which each patient experienced the first hospitalization episode due to DKA.

New Intervention	Standard Care	Hospitalization by DKA (in months)
Patient 1		5
Patient 67		8
Patient 198		12
	Patient 4	2
	Patient 152	4
	Patient 178	3
...	...	...

After analyzing the time until the first hospitalization, the outcome shows that the median survival time for patients that benefited from the new education intervention had a median survival time of 8 months, while the other group had a median survival time of 3 months. Therefore, depending on the research question, survival analysis may be also be a more effective test to analyze data dependent on events (yes/no).

MEDIAN SURVIVAL TIME

The median survival time is the first important concept to understand in survival analysis. The median survival time is the time point in which 50% of patients developed the event. In the DKA example, 50% of patients that benefited from the new intervention were hospitalized 8 months after the intervention; and 50% of patients under standard care were hospitalized after 3 months. The remaining 50% could be hospitalized at a later point, or not at all.

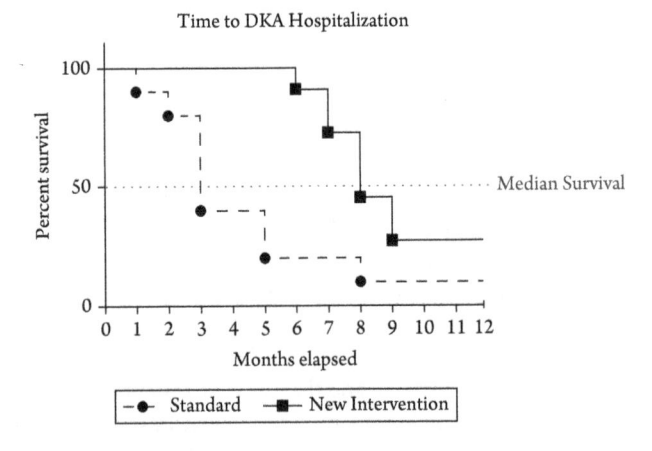

The concept of median survival time then allows us to have an estimate of when 50% of the subjects in our sample develop the outcome of interest. And thus it is an especially useful metric when assessing time until death, reoccurrence of an important clinical outcome, time from exposure until a specific outcome, among others.

Nonetheless, by itself, the median survival time is unable to tell us if the new intervention is superior to the standard of care. Median survival time can be considered along the Kaplan-Meier curve (see the following) as descriptive statistics, similar to mean and standard deviation, respectively, for continuous data.

KAPLAN-MEIER SURVIVAL PROBABILITY ESTIMATORS

This is another important concept of survival analysis that estimates the cumulative probability of survival at specific time points. For instance, imagine that in the group that benefited from standard care, 10 patients were hospitalized in the first month. This means that each patient will have 90% chance (90 that survived the event/100 patients in the group = 0.90) of not being hospitalized (i.e., survival) due to DKA in the first month following standard care (i.e., survival rate for first month). On the second month, 10 were already hospitalized, so the number of subjects that could be hospitalized due to DKA complications was reduced to 90. If 8 other patients were hospitalized due to DKA complications on the second month, the cumulative survival rate will be the multiplication of the survival rate in the second month (82/90 = 0.91) by the product of the previous month (i.e., survival rate for first month = 0.90), which will then be (0.91*0.90 = 0.82). So if a patient survives the first month, the probability of not being hospitalized due to DKA at two months will be 82%.

The Kaplan-Meier [2] survival probability estimates then the cumulative probability for that specific time point, taking into consideration the survival probability in the previous time point.

Month	At Risk	Not Hospitalized	Survival Probability	Cumulative Survival Probability
1	100	90	$\frac{90}{100} = 0.90$	**0.90**
2	90	82	$\frac{82}{90} = 0.91$	0.90*0.91 = **0.82**
3	82	46	$\frac{46}{82} = 0.56$	0.82*0.56 = **0.46**

Survival analysis focuses on something that is called the survival function—which is the cumulative probability of surviving the event. The Kaplan-Meier estimator is an easy function that can be calculated by hand to provide an estimate of the cumulative probability of surviving an event. As aforementioned, it is an important method to describe the data and provide an overall picture of what happened in the trial for all subjects.

THE LOG RANK TEST (MANTEL–COX)

In order to estimate if one treatment (or exposure) leads to a significant longer survival period until an event, survival functions need to be compared. In our analogy, this would be similar to conducting a t-test when comparing the means of two groups (as measured with continuous data). This can be performed using the log rank test [3]. In this test, survival curves are estimated against the null hypothesis that there are no differences between them. Thus, a p-value of less than 0.05 is interpreted as a null hypothesis rejection, and thus the survival functions are assumed to be statistically significantly different.

In the trial that aims to compare the new educational intervention against standard of care in DKA prevention, the new intervention seems to statistically significant increase the time until DKA hospitalization, when compared to standard of care $[\chi^2(1) = 6.64, p = .01]$. In this case, we state that the difference between survival functions is statistically significant because the p-value (.01) is less than .05, and thus the null hypothesis is rejected.

The log rank test is usually the standard test to compare survival functions and is powerful if the survival function (sometimes also called hazard function) has proportional hazards (the number of events is kept the same at all the time points). If this is not true, then there is another method, the Gehan-Breslow-Wilcoxon, which is more suitable if there is no consistent hazard ratio [4]. Nonetheless, the Gehan-Breslow-Wilcoxon requires that one group has a consistently higher survival than the other. Moreover, this second method gives more weight to events at early time points, which can be misleading, especially with censoring at early stages.

CENSORING

So far we have been addressing survival analysis as if the time to event observations are complete. In some cases, the variable of interest (i.e., event) will not be possible to assess during the period of the study. For instance, from our research question, if a patient has a hospitalization due to DKA complications after the 12-month period following the intervention, that occurrence will not be available. This is not considered to be missing data. Instead, this occurrence is considered to be out of the specified time window (i.e., 12 months) and is a specific type of censoring—*right censoring*. This is the most common type of censoring. And it happens when the occurrence of an event is after the specified time for the survival analysis.

There are other types of censoring [5]. For instance, left censoring occurs when an event stops from occurring before the analysis period. We don't know exactly when it happened, but just that the event occurred prior to study entry. For instance, imagine that one patient is enrolled, but no hospitalizations due to DKA have occurred in the 12 months prior to the enrollment. It seems that hospitalizations due to DKA stopped before, but we don't know when, and thus this can be an example of *left censoring*.

The last type of censoring is called *interval censoring*. It usually happens when the event occurs between survey intervals. For instance, imagine that in the DKA example, instead of using hospital records, we were using questionnaires to assess the DKA occurrence. A possibility is that the event of interest could happen between visits. Then it would not be possible to accurately know when it actually happened. This interval censoring occurs when the occurrence of the event is between assessment periods, and there is no way to know exactly when it did happen.

HOW TO DEAL WITH CENSORING

So far, we have been assuming that for all time points, we have the correct observation for hospitalization due to DKA. We now are going to assume that instead of using the hospitalization record, the trial was designed to survey diabetic patients once a month, for the 12 months following the intervention. By doing so, it is possible to have censored observations (i.e., hospitalization due to DKA) between surveys.

One way of dealing with censoring in the Kaplan-Meier estimate is, following a censored observation, remove it from the population at risk at the following time point. For instance, we have 100 at risk of hospitalization in the first month. At the first month survey, 10 were hospitalized at that point, but 3 were hospitalized at some point before the survey. So the survival probability for the first month would be 0.90 (90/100). At this point the censored observations would not impact the results, but they will be removed from the population at risk for the second month—instead of 90, the population at risk would then be 87 (90–3 censored).

Month	At Risk	Censored	Not Hospitalized	Survival Probability	Cumulative Survival Probability
1	100	3	90	$\frac{90}{100} = 0.90$	**0.90**
2	87	8	82	$\frac{82}{87} = 0.94$	0.90*0.94 = **0.85**
3	74	12	46	$\frac{46}{74} = 0.62$	0.85*0.62 = **0.53**

Please note that censoring does not impact the survival function at the first time point, as the probability is the same with or without censoring. But after that time point, censoring will change the survival function. For instance, at the end of the second month the three observations that were previously censored in the month before will not count toward the population at risk, and thus cumulative probability will change. Please note that from the first example, a patient at the end of the second month has an 82% probability of not being hospitalized due to DKA complications. But with censoring, the probability increases to 85%.

There are other options to deal with censored data. These options include setting the censored observation to missing, or replacing it with zero, minimum, maximum, mean value, or a random assigned number. Although the use of such methods can be sound in some cases, a small number of censored data is required. If not, these methods can produce undesirable effects, such as bias in statistical estimates, samples that are not representative of the general population, and even important information could be potentially discarded from the study.

ADJUSTING FOR COVARIATES: THE USE OF COX PROPORTIONAL HAZARDS (COX REGRESSION MODEL)

So far we have been discussing survival analysis as if the hospitalization events are solely due to the intervention. But commonly, there are several interrelated factors that can contribute to the increase or decrease of survival probability, especially for non-randomized studies. Imagine, for instance, that you want to explore the importance of risk factors, such as diabetes type, or miss of an insulin dose in hospitalization due to DKA. These two factors can be covariates to the intervention, as they are also associated with the risk of developing the hospitalization event. These covariates can then influence the outcome and need to be accounted for in the analysis. This is often done by using a specific statistical procedure, the Cox Proportional Hazards model (or Cox regression model; indeed regression or multivariate analysis is used with different types of outcomes [e.g., linear regression for continuous variables and logistic regression for categorical variables; and here Cox Proportional Hazards for time to event variables]). In the chapter introducing linear regression (Chapter 9), you learned that when the outcomes are binomial, the appropriate model to use is the logistic regression. In this case, hospitalization due to DKA is also a binomial variable, thus it will be possible to use a logistic regression model to compare the presence or absence of hospitalization due to DKA at a specific time point, but not to compare survival curves based on time to event—the focus of survival analysis. Thus, in order to compare the influence of one or multiple predictors in a time to event analysis, the most suitable regression model is the Cox Proportional Hazards model [6].

In this model, the aim is to construct the *hazard function*, which can be defined as the probability that if a subject survives t, he or she will experience the event in the following instant. The logistic regression estimates instead the proportion of cases that develop the event at a specific time point. Thus, if logistic regression estimates odds ratios, Cox regression estimates hazard ratios. In simple terms, Cox regression model is a function of the relative risk of developing the event at a specific moment (i.e., t).

Although the focus of this chapter is not to have an extensive explanation regarding the underlying assumptions to regression modeling, there is one important concept: the proportionality. In this model, the hazard function for one subject is a fixed proportional of the hazard function of another subject. Also, if all the covariates of a subject are set to zero ($\lambda_0(t) = 0$), and for another subject the ($\lambda_1(t) = \exp(\beta_1 X_{1i} + \beta_2 X_{2i} + \ldots)$), then the hazard function will not be dependent on time, but only on the effects of predictor variables. This means that if, for instance, a predictor triples the risk of an event on one day, it will also triple the risk of an event on any other day.

CASE STUDY: USING SURVIVAL ANALYSIS IN A RETROSPECTIVE STUDY FOR MITRAL VALVE SURGERY

Munir Boodhwani and Felipe Fregni

Maria hesitated for a second before walking through the door. She looked up at the sign on the door. It read "Dr. Christof Feldman—Johnson and Johnson Endowed Chair of the Department of Surgery." It was her first week at her new job as a clinical research consultant at the University of Pennsylvania. She had completed her PhD in clinical epidemiology at the University of Colorado and had been hired immediately by the University of Pennsylvania. Her role was to serve as a consultant to the various clinical departments that needed support to perform their clinical research studies. This was her first meeting with a clinical team—her first assignment.[1]

She had heard about Dr. Feldman even before she came to the University of Pennsylvania. It had been about six months before her graduation. It was a news story, she recalled, that discussed the latest developments in heart valve surgery, and they had interviewed Dr. Feldman to get his opinion on the new "keyhole" or minimally invasive mitral valve repair procedure. Apparently, he had a national reputation for what he did and, from what she had heard; he had a pretty intimidating personality. Today's meeting was with Dr. Feldman, Dr. James Sunder (Dr. Feldman's research associate), and Dr. David Kurdy (a junior surgery resident).

From talking to her colleagues, Maria had learned that Dr. Feldman was the best cardiothoracic surgeon in the city, and one of the best in the country. Although over the age of 60, he was known to have a busy practice, excellent technical skills, and a keen sense of clinical intuition. When he made a diagnosis or a clinical observation, he was usually right. But he didn't know the first thing about research or data analysis. Dr. Sunder, his younger colleague, had been in practice for about six years and was Dr. Feldman's understudy. He had some basic training in clinical research but lacked Feldman's clinical acumen. David Kurdy was a recent graduate from medical school, now a first year resident in surgery, who had spent most of his weekends and summers working with the department over the past two years, trying to build a database of patients who had undergone mitral valve surgery at this institution.

Introduction: The Trial

Maria knocked softly and then walked through the door and took a seat at the conference table where the other three were already seated.

"For this study that we are working on and want you, Maria, to join us on, I want to show that patients do better after mitral valve repair than replacement," Dr. Feldman said in his booming voice. In response to the puzzled look on Maria's face, Dr. Sunder

---

[1] Munir Boodhwani and Felipe Fregni prepared this case. Course cases are developed solely as the basis for class discussion. The situation in this case is fictional. Cases are not intended to serve as endorsements or sources of primary data. All rights reserved to the author of this case. Reproduction and distribution without permission from authors is not allowed.

began to explain, "The classical treatment for severe mitral valve insufficiency has been replacement of the valve either with a biologic or mechanical prosthesis. Over the past 15–20 years, under Dr. Feldman's leadership, surgical techniques have been developed to repair the mitral valve preserving the native valve tissue. We prefer repair over replacement because the biologic prostheses degrade over time and don't seem to last more than 10 years or so and then the patients require reoperation for a re-replacement of the valve. On the other hand, mechanical valves last for a long time but interact with the blood and increase the chance of blood clots forming on the valve, which can then go to different parts of the body and can lead to stroke or ischemia of the different parts of the body. So, we have to give them blood thinners to prevent that, but then there is a risk of bleeding complications. What we are interested in finding out is whether valve repair has a long-term advantage over replacement, particularly in terms of survival." Dr. Sunder went on to explain in more detail the nature of mitral valve disease and the history of mitral valve surgery at the University of Pennsylvania.

After understanding the main clinical characteristics associated with mitral valve repair, Maria asks, "That is a quite interesting clinical problem, but are we talking about a prospective randomized study—my guess is that would be difficult due to ethical issues and also long follow-up time until patients start having issues related to the previous operation—or a retrospective study?" James Sunder quickly responds, "That is a good point, Maria. You are right; a prospective study would not be feasible. We want to analyze our data retrospectively. We have data from 3,728 patients who underwent either mitral valve repair or replacement and we actually could follow most of these patients as we are a renowned cardiac center in the area and patients rarely move to other services. If they move to other cities, it is common that they maintain appointments with their doctors in our hospital. In addition, we have a detailed electronic database that goes back to the 1980s."

"That is wonderful," Maria comments. In fact, this is what epidemiologists need—large databases and an interesting and important clinical question. She then comments, "Now we need to decide how we are analyzing the data. We have some challenges ahead of us. The main question for us is how to analyze the data: using other outcomes (such as quality of life and simple methods of analysis) or the use of survival and more complicated models."

Survival Analysis

Survival analysis is commonly used in medicine. In fact, its use has been increasing in recent years. The main advantage of survival analysis is that this method allows you to compare groups in which individuals have different lengths of observation. For instance, if an investigator is measuring survival associated with cancer, but length of follow-up is variable across patients, this would create a problem if this investigator uses traditional methods of data analysis. In addition, treatments might have survival rates that vary across time—for instance, surgical versus medical treatments. While mortality would be higher initially for the surgical treatments, it might be smaller after the first year as compared to medical treatments (which would be associated with a more stable mortality over years). Therefore, a method such as survival analysis, which can take into account variable lengths of follow-up (including cases of censoring and loss to follow-up) and change in survival rates across time, is important in medicine.

More about Mitral Valve Repair

During the 1980s, replacement was the exclusive surgical treatment of mitral valve insufficiency. In the early 1990s, repair techniques were slowly adapted, and over time, the repair rate of mitral valves has improved to close to 90%. The volume of cases of mitral valve disease has also been increasing over the past decade and because of improved outcomes with this surgery, less symptomatic patients (who are earlier in their disease process) are being referred for surgery in recent years.[2]

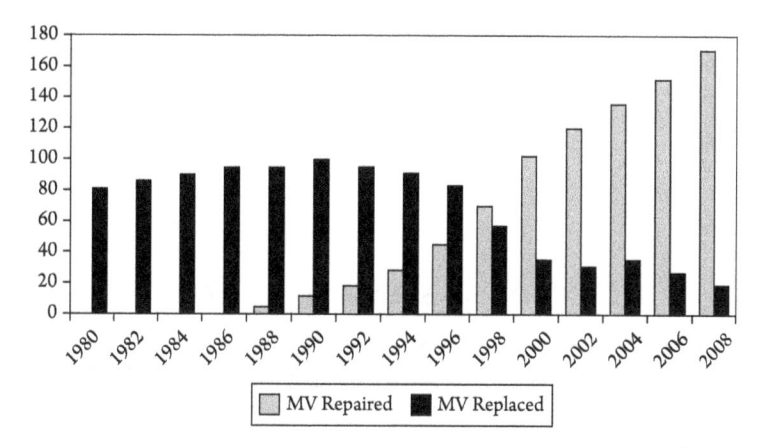

Mitral valve disease can be due to four causes: Barlow's disease (occurs in young patients), degenerative disease (older patients), endocarditis (valve infection), and rheumatic valve disease. Endocarditis and rheumatic valve disease are significantly less common, but these valves are much more difficult to repair and consequently have a higher failure rate. Patients typically enjoy a good overall survival after mitral valve surgery (~80%–90% at 10 years). There is a small rate of recurrent mitral insufficiency requiring reoperation (~1%–2%/year). Other important determinants of outcome after mitral valve surgery include the following:

- Left ventricular function
- Presence of other cardiac disease (coronary disease, other valve disease)
- Severity of pre-operative symptoms.

Twenty minutes into the meeting, Dr. Feldman's pager went off. It was an emergency in the operating room. As he was leaving, he said, "Hey Maria. Can we look at some raw results tomorrow?" Before she could reply, he was gone.

---

[2] All graphs in this case study were created solely for educational purposes and the data are fictional.

Table 12.1 Baseline Characteristics of MV Repair versus Replacement

Variable	MV Repair (n = 1711)	MV replacement (n = 2017)
Age	58.6 ± 8.4	61.2 ± 9.8
Sex (% male)	72	74
Etiology (%)		
Barlow's	31	29
Degenerative	53	25
Rheumatic	9	27
Endocarditis	7	19
LVEF < 30%	14	18
Concomitant Coronary/Vale Disease (%)	12	36
Preoperative Severe Symptoms (NYHA ≥ 31) (%)	10	24
Type of Valve Prosthesis (%)		
Biologic		32
Mechanical		68

THE NEXT DAY: ASSESSING THE OPTIONS

In the conference room, they awaited the arrival of Dr. Feldman. When Dr. Feldman entered the room, they began to talk about the results. Maria had prepared first a table of baseline characteristics between the two groups (repair and replacement) (Table 12.1) and also raw unadjusted Kaplan-Meier curves[3] of the two groups.

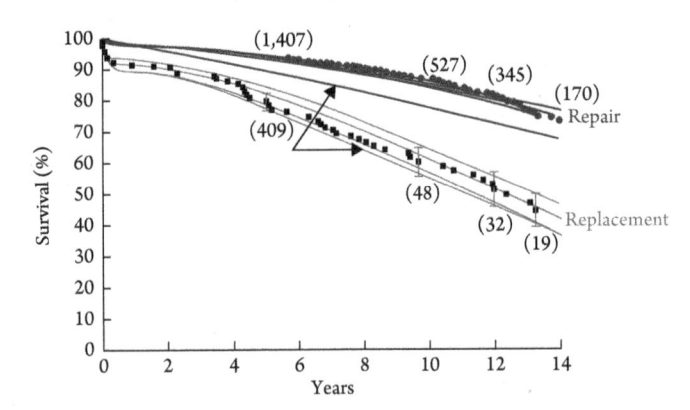

Dr. Feldman is extremely happy with the results presented. "I knew the patients were doing better with the repair," he commented. "This is going to be a great paper—we should be able to publish in a top tier cardiovascular journal. So how should we proceed?"

---

[3] Please see the definition of Kaplan-Meier curves in Appendix 1.

First Option: Using Another Outcome—Quality of Life—and a Simpler Analysis Method (ANOVA or Linear Regression Model)

James decided to give his opinion first, as he was extremely interested in the results of this study as well. He begins, "I think we should opt for simplicity and choose another outcome and method of analysis so readers and doctors can understand easily. I would suggest choosing quality of life as we also measured this yearly in these patients using SF-36 quality of life scale. We could therefore compare quality of life scores between the two groups using an ANOVA model or a regression model if we want to adjust to covariates. Although using the outcome of death (survival) might increase the clinical significance, I am not comfortable with survival analysis. To be honest, I do not understand this method and I am afraid that results would not be easily interpretable."

Dr. Feldman then concludes, "Good point, James. I also like simplicity, but let us see what David has to say."

Second Option: Using Survival Analysis and Comparing the Two Groups Using Log Rank Test

Although David was at the beginning of his residency, he had a considerable exposure to survival analysis techniques during college and he was familiar with this technique. He then starts, "Well, I agree with James, regarding the point that survival analysis is a technique that is not extremely easy to understand; however, it is also not very complicated. In fact, what this technique does is to divide the data set in small periods to be able to capture information of every patient including those with censoring and those who are lost to follow-up. Actually, we can calculate mean survival using the Kaplan Meier method by hand. I would therefore use death as an outcome and show the survival using Kaplan-Meier curves and then compare the two groups using the method of log rank test. This method (log rank test) is also a relatively simple method based on the notion that if two groups have a similar event rate (in this case, death), then at each time point (called as failure time), the number of deaths in each group should be proportional to patients at risk. This test is a non-parametric test that has resemblance to chi-square test."

It is now Dr. Feldman's turn again. "Well, at the end, it might be feasible, but now I want to hear from Maria."

Third Option: Adjusting for Covariates Using Survival and Cox Proportional Model

Maria is actually eager to speak, and now it is her turn. "Those are all valid options. But I would say that we need to complicate it a bit and besides using survival (death as outcome), we also need to use Cox regression model[4] to adjust for covariates. In my little research experience, I found out that it is not fair to compare these patients in these two groups. Do you know how many things have changed since the 1980s? It seems that surgery methodology now is different compared to the 1980s.

---

[4] Please see the definition of Cox regression model in Appendix 1.

Anesthesia is different, post-op care is different, even patients' selection seems to be quite different. And what about confounding by indication? This is a very important confounding factor for observational studies, and in fact these are unadjusted data and many important variables are unevenly distributed between groups. This is the main problem of observational studies; if this were a randomized study, then I would be comfortable with other suggestions. As this is a large sample, we will probably be able to adjust for several confounders without losing power or validity of the test. We must keep in mind, however, that we may show a small difference in survival, that is not clinically relevant, but, due to this large sample, may be statistically significant."

Dr. Feldman responds with a smirk, "You can do all the adjusting you want—I know repair will eventually win out."

Maria leaves the meeting starting to understand the task in front of her—to consider and account for all the possible ways to explain the differences in outcome between the repair versus replacement groups. It will not be an easy task, but she is thrilled with this new challenge.

APPENDIX 1

Kaplan-Meier Estimates: "[T]he Kaplan-Meier Estimates is the most common method of determining survival time, which does not depend on grouping data into specific time intervals. This approach generates a step function, changing the survival estimate each time a patient dies (or reaches the terminal event). Graphic displays of survival functions computed as a series of steps of decreasing magnitude. This method can account for censored observations over time. Confidence intervals can also be calculated." Source: Portney L, Watkins M. *Foundations of clinical research: applications to practice*, 3rd ed. (pp. 721–724). Pearson International Edition; 2009.

Cox Proportional Hazards Model: "Survival time is often dependent on many interrelated factors that can contribute to increased or decreased probabilities of survival or failure. A regression model can be used to adjust survival estimates on the basis of several independent variables. Standard multiple regression methods cannot be used because survival times are typically not normally distributed—an important assumption in least squares regression. And of course, the presence of censored observations presents a serious problem. The Cox proportional hazards model, which conceptually similar to multiple regression, but without assumptions about the shape of distributions. For this reason, this analysis is often considered a nonparametric technique." Source: Portney L, Watkins M. *Foundations of clinical research: applications to practice*, 3rd ed. (pp. 721–724). Pearson International Edition; 2009.

CASE DISCUSSION

Dr. Feldmann, the chair of the surgery department of University of Pennsylvania, wants to "show that patients do better after mitral valve repair than replacement." To accomplish that, he plans to analyze retrospectively the data of 3,728 patients who underwent mitral valve replacement or repair.

This is an important and valuable research question that can be approached in different ways. One of them is to simply use a quality of life scale and use an ANOVA or a linear regression to control for some covariates—in this case, a linear regression would be more suitable than an ANCOVA because the focus would be on the outcome and not on the difference among groups.

This will be a simple and straightforward way of assessing the impact of mitral valve replacement or repair, which will certainly be very welcomed by clinicians. However this type of analysis focuses on one or several specific time points, but does not provide information about time to event. An important event after mitral valve replacement or repair is death. An intervention can be considered more effective than the other if, after the procedure, patients live longer.

The Kaplan-Meier method is easy to calculate by hand and, the survival curves can be compared using a method such as the log rank. In this method, the null hypothesis is that the survival curves are not statistically different one from the other, so a p-value of less than 0.05 is used to reject the null hypothesis. By using this method, interventions that have a similar event rate, the number of events (in this case, death) in a given moment should be proportional to the number of elements in the population at risk.

Also it is possible to include some covariates in order to control for potential effects of such predictors on the time to event analysis. This can be achieved by performing statistical modeling, using the Cox Proportional Hazards regression. In this mode, the proportional impact of predictor factors is analyzed, and then survival times are adjusted based on those factors. The main difference between logistic regression and the Cox Proportional Hazards regression is that the first accounts for the possible influence of covariates at a specific time point, while the latter assumes the relative risk of developing the event at each time point.

CASE QUESTIONS FOR REFLECTION

1. What are the challenges this team of researchers is facing for choosing the best analytical method?
2. What are the advantages and disadvantages of using a univariate analysis (log rank test) versus a multivariate analysis (Cox Proportional Hazards model)?

FURTHER READING

Online Resources

http://vassarstats.net/survival.html
http://www.ats.ucla.edu/stat/sas/seminars/sas_survival/
http://data.princeton.edu/pop509
http://sphweb.bumc.bu.edu/otlt/MPH-Modules/BS/BS704_Survival/BS704_Survival_print.html

REFERENCES

1. Bewick V, Cheek L, Ball J. Statistics review 12: Survival analysis. *Critical Care.* 2004; 8(5): 389–394.
2. Kaplan EL, Meier P. Nonparametric estimation from incomplete observations. *JASA.* 1958; 53(282): 457–481.
3. Bland JM, Altman DG. The logrank test. *BMJ.* 2004; 328(7447): 1073–.
4. Machin D, Cheung YB, Parmar M. *Survival analysis: a practical approach.* 2nd ed. Wiltshire, UK: Wiley; 2006.

5. Prinja S, Gupta N, Verma R. Censoring in clinical trials: review of survival analysis techniques. *Indian Journal of Community Medicine.* 2010; 35(2): 217–221.
6. Armitage P, Berry G, Matthews JNS. *Statistical methods in medical research.* 4th ed. Oxford: Blackwell Science; 2001.

13

OTHER ISSUES IN STATISTICS I
MISSING DATA, INTENTION-TO-TREAT ANALYSIS, AND COVARIATE ADJUSTMENT

Authors: *Tamara Jorquiera and Hang Lee*

Case study authors: *Felipe Fregni and André Brunoni*

INTRODUCTION

This chapter begins with an explanation of what is considered incomplete or lost data and how to handle this issue using an intention-to-treat (ITT) approach, followed by another topic (covariate adjustment). The next chapter will complete the statistics unit, covering subgroup analysis and meta-analysis.

The previous chapters introduced you to statistics, covering hypothesis testing, how to handle data, how to perform data analysis depending on the type of data you collected (parametric vs. non-parametric tests), and sample size calculations. You need to remember that without an adequate number of subjects in your study, you will not have enough power to reach statistical significance. But what if you started your study with a sufficient sample size and then had dropouts, problems with adherence (cross-overs), missed appointments, data entry/acquisition problems? This leads us to the first part of this chapter: what to do if we have incomplete or lost data.

When reporting a randomized controlled trial (RCT), you will need to clearly state and explain the method used to handle missing data and you should use a flowchart diagram to document how participants progressed throughout each phase of the study (see Figure 13.1).

MISSING DATA

Missing data have been defined as "values that are not available and that would be meaningful for analysis if they were observed" by the members of an expert panel convened by the National Research Council (NRC) [1]. It is very common in clinical research to have missing data. The most important thing is to account for all losses, stating when and why they happened whenever this is possible.

Missing data can happen for several reasons:

- Participants drop out, or withdraw from the study before its completion. Usually those who remain in the study are different from the ones who left (biasing

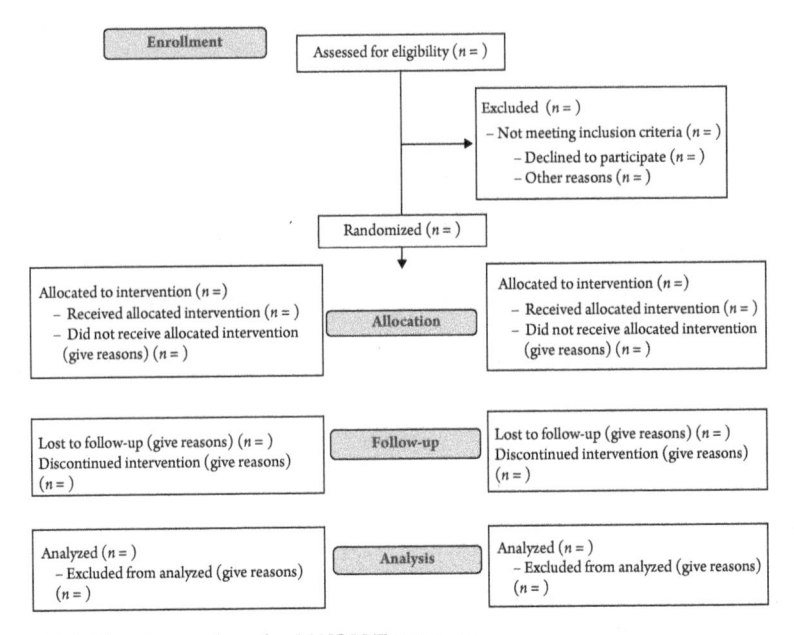

Figure 13.1. Flow diagram from the CONSORT statement.
Source: http://www.consort-statement.org/consort-statement/flow-diagram0/)

analysis). Participants may leave the study for several reasons (e.g. death, adverse reaction, unpleasant procedures, lack of improvement, or early recovery).
- Participants refuse the assigned treatment after allocation. Even if they signed the informed consent and were aware of the possible treatments, they must be allowed to withdraw at any time.
- Participants do not attend an appointment at which outcomes should have been measured.
- Participants attend an appointment but do not provide relevant data.
- Participants fail to complete diaries or questionnaires.
- Participants cannot be located (lost to follow-up).
- The study investigators decide, usually inappropriately, to cease follow-up.
- Data or records are lost, or are unavailable for other reasons, despite being collected successfully.
- Some enrolled participants were later found to be ineligible. This may happen if the random assignment is prior to the point where eligibility can be determined.

There are two patterns of missing data:

1. *Monotonous missing data*: Each participant with a missing value has all subsequent measurements missing as well.
2. *Non-monotonous missing data*: A participant may have one missing value, but has some observed values after that.

Missing data are an important source of bias, unbalancing the groups, decreasing the sample size, and reducing precision and study power, which could all lead to invalid or non-significant results.

Your challenge to deal with missing data has three parts. First of all you will need to design a clinical trial so as to limit the occurrence of missing data (also see Chapter 7 on recruitment and adherence). Then you can employ methods during the data collection process to prevent more losses. The expert panel convened by the NRC also emphasized the importance of strategies in design and conduct of a study to help minimize missing data. Finally, anticipating that you will have some missing data nevertheless, you should plan a way to control or assess its potential impact on the trial outcome. In the following, we present strategies for addressing this issue at three different stages of the study.

Addressing the Issue of Missing Data at the Study Design Stage

There are several strategies you can include in your study design to minimize missing data and in this way maintain the scientific integrity of your research:

- Use a straightforward design, collecting sufficient data to address the research questions. Focus on your objectives and do not use unnecessary time and resources on data that will not contribute to them.
- Target the appropriate patient population. While a broad population will improve generalizability, if you end up with too many missing data, you may irreversibly compromise your study.
- Use basic data collection strategies, rather than complex ones that are difficult to teach and use.
- Try to obtain institutional review board (IRB) and participants' permission to contact them even after they withdraw from the study, or to review their medical charts.
- Ensure proper allocation of resources to facilitate the collection of data. This is more than having an accurate budget to finish the study. Consider travel reimbursement and meals for participants when they need to have evaluation appointments.
- Consider a data-monitoring committee to monitor missing data during all phases. This will ensure that timely actions can be taken.
- Estimate a genuine amount of missing data and account for it in your sample size calculation. This will minimize the probability of having an underpowered study.
- Specify a priori the strategies you will use for handling the missing data; if more than one method will be considered depending on the different situations, they should all be clearly explained. Most post hoc approaches will negatively affect the validity of results.

Addressing the Issue of Missing Data during Data Collection

Missing data occur frequently due to the burden of evaluation on participants. Here are a few recommendations you should follow to minimize the inconvenience and burden of study procedures:

- Limit the number of evaluations to the minimum to reach your objectives.
- Consolidate instruments by exploiting redundancy of questions or assessments. This will take less time and make visits more efficient.
- Provide a flexible schedule for visits.
- Compensate participants for their time and effort.

- Provide increasing incentives to participants in long-term follow-up studies.
- Choose researchers and sites with a good rate of patient follow-up and study completion.
- Use straightforward instruments and questionnaires with simple, unambiguous language.
- Record the reasons for dropping out of the study; this will help in determining the type of missing data.
- Use electronic data collection strategies and take advantage of their characteristics, like temporary storage of data and offline completion of questionnaires.
- Site investigators should emphasize the importance of completing the study when explaining the informed consent and at every other visit.
- Sites should be welcoming to participants and their families, providing a comfortable atmosphere, where they feel their well-being is important, not only the study completion.
- Provide timely reminders to participants of their next visit and encourage communication between visits; this will improve patient-clinician bond.

Addressing Missing Data at the Analysis Stage

Types of Missing Data

In order to address how to deal with missing data problems using an appropriate method, we need to classify the types of missing data mechanisms. Little and Rubin (1987) defined three types of missing data mechanisms: missing completely at random (MCAR), missing at random (MAR), and missing not at random (MNAR) [2]. This categorization depends on whether the reason for the loss of data is related to the dependent variable (non-observed data, performance at follow-up) or the independent variable (observed data, demographic and baseline characteristics) (see Table 13.1).

Before we actually address methods of dealing with missing data problems, we would like to introduce the concept of intention-to-treat (ITT) and per-protocol (PP) analysis

ITT analyzes all patients based on how they were originally allocated based on randomization, regardless of

- whether they actually started the allocated treatment,
- subsequently withdrew from treatment,
- deviated from the treatment protocol,
- or received a different treatment.

Per-protocol analysis (or also called *modified ITT* [mITT], which may not be the best term to use) analyzes only subjects who did not deviate from the protocol. For instance, if a subject is included in a trial but later the investigator realizes (after randomization) that the subject does not have the disease being treated, in the PP analysis, this subject is excluded, but all other subjects are included. There are other types of mITT that include analyzing subjects who received at least a certain amount of the intervention or who had one baseline assessment. Regardless of the method, mITT can lead to bias as it may analyze different groups.

Table 13.1 Three Types of Missing Data

Missing Completely At Random: MCAR

Completely unrelated to observed (indicates independent variables (e.g., age, gender) or unobserved data of any variables (indicates the outcome) in the analysis.

This can happen if a rater gets sick or study files get lost.

Perfect scenario. Balance through randomization is maintained. Non-missing data constitute effectively a random sample. Per protocol analysis could be used but power may be affected

Missing At Random (less stringent): MAR

Pattern of missing data is related to the value of observed variables (e.g., age), but it is not related to unobserved values. Missing data pattern can be fully explained.

This could happen if old subjects drop out of a treatment because they have more difficulties going to the clinic center. However, among older subjects, the likelihood of dropping out does not relate to the outcome.

Imputation methods should be used to allow ITT analysis.

Missing Not At Random: MNAR

Occurs when the pattern of missing data is related to unobserved values of the variables (or the outcome), therefore it is impossible to estimate data from other values of the variables in the analysis.

There is no good method of handling these data. The best you can do is use maximum likelihood method, if you have a correct model for missing mechanism.

PP analysis is *not* the same as complete-case analysis, as in complete-case analysis only the data that are not missing are analyzed.

You could argue that when using ITT analysis you will have to deal with missing data problems if you had dropouts; thus proper methods of dealing with the problem would be recommended. Note that ITT itself is not a method of handling missing data; it means that all subjects who were randomized will be analyzed.

An RCT is considered to produce the highest level of evidence to provide inference for causality. The most important characteristic of the RCT is its ability to avoid bias by randomization. If this was perfect, it would mean that groups have the same characteristics at baseline, so any difference found between groups at the end of the trial can be attributed to the intervention itself and not to a prior difference between the groups (see Chapter 6 for more on randomization).

The most important upshot of the randomization is that it balances groups regarding their covariates at baseline.

Intention to Treat

In order to keep the benefit of randomization, we must adhere to it. This means that all participants who were randomized need to be included in the analysis. We will later explain several methods used to handle missing data. However, the analysis must also include participants in the same group they were randomized to, regardless of what happened to them afterward, even if they never started their allocated treatment or crossed over to the other group. This approach is called *intention to treat* (ITT). But if some participants do not have measurements, how can we use them in our analysis? You will need to use imputation methods to complete the lost data [3].

ITT analysis may lead results toward the null hypothesis, against a treatment difference, therefore minimizing type I error. It has been said to be too cautious, increasing the possibility of type II error, but it also reflects the "real world" of clinical practice by accounting for non-compliance and protocol deviations, which happen with regular patients.

Note that if ITT analysis tend to bias the results toward no difference, it might not be appropriate when doing equivalence or non-inferiority trials.

You could find it useful to do both PP and ITT analysis. If the results are both similar, then it is possible to have more confidence in your inference. If the results are opposite, then you should try to consider what factors might be biasing this results [4].

Advantages of Using ITT

- The Consolidated Standards of Reporting Trials (CONSORT) guidelines to help authors improve their reports of RCTs state that the number of participants in each group should be analyzed by the "intention-to-treat" principle.
- It reflects the reality of clinical practice. In a clinical scenario we will always have a group of patients who are not compliant with our indications. ITT will get results based on the initial random allocation and therefore will give us an estimate of treatment effect. In an RCT, non-compliance may be due to their response to treatment, such as non-response or adverse effects.
- It keeps the sample size necessary for the analysis, maintaining the desired power.
- It helps investigators to become aware of the reasons for non-compliance and emphasizes the importance of good accountability of all the enrolled patients.
- It minimizes type I error; it is more conservative with results, and will therefore be easier to generalize results. However, this may also depend on the method utilized.

Disadvantages of Using ITT

- If a non-compliant patient who did not really receive the treatment is analyzed in the group where patients were supposed to get treatment, results based on him do not really indicate any efficacy.
- We usually have a dilution effect from the non-compliant participants, so type II error increases; it has been said to be too cautious.
- Variance of results will be greater because compliant participants are grouped together with dropouts and non-compliant ones for the analysis [5].

METHODS OF HANDLING MISSING DATA

There are basically four main strategies to deal with missing data:

1. CCA/ACA (no replacement of missing data)
2. Single imputation/LOCF/rank-based tests (assigning patients a worse rank than those with observed data)

3. Multiple imputation
4. Maximum likelihood techniques.

Complete Case Analysis (CCA)

Any loss of data causes a problem during data analysis, because the groups will not be composed as initially planned with randomization. This problem will be greater if there is a big loss of data. CCA excludes all patients who did not get or did not complete the specified treatment. Also cases that have missing observations (e.g., in a repeated measure design) will be excluded (important distinction from available case analysis). This method has also been called *completer analysis*. It is the most common and basic approach. Data are analyzed without being manipulated. However, this approach should only be used if missing data can be considered missing completely at random. You need to remember to always report all reasons for the loss of data. If data are not MCAR and you use this approach, it will tend to overestimate the treatment effect [6].

CCA is the default for most of the statistical software packages.

Advantages:

- There is no manipulation because it analyzes only real data.
- There are no assumptions.
- It is simple to perform.
- It may be acceptable to use if there is less than 5% of missing values.

Disadvantages:

- It reduces power because of a reduced sample size, especially if there is a high dropout rate, and may lead to a loss of precision.
- It may bias the outcome if the incomplete cases differ from the complete cases.
- Dropouts may be unbalanced across groups, loosing the balance between groups initially achieved via randomization.
- It may increase type I and II errors.

Weighted Complete-Case Analysis

This is used in surveys because it gives a weight for responses based on likelihood of response for each question.
   Example: survey with five questions

$Q1 - 100\%, Q2 - 80\%, Q3 - 60\%, Q4 - 80\%, Q5 - 80\%$

$Total = 1*Q1 + 0.8*Q2 + 0.6*Q3 + 0.8*Q4 + 0.8*Q5 / (1+0.8+0.6+0.8+0.8)$

Disadvantage:
- It might introduce bias, depending on the reason for missing data.

Single Imputation (Replacement of Missing Values)

There are several procedures of single imputation, which we discuss in the following:

Mean and Median Imputation

This method replaces all the missing values with the mean or median of the observed values.

Advantages:

- It is a basic method.
- It has a potential to reduce bias by using all study data to estimate the response of missing participants.

Disadvantages:

- It significantly decreases variance and standard deviation, giving a false sense of precision.
- It has an increased type I error and overestimation of effect.
- It is rarely used.

Regression Imputation

This method replaces each missing value with one estimated using a regression model performed on the non-missing ones. The imputation is different in each case based on the baseline characteristics of each participant.

Advantages:

- It is a basic method.
- It has a smaller impact on variance, but still reduces it.
- It has the potential to reduce bias by using all study data to estimate the response of missing participants.

Disadvantages:

- It is a more complicated method than those explained earlier.
- It has a decreased standard deviation, although not as low as when using mean or median imputation.

The regression model can consider several baseline characteristics in the equation to get the outcome most appropriate for each case considering the available data. For example:

$$Y = \beta_0 + \beta_1 * age + \beta_2 * gender + \beta_3 * duration\ of\ disease + \ldots$$

Stochastic Regression Imputation

This is a basic variation of the regression imputation; it adds a residual error so it has an increased variance. This means it has the same issues for advantages and disadvantages but with somewhat higher standard deviation (closer to reality). For example:

$Y = \beta_0 + \beta_1 * age + \beta_2 * gender + \beta_3 * duration\ of\ disease\ ... + e$

Increased Random Variability Method

In this case, an error is added to the estimated value. But the error is chosen at random, by software, to replace each missing value.

Advantages:

- It has a potential to reduce bias by using all study data to estimate a response for missing participants.

Disadvantages:

- It is a complicated statistical model that requires specific training.
- Because it is not commonly used, reviewers might question it.

Hot and Cold Deck Imputation Method

Hot: A missing value from a participant is replaced with the value of a case with similar characteristics.
Cold: similar to hot but the replacement value is chosen from another dataset.

Last Observation Carried Forward

Here, the missing value is replaced with the last observed value for that subject, using the assumption that the value did not change from the previous one. The analysis that follows does not distinguish between the observed and the "carried forward" data.

Advantages:

- It is a basic method.
- It is widely accepted.
- It is the most commonly used method.
- It is accepted and even recommended by the US Food and Drug Administration (FDA) as a conservative method; however, this method is being less frequently used.
- It mimics real-life scenarios of non-compliance.

Disadvantages:

- It may lead to biased estimates, which tend toward the null hypothesis or even inflate results.
- Dropouts may be unbalanced across treatment groups.

- Dropouts may occur early during the intervention, so the last observation may not really reflect what would have happened if the participant had finished.
- It assumes that patients who drop out maintain same outcome result, not improving or getting worse.
- Time trends in the data, when combined with differential dropout rates between groups, can introduce severe bias.
- This method also ignores the fact that, even if a participant's disease state remains constant, measurements of this state are unlikely to stay exactly the same, introducing a spurious lack of random variability into the analysis [6].

Worst- (and Best-) Case Scenario Carried Forward

In worst-case scenario, you substitute all the missing values for the less favorable outcome. If results show significant values, then your data is robust.

For best-case scenario, you substitute all the missing values for the most favorable result.

Advantages:

- Positive results obtained using worst-case can be trusted; it is a very conservative method.

Disadvantages:

- It should not be used in cases with a high number of dropouts.

Baseline Carried Forward

Here you assume that patients who drop out return to baseline; therefore there is no change.

Advantages:

- It is a conservative method.

Disadvantages:

- It biases results toward the null hypothesis, underestimating the effect of treatment [7].

Single imputation methods are easier to perform; they will only replace missing values using the known characteristics of the rest of the available data [8]. Using various methods, for example regression, will calculate predicted values for the missing ones [9]. However, since we would be using the known values, the variance with those predicted values is smaller than the real one. This smaller variance may introduce bias in other estimates [10].

Multiple Imputation

This is a more complex approach to the analysis of missing data, as is it involves multiple calculations. In multiple imputations (MI), each missing value will be replaced by a simulated value. This will be done several times (3 to 10 times), obtaining multiple sets of completed data by imputation. All data will be analyzed by standard methods, and the results will be combined to produce a unique result for inference. This result incorporates missing data uncertainty, having a standard deviation and standard error closer to the one obtained with a complete sample.

When we use MI, we incorporate an error into the equation for prediction. This error is drawn randomly from a standard normal distribution. This random error added to the prediction will increase the variance and make it closer to the real one (when there are no missing values). Ultimately, this avoids the inclusion of biases, which happens from having too small a variance.

To carry out MI there are three basic steps:

1. In the prediction of the missing values, we introduce a random error. Instead of using this unique data set with one set of imputed values, we create several data sets, with different imputed missing values, due to the use of a random error in each case.
2. Once we have several different data sets (different imputed vales in each set), we analyze each set with the planned statistical analysis, obtaining several results.
3. Now we combine the results to get only one set of parameters.

It is important to know that most of the software available to handle missing data using either multiple imputation or maximum likelihood need the assumption that data are missing at random [9].

Advantages:

- Estimates have almost optimal statistical properties.
- Results are mostly consistent, therefore generally unbiased in large samples.
- Almost perfect efficiency (gets better with larger sample size, tending to 1, perfect). To get perfect efficiency we would need to analyze an infinite number of data sets. Using five data sets achieves over 90% efficiency. If the sample is small or there are too many missing values, more data sets would be needed to achieve efficiency.
- It can be applied to most data or models.
- It uses conventional software.

Disadvantages:

- It produces different results each time, because of the random error used.
- It requires a few decisions:
  - Which method to use: There are various ways to perform MI, so it can be confusing. The two most common methods used are Markov Chain Montecarlo (MCMC) algorithm, which is based on linear regression, and the Fully Conditional Specification (FCS) algorithm, which can also be called Multiple Imputation by Chain Equation (MICE).
  - If you choose FCS, you need to choose a model for each variable.
  - You need to decide how many data sets to create.

- Is the model used for the imputation of each variable compatible with the model for the final analysis? The analysis may be using a variable as categorical, but the imputation model may be using it differently, maybe as quantitative. This is called *model congeniality*.

Maximum Likelihood Techniques

Maximum likelihood (ML) techniques have good statistical properties and rely on weaker assumptions. However, they are not commonly used by most researchers, because most researchers do not know of them, and, even if they do, because these techniques can take more time and effort to perform. This method also produces estimates that have nearly optimal statistical properties. They are consistent and therefore mostly unbiased in large samples, asymptotically efficient, and asymptotically normal. The principle of ML is to use the available values in order to find parameter estimates (the measures describing a population) that would be the most fitting to the already observed data. ML does not impute missing values, so your result will not be a complete data set. However, it uses the known characteristics of the individuals to better estimate the unknown parameters of the incomplete variable.

To carry out ML, you need to define the likelihood function, which will quantify how well the data fits to the parameters.

Advantages:

- It can even be used for cases with MNAR data, if you have a correct model for the missingness mechanism. It is more efficient than multiple imputation.
- For the same data set, it always gives the same result. On the contrary, multiple imputation has a different result every time you perform it, because of the use of random numbers. There will always be a possibility of reaching different conclusions based on the same data.
- It has fewer decisions to make than multiple imputation before performing the technique. The results will not depend on your decisions.
- It uses a single model, so there will be no incompatibility between the imputation and analysis model. All variables will be taken into account, as well as the linear or nonlinear relations between them.
- ML is said to be more efficient than MI because it has smaller standard errors, and for small samples or large amounts of missing data you would need too many data sets in MI.

Disadvantages:

- It requires specialized software.
- It needs a parametric model for the joint distribution of all the variables with missing data. This model can be difficult to achieve.
- It needs large samples.
- Most software assumes MAR [11].

Sensitivity Analysis

Other recommendations of the NCR expert panel, apart from the preventive strategies cited earlier, were to recommend a sensitivity analysis, where you would compare your analysis to an extreme method and see how results change. This will give you an idea of how robust (sensitive) your findings are. The analysis measures the impact on the results from different methods of handling missing data, and it helps to justify the choice of the particular method applied. It should be planned and described in the protocol. If the sensitivity analysis shows consistent results and leads to reasonably similar estimates of the treatment effect, then you would say you have robust findings. Also recommended are model-based methods of analysis, or those that use appropriate weighting, as superior to complete-case analysis or single imputation methods such as last observation carried forward, because they require less restrictive assumptions about the missing data mechanism. One more important question is that the issues raised by the panel also apply to observational studies.

MISSING DATA IN OTHER SITUATIONS

Missing Data in Observational Studies

As you know, RCTs are not the only type of research, and certainly, they are not the only type to have the problem of missing data. Survey analysis, epidemiological studies and observational studies in general also need ways to handle missing data. In all cases, current standards require an ITT method to avoid bias and maintain power in order to make valid inferences. More often now, reviews of missing data methods are recommending multiple imputation methods, as they appear to be superior by giving a variability closer to that of a complete data set [12].

Missing Data in Meta-analysis

In this case, a whole study may be missing from the review, an outcome may be missing from a study, summary data may be missing for an outcome, and individual participants may be missing from the summary data (Table 13.2).

Table 13.2 Types of Missing Data in a Meta-analysis

Type of Missing Data	Some Possible Reasons for Missing Data
Missing studies	Publication bias
	Search not sufficiently comprehensive.
Missing outcomes	Outcome not measured
	Selective reporting bias
Missing summary data	Selective reporting bias
	Incomplete reporting
Missing individuals	Lack of intention-to-treat analysis
	Attrition from the study
	Selective reporting bias
Missing study-level characteristics (for subgroup analysis or meta-regression)	Characteristic not measured
	Incomplete reporting

Source: *Cochrane Handbook for Systematic Reviews of Interventions*, Part 3: Table 16.1.a.

Whenever possible, contact the original investigators to request if they have the missing values. You should also consider performing a funnel plot analysis (a method to see whether positive and negative studies were equally published; see Chapter 14)

Missing Data in Longitudinal Studies

Longitudinal studies usually have repeated observation over time; lost values in one observation or from one observation onward will generate a complication for the analysis of data. Standard analysis will generally yield inappropriate results by loss of power and introduction of bias. Some recommended approaches are univariate analysis with adjustment for variance estimates, two-step analysis, and likelihood-based approaches [13].

Missing Data in Survival Analysis: Censoring

Censoring is a special type of missing data; it occurs when the value of a measurement or observation is only partially known, so not all the information of that value is missing (see also Chapter 12). For example, you might be doing a study where participants need to be weighed and your scale has a top weight of 200 kg, but one of your participants weighs more than that. In this case, you will not know the exact value, but you know he weighs more than 200. In longitudinal studies, you could have an endpoint of age at death, but a participant dropped out after the first year of follow-up. In this case, if you know the participant was alive at the first year evaluation, and he was 70 years old, so you will know he was at least 70 years old at death. It could also happen that your study ended before a participant died, but he was 80 years old at that time, so you will know he will be at least 80 when he dies.

- Daniel Bernoulli analyzed smallpox morbidity and mortality data to demonstrate the efficacy of vaccination in 1766. His paper was one of the first to use censored data in a statistical problem [14].

COVARIATE ADJUSTMENT

Covariate adjustment is used because, even with randomization, the groups of your study may be imbalanced for certain characteristics, also called covariates [15], or it can also be used to improve the efficiency of data analysis.

Randomization does not guarantee perfect balance across treatment arms with respect to one or more baseline covariates, especially in small trials [16].

You can avoid imbalances and plan for adjusted analysis at the design stage of your study. First, by performing a stratified blocked randomization, you can ensure a reasonable balance across treatment groups in some of the baseline factors known to be strong predictors (see Chapter 6). These blocks should be entered into the analysis, unless there are too many blocks. You should also pre-specify in the protocol which baseline covariates will be adjusted for and why. This planned approach is preferred over doing it post hoc, because any unplanned analysis has to be declared as exploratory. If not declared as exploratory, then it may be considered a "fishing expedition," meaning you are playing with data to get the results you want. Multiple analyses may yield a positive result simply by chance (see Chapters 9, 10, and 14), increasing the chance of type I error. The FDA and the International Conference on Harmonization of Technical Requirements for Registration of Pharmaceuticals for Human Use (ICH) guidelines for clinical reports require that the selection of and adjustment for any covariates should be an integral part of the planned analysis, and hence should be set out in the protocol and explained in the reports.

In an unadjusted analysis, the baseline characteristics of participants (covariates) are not taken into account to assess the outcome. In an adjusted analysis, the covariates are taken into account, because it is possible that the estimates of treatment effect will be influenced by these baseline differences between groups.

The final effect on the outcome will depend on

- The magnitude of these differences
- The strength of the correlation between the outcome and the covariate in question, which is the most important contributing factor.

You should also note that if the baseline covariate is strongly correlated with the outcome, there is still an advantage in adjusting for a baseline covariate, even if this is balanced across the treatment arms [17].

Another effect of this adjustment is an increase in precision of the estimated treatment effect. This, however, only applies to linear regression models [16,17].

Objectives and Advantages

- Achieve the most appropriate *p*-value for the treatment difference.
- Improve precision of the estimated treatment difference.
- Increase statistical power.
- It reduces bias.
- It increases statistical efficiency.

You should note that by using covariate adjustment we are *not* interested in learning how groups respond to treatments; the purpose is only to increase power. Thus it is important for the reader to understand also that the goal of covariate adjustment is to make the statistical analysis more efficient; but also this only happens if the covariates are associated to the response to the treatment being tested.

Common Covariates to Adjust

Prognostic or risk factors

- In randomized trials, the better therapy may depend on values of a baseline risk or prognostic factor. You can adjust for them by subdividing the target population into subsets. In a two-arm randomized trial setting, it is customary to use subsets: two regions of superiority of the treatment arms (i.e., one region for each arm), and the third region of uncertainty. The goal is to detect treatment efficacy by prognostic factor interaction.

- In multicenter trials and sites, because centers differ in their demography of participants, medical practice, and adherence to all aspects of the protocol, causing a variation across centers.

When should you do the covariate adjustment?

1. In the planning phase of your study, by using a stratified randomization technique, and planning for covariate adjustment.
2. After the data are collected, in the analysis phase, there are a few methods you can use.

Methods for Covariate Adjustment Depending on the Analysis Being Performed

See chapters 9, 10, and 12 for more information on how to run each test.

For ANOVA

In an analysis where you would run ANOVA, you should add another variable, therefore effectively using ANCOVA.

In STATA if you wanted to adjust for gender, the command would be changed from *anova pain changes treatment* to *anova pain changes treatment gender*. ANCOVA tests whether certain factors have an effect on the outcome variable.

For Regression

In an analysis where you would run a regression, you should add another variable into the equation.

In STATA if you wanted to adjust for gender, the command would be changed from *regress pain changes treatment* to *regress pain changes treatment gender*. This allows you to control for important covariates or potential confounders.

For Survival Analysis

In an analysis where you would run survival (see Chapter 12), you should add another variable, therefore effectively performing the Cox proportional model. This is a complex statistical analysis that allows for covariates in survival analysis.

For Categorical Data

This method adjusts for covariates using categorical data by averaging several strata. It is the comparison of two groups of categorical response, allowing to adjust or control for important covariates.

So far, we have evaluated the use of covariate adjustment in randomized controlled trials, because even randomization may not adequately balance groups. But what happens in observational studies, where there is no randomization to begin with? In this type of study, the compared groups are usually very different on the covariates. If you do not adjust for this, your treatment effect will be biased.

Besides the method of addressing confounders using modeling or multivariate analysis (which is the most common method), another method is called *propensity scores*. We will briefly mention this method, as it is a way to help with covariate adjustment in observational studies (for more details, see Chapter 19).

The method of propensity scores (PS) is defined as a conditional probability of being treated given the individual's characteristics or covariates. This means it will always be a fraction or percentage. PS is also considered a score, which summarizes all the used covariates in only one number (it is usually estimated using logistic regression where the outcome is the treatment and the covariates are the predictors). Once estimated, the propensity score can be used to reduce bias through matching, stratification, regression adjustment, or some combination of all three.

However, you must remember that, unlike randomization, propensity scores will only balance known covariates, but not unobserved ones; so only covariates that will be measured before the treatment is given should be included in the propensity score.

The value of propensity is that it gives us one number with which we can compare treatment and control groups, instead of having to compare for several different covariates.

CASE STUDY: WISH YOU WERE HERE— HANDLING MISSING DATA

André Brunoni and Felipe Fregni

While looking at the beautiful fireworks lighting Fort Lauderdale's sky on New Year's Eve, Professor Strong could not avoid a feeling of relief that 2008 was over. No, it was not economics or the world crisis that made 2008 a very complicated year for Prof. Strong, but the weight-loss trial he had been conducting since 2006. As an endocrinologist and active researcher at Bernard A. Mitchell, a teaching hospital of the University of Chicago Medical School, he has been leading several clinical trials for the past 20 years, and he was the principal investigator (PI) of the W-WELT (Women's Weight Loss Trial) study, a randomized clinical trial that enrolled 70 post-menopausal women for two interventions: standard (low-fat, low-calorie, and high-carbohydrate) versus Atkins (low-carbohydrate, high-fat, and high-protein) diet. The trial finished one month ago. Prof. Strong recalled how he and his team carefully designed the trial, setting the eligibility criteria and the primary outcome (weight at 12 months, adjusting for baseline weight through an ANCOVA model), the randomization and blinding method, weighing the first patients at the research center—but then, everything started to fall apart.

Two research assistants went to private companies, one NIH grant for analyses of secondary outcomes (genetic polymorphisms related to obesity) was denied, and, most important, several patients were lost to follow-up. He realized it would have been a good idea to include methods for handling missing data in the protocol. Prof. Strong was apprehensive, checking his emails every five minutes. He knew Melissa MacGyver, the statistician of W-WELT, would be finishing the database at any moment and soon he would know the amount of damage—due to missing data. He was preparing in his head some damage-control strategies.

His wife, calling for him, interrupted his thoughts, "Robert, please! I know you are upset, but could you just forget this trial today? It's New Year's Eve!" He then stopped for a couple of minutes and they kissed and hugged and wished each other a happy 2009. He then tried not to think about W-WELT anymore—at least for that night

Introduction: When the Conventional Methods of Data Imputation Fail

A few days later, Prof. Strong received an email from Ms. MacGyver. He became anxious even before reading the message, as the email subject was "final dataset":

Dear Prof. Strong, the database is complete. We had only 60% patients finishing the study—42 patients: 22 on Atkins diet and 20 on standard. I would like to discuss with you the methods of missing data imputation as I did not find it in the protocol. I think we can assume the data missing as at random2. I am in Dallas with my family for the holidays.

My phone number is . . .

The simplest—and often, the worst—approach of handling missing data is to analyze only the patients who completed the study (i.e., "to do nothing"). This approach is known as complete-case analysis (CCA) or listwise deletion. CCA has the advantage of not involving any data manipulation, thus using the raw data. In fact, readers (and sometimes, reviewers) unfamiliar to statistics often consider CCA as the fairest method for this reason; however, this assumption is quite naïve, because even CCA might lead to biased results, as patients who dropped out are excluded from all analysis and thus the initial advantage of randomization of generating balanced groups is lost. Also, CCA decreases study power significantly, especially when dropout rates are high, therefore increasing significantly the type II error. If a researcher wants to use this method, the reasons for dropouts need to be justified and they need to be balanced across treatment groups.

In fact, the mechanism of missing data is extremely important to determine how to handle missing data. There are three types of missing data. The first type of missing data is *missing completely at random* (MCAR). In MCAR, missing data are not related to the outcome or to the independent variables (e.g., demographics). The second is the *missing at random* (MAR). In MAR, missing data are not related to the outcome (in other words, e.g., patients did not drop out of the study because of not improving (outcome), but rather it is related to the independent variables (e.g., age—older patients may drop out more frequently). Finally, the third type is *missing not at random* (MNAR). In this case, missing data are related to outcome. This is the worst case, and there are no simple and effective methods of addressing missing data of this type. For instance, for the CCA method, the data must be MCAR. When data are MAR, methods of intention to treat (ITT) should be used.

The ITT method is frequently used, as it tries to preserve the original groups created by the randomization. It means that patients randomized to a given group should be analyzed as the initial "intention." One ITT method often used is the last-observation carried forward (LOCF)—in which missing data at endpoint are imputed from the last observation method (e.g., if weight data at 12 months—end of trial—was missed but not at the last observation, then the last observed value is imputed at 12 months). The basic idea here is that participants should have a gradual improvement over time and therefore if we consider that after leaving the trial they would not improve further, then this is a conservative method. Almost all reviewers accept it and, traditionally, LOCF is the only imputation method accepted for US FDA drug approval trials. Another advantage of LOCF is that it is very simple and does not require complex statistical methodology. However, it is also a conservative method of data imputation (depending on the mechanism of missing data) and can lead to biased estimates, especially for patients lost just after the trial started and for imbalanced losses. It can also decrease the statistical power of a study, especially those with small samples.

As mentioned, an important advantage of LOCF is that this method uses the principle of ITT analysis, meaning that all subjects that were randomized to the study are analyzed. The advantage of this method is that it includes all the subjects and also mimics real-life scenarios better since an important proportion of patients in clinical practice are non-compliant. The disadvantage of this or other ITT methods is that they depend on data imputation that usually makes statisticians and other researchers nervous.

After reading Melissa's email, Prof. Strong did not know which statistical approach to choose. He was now sure that he should have decided the method for missing data approach when he designed the trial, but he was too optimistic and considered that only 5% of patients would drop out from this study and therefore this would not be a critical issue. In the case of this study, CCA seemed very problematic, as they had 40% dropouts, implying a huge loss of study power. Also, it would be possible that patients who dropped out were those who started to regain weight, became unmotivated to continue the diet, and finally left the study. LOCF, on the other hand, would assume that patients who dropped out would maintain the same weight, which might be too optimistic. Therefore, he also agreed with her that perhaps more sophisticated statistical methods for data imputation could be interesting. Fortunately, Ms. MacGyver was an expert on these methods.

The Trial

The Atkins diet that has been developed in the 1970s is one of the most popular types of diets. Several books have been published on this diet, and millions of subjects have tried it. However, despite the popularity, very few studies have been performed on this subject, and it is still not clear whether or not this diet is effective. Based on this important question, Prof. Strong designed and ran a one-year, multi-center, randomized controlled trial in which 70 patients were randomly assigned to receive the Atkins diet or the conventional diet (low-calorie, high-carbohydrate, and low-fat diet). The main outcome was weight at one year, and the hypothesis was that the Atkins diet would induce a larger weight reduction as compared to the conventional diet.

Prof. Strong called Melissa: "Hi, Melissa! How are you? Happy 2009!"

She replied, "Happy 2009, Professor!"

After a few minutes chatting, they realized they would be on the same flight back to Chicago, as Prof. Strong would make a connection in Dallas. They settled that they would meet at the airport to discuss the potential method for handling the missing data, so they could discuss their trial while flying back to Chicago.

A Brainstorm—and a Thunderstorm

A few days later, Prof. Strong and Ms. MacGyver met while boarding the airplane at Dallas Airport.

"Hi, Melissa! How are you? Are you prepared for the cold weather? I heard the temperature in Chicago is around zero Fahrenheit plus the chill factor—that would be near −15 F."

She replied, "I heard about that too! But that's fine for me. I prefer cold to warm. I grew up in Minnesota! And how about you, Professor? How was it in Miami? And where is Mrs. Strong?"

He said, "It was fine, thank you! She stayed with the kids; she has family in Fort Lauderdale."

They paused their conversation while the plane took off. After the announcement that it was safe to use portable electronic devices, they did not hesitate and both got their laptops out and started talking about their trial.

Common Approaches: Completers Only and Last Observation Carried Forward

Prof. Strong then starts the conversation, "Melissa, why don't we simplify and use the completers only? With this approach, no one will accuse us that we are manipulating the data, and we would be showing what we have, instead of making assumptions about the values for the patients who dropped out of the study."

Melissa, after a small pause, responds, "It is certainly an option, but in this case, we have a large number of dropouts—almost half of the initial sample—and we do not know if the patients in the study are similar to the original randomized sample. This is a risky approach when the attrition rate is large. In addition, with the small sample, the power would be significantly affected and the type II error would be increased."

Prof. Strong knows this will be a long conversation. "That is a good point, Melissa. Let us explore the method of last observation carried forward. I know this is a conservative method and is recommended by the FDA. Also, using this method, we would be doing an intention-to-treat analysis since all the patients would be included. This might be our salvation."

"Well, it is not so simple," Melissa quickly responds, "We also have a big problem here. The method of LOCF was built with the main assumption that patients, after dropping out of a trial, would either not improve or continue to get better. But this is not the case for a weight-loss trial in which subjects might have a rebound of their weight after stopping a diet. But it is still an option."

They then stopped for 10 minutes, as Prof. Strong wanted to drink something and the flight attendant was passing in the aisle, offering beverages.

Other Methods of Data Imputation: Regression Substitution

They then restart, with Melissa describing other methods of data imputation for Prof. Strong: "I think we could use some mathematical approaches to input data on the dependent variables missing as to keep the initial randomized groups and analyze all the subjects by predicting the main outcome for the missing data. The simplest approach is called *mean substitution*, in which the missing values are replaced by the mean of non- missing values. However, I am not so enthusiastic about this approach. The problem of this approach is that it is very liberal, as it greatly decreases the standard deviation of the sample on both groups. In fact, it is very good to decrease the standard deviation of endpoint results as the "noise" is decreased and the "signal" is amplified—but artificially as in this case. Thus, such an approach increases the probability of type I error."

Then she continues: "A more sophisticated method is called "regression substitution," in which the missing values are replaced by values estimated from regression models performed on the non-missing values. That is, instead of just imputing the same value (the mean) in all missing data, we can input different values based on the baseline characteristics of each patient. There are other very sophisticated techniques, in which we can add to the formula even a random error (based on the residual distribution of our regression models) before the final value is calculated—as a statistician, I like this technique very much, but it would take some time to estimate a good model, and I would have to use a special statistics software to do it. However, the advantage of these tools is the potential to reduce bias by using all the study data to estimate response for missing subjects.

"In our example, it is possible that a generalized regression model for the non-missing variables showed something like that:

$$\begin{aligned}\text{Final Weight} = {} & \text{Baseline Weight} + 0.25^* \left(\text{Age-65}\right) \\ & + 1.5^* \left(\text{Hypothetical Sedentary Scale}\right) \\ & - 2.25^* \left(\text{Standard Diet Group}\right) - 5.5^* \left(\text{Atkins Diet}\right) \\ & + 0.33^* \left(\text{Baseline Cholesterol Levels}\right)\end{aligned}$$

In this case, the final values for each missing value would be replaced by a value calculated from this formula. This approach is an advance, as it increases slightly the standard deviation when compared to the *mean substitution*; however, even this approach is optimistic as the SD would still be underestimated because the missing values are still estimated from the non-missing values (in fact, there is no possibility to *increase* SD using this technique).

"Thus, a third approach would be to increase random variability to the inputted values. There are modern statistical methods that generate thousands of values, adding error to the estimated value, and then one of these values is chosen at random by the statistical software to replace the missing values. However, this approach is not commonly used and might be questioned by reviewers. Moreover, it requires familiarity with statistics and involves specific training for using software that can generate simulation methods."

After seeing all of these methods, Prof. Strong concludes, "Oh, well, it seems that these methods decrease the standard deviation but might also give better estimates depending on our assumptions. What else, Melissa?"

The Other Options: Worst-Case Scenario and Baseline Carried Forward

During the discussion, the airplane starts to shake. The captain's voice is heard, "Hi folks, we are flying over an area of instability—there is a thunderstorm formation ahead of us—I contacted traffic control and we are trying to get smoother areas, but there are not many options. It will be bumpy for several minutes and heavy turbulence is expected—so please, fasten your seatbelts, folks, we are going to land as soon as the weather conditions allow." Prof. Strong and Melissa turn off their laptops and remain in silence for a while. They can see tremendous flashes of lightning in the sky, and Prof. Strong somehow remembers the fireworks during New Year's Eve. He breaks the silence: "I was reading about an imputation technique called the worst-case scenario. I was also reading about a technique called baseline carried forward, in which we can assume that all patients who dropped out regain their weight. What do you think?"

Melissa answers, "The worst-case scenario method substitutes the missing values for the less favorable result. If the outcome under study is mortality, for instance, then all missing values are imputed as "death" on the experimental treatment and as "alive" on the standard treatment. The advantage of this approach is that if the results are positive, they can be trusted, since they were obtained under the "worst-case scenario." However, this approach cannot be used in studies in which a high number of dropouts was observed.

"Another technique is the baseline carried forward—it assumes that all patients who dropped out, regardless of the treatment received, returned to their baseline levels: in our case, regained the baseline weight. This approach is not commonly used and might underestimate the effects of treatment, as it introduces a bias "toward the null hypothesis" because in this technique, the same values are inputted for both groups—therefore getting both means closer. However, it may be interesting for this trial as it is based on the idea that patients after dropping out of the study will regain the weight and return to their baseline levels.

"But Professor Strong, there are two more options to consider. Although they are more complicated, they yield the best results."

Professor Strong replies, "Even more options and more complicated? I have not heard of anything else than what we have discussed already!"

"Yes, Professor, although these methods are better, they are not well known. We can go over the basics now and then you can decide."

"Ok, Melissa, tell me about these new methods."

"The first is multiple imputation, or MI. With this, each missing value will be replaced by a simulated value. This will be done several times (3 to 10 times), obtaining multiple sets of completed data by imputation."

Prof. Strong interrupts her: "So I would have 3 to 10 sets of data? Which one would I use for the final analysis?".

Melissa continues, "All data sets will be individually analyzed by standard methods, and the results will be combined to produce a unique result for inference. This result incorporates missing data uncertainty, having a standard deviation and standard error closer to the one obtained with a complete sample."

"So, Melissa, you would like to work 10 times more?" asks the professor.

"Fortunately, there are now better versions of software for this, and they are not as difficult to find as before. So, although it is more elaborate to do, it is not 10 times more difficult. But there is still one more method to consider, the maximum likelihood, or ML. The principle of ML is to use the available values in order to find parameter estimates (the measures describing a population) that would be the best fit to the already observed data. ML does not impute missing values, so your result will not be a complete data set. However, it uses the known characteristics of the individuals to better estimate the unknown parameters of the incomplete variable. To carry out ML you need to define the likelihood function, which will quantify how well the data fit to the parameters. But, this you do not need to know, you will only need to help me find the most appropriate variables to use. I would take care of the rest."

Prof. Strong once more interrupts her, "There is a lot to consider, Melissa." Fortunately, the airplane was soon able to land after a missed approach that scared many of the passengers. Despite the bumpy ride they had, they considered that the discussion was very productive. One important issue they know is that they need to decide the method before testing it in the data so as not to increase type 1 error. Though sensitivity analysis is a possible option, it is also difficult to make a decision when discordant results are seen. They planned to meet one day later to finally decide the best approach to use. There was a light at the end of the tunnel.

CASE DISCUSSION: CHOOSING THE STATISTICAL TEST

First of all, Prof. Strong should have considered some methods to help avoid the loss of follow-up. Also, he did not plan for any method of handling missing data, so this is the first challenge he will face: to choose a method. It is important to know that both FDA and ICH guidelines say you should consider this in the protocol.

The next important challenge is that he has a big (40%) loss of patients in the follow-up; he will need to keep this in mind in order to decide on the method of imputation.

The next step in choosing the strategy is to find the mechanism of missing data: is it MCAR, MAR, or MNAR? Should he just see the reasons for missingness, or should he use a formal approach? Ms. MacGyver says they can assume data as MAR, but why?

In order to assume MAR, lost data can be related to independent variables, but not to outcome. So Prof. Strong needs to decide if the patients who left the study were those who did not see as much weight loss, or those who did see weight loss (is it related to the outcome?). For this, it would be necessary to know the reasons for dropping out, apart from knowing the baseline characteristics of patients. Also, he could consider a formal method to decide on MCAR, MAR, or MCAR.

Only MCAR data can use a CCA analysis. If we assume MAR, then we cannot choose CCA; we should use a method of ITT. But if our data are MNAR, then we have only one method we can use: maximum likehood, which, as noted earlier, is not really an imputation method, as you will not end up with a completed data set. The principle of maximum likelihood is to use the available values in order to find parameter estimates (the measures describing a population) that would be the most fitting to the already observed data. ML does not impute missing values, so your result will not be a complete data set. However, it uses the known characteristics of the individuals to better estimate the unknown parameters of the incomplete variable.

Now that we know we should use ITT, we need to decide on one. Single imputation methods are simple, but most are not adequate for use when there is a large loss of data, or can cause a loss of power, or increase the probability of type I error.

Planning in the protocol is very important because it will give you the opportunity to collect all the information needed to make a good decision of the type of missingness and ITT methods. For instance, if you want to use a regression model, they would need to collect the baseline characteristics they think would influence the type of missingness.

CASE QUESTIONS FOR REFLECTION

1. What are the challenges faced by Prof. Strong in choosing the best analytical method?
2. What are his main concerns?

3. What should he consider to make the decision?
4. One of the methods that is frequently used in missing data is the worst-case analysis. What are the potential issues of this method? When is this method useful? Worst-case analysis can be used as a method of sensitivity analysis. Have you used sensitivity analysis before?

FURTHER READING

Papers

- Altman DG. Adjustment for covariate imbalance. In: *Biostatistics in Clinical Trials*. Chichester, UK: John Wiley & Sons, 2001.
- Bernoulli D, Blower S. An attempt at a new analysis of the mortality caused by smallpox and of the advantages of inoculation to prevent it. *Rev Med Virol*. 2004; 14: 275–288.
- Donders ART, et al. Missing data review: A gentle imputation of missing values. *J Clin Epidemiol*. 2006; 59: 1087–1091.
- Frison L, Pocock SJ. Repeated measures in clinical trials: analysis using mean summary statistics and its implications for design. *Stat Med*. 1992; 11: 1685–1704.
- Gupta SK. Intention-to-treat concept: a review. *Perspect Clin Res*. 2011; 2: 109–112.
- Haukoos JS, Newgard CD. Advanced statistics: missing data in clinical research—part 1: an introduction and conceptual framework. *Acad Emerg Med*. 2007 Jul; 14(7): 662–668.
- Hollis S, Campbell F. What is meant by intention to treat analysis? Survey of published randomised controlled trials. *BMJ*. 1999; 319: 670.
- Laird NM. Missing data in longitudinal studies. *Stat Med*. 1988 Jan–Feb; 7(1–2): 305–315.
- Molenberghs G, Thijs H, Jansen I, et al. Analyzing incomplete longitudinal clinical trial data. *Biostatistics*. 2004; 5: 445–464.
- Newgard CD, Haukoos JS. Advanced statistics: missing data in clinical research—part 2: multiple imputation. *Acad Emerg Med*. 2007 Jul; 14(7): 669–678.
- Pocock SJ, Assmann SE, Enos LE, et al. Subgroup analysis, covariate adjustment and baseline comparisons in clinical trial reporting: current practice and problems. *Stat Med*. 2002; 21: 2917–2930.
- Senn SJ. Covariate imbalance and random allocation in clinical trials. *Stat Med*. 1989; 8: 467–475.
- Ware JH, Harrington D, Hunter DJ, D'Agostino RB. Missing data. *N Engl J Med*. 2012; 367: 1353–1354.

Online Statistical Tests

http://handbook.cochrane.org/index.htm#chapter_16/16_2_intention_to_treat_issues.htm
http://statpages.org/

Books

- Cochrane Handbook for Systematic Reviews of Interventions. Version 5.1.0 [updated March 2011]. The Cochrane Collaboration, 2011. Available from www.handbook.cochrane.org.

- European Agency for the Evaluation of Medical Products (EMEA). Committee for Propietary Medicinal Products. Points to consider on missing data. Available from: http://www.ema.europa.eu/docs/en_GB/document_library/Scientific_guideline/2009/09/WC500003641.pdf
- FDA, Section 5.8 of the International Conference on Harmonization: Guidance on Statistical Principles for Clinical Trials. Available from: http://www.fda.gov/cber/gdlns/ichclinical.pdf. Accessed April 19, 2005.
- Little RJA, Rubin DB. *Statistical analysis with missing data.* New York: Wiley; 1987.
- Ting N. Carry-forward analysis. In: Chow SC, ed. *Encyclopedia of biopharmaceutical statistics.* New York: Marcel Dekker; 2000: 103–109.
- Wang D, Bakhai A. *Clinical trials: a practical guide to design, analysis and reporting.* England: Remedica Publishing; 2006.
- Weichung JS. Problems in dealing with missing data and informative censoring in clinical trials. *Curr Control Trials Cardiovasc Med.* 2002; 3(1): 4. https://doi.org/10.1186/1468-6708-3-4.

REFERENCES

1. Ware JH, Harrington D, Hunter DJ, D'Agostino RB. Missing Data. *N Engl J Med.* 2012; 367: 1353–1354. http://www.nationalacademies.org/nrc/
2. Little RJA, Rubin DB. *Statisical analysis with missing data.* New York: John Wiley & Sons; 1987.
3. Hollis S, Campbell F. What is meant by intention to treat analysis? Survey of published randomised controlled trials *BMJ.* 1999; 319: 670.
4. Haukoos JS, Newgard CD. Advanced statistics: missing data in clinical research—part 1: an introduction and conceptual framework. *Acad Emerg Med.* 2007 Jul; 662–668.
5. Gupta SK. Intention-to-treat concept: a review. *Perspect Clin Res.* 2011; 2: 109–112.
6. Molenberghs G, Thijs H, Jansen I, et al. Analyzing incomplete longitudinal clinical trial data. *Biostatistics.* 2004; 5: 445–464.
7. Frison L, Pocock SJ. Repeated measures in clinical trials: analysis using mean summary statistics and its implications for design. *Stat Med.* 1992; 11: 1685–1704.
8. Ting N. Carry-forward analysis. In: Chow SC, ed. *Encyclopedia of biopharmaceutical statistics.* New York: Marcel Dekker; 2000: 103–109.
9. Haukoos JS, Newgard CD. Advanced statistics: missing data in clinical research—part 1: an introduction and conceptual framework. *Acad Emerg Med.* 2007 Jul; 14(7): 662–668.
10. Donders ART, et al. Missing data review: a gentle imputation of missing values. *J Clin Epidemiol.* 2006; 59: 1087–1091.
11. Allison PD. Paper 312-2012. Handling missing data by maximum likelihood. SAS Global Forum. Haverford, PA: Statistical Horizons; 2012. http://www.statisticalhorizons.com/wp-content/uploads/MissingDataByML.pdf
12. Allison PD. Missing data. Series: A SAGE University Papers Series on Quantitative Applications in the Social Sciences, 07-136. Thousand Oaks, CA: Sage; 2001.
13. Laird NM. Missing data in longitudinal studies. *Stat Med.* 1988 Jan–Feb; 7(1–2): 305–315.
14. D Bernoulli, S Blower. An attempt at a new analysis of the mortality caused by smallpox and of the advantages of inoculation to prevent it. *Rev Med Virol.* 2004; 14: 275–288.
15. Altman DG. Adjustment for covariate imbalance. *Biostatistics in clinical trials.* Chichester, UK: John Wiley & Sons, 2001.

16. Senn SJ. Covariate imbalance and random allocation in clinical trials. *Stat Med*. 1989; 8: 467–475.
17. Pocock SJ, Assmann SE, Enos LE, et al. Subgroup analysis, covariate adjustment and baseline comparisons in clinical trial reporting: current practice and problems. *Stat Med*. 2002; 21: 2917–2930.

14

OTHER ISSUES IN STATISTICS II
SUBGROUP ANALYSIS AND META-ANALYSIS

Authors: *Jorge Leite and Munir Boodhwani*

Case study author: *Felipe Fregni*

INTRODUCTION

Clinical studies can provide invaluable information on the effects of particular treatment on a population of research subjects. However, in the translation process of applying data from clinical trials to the management of patients, clinicians frequently face a very specific challenge: Among all the various available treatment options for a disease, what specific therapeutic approach would be best for the individual patient? And what should be done when a clinician has to interpret conflicting data from different clinical studies on a particular subject? These questions form the basis of this chapter in which subgroup analysis and meta-analysis will be discussed.

The first section of this chapter will provide a step-by-step discussion of subgroup analysis and meta-analysis. The second section will invite the reader to critically think about one case study.

SUBGROUP ANALYSIS

Subgroup analysis is especially concerned about variability and how treatment effects can differ due to specific characteristics of the population (e.g., gender, age, smoking status).

> The International Subarachnoid Aneurysm Trial (ISAT) ($n = 2,143$) suggested that endovascular coiling was superior to neurosurgical clipping in patients with ruptured intracranial aneurysms, who were eligible for both interventions [1]. But a later subgroup analysis ($n = 278$) suggested that older patients with middle cerebral aneurisms (MCA) may indeed benefit more from clipping [2].

A subgroup analysis can then be defined as the assessment of specific treatment endpoints (both safety and efficacy) in a defined group (or groups) of patients that share certain specific characteristics [3].

The example from the ISAT trial suggests that the effect of one treatment in the overall sample population may not be the same for all the subsets in that sample. For instance, although endovascular coiling was superior in the trial for patients with ruptured intracranial aneurysms, indeed it seemed that older patients with MCA aneurisms indeed benefited more from clipping.

It is important to distinguish subgroup analysis from covariate adjustment. Covariate adjustment aims to decrease variability between groups by adjusting for possible confounding effects of other variables, thus improving the precision of the estimated overall treatment effect for the *entire* study population. Subgroup analysis, on the other hand, aims to assess the effects of the intervention in *specific subgroups*, in which there could be potential heterogeneous effects of a treatment related to demographics, pathophysiology, risks, response to therapy, potential clinical applications, and even clinical practice [4].

Subgroup analysis can be the primary objective of a study, or can alternatively be used to generate hypotheses for future studies. And usually are tested as an interaction term, namely when the effect on one independent variable may depend on the level of another independent variable.

An interaction term can be tested using a regression model, in order to consider the effects separately, as well as the interaction between them, as can be seen in the following equation.

$$Y = \beta 0 + \beta 1(x1) + \beta 2(x2) + \beta 3(x1 * x2) + e$$

If the variables in the model were gender and age, the equation could be coded as

$$Y = intercept + \beta 1(gender) + \beta 2(age) + \beta 3(gender * age) + e$$

The interaction term here is $\beta 3$ (x1*x2) (e.g., gender * age). In the absence of interaction effects, fit lines for each variable will be displayed as parallel lines (Figure 14.1 A). However, if an interaction effect exists, $\beta 3$ will be significantly different from 0, and fit lines can cross (Figure 14.1 B) (see Chapter 9 for linear regression).

There is a special consideration concerning qualitative heterogeneity, in which treatment effects on opposite directions are due to specific group characteristics

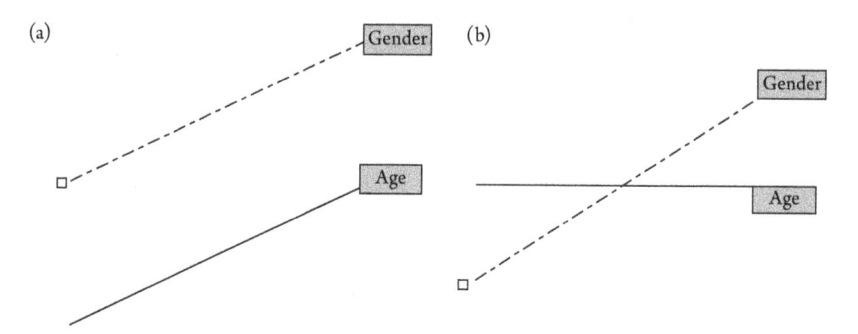

Figure 14.1. A: Parallel lines suggesting no interaction. B: Age and gender cross, thus suggesting a potential interaction.

[e.g., 5], although the treatment effects are on opposite directions that cannot be directly translated to risks, or even impact on quality of life.

TYPE I ERROR: DEALING WITH FALSE POSITIVES

An important issue to consider when performing subgroup analysis is the increased chance for type I error (false positive). The probability of type I error increases as the number of tests increases. For instance, if we set alpha (α) to 0.05 (i.e., 5% probability of a false positive), and then 20 comparisons are performed, the probability of having at least one of them defined as statistically significant ($p < 0.05$) due to chance is 100%. This is considered to be a false positive or type I error. If we increase the number of comparisons, we will increase the likelihood of having even more false positives.

The second important potential issue in subgroup analysis is to be unable to detect the effect when in fact there is an effect. This is called type II error. Thus it is important to carefully plan the subgroup analysis, as even a clinically important difference in a particular subgroup may be statistically non-significant if the number of subjects in that particular subgroup is small. In order to prevent that, several considerations need to be addressed. First, the number of subgroups should be kept to the minimum possible. The choice of subgroups should be driven by biological plausibility and, when possible, by preexisting data. Second, these analyses should also be defined a priori in the study protocol. One strategy to ensure equal distribution within subgroups of the variables of interest is by using stratified randomization methods, whereby randomization to the treatment is performed within each strata of the subgroup. Third, post hoc definition of subgroups to be analyzed should be avoided. Plan your analysis carefully before running the trial.

THE BONFERRONI CORRECTION

Even when subgroup comparisons are minimized and subgroups are carefully chosen, it may be possible in some situations that some statistical correction is required to avoid the inflation of type 1 error. One of the simplest methods available to perform multiple comparisons correction is to divide the alpha (α, usually .05) by the total number of comparisons to be performed. This is the Bonferroni correction method. In simple terms, if we are comparing three subgroups (A, B, and C) for a given treatment, we can have the following pairwise comparisons: A versus B, A versus C and B versus C. The most conservative and simple approach it to divide α by 3, and set the α value cut-off to approximately 0.017. If none of the three dyads has a p-value $<.017$, none of them will be stated as statistically significant.

The following equation is the mathematical representation of the Bonferroni method for α correction (α usually set to .05; k number of comparisons to be performed):

$$\frac{\alpha}{k} = \alpha^{corrected}$$

OTHER METHODS FOR DEALING WITH MULTIPLE COMPARISONS

The previously mentioned Bonferroni correction is probably one of the most conservative and widely disseminated methods of performing correction for multiple testing. But is not the only option available. There are several other methods available that follow more or less restrictive assumptions. These methods include the Tukey's Honestly Significant Difference (Tukey's HSD) or the Fischer's Least Significant Difference (Fischer's LSD) [6].

When employing correction for multiple comparisons, it is important to note that with the increase of the number of corrected multiple comparisons, the chance of type II error also increases (i.e., chance of false negatives). Therefore, it is important to be aware that there is a trade-off between the probability of type I and II errors, in which a decreased probability of type I error may increase the probability of a type II error.

There have been some interesting methods to deal with these issues, including the method proposed by Jackson et al. [7], in which instead of correcting for multiple comparisons, they disclosed the *error rate*. The rationale underlying this method is that if each comparison has a 5% probability of type I error, by multiplying that value by the total number of comparisons, the product will reflect the probability of having at least one false positive. Please note that in this method it is not possible to assess which comparisons are more likely to result from a type I error, but only that we have a certain probability.

For instance, if in total there are 40 statistical tests (i.e., multiple comparisons), multiplying 5% by 40, we have a 200% chance of having a type I error. In other words, we have 100% chance of having at least 2 tests that are statistically significant, due to chance alone.

Another possibility is *pre-specifying the comparisons to be made*. In this method, not all possible comparisons will be tested. Instead, contrasts are planned before data analysis in line with the study objectives. For instance, instead of testing all the possible comparisons between three subgroups, it is possible to pre-specify two contrasts that are clearly stated in the study objectives (e.g., subgroup A versus B, and subgroup B versus C; but not subgroup A versus C).

OTHER ISSUES WHEN COMPARING SUBGROUPS

One important issue when performing a subgroup analysis is that subgroups need to be comparable. This applies to the subsample size, as well as to the outcomes. For instance, due to randomization, subgroups may not be comparable due to differences in baseline characteristics differences. This can emerge when subgroups are analyzed even if those differences are not present in the broader study cohort, due to successful randomization.

HOW TO DEAL WITH UNEXPECTED RESULTS

Subgroup analyses can often yield unexpected outcomes. The question of whether these findings are real or not can be daunting. When this happens, the first step is to analyze thoroughly the study protocol and address several questions, such as the following: *Were there any differences in the sample size between the treatment and control arms within the subgroup? Could a covariate that is unequally distributed explain part of the results? Was the statistical analysis the most appropriate?* If no issues with the protocol are exposed, or other confounding variables do not explain the unexpected results, one should then examine the literature to determine if this finding (or trend) has been previously observed in other studies. Finally, the finding has to be assessed for biological plausibility. Nonetheless, there is often the real danger of ascribing a biological explanation to a spurious statistical finding.

This chapter has focused so far in dealing with the heterogeneity across subgroups. Analysis of data from subgroups of patients with certain baseline characteristics is typically insufficient to change general clinical practice. Often the sample size of a subgroup is small and therefore lacks the required statistical power, which will impose serious limitations to the generalizability of the study results. Thus, these analyses will often be exploratory in nature, and will mainly launch the basis for future studies, focusing on the particular subgroup.

META-ANALYSIS

Meta-analysis is a method of pooling data from several studies in order to quantify the overall effect of an intervention or exposure. The advent of evidence-based medicine and the general acknowledgment of meta-analysis as the apex level of evidence has led to an increasing interest in this specific type of quantitative systematic reviews. Meta-analysis can increase the precision of information on a specific topic, by addressing the variability between multiple studies and by adjusting for the limitations of individual studies, and ultimately they can contribute to changing clinical practices.

A meta-analysis can be seen as a two-step literature review: qualitative and quantitative. The first critical step is the qualitative assessments of a given topic. Such assessment usually shapes into a compendium of relevant studies in that particular area, exploring thoroughly the topic at hand. Nonetheless, there are several areas (and the clinical area is one of them) in which a quantitative assessment of a phenomenon is critical (e.g., when choosing the most appropriate treatment for a certain disease). This quantification of the magnitude of the effect of the intervention or exposure is what distinguishes meta-analysis from other types of literature review.

Thus, a meta-analysis is an integrative summary of the relevant studies in a particular topic, analyzing potential differences among studies, while simultaneously increasing the precision in the estimation of effects, evaluating effects in subsets of patients, overcoming the limitations of small sample size studies, as well as analyzing the clinical endpoints that require larger sample sizes, ultimately developing hypotheses for future studies [8].

IS THE RESULT FROM A META-ANALYSIS MORE ACCURATE THAN THE ONE FROM A RANDOMIZED CONTROLLED TRIAL?

There has been some controversy surrounding the discrepancies between results from meta-analyses and large randomized controlled trials (RCTs). For instance, LeLorier et al. [9] showed that the outcomes from 12 large randomized trials were not predicted accurately in 35% of previously conducted meta-analyses. Nonetheless, statistically significant differences between results from RCTs and the predicted result from meta-analysis were shown only for 12% of the outcomes analyzed (5 in 40 comparisons). If by chance alone a 5% difference is expected, these discrepancies are smaller than one could have anticipated. Also, as Ioannidis et al. [10] pointed out, the results showed in previous studies could be overestimations of the true effect, due to the fact that the 12 major RCTs included in the meta-analysis were all from four major journals. These studies usually have a high impact in the field, and commonly change clinical practice; thus they are not as easily predictable by other studies in the same topic. Therefore, it is reasonable to assume that the results derived from a meta-analysis are not that different from those derived from an RCT in the same topic.

The gold standard for clinical research will continue to be the large RCT, by continuing to provide the most reliable information within the specific population in which it was conducted. But in a meta-analysis, even studies with small sample size and/or varying degrees of heterogeneity are able to provide clinicians and researchers with fairly precise and accurate information, without the costs associated with large RCTs.

CONDUCTING AND UNDERSTANDING A META-ANALYSIS

In order to conduct a meta-analysis, it is important to have a clear definition of the criteria that will be applied to the selection of relevant studies to be included (or excluded); how potential heterogeneity among studies will be dealt with; the availability of information; how to perform data analysis; and ultimately how to disseminate the results to the scientific community. We will explore these points on the next pages.

What Studies Should Be Included?

The first step to conduct a meta-analysis is to assess if there is a real gap in the knowledge about that specific topic. How many meta-analyses were conducted on that topic? Has the literature evolved significantly to justify an up-to-date meta-analysis? Are there any relevant studies missing in the already published meta-analyses? All of these questions can only be addressed by a search of the available literature. This search should be as through as possible, using a systematic and accurate method of selection, as will be discussed later in this chapter.

Initial Search of Relevant Studies

Upon choosing a specific topic, the search strategy to retrieve relevant studies will consist of cross-referencing relevant keywords in at least two different databases (e.g., PubMed, Scopus, Google Scholar, PsycINFO). The number of relevant keywords should be maximized, as it has already been shown that even small differences in the data-gathering strategies can yield very different results [11].

In this stage, this initial search of the literature could suffer from search bias (see Chapter 3 for review). Even in an ideal scenario, in which all relevant articles are retrieved, there is still a potential source of bias: the publication bias [12]. The publication bias refers to a phenomenon in which positive studies are more likely to be published than negative ones. This will cause a bias toward an overall positive effect. Turner and colleagues analyzed this phenomenon in trials with antidepressants agents, and showed that 97% of positive outcome studies were published against 12% of negative ones [13]. Similarly, journals are more likely to accept a manuscript that shows an effect than a study that was "unsuccessful." Additionally, in some industry-sponsored trials, the sponsor retains the publication rights, and will not be very sympathetic toward publishing negative results. There can also be a language bias (e.g., only articles published in English), multiple publication bias (i.e., same study published more than once), or citation bias (i.e., more likely to be cited).

In order to minimize potential publication bias, efforts to include the maximum number of studies should be made, even the ones that were not published. This can be especially tricky if there is no way of obtaining information about them. That is why in recent years there has been an effort to have all clinical trials included in a registry, prior to the enrollment of participants.

Study Selection

There are not that many differences from selecting a study or a study population. In both scenarios, the inclusion and exclusion criteria need to be clearly defined. In the case of studies, objectives, study population, sample size, study design (randomized vs. non-randomized), choice of treatment, criteria for enrollment of patients and controls, endpoints, length of follow-up, analysis and quality of the data and, finally, a quality assessment of the study are used to define the inclusion and exclusion criteria.

Assessment of the quality of a study is essential when assessing the quality of the evidence and even more so when performing a meta-analysis [14], despite the fact that it is not hazard free [15]. Moher et al. [16] showed that incorporating the quality assessment in a meta-analysis drastically changes the results, which can improve our understanding of the "true results." However, as mentioned before, this approach is not hazard free, and thus, relevant methodological issues should be assessed individually, in order to allow a better understanding of their "real" contribution to the overall outcome [15].

In order to overcome this issue, several studies scoring systems were developed, allowing relevant studies to be stratified according to pre-specified criteria, enforcing studies' "coherency" within the strata. Then comparisons regarding randomization, blinding, patient selection, sample size, type of analyses, and outcomes, among others, can be performed.

The critical step when performing a literature search and study selection is to develop a process that will provide enough information about the decision tree process that will also be reproducible. The keywords are part of this process, as well as the flow diagram. This flow diagram can be built upon several "yes or no" questions that will determine if the study is to be included or not (see Figure 14.2). For instance, if a retrieved manuscript is a literature review or an observational study, and the question is "Is this study an RCT"? the answer will be no, and then that study will be dropped from further analysis. Usually at this stage, only abstracts are analyzed. Full manuscripts are only analyzed in the last stages, when study quality is to be assessed.

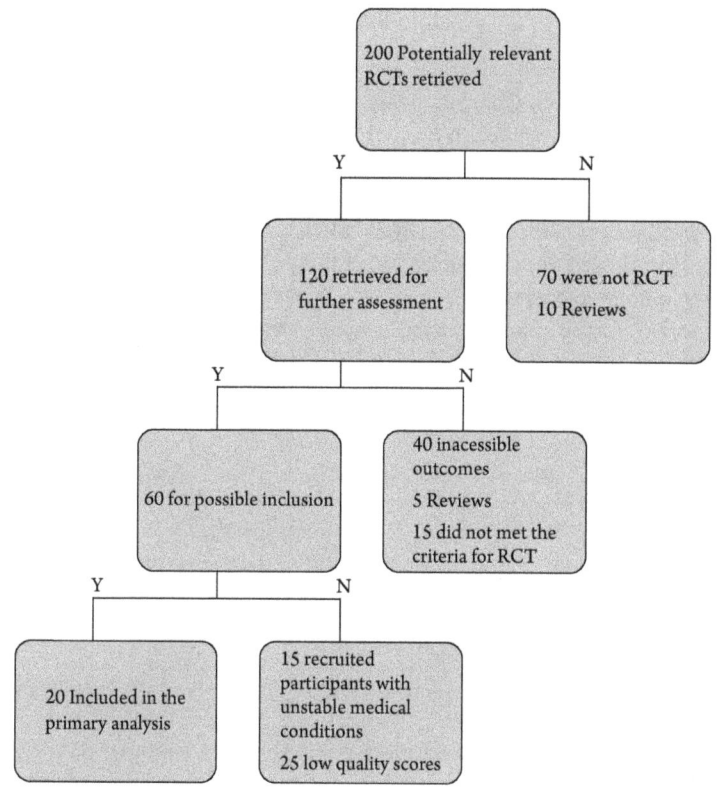

Figure 14.2. Flow diagram: Y = Yes; N = No. From 200 potentially relevant studies, only 20 were included in the primary analysis.

Figure 14.2 provides an illustration of the decision-making process involved in the inclusion/exclusion criteria of a meta-analysis. In order to standardize this process of study selection, several guidelines were already published. Please refer to the Preferred Reporting Items for Systematic Reviews and Meta-Analyses (PRISMA) statement for further information [17].

Problem of the Availability of Information

There are several examples in the literature when there is not enough information in the published study to perform a proper data collection for a meta-analysis. Frequently, only a summary of the results is displayed, such as means, standard deviations, odds ratio, or relative risks. The choice of data to present also varies from study to study. If the data from individual studies are not comparable, then the meta-analysis could be jeopardized. This problem can be even more serious if specific subgroups are to be analyzed. Therefore, it is important that published studies provide complete and factual information, which will help for better understanding of the results. Also, the harmonization of outcome reporting across studies is very desirable, as it facilitates the comparison between studies.

Data Synthesis

A critical issue when conducting/understanding a meta-analysis is to make realities across studies comparable. Comparing "apples and oranges" should ideally be avoided, and the chosen outcomes need to be comparable in order to be pooled in an overall effect. In some situations, outcomes across the studies are the same, and thus the comparison between them is straightforward. But sometimes, metrics that are being used are different and a common metric is required—this is called *standardization of outcomes*.

On way to do this is to transform the data into the same type of outcome (e.g., death), or combine scores into a Z score. The Z score is calculated based upon the individual score and how many standard deviations that individual score deviates from the mean:

$$Z = \frac{x - \mu}{\sigma}$$

> Imagine that the individual score in a self-report questionnaire for depression is 36 (in a maximum of 100 points), with a population mean of 24 and standard deviation of 12. Using the previous equation, Z score could be calculated as
>
> $$Z = \frac{36 - 24}{12} = 1$$
>
> Now imagine that you have a second questionnaire for depression (maximum of 50), in which the score is 18 (population mean of 12 and standard deviation of 4.5). The new Z score can be calculated as
>
> $$Z = \frac{18 - 12}{4.5} = 1.33$$

As the Z scores are unit free, they can then be combined into a global score for that individual, or as a comparison score across different metrics. If in the preceding example it will not be possible to compare directly the questionnaires (because of the different scales), the Z value represents how many standard deviations that particular individual deviates from the population mean, and thus allows a direct comparison. For the first questionnaire, that subject deviated 1 SD from the mean (Z = 1) and for the second, the same subject deviated 1.33 SD from the mean (Z = 1.33), which now allows a direct comparison between the two scores. It is also possible to attribute different weights to those global scores based upon the strength of association with an endpoint (e.g., ORs <1 = 0; 1≤ ORs ≤1.4 = 1; ORs >1.4 = 2).

The Pooled Effect Size

The effect size is a standardized measure of the magnitude of an observed effect [18]. The process in a meta-analysis depends on the estimation of the magnitude of an effect, prior to the combination (pooling) of the effects from several studies into one score. Typically, this pooled score can be found in the forest plot (see Figure 14.3,

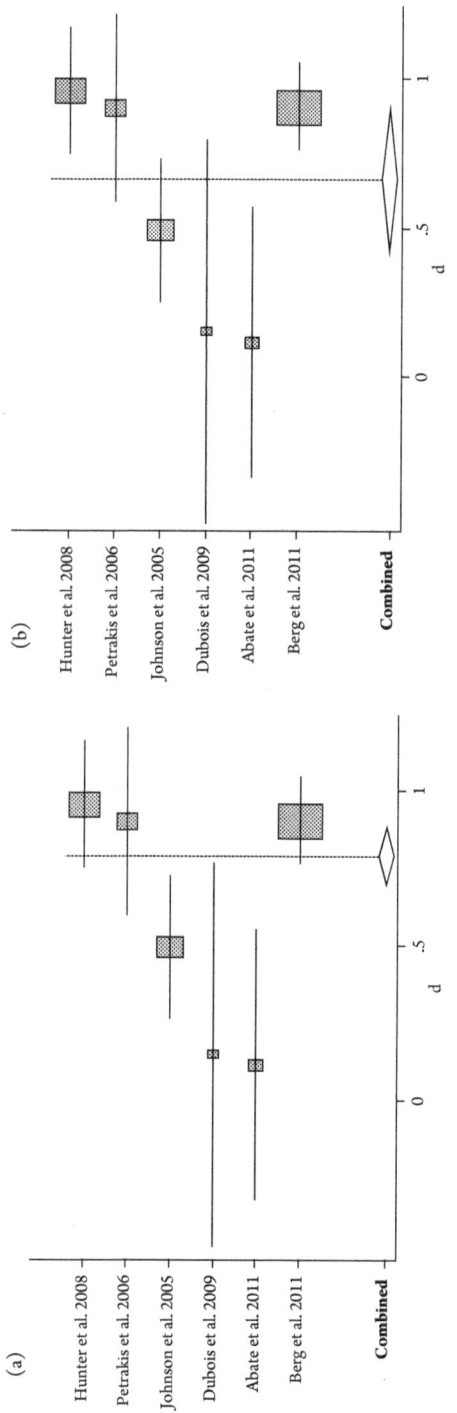

Figure 14.3. Forest plots comparing fixed (A) and random (B) effects model.

overall score, later in the chapter) along with the 95% confidence interval. The use of effect sizes has increased in the recent years, especially after the harsh criticism surrounding p-values.

There are several methods for estimating effect sizes depending on the nature of the variable. One of the most well-known and used method for continuous outcomes is the Cohen's d (also called standardized mean difference). The calculation of this score is easy to perform, and relies on obtaining the mean difference between populations ($\mu1$ and $\mu2$) and dividing by the pooled standard deviation.

$$d = \frac{\mu1 - \mu2}{\sigma}$$

The magnitude of the effect is considered to be small (0.2), medium (0.5), or large (0.8). Please beware that these cut-off points are arbitrary; thus the quality of the study and the uncertainty of the estimate need to be carefully addressed prior to their use.

> Meta-analyses can be performed using several outcomes. For dichotomous outcomes risk ratios, odds ratios or even risk differences can be used. Ordinal outcomes can be analyzed using the same strategy as dichotomous if the outcomes are summarized by the means of dichotomous categories, or by continuous methods if the intervention is summarized using means, or standardized mean difference.

Forest Plot and Heterogeneity

Heterogeneity in a meta-analysis is the variation in study outcomes among studies. Heterogeneity per se is not bad, as it can increase the external validity of a meta-analysis. But sometimes heterogeneity can be problematic when there are large dissimilarities in the results between studies. Sometimes these differences are attributable to a particular aspect of a study (which strengthens the argument for the quality scoring system), but this is not the most common scenario [8].

Heterogeneity should not be mistaken for the "oranges and apples" problem. Heterogeneity does not arise from combining realities that are dissimilar, but from differences between individual studies.

Heterogeneity can be tested using the Cochran's Q. It is calculated as the weighted sum of squared differences between the individual studies and the pooled effect. The null hypothesis in this test is that there is no heterogeneity among studies. If the p-value is less than 0.05, then the null hypothesis is rejected and thus heterogeneity is assumed. So a significant p-value in Cochran's Q usually means statistical significant heterogeneity among studies. But beware, this test typically has a low power, especially when the number of studies in the analysis is small.

Fixed versus Random Analysis

The decision between a fixed or a random model is dependent on the degree of heterogeneity. The fixed effect assumes that there is one true effect size, and all the studies included in the analysis share similar magnitudes and directions. In the random effects model, it is assumed that the true effect size can vary from study to study, but they follow a given distribution. So fixed effects models should be used preferentially when the heterogeneity is low. But if heterogeneity is high, random effects models should be used.

In detail, a fixed effects model assumes that all the studies share a common pooled effect size, which will have a mean (μ) and a variance of σ^2. In this case there is only one source of error in the estimates of the random error within studies. If the sample size is large enough, this error will show a trend to zero. As the random effects model assumes a distribution, has two sources of potential errors: as it tries to assess the "real" effect for the specific population, it is prone to the same within-study error that appears in the fixed effect; but it has also to weight the mean across studies, therefore it is also prone to random error between studies.

Figure 14.3 shows a fixed and a random effects model. Please note that pooled effect size is slightly higher in the fixed model (Figure 14.3 A), along with the wider confidence intervals in the random effects model (Figure 14.3 B).

Another important issue when conducting a meta-analysis is the sample size. The sample size of a study can influence the results of a trial. For instance, a smaller study could lack power (type II error) to detect an effect. Or can overinflate it. If 1:1 comparison between small and large sample studies is to be performed, the sample size is incorporated in the calculation. This means that in meta-analysis rather than using a simple mean, we often calculate a *weighted mean* of the effect size, in which larger studies carry more weight in the proportion of their sample size. In other words, if the pooled sample size from a given number of studies is, for instance, 10,000, if one large RCT enrolled 3,000, in the meta-analysis that study will carry 30% of the weight. This can introduce bias into the model, because larger studies will have more weight than the smaller ones, which is why sometimes in order to reduce bias, there is a stratification by sample size.

It is important to note that weighting studies by sample size or choosing random models with high heterogeneity does not solve the issue related to the source of the heterogeneity. As heterogeneity among studies is "inevitable" in meta-analysis, its quantification has been strongly recommended [12].

Quantifying Heterogeneity

Since there are clinical and methodological differences across studies, heterogeneity has been suggested as being inevitable [19]. Thus, instead of choosing models based on heterogeneity, test for variability in the sample estimates that is not due to change [12]:

$$I^2 = \frac{Q - df}{Q} * 100$$

in which Q is the chi-square statistic and df its degrees of freedom. Although there are no rules of thumb, and each analysis should be thoroughly assessed for magnitude and direction of the effects, the convention is that a score below 40% does not represent significant heterogeneity. Moderate heterogeneity can occur when he I^2 is between

30% and 60%. Between 50% and 90% may be a sign of substantial heterogeneity, and if the values range from 75% to 100%, then there is considerable heterogeneity among the studies included in the meta-analysis [12].

Sensitivity Analysis

An additional method of exploring heterogeneity, or if a study is of doubtful interest to be included in a meta-analysis, is to conduct a sensitivity analysis. In this analysis the pooled effect size is systematically plotted with or without a given study, along with the confidence interval (CI). This will provide a more accurate estimate of the effects of a single study on the overall results.

The CI is as important as the pooled effect size estimate for sensitivity analysis. The CI is calculated based on the sample mean (μ) and standard error (SE).

When CIs from individual studies overlap, effects sizes are similar and the heterogeneity is low. In some cases, there could be a line drawn at "no effect," with scores on the left favoring controls, and scores on the right side favoring treatment. If some results are on opposite sides of the "no effect line," these results are considered to be inconsistent, and therefore the heterogeneity is high. Even in the absence of results on opposite sides, usually random effects model has wider CIs than the fixed effects model due to the specific assumptions underlying each model (see Figure 14.4).

In order to conduct a sensitivity analysis, the forest plot can be used to calculate the pooled effect estimate along with the pooled confidence interval. This allows further testing of heterogeneity, by allowing each study to be removed sequentially, assessing the impact of each study on the pooled effect estimate.

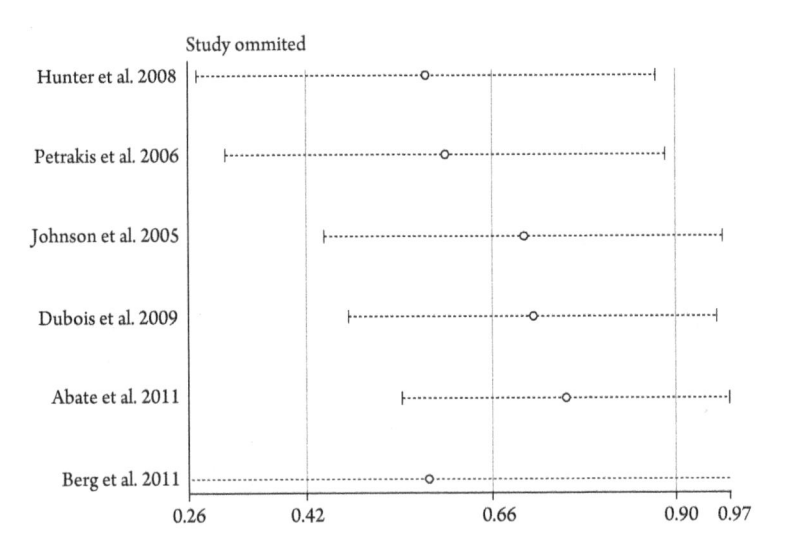

Figure 14.4. Sensitivity analysis: Each horizontal score represents the mean (with the 95% CI) if that particular study is removed. The vertical bar at 0.66 represents the overall pooled effect (i.e., all studies), with 0.42 and 0.90, representing the 95% CI. As can be seen, omitting one study sequentially does not seem to change the effect, as the 95% CI seem to overlap.

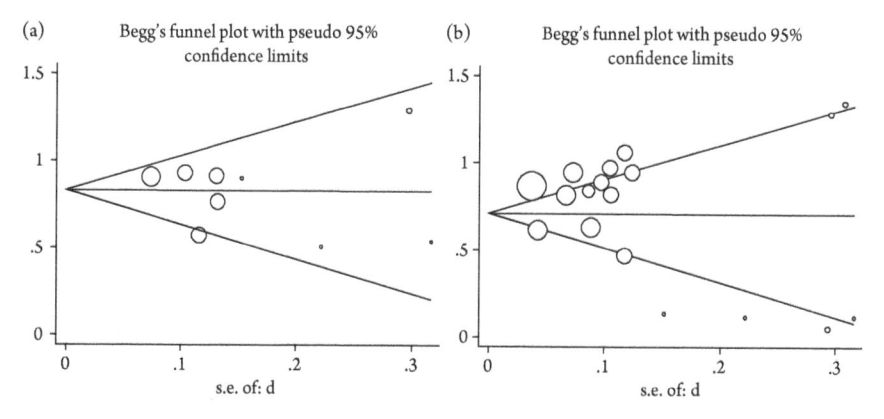

Figure 14.5. Funnel Plot: A: symmetrical funnel plot; B: Asymmetrical funnel plot. The y axis represents the effect size and the x axis the standard error. Larger studies have smaller standard error, therefore larger studies are distributed to the left of the x axis, while smaller studies will be progressively distributed more on the right. Also positive studies will be above the horizontal line (this means increased effect size), and negative studies will be bellow (i.e., with smaller effects).

Understanding a Funnel Plot and Publication Bias

The last critical step is to assess publication bias. As mentioned earlier, this type of bias can occur, especially because positive findings are more likely to get published than negative ones (sometimes named "the file drawer problem"). The effect on a meta-analysis is highly dependent on the studies that were included, thus assessment of potential bias is critical. The *funnel plot* was developed as a way of displaying potential publication bias. If the studies presented in a funnel plot have an almost symmetrical distribution (see Figure 14.5 A) there is no evidence that suggests publication bias. But if the distribution instead shows signs of asymmetry, then publication bias can be a possibility (see Figure 14.5 B).

In Figure 14.5, there are five positive and four negative studies in Figure 14.5 A. The studies with larger sample sizes are distributed to the left, while the smaller ones are distributed toward the right. Studies with positive effects are represented above the horizontal line, while the ones with negative effects are below that line. From a quick analysis, it seems that the distribution of studies follows a symmetrical pattern, and thus there is no suggestion of publication bias. While in Figure 14.5 B, most of the studies with larger sample sizes are positive, and cumulatively are outside the 95% CI in an asymmetrical distribution, which strongly suggests publication bias.

CASE STUDY: CHANGING MEDICAL PRACTICE AFTER KNEE SURGERY—USE OF META-ANALYSIS

Felipe Fregni

Professor Turner just hung up the phone—it was a call from the office of the Ministry of Health. The reason for this important phone call is that the new government is planning extensive changes in the health-care system, and one of these measures is to reassess the effectiveness of interventions aimed at the treatment of chronic diseases. This new administration wants to use evidence-based medicine for health policies. As Professor Turner is a renowned physical therapist and his specialty is knee rehabilitation, he was being recruited to assess the question of whether physiotherapy exercise after an elective unilateral total knee arthroplasty is effective and therefore should be supported by the government. He was being asked to come up with a final report in four weeks and the message was clear: he needed to get the best level of evidence.[1]

Professor John Turner is a full professor at the University of Sydney. He moved to Australia from the United Kingdom 16 years ago and he now has a privileged position in which he can dedicate almost all of his time to research, which he does in his laboratory at the university and from his house on the coast of Manly. He is particularly excited about this project since he has been a long-time defender of physiotherapy for rehabilitation after knee arthroplasty. In his clinical practice, he has seen the difference in terms of quality of life when comparing patients who did with those who did not undergo physiotherapy exercises after hospital discharge. He now has the chance to delve into this matter and collect all the evidence for this final report to the government. He knows his report will change clinical practice in Australia and he is thrilled to be part of this project.

He then calls his colleague, Dr. Richard Hamilton, an epidemiologist in Canberra, to discuss this project. "Richard, I need your help—I just got a call from the Ministry of Health requesting me to prepare a report on the effectiveness of physiotherapy exercise after total knee arthroplasty. This document will be used for the new guidelines of our health system to be adopted soon. How should I do that?" Dr. Hamilton is direct and short, "John, you do not have too many options here—the best way is to perform a well-conducted meta-analysis. By the way, if you are interested, I can go to Sydney next week and we can plan and start doing the first steps of this meta-analysis together. I would be pleased to be part of this project." Prof. Turner is happy with this offer, as he knows he may need additional expertise to conduct this report for the government. Meanwhile, he decides to perform a preliminary review of the literature on this subject.

---

[1] Professor Felipe Fregni prepared this case. Course cases are developed solely as the basis for class discussion. The situation in this case is fictional. Cases are not intended to serve as endorsements or sources of primary data. All rights reserved to the author of this case. Reproduction and distribution without permission are not allowed.

The Topic: Physiotherapy Exercise after Knee Surgery

Osteoarthritis (OA) is a common disease and a common cause of disability, especially with the aging of the population. There are several types of treatments—surgery being one of them. For cases in which surgery is indicated, physiotherapy may play a critical role for the rehabilitation of these patients. In addition, the length of hospital stay after joint arthroplasty surgery has markedly and rapidly decreased, thus decreasing the opportunity for in-hospital physiotherapy. Given that patients who undergo knee arthroplasty may still experience considerable functional impairment postoperatively, the effectiveness of physiotherapy after discharge is an important and valid question.

The Technique of Meta-analysis

Meta-analysis is a technique developed recently and comes from the need to have a tool to summarize results from several studies in a systematic way—in addition to providing quantitative measures for the combined results. Although reviews (descriptive) of the literature have been performed for many decades, their results are often confusing and difficult to interpret. For instance, if you perform a review on a given treatment and see that 70% of the studies show positive results and 30% show negative results, what is your main conclusion, especially if the negative studies are the largest ones? Even when you conclude that a treatment is effective for a given condition, how can you conclude the magnitude of the effects based on the analyzed studies? Meta-analysis can deal with these issues.

One important concept of meta-analysis is that studies might not necessarily be equal in their designs, but they need to have similar hypotheses or test the same treatments. Although this can be viewed as a limitation, meta-analysis techniques can assess the differences (or heterogeneity) between treatments, and there is a notion that RCTs can be generally externally valid even if the cohort studied is atypical. In addition, RCTs are expensive, and therefore being able to merge results from different studies is certainly very useful.

The main steps of meta-analysis are: "(1) formulation of the research question; (2) identification of relevant studies; (3) establishing inclusion and exclusion criteria; (4) data abstraction and acquisition; (5) data analysis; and (6) dissemination of results and conclusions."[2]

First Day of Work: Data Retrieval and Eligibility Criteria

In preparation for Dr. Hamilton's visit, Prof. Turner has worked together with his PhD student—Cara Lee, a student from mainland China who has arrived in Sydney only a couple of months ago but has demonstrated a great deal of energy. Both of them

---

[2] Piantadosi, S. (2005). *Clinical trials: a methodologic perspective* (2nd ed.). New York: NY, John Wiley & Sons, 720 p.

had collected preliminary information on the trials of exercises following total knee arthroplasty and are ready to discuss it with Dr. Hamilton.

Dr. Hamilton arrived, and after leaving his bags at the hotel near the university—a beautiful residential area in the heart of Sydney—he is ready for the challenge. He goes to the university to meet Prof. Turner and his fellow. They decide then to take the initial meeting to a nice restaurant in the harbor near the opera house. It is a beautiful and warm evening in Australia.

"So, John, let us not waste too much time and go directly to the point as we have a tight schedule ahead of us. I understand that the research question is decided: to determine whether physiotherapy after discharge following a total knee arthroplasty is effective. Well, now the work starts! First, we need to decide the retrieval method. As you know we can—and should!—select a bunch of electronic databases. I would suggest MEDLINE, EMBASE and Cochrane Controlled trials registry. However, this is not enough; we also need to look at the reference lists of the retrieved papers and also check the abstract lists of conferences on the topic. But this still cannot address the issue of publication bias—in other words, negative trials (especially small trials) are often not published, and this might severely bias the results of a given meta-analysis. To address this issue, alternatives are contacting experts in the field, writing to authors of previous trials and asking them for any unpublished data and, in the case of drug trials, even contacting the drug company for unpublished internal trials. Besides that, it is also possible to run some tests to assess publication bias—such as the funnel plot. So my first question to you: based on your resources and timeline, do you want to search only on the electronic databases or do you want to perform an extensive search?"

But even before Prof. Turner has a chance to talk, Dr. Hamilton continues, "The second important issue is the eligibility criteria for the inclusion of studies. This is an important step, John. As you also know, it is important to be as inclusive as possible but the risk is that by including small studies with low quality you might bias your analysis."

"What do you think, Cara?" Prof. Turner quickly turned the conversation to her to get her more involved. Cara is still used to the hierarchical Chinese system and hesitates before speaking, but as she was asked, she then starts, "Thank you very much, Professor, for the honor of participating in this study. In the quick research I performed, I see that a good option is to include trials that investigated physiotherapy intervention compared with usual or standard care or compared two different types of relevant physiotherapy intervention. The usual therapy consists of isometric or simple strengthening exercises to regain range of movement, and stretches." It is Prof. Turner's turn again, "Thank you, Cara. I think the challenge here is whether we will also include the open label trials and whether we will include studies that have different control groups."

"Well—" Dr. Hamilton intervenes, "this is an important issue in meta-analysis: limiting the inclusion criteria to have a more homogeneous group versus broadening the inclusion criteria to have more data and a greater generalizability. Both options are correct and have their advantages and disadvantages. Another option is to include studies based on assessment of study quality, but although this is usually done in meta-analyses, I think there are some problems with it, as it is difficult to assess study quality, and excluding studies based on methodological issues might also bias the results of the meta-analysis." They stopped as the food just arrived and Prof. Turner decided to take a break, "Let us have our dinner and we can restart our discussions tomorrow." As Dr. Hamilton was also tired, he quickly agreed with this suggestion.

Second Day: A Beautiful Day in Sydney and the Controversy of the Main Outcome

After a breakfast at the university cafeteria, the three researchers went to Prof. Turner's lab in the main quadrangle of the University of Sydney to reinitiate the work. Prof. Turner begins, "Well, now that we have decided the inclusion criteria, we need to decide which scale we will use. This will not be easy as studies used different scales. For instance, they used the Oxford knee score, the American Knee Society clinical rating score, the Western Ontario and McMaster Universities osteoarthritis index, and the Bartlett patellar score. In addition, they also measured the degree of motion and also quality of life. What should we do now?"

"This is a common problem," Dr. Hamilton responds. "Usually, studies use different scales and the meta-analysis is a technique that allows analysis of the data of studies using different scales for each study. This technique calculates the effect size, which is a measure with no units that represents the magnitude of the effects; however, you can only do this for the outcomes measuring the same domain, for instance, quality of life or measures of knee function. Then the question here is whether you want to choose one domain as the main outcome or to use several domains and show all of them in this meta-analysis." Prof. Turner then asks Cara to show the list of studies with the respective scales they used. That would be another long day and they needed to be efficient, as Prof. Turner had to catch the ferry to his house in Manly at 5 p.m.

Third Day: The Challenge Continues to Decide Methods of Statistical Analysis

Dr. Hamilton packs his bags and prepares to go back to his laboratory in Canberra after the final meeting in the morning when the group will decide the main directions for the data analysis. They therefore skip the breakfast in order to have more time for discussion, which is initiated by Dr. Hamilton. "Now we need to decide the main methods of analysis. First, we need to decide whether we are using categorical or continuous outcomes. Although this might also depend on how the studies report their findings. If we use continuous outcomes, then we would need the mean improvements and standard deviation for each group of treatment in each study as to calculate the pooled effect size. After that, we can run some additional analyses such as cumulative meta-analysis—which gives the changes in the effect size over time; sensitivity analysis—which gives estimates with exclusion of one study at a time as to assess whether the results are being driven by one study in particular; and funnel plot—which assesses whether there is likely publication bias in the analyses with the idea that studies should be distributed symmetrically in this plot if there is no publication bias."

After a long and productive discussion, the group seemed to agree with the main methods for this study, and Prof. Turner is feeling particularly glad for having accomplished this initial step, since he believes that these results will change the use of physiotherapy after knee surgery.

CASE DISCUSSION

Prof. Turner plans to perform a meta-analysis because "patients who undergo knee arthroplasty may still experience considerable functional impairment postoperatively, the effectiveness of physiotherapy after discharge is an important and valid question." After the initial stage of the formulation of the research question, Prof. Turner and his team face the first challenge: how to identify and select relevant studies in order to minimize the possibility of bias. This can be achieved by several methods that are discussed, including the inclusion and exclusion criteria, and by assessing the quality of the studies. After all these points are established, it is important to define the outcomes, and how the variables will be defined: this can have a clear impact on the possibility of statistical analysis. Finally, the best strategies for results and conclusions dissemination throughout the scientific and clinical community, and thus possibly changing the practice, must be decided.

CASE QUESTIONS FOR REFLECTION

1. What strategies might help include more trials in the meta-analysis?
2. How can unpublished data be found?
3. Discuss the pros and cons of including trials with different designs and qualities in the analysis, and how to deal with the problems.
4. How can we compare different scales? How can we convert effect sizes into clinical significance?
5. What is the Cochrane Collaboration and how might it help Prof. Turner?

ONLINE RESOURCES

For more information about trial registry, go to http://www.clinicaltrials.gov/. For a database of systematic literature review, consult the Cochrane Collaboration at http://www.cochrane.org/cochrane-reviews. Also for the PRISMA guidelines and supporting material, consult http://www.prisma-statement.org/.

REFERENCES

1. Molyneux AJ, Kerr RS, Yu LM, Clarke M, Sneade M, Yarnold JA, et al. International subarachnoid aneurysm trial (ISAT) of neurosurgical clipping versus endovascular coiling in 2143 patients with ruptured intracranial aneurysms: a randomised comparison of effects on survival, dependency, seizures, rebleeding, subgroups, and aneurysm occlusion. *Lancet.* 2005; 366(9488): 809–817.
2. Ryttlefors M, Enblad P, Kerr RS, Molyneux AJ. International subarachnoid aneurysm trial of neurosurgical clipping versus endovascular coiling: subgroup analysis of 278 elderly patients. *Stroke.* 2008; 39(10): 2720–2726.

3. Wang R, Lagakos SW, Ware JH, Hunter DJ, Drazen JM. Statistics in medicine: reporting of subgroup analyses in clinical trials. *N Engl J Med*. 2007; 357(21): 2189–2194.
4. Rothwell PM. Subgroup analysis in randomised controlled trials: importance, indications, and interpretation. *Lancet*. 2005; 365(9454): 176–186.
5. Collins R, MacMahon S. Reliable assessment of the effects of treatment on mortality and major morbidity, I: clinical trials. *Lancet*. 2001; 357(9253): 373–380.
6. Gopalan R, Berry DA. Bayesian multiple comparisons using Dirichlet process priors. *J Am Stat Assoc*. 1998; 93(443): 1130–1139.
7. Jackson RD, LaCroix AZ, Gass M, Wallace RB, Robbins J, Lewis CE, et al. Calcium plus vitamin D supplementation and the risk of fractures. *N Engl J Med*. 2006; 354(7): 669–683.
8. Walker E, Hernandez AV, Kattan MW. Meta-analysis: Its strengths and limitations. *Cleve Clin J Med*. 2008; 75(6): 431–439.
9. LeLorier J, Grégoire G, Benhaddad A, Lapierre J, Derderian F. Discrepancies between meta-analyses and subsequent large randomized, controlled trials. *N Engl J Med*. 1997; 337(8): 536–542.
10. Ioannidis J, Cappelleri J, Lau J. Meta-analyses and large randomized, controlled trials. *N Engl J Med*. 1998; 338(1): 59–62.
11. Dickersin K, Scherer R, Lefebvre C. Systematic reviews: identifying relevant studies for systematic reviews. *BMJ*. 1994; 309(6964): 1286–1291.
12. Higgins JPT, Green S, eds. *Cochrane handbook for systematic reviews of interventions*. 1st ed. Chichester, UK: Wiley-Blackwell; 2008.
13. Turner EH, Matthews AM, Linardatos E, Tell RA, Rosenthal R. Selective publication of antidepressant trials and its influence on apparent efficacy. *N Engl J Med*. 2008; 358(3): 252–260.
14. Pogue J, Yusuf S. Overcoming the limitations of current meta-analysis of randomised controlled trials. *Lancet*. 1998; 351(9095): 47–52.
15. Jüni P, Witschi A, Bloch R, Egger M. The hazards of scoring the quality of clinical trials for meta-analysis. *JAMA*. 1999; 282(11): 1054–1060.
16. Moher D, Pham B, Jones A, Cook DJ, Jadad AR, Moher M, et al. Does quality of reports of randomised trials affect estimates of intervention efficacy reported in meta-analyses? *Lancet*. 1998; 352(9128): 609–613.
17. Moher D, Liberati A, Tetzlaff J, Altman DG. Preferred reporting items for systematic reviews and meta-analyses: the PRISMA statement. *BMJ*. 2009; 339: b2535.
18. Field A. *Discovering statistics using SPSS*. London: Sage Publications; 2009.
19. Higgins JP, Thompson SG, Deeks JJ, Altman DG. Measuring inconsistency in meta-analyses. *BMJ*. 2003; 327(7414): 557–560.

UNIT III
Practical Aspects of Clinical Research

15

NON-INFERIORITY DESIGN

Authors: *Raquel Ajub Moyses, Valeria Angelim, and Scott Evans*

Case study authors: *Rui Imamura and Felipe Fregni*

INTRODUCTION

Clinical trials are the gold standard of study designs to implement new therapies into practice. The placebo-controlled trial is considered by many to be the ideal model to demonstrate and estimate the effect of a new intervention. For many conditions, however, it is not ethically adequate to use placebo, so the standard of care is therefore used as an active control over which the superiority of a new drug is shown. However, superiority of effect is not the only purpose of a new treatment. More and more, lower costs, less side effects, and lighter dosing regimens (with possible better adherence) are also important goals to be sought, as long it is possible to preserve the effect at a reasonable magnitude. A non-inferiority trial is the ideal design to address this issue. It is possible to show that a new intervention (with presumable other advantages) is not inferior in effect to the standard of care, which has been previously proven effective over placebo [1].

This chapter will begin with the main aspects of three basic study designs: superiority, equivalence and non-inferiority trials. The main guiding principles of the latter will be reviewed.

SUPERIORITY TRIALS

The aim of this design is to demonstrate the superiority of a new intervention over placebo or the current standard of care. As already demonstrated in previous chapters, the classical null hypothesis of this design states that there is no difference between treatments, while the alternative hypothesis states that the difference is statistically different from zero, i.e. not only the point estimate but also the 95% confidence interval (see Chapter 9) (see Figure 15.1, Table 15.1).

For sample size estimation, the predicted difference in effect and the estimated variance are important factors to consider (see Chapter 11). When analyzing results, the more conservative and usually preferable strategy is intention to treat (ITT), because considering protocol violators and withdrawals in the analysis will make the treatments look more similar, making it more difficult to reject H_0. Per-protocol analysis, on the other hand, tends to increase the estimate of effect, leading to an increased type I error [2].

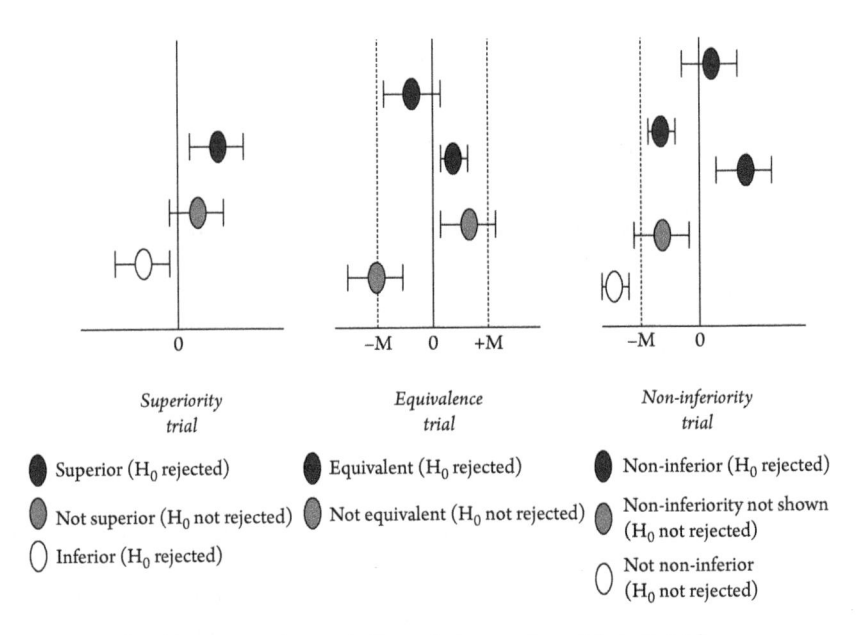

Figure 15.1. Possible outcomes in superiority, equivalence and non-inferiority trials. M = equivalence or non-inferiority margin. H_0 = null hypothesis.

Table 15.1 Main Differences Between Superiority, Equivalence and Non-Inferiority Trials

	Superiority	Equivalence	Non-Inferiority
Desired conclusion	New treatment is superior to old treatment (or placebo)	Both treatments are the same or not unacceptably different	New treatment not unacceptably worse than old treatment
H_0	Difference = 0	Difference ≠ 0 (difference <−M or difference >+M)	Difference ≤−M (or ≥M)
H_A	Difference ≠ 0	Difference = 0 (−M≤ difference ≤+M)	Difference >−M (or <M)
95% CI of the difference in effect	CI must not include 0 (or 1, in case of ratios)	The entire CI must lie between −M and +M	Lower limit must lie above −M (the position of the upper limit is not of interest)
Sample size	+ (depends on predicted difference)	++++ (depends on M)	+++ (depends on M)
Type of analysis	ITT preferable	Both ITT and PP should be performed	

H_0: null hypothesis; H_A: alternative hypothesis; 95% CI: 95% confidence interval; M: equivalence or non-inferiority margins; ITT: intention to treat; PP: per-protocol

Not showing superiority or inferiority of a treatment over another, however, does not imply that they are somehow equivalent. That is, unfortunately, a common interpretation mistake that may lead to false conclusions when comparing treatments.

EQUIVALENCE TRIALS

The aim of this design is to show that a new intervention is equivalent to another. It is a useful design to demonstrate, for instance, that a generic and an original drug are equally effective, or that a new formulation of a compound does not change the efficacy of the original one. It may be also desirable that it is not superior, because it may result in increased toxicity. In this setting, however, the null and alternative hypotheses are the opposite of the ones usually considered for superiority trials. While the null hypothesis states that both treatments are different in effect, the alternative hypothesis states that there is no difference in effect of both treatments, or difference = 0. Because a statistical difference of zero is virtually impossible due to variance of estimations, an equivalence margin (M) is established both under and above zero, between which the point estimate and variance of the effect of the new intervention over the standard will be (Figure 15.1, Table 15.1). Establishing an adequate M is not a simple task. It should ideally be smaller than any value that is considered a clinically meaningful difference. However, a very tight M would imply in an unfeasibly large sample size. That is because in equivalence trials, the estimated margin of equivalence is the main factor for sample size estimation. Equivalence studies are often very large trials.

When analyzing equivalence trials, ITT is not considered a conservative approach as in superiority trials, because making treatments look more similar will, in this setting, increase type I error [3]. Per-protocol analysis, although less conservative, may result in wider confidence intervals, because it is based on fewer study participants. For the previously mentioned reasons, both ITT and per-protocol analysis should be carried and, ideally, equivalence should be demonstrated in both analyses.

NON-INFERIORITY TRIALS

In this trial design, the main purpose is to demonstrate that a new intervention is at least as good as or not worse than the control treatment. Similarly to equivalence trials, other advantages of the new treatment may justify its use, even if it is necessary to sacrifice a small (and clinically non-significant) fraction of the effect of the standard treatment. This fraction is termed the *non-inferiority margin* (M), and, in other words, means how much the active control can exceed the new treatment, with the new treatment still being considered as non-inferior to the active control [4].

In this study design, the null hypothesis states that the difference between the treatments is larger than the non-inferiority margin (i.e., the point estimate and 95% CI of the difference between control and treatment is less than –M, or more than M) (see Figure 15.1, Table 15.1). The alternative hypothesis is that the difference between treatments is smaller than the non-inferiority margin or, in other words, the point estimate and 95% CI of the difference between control and treatment is more than –M (or less than M). Note that the new treatment can even be superior to the control, but this is not the primary concern of this study design. However, this particular feature of this design may lead to doubts when interpreting trial results. The same difference in treatment effects may be interpreted as non-inferior or inferior, depending on trial design, if the point estimates and 95% CI stay completely between 0 and –M (Figure 15.2). The key point in understanding that controversy is to consider that a statistically relevant difference (superiority trial) may not be a clinically relevant difference (non-inferiority trial).

Although non-inferiority trials are generally believed to require larger sample sizes than superiority trials, it will strongly depend on the magnitude of M. The smaller M, the greater sample size. Other parameters are also important, such as stratification (because smaller variance of data may require smaller samples) and type of analysis (ITT versus per-protocol). However, the same considerations made for equivalence trials regarding type of analysis are valid for non-inferiority trials, and the study should be powered for both strategies [5].

Important Considerations in Non-Inferiority Trials
Goals of Non-inferiority Designs

There are two main objectives of non-inferiority trials, which may be accomplished by proper study design:

1. Directly demonstrate that the new intervention is not inferior to the active control
2. Indirectly demonstrate that the new intervention is superior to placebo.

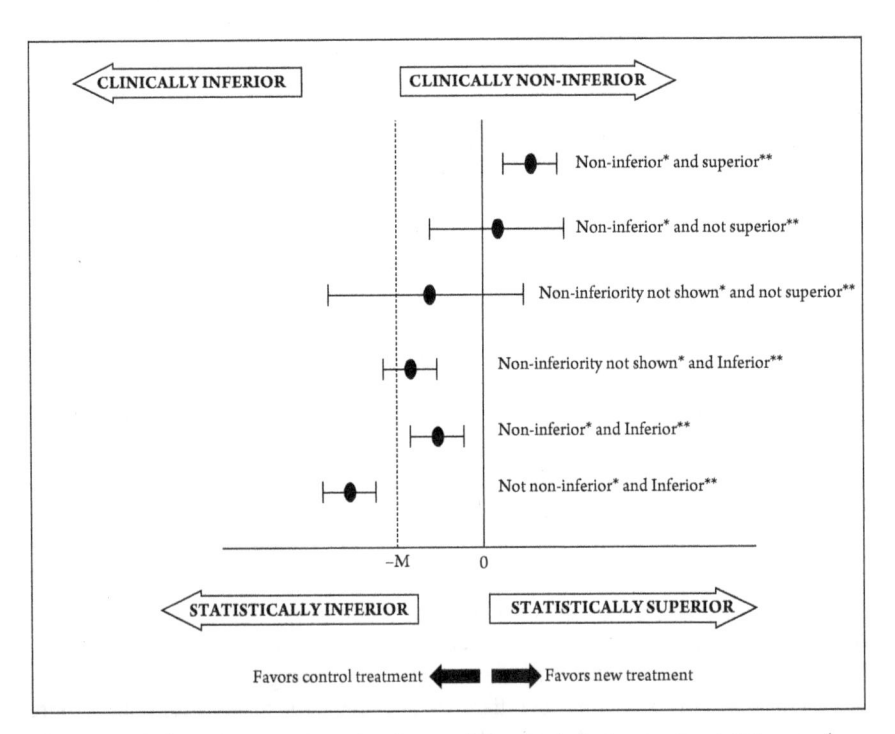

Figure 15.2. Different interpretation of results according to study design: treatment differences (new treatment; control treatment).

* In the context of a non-inferiority trial; ** In the context of a superiority trial.

To properly reach these goals, several assumptions and strategies must be taken, which will be further explained in this chapter [6].

Assay Sensitivity

This refers to the ability of the trial to distinguish differences between treatments if they actually exist. It may lead to false conclusions in two ways:

- If there are clinically meaningful differences between the new treatment and the active control, but the trial is unable to detect it, it will result in a false claim of non-inferiority.
- If the differences between the active control and placebo are no longer detectable by this trial, the new intervention may be claimed non-inferior when, in fact, it is ineffective if compared to placebo.

This is a concern in non-inferiority trials because a successful (positive) superiority trial has, by definition, assay sensitivity, whereas a successful non-inferiority trial may or may not have assay sensitivity. The ideal way to avoid this problem is to include a third arm with placebo (if ethically acceptable). In this setting, it is possible to test non-inferiority of the new treatment over the active control, as well as superiority of the new treatment and active control over placebo [7].

Constancy Assumption

An important premise of non-inferiority trials is that the active control was superior to placebo in previous trials. However, this superiority may have changed over time due to several reasons, like resistance development (in case of antibiotics), better medical practice, and so on. It is important to ensure that the active control would also be superior to placebo in the setting of the new trial, because even if showing that the new treatment is not inferior to the active control, this may just mean that both are equally uneffective.

Again, a three-arm design including placebo would address this question. If it is not possible due to ethical concerns, a way of minimizing this issue would be conducting the non-inferiority trial using a method as similar as possible to the one used for the trials that established the superiority of the active control over placebo. Inclusion/exclusion criteria, blinding and randomization strategies, the treatment scheme, and measuring methods are important parameters to consider [8].

CHOOSING THE NON-INFERIORITY MARGIN

The most critical problem of non-inferiority trials is choosing the margin. It is not statistically calculated, but instead, it must be assumed based on the performance of the active control in previous trials [9]. It will directly impact the design, conduct, and interpretation of the study findings. Two concepts are important:

1. The margin cannot be larger than the entire effect of the active control over placebo, generally referred to as M_1. Historical data of the effect of the active control

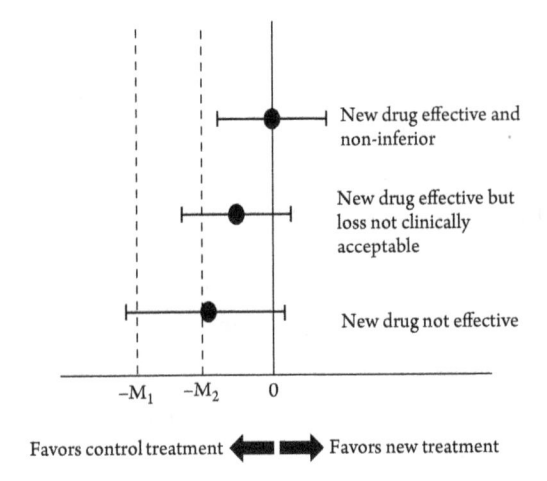

Figure 15.3. Non-inferiority margins.
M_1: the entire effect of the active control over a placebo, if a placebo was used in the trial; M_2: largest clinically acceptable loss in effect of the new drug compared to the active control.

over placebo, as well as within- and across-trial variability in estimates are key components to define M_1.

Here, it is essential to guarantee that the effect of the active control over placebo remains the same, otherwise, using M_1 as a non-inferiority margin when in the current non-inferiority trial the effect over placebo would be smaller, the new drug could be claimed non-inferior when possibly non-effective. Showing that the new treatment is non-inferior than M_1 will tell us that its effect is greater than zero. However, it does not assure that the drug has a clinically meaningful effect.

2. It is usual and desirable to choose a smaller value than M_1, in order to preserve some estimate of the effect of the active control. This other estimation of the margin (M_2) represents the largest loss of effect of the active control that would be acceptable (i.e., not clinically meaningful). If the lower bound of the 95% CI for the effect of the new drug over the active control is above $-M_2$, non-inferiority is demonstrated (Figure 15.3). Some strategies for estimation of M_2 are the following:

    Clinical judgment: reflects how much of the effect of the active control over placebo should be kept by the test drug in order to be considered non-inferior. Investigators may ask a panel of experts—or even patients—how much would they would be willing to sacrifice in effect in order to get other potential benefits. In a regulatory setting, however, this choice may be subjected to criticism.

    Fixed margin approach: Set the non-inferiority margin (M_2) to a proportion of M_1. So, if investigators concluded that it would be necessary for the new drug to preserve 80% of the effect of the active control, then M_2 should be set at 20% of M_1. However, one must keep in mind that this method does not consider that M_1 is a point estimate of the effect of the active control over placebo, which is subject to uncertainty.

95%–95% method: Set the non-inferiority margin ($-M_2$) to the upper bound of the 95% CI of the estimation of the effect of active control over placebo. Although this method addresses the issue of variability, it is usually very stringent.

Sometimes, it is interesting to change the non-inferiority margin. No concerns are usually raised if the margin is decreased, because it will result in a higher degree of certainty of non-inferiority. However, if the margin is increased, it must be strongly based on external data (e.g., new evidence) and never on data from the trial, otherwise the suspicion of manipulating the margin to fulfill the alternative hypothesis will be raised.

CHOOSING THE ACTIVE CONTROL

The active control chosen for non-inferiority trials must be carefully selected. If the standard of care does not have a high evidence of efficacy over placebo based on available supportive data, trial design may be unfeasible. Small magnitude of effect and low precision of the estimate also represent challenges to the study concept [10]. It is essential to assure that the active control would be superior to placebo in the current study, if a placebo were used. Investigators should search for the best active control available that fulfills these conditions. The fact that it has regulatory approval does not mean that it will be an appropriate active control.

Biocreep

Consider that for a given disease there is a standard treatment (A), previously proven effective against placebo, which is used as an active control in a non-inferiority trial for a drug B, with fewer side effects. After the non-inferiority is shown, drug B becomes the standard of care for some time, until a new drug C is developed. Investigators believe drug C has a lighter dosing regimen and want to test it against the standard of care (drug B) in a non-inferiority trial. Non-inferiority is shown and drug C becomes the standard of treatment. *Biocreep* is the term given to this effect, by which multiple generations of non-inferiority trials—that used drugs that were not tested against placebo as active controls—can result in demonstrating non-inferiority of a therapy that is actually not superior to placebo. It means B is not inferior to A; C is not inferior to B, but maybe C is neither inferior to A, nor superior to placebo. The term *technocreep* is also used to refer to the same effect in the case of medical devices.

INTERIM ANALYSIS

The reasons to perform an interim analysis in superiority trials, as well as advantages and disadvantages of doing so, are discussed in Chapter 18. These reasons may not always apply to non-inferiority trials.

1. *Efficacy*: In superiority trials, showing efficacy during interim analysis is an ethical issue, since it is not acceptable to keep randomizing patients to an inferior/placebo arm, and the drug should be available in the market as soon as possible. In non-inferiority trials, however, if during the interim analysis non-inferiority is shown, then there is no ethical imperative to stop the trial for any of the reasons

noted earlier. In fact, it is interesting to continue the trial, because superiority of the new drug may be further demonstrated.
2. *Safety*: The same concerns of superiority trials (new drug doing more harm than good, more side effects, etc.) are present in a non-inferiority trial, so this may be a motivation for performing an interim analysis and early terminating the trial.
3. *Futility*: Also the same concerns as superiority trials, as during interim analysis the new drug shows that it is unlikely to be non-inferior to the active control at the end of the trial.

MISSING DATA

While in superiority trials missing data may lead to failure to show superiority because of increased variance (type II error), in non-inferiority trials the effect may be making treatments look more similar and so increase type I error (claiming non-inferiority when it does not exist) [11]. Approaches for handling missing data in non-inferiority trials tend to be conservative:

1. Imputing success to active control and failure to new drug
2. Imputing expected values for the active control and for the new drug: for the new drug, the value imputed is the value measured for the active control less the value of M (favoring the null hypothesis) and vice versa.

SWITCHING DESIGNS

From Non-Inferiority to Superiority

Showing a possible superiority of the new treatment is not a primary concern of non-inferiority trials. However, once non-inferiority has been demonstrated, if the lower bound of the 95% CI is also above zero (Figure 15.2), superiority is also shown. Because the analysis is made examining the same single confidence interval, no penalty for multiple testing is necessary [12]. One should remember, however, that an ITT analysis should be preferred in the setting of a superiority trial [13].

From Superiority to Non-Inferiority

Switching from a superiority to a non-inferiority trial is generally less acceptable, but may also be appropriate, as long as some important requirements are met:

1. The non-inferiority margin must be planned a priori, otherwise, results may influence the clinical judgment of an adequate margin.
2. The active control group fulfill the criteria of an appropriate control for non-inferiority trials.
3. Assay sensitivity and constancy are satisfied.
4. Both ITT and per-protocol analysis are performed.
5. A high-quality trial is conducted (because poor quality may falsely claim non-inferiority).

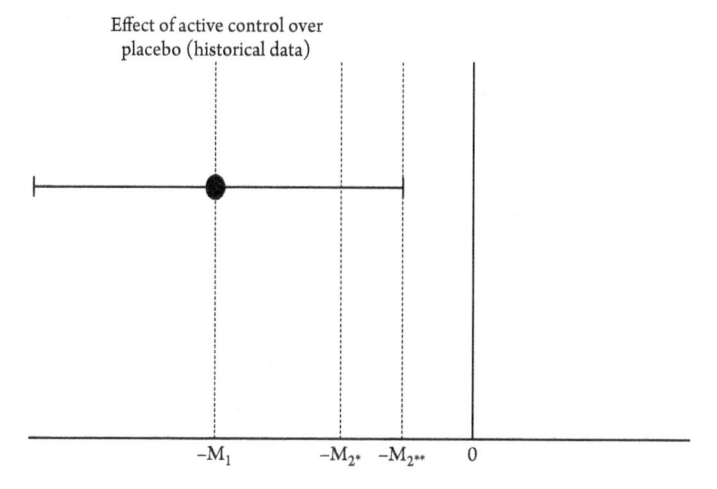

Figure 15.4. Strategies for determining the non-inferiority margin. $-M_{2*}$: M_2 set at 50% of the point estimate of the effect of active control over placebo (M_1); $-M_{2**}$: M_2 set at the upper bound of the 95% CI of the estimation of the effect of active control over placebo.

APPLYING RESULTS FROM NON-INFERIORITY TRIALS TO PATIENTS

As for any trial design, it is important to assure that patients from the trials (either the non-inferiority or the original trial that stated the active control superiority) are similar to patients to whom trial results shall be applied. Moreover, are the potential risks and benefits offered by the new drug relevant to a given patient? For instance, should a patient using the active control without side effects be offered the non-inferior drug, advocated for causing fewer side effects than the active control?

CASE STUDY: NON-INFERIORITY AND EQUIVALENCE TRIALS: PLAYING CHESS WITH REVIEWERS

Rui Imamura and Felipe Fregni

Professor Daniel Perkins has just moved to Toronto, Canada, to assume a new position as dean of research at a large university. This morning had started with exciting and challenging news. After turning on his computer, he saw this message in his mailbox:

Subject: Your Submission to *The Lancet*
Dear Dr. Perkins,
Thank you for submitting your manuscript to *The Lancet*. Your submission has now been assessed by external advisers and discussed by the editorial team. We would like to invite you to REVISE your paper in light of the reviewers' comments below.

Best wishes

Prof. Perkins was excited by this news. He had dedicated his life to academia and this recent study he had submitted to *The Lancet* had a special meaning for him. He and his team had spent several years conducting this study and the results could have a significant impact on the field. But after reading the reviewers' comments, he realized that the challenges to get this published were not over: it would not be easy to address reviewers' comments. But one thing he enjoys is the intellectual debate with reviewers, as he compares it with chess play. In this case, he wanted to be the one to make the "checkmate" move.[1]

The Study: A New Drug for Anticoagulation during Percutaneous Coronary Intervention

One of the complications of percutaneous coronary intervention is the risk of thrombosis during the procedure or the short-term follow-up that can lead to fatal outcomes. One potential solution to mitigate this risk is the use of anticoagulants; but the trade-off is the increased risk of bleeding, especially considering the invasive procedure of percutaneous coronary intervention.

For the current study, a big pharmaceutical company invited him and his team to run a large phase III multicenter trial, testing a new drug (Thrombase) for anticoagulation during percutaneous coronary intervention in individuals with moderate- and high-risk acute coronary syndromes. The advantages of this new drug were fewer side effects than heparin, notably lower risk of significant hemorrhagic episodes.

The aim of the study was therefore to assess anticoagulation with a new thrombolytic agent (Thrombase) during percutaneous coronary intervention in individuals with moderate- and high-risk acute coronary syndromes. The primary

---

[1] Dr. Imamura and Professor Fregni prepared this case. Course cases are developed solely as the basis for class discussion. Although cases might be based on past episodes, the situation in this case is fictional. Cases are not intended to serve as endorsements or sources of primary data. All rights reserved to the author of this case. Reproduction and distribution without permission is not allowed.

endpoint would be 30-day composite ischemia (death, myocardial infarction, or unplanned revascularization for ischemia). The main issue when designing this study was whether to compare this new drug against placebo or against the standard treatment. After intensive discussion during the planning stages, the team of researchers decided to use the active control and therefore use a non-inferiority design. As Prof. Perkins just realized after reading comments from reviewer 1, this has proven to be a controversial decision.

Non-Inferiority and Equivalence Trials: An Interesting Alternative?

The non-inferiority margin trial aims to show that a given new treatment is as good or better than a standard treatment—this can be concluded if the new treatment is not worse than a specified amount, called a non-inferiority margin. Therefore, the lack of a statistically significant difference in a superiority trial does not indicate non-inferiority, as the difference between two treatments might still be larger than the specified margin.

One important point here is that a non-inferiority trial is not the same as an equivalence trial. In an equivalence trial, the new treatment is not only not inferior to a standard treatment but also not superior; therefore, the difference between two treatments is either +d or –d (d represents the margin). The margin in equivalence trials is a value that would not be considered clinically meaningful; in other words, this value would indicate an equivalent clinical effect between the treatments being compared.

One of the main reasons to use non-inferiority designs is when it is unethical to carry out randomized placebo-controlled clinical trials. Another potential application is when there is a question of whether a new treatment that has fewer side effects has at least the same efficacy as the standard treatment.

Although it is an attractive design, non-inferiority designs raise several important issues, such as how to calculate the margin (or the minimal difference that is acceptable between the two treatments) and two other important issues: (1) assay sensitivity and (2) constancy assumption. Assay sensitivity indicates whether the trial in which the standard drug is being used can show that this standard intervention is better than an ineffective intervention such as placebo. One important issue is that regardless of historical data showing that, for instance, aspirin is beneficial for myocardial infarction as compared to placebo, there is no assurance that in a trial comparing aspirin to a new drug, aspirin in this trial would be better than placebo. The other point is constancy assumption. The point here is that with rapid changes in medical practice, the historical difference between placebo and a given treatment might not be applied in the current medical practice.

First Look at the Reviewers' Comments

That morning was a chilly autumn morning and after reading that email, Prof. Perkins was preparing to leave home for his 30-minute jog in his quiet neighborhood. That has been his habit for the past 15 years, and now he really enjoys doing this in Toronto, especially during the fall with the beautiful scenery from the foliage color change.

It was dawn and the sky was just turning from orange to light blue. Old maple trees that were particularly beautiful this time of year adorned his path. This morning he had a lot to think about. Although the reviewers were positive regarding his trial, they also had several comments and criticisms.

He had already sent an email to schedule a meeting with his research team—he had taken almost his entire team to Toronto, and for this study, he had one postdoc student and two junior faculty members working with him. He abbreviated his jog and went quickly to his office.

Reviewer 1: Was the Non-Inferiority Trial the Best Design?

After arriving at the office, Prof. Perkins goes directly to his office to meet with his research team and starts the discussion, "Gentlemen, we need to go over a couple of issues that are more difficult to respond to. Let us start with reviewer 1, who was the pickiest—although he made clever suggestions. His main criticism was—(he then reads the comment from reviewer 1):

> The main issue I have with this trial is its design—I am not convinced that non-inferiority trial is the best design—the problems I have with this design are (i) we do not know in this case whether the drug is equally good or equally ineffective—as the authors know the assay sensitivity is extremely important. Given that this trial was performed using state-of-the-art percutaneous intervention that we know is associated with a smaller rate of thrombotic events, the lack of differences between two treatments might be due to the fact that the standard drug (heparin) in this case is not different from placebo, as patients did not have an excess of thrombotic events, and (ii) because of this issue, I believe that this was a waste of resources as the trial was extremely large. For these reasons the authors should have pursued a superiority trial.

Jan Klose, a postdoctoral fellow who has been working with Prof. Perkins for many years, is the first to speak. He has always been proactive and he quickly begins:

> He is certainly clever in his comments, but according to the Declaration of Helsinki, "The benefits, risks, burdens and effectiveness of a new method should be tested against those of the best current prophylactic, diagnostic, and therapeutic methods." That is an important consideration when we designed this study. It is not ethical to use placebo controls since that would require withholding the proven therapy (heparin). Also we do know that the standard care, heparin, is very effective. Although it would be easier to demonstrate efficacy over placebo, that would lead to ethical concerns.

Sunil Kumar, an instructor from India who is very knowledgeable about clinical trials, adds some considerations:

> Well, this reviewer has a good point, we cannot prove assay sensitivity in our study. Therefore our new drug might be similar to placebo if heparin (the standard drug) had no significant effect in our study. Therefore, patients in the future might use our

drug when in fact it is ineffective. We certainly do not want this. I wonder now if we should have considered another trial design—for instance, conduct a superiority trial in patients who have an allergic reaction to heparin and therefore cannot take it. This is certainly an important limitation of our study.

"Excellent points, Sunil and Jan. We should add some comments in the limitations section in which we discuss the ethical issue of using placebo in this case and also the potential limitation of assay sensitivity." After a small pause, Prof. Perkins continues, "Although he might have put our 'king' on 'check', this was not a 'checkmate.' Let us review now the main comment of reviewer 2."

Reviewer 2: Defining the Non-Inferiority Margin

Prof. Perkins then proceeds, "Well, I think I know who reviewer 2 is; although he is a colleague, he made sharp comments—here he goes:

> My main concern here is with the non-inferiority margin that was chosen for this study. As the authors know, the non-inferiority margin is a critical piece for the non-inferiority design, as a large margin might invalidate the results of a given study. In the case of the current study, I think the margin is excessively large. In fact, this non-inferiority trial provides a direct comparison of T (Thrombase), to C (heparin), but not of Thrombase to placebo. Thus, one hopes to choose a non-inferiority margin that will provide assurance that Thrombase is better than placebo. That concern is especially true when the comparator drug C has small effect size over placebo. Please address this important issue, especially because the new drug was in the inferior rather than superior side when compared to heparin.

This time, Michelle Beck, an active clinician and researcher, starts:

> This is the main issue in the previous non-inferiority studies in which I have participated: defining the NI margin. Although heparin (our standard drug) has a large effect size as compared to placebo in historical controls, the issue of the non-inferiority margin is still a challenging one. We have seen some non-inferiority studies which were criticized for the use of margins that were considered inappropriately high (TARGET trial).[2] And a very small margin means too many patients; that would be unfeasible. But because we used the clinical judgment, which is an acceptable method but is subjective, how do we justify that our margin was adequate?

Jan has been listening attentively and then decides to add:

> I believe that clinical judgment was adequate. We as clinicians might consider what difference in event rates would make the two treatments no longer "therapeutically

---

[2] Moliterno DF, Steven J Yakubov SJ, DiBattiste PM et al. Outcomes at 6 months for the direct comparison of tirofiban and abciximab during percutaneous coronary revascularization with stent placement: the TARGET follow-up study. *Lancet*. 2002; 360: 355–360.

equivalent." Of course this judgment varies from setting to setting and it may not be easy to reach a consensus. However, I believe that our number for the margin was conservative and okay.

Sunil, the savvy clinical researcher, has been waiting to give his remarks:

I kind of predicted this issue when we designed our study; but most of you wanted the clinical judgment to define the margin. But as Prof. Perkins likes to say: our king has not been killed yet—we still have a chance. If we calculate the margin again using other methods and show that our results do not change, we would be all set—this would be a sensitivity analysis. The two methods I propose are: (i) using the effect size (ES) of C (heparin) compared to P (placebo). So we can combine all available evidence, a meta-analysis if possible, to obtain an estimate of the ES of C (over placebo) with a confidence interval. We may, then, choose the NI margin based on the estimate of this effect size (ES). For example, we may set M equal to half the point estimate of ES. The intent of this approach is to provide assurance that T (new drug) provides at least half as much benefit as C (heparin), compared to placebo. My concern with this approach is that large point estimates of ES may lead to unacceptably large M as well. We know that estimates of ES are subject to uncertainty even if they are obtained from meta-analysis. The actual ES may be smaller than stated, and if that is the case, the use of a large M could lead to a false claim of non-inferiority. Another option (ii) is to set the NI margin equal to half the lower limit of the confidence interval for ES of C (also obtained from a meta-analysis of previous studies). This is known as the 95–95 method and is usually suggested by FDA statisticians. This is conservative in that it provides strong assurance that T (new drug) is superior to P (placebo) if the NI trial is successful.

The problem with these methods, as I mentioned before, is that the lower the margin, the more difficult to establish non-inferiority and the larger the sample size needed. For example, reducing the NI margin from 25% change in event rate to 20% increases the sample size by about $(5/4)2 = 1.56$. The 95–95 method, in particular, not uncommonly requires sample sizes that are impossible to reach.

After listening to all the comments, Prof. Perkins concludes, "Well these are all important issues that need to be addressed. What we can do here is to do a sensitivity analysis—see how the results would change if we change the method of defining the margin and also mention that using these other methods, we would need a much larger sample size that would be unfeasible. Also we should point out that the best method is not established yet and point out that the method we used is often used in the literature."

Prof. Perkins was happy with the outcome of this meeting—he thought to himself, "Checkmate, reviewers!"

CASE DISCUSSION

Motivation of the Investigators to Run This Trial

Thrombase may have fewer side effects than heparin; it is also unethical to have a placebo arm.

Drawbacks Presented by the Reviewers

What could be done to address these drawbacks?

1. Choice of the trial design—is there enough assay sensitivity? Is the current trial sensitive enough to detect a difference in effect of heparin over placebo if a placebo would have been included? Another point: is this trial sensitive enough to detect differences between heparin and Thrombase? If a difference does exist but cannot be detected by this trial, a false claim of non-inferiority will be made.

   Possible ways to address this issue:
   - Include a third arm with placebo? Is it ethical?
   - Run this trial as similarly as possible to the trials that have shown superiority of heparin over placebo.
   - Constancy assumption: since the trials that showed superiority of heparin over placebo were run, standards of care of these patients might have improved and, in the current setting, heparin may not demonstrate such a benefit over placebo as before. If this is true, showing that Thrombase is non-inferior to aspirin might just mean that they are both ineffective. One point to consider is that if the effect of heparin over placebo is large (impressive risk reduction in ischaemia), it is unlikely that it would not be still superior to placebo in the current trial.

2. Choice of the non-inferiority margin—selecting the margin: To better understand the two options given in the case, we can suppose that, in a previous meta-analysis, the relative risk of ischemic events for placebo over heparin was, for instance, 2.30 (95% CI 1.95–2.75). The interpretation would be: given an RR = 2.30, placebo increases the rate of ischemic events in 130% (CI 95%–175%).
   - *First method* (fixed margin approach): Set the NI margin at half the point estimate of the effect size of placebo over heparin: so, to be claimed non-inferior, the NI margin for Thrombase would have to be: Half the effect size of placebo over heparin: 130%/2 = 65%, which means an RR of 1.65 or, using the formula: $1+[(x-1)/2]$.
   - *Second method* (95–95 method): Set the NI margin at the lower bound of the 95% CI of the effect size of placebo over heparin: 1.95. The upper bound of the 95% confidence interval of the effect of Thrombase over heparin must be less than the selected NI margin (Figure 15.5). Note that the 95–95 method assumes a smaller loss of effect to claim for non-inferiority.

CASE QUESTIONS FOR REFLECTION

1. What are the issues involved in this case that should be considered in order to respond to reviewers?
2. What are the concerns?
3. Was non-inferiority design the best one? Why? Why not?
4. Have you seen a similar situation? If you know similar cases (that can be disclosed), please share with the group.

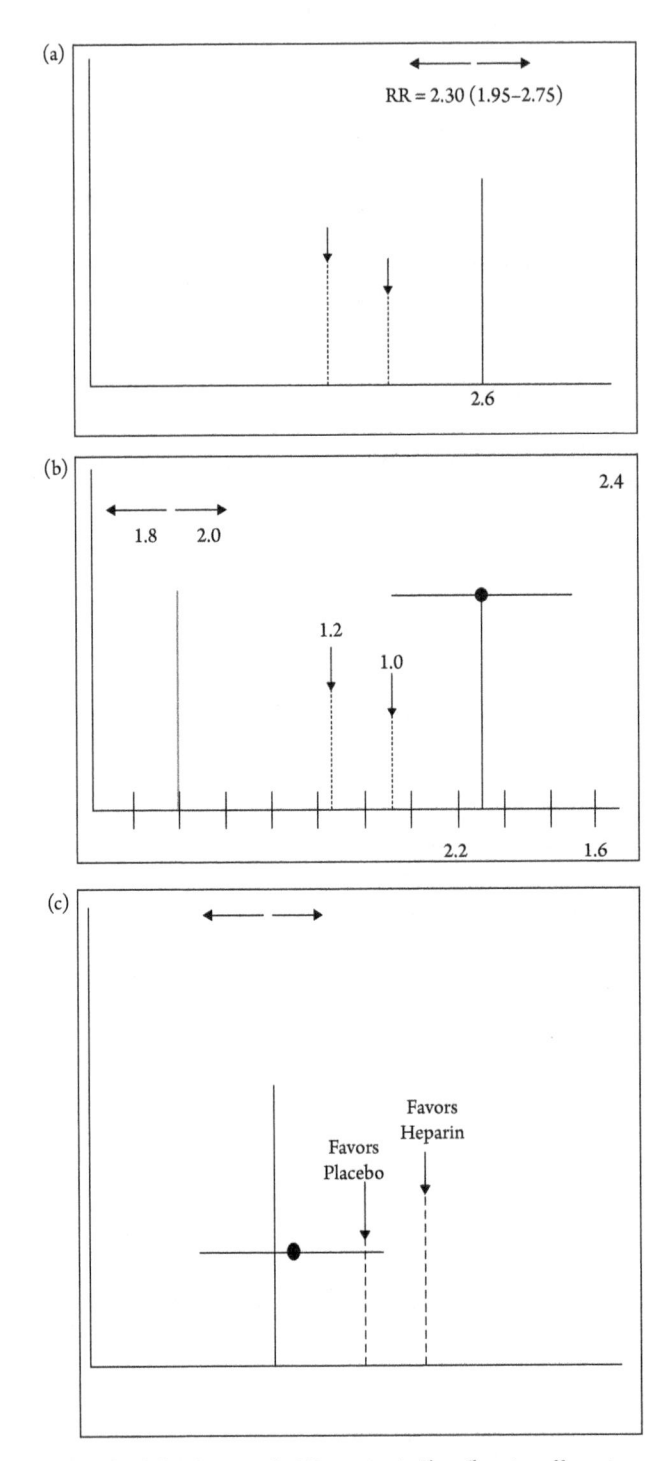

Figure 15.5. Two methods for choosing the NI margin. A: The effect size of heparin over placebo and the non-inferiority margins: M_a: set at half the point estimate of the effect size; M_b: set at the lower bound of the 95% CI. B: Transposing the margins to the NI trial with thrombase and heparin. C: Fictitious result of the non-inferiority trial: non-inferiority would have been claimed if M_a would be the chosen non-inferiority margin, not M_b.

FURTHER READING

UnitedStates Food and Drug Administration: Guidance for Industry Non-Inferiority Clinical Trials 2010: focuses on a deeper understanding of the methods for determining a non-inferiority margin that are recommended by FDA.

Reporting of Noninferiority and Equivalence Randomized Trials. An Extension of the CONSORT Statement: check-list for elaboration and reporting of Non-inferiority trials.

REFERENCES

1. Christensen E. Methodology of superiority vs. equivalence trials and non-inferiority trials. J Hepatol. 2007 May; 46(5): 947–954.
2. D'Agostino RB, Sr., Massaro JM, Sullivan LM. Non-inferiority trials: design concepts and issues—the encounters of academic consultants in statistics. Stat Med. 2003 Jan 30; 22(2): 169–186.
3. Evans SR. Clinical trial structures. J Exp Stroke Transl Med. 2010 Feb 9; 3(1): 8–18.
4. Evans S. Noninferiority clinical trials. CHANCE. 2009; 22(3).
5. US Department of Health and Human Services; Food and Drug Administration; Center for Drug Evaluation and Research (CDER); Center for Biologics Evaluation and Research (CBER). Guidance for industry non-inferiority clinical trials 2010.
6. Fleming TR, Odem-Davis K, Rothmann MD, Li Shen Y. Some essential considerations in the design and conduct of non-inferiority trials. Clin Trials. 2011 Aug; 8(4): 432–439.
7. Schumi J, Wittes JT. Through the looking glass: understanding non-inferiority. Trials. 2011; 12: 106.
8. Nathan N, Borel T, Djibo A, Evans D, Djibo S, Corty JF, et al. Ceftriaxone as effective as long-acting chloramphenicol in short-course treatment of meningococcal meningitis during epidemics: a randomised non-inferiority study. Lancet. 2005 Jul 23–29; 366(9482): 308–313.
9. Yonemura M, Katsumata N, Hashimoto H, Satake S, Kaneko M, Kobayashi Y, et al. Randomized controlled study comparing two doses of intravenous granisetron (1 and 3 mg) for acute chemotherapy-induced nausea and vomiting in cancer patients: a non-inferiority trial. Jpn J Clin Oncol. 2009 Jul; 39(7): 443–448.
10. The Italian Group for Antiemetic Research. Dexamethasone, granisetron, or both for the prevention of nausea and vomiting during chemotherapy for cancer. N Engl J Med. 1995 Jan 5; 332(1): 1–5.
11. Flandre P. Design of HIV non-inferiority trials: where are we going? AIDS. 2012 Oct 17.
12. Schiller P, Burchardi N, Niestroj M, Kieser M. Quality of reporting of clinical non-inferiority and equivalence randomised trials: update and extension. Trials. 2012 Nov 16; 13(1): 214.
13. Wangge G, Klungel OH, Roes KC, de Boer A, Hoes AW, Knol MJ. Room for improvement in conducting and reporting non-inferiority randomized controlled trials on drugs: a systematic review. PLoS One. 2010; 5(10): e13550.

16

OBSERVATIONAL STUDIES

Authors: *Minou Djannatian and Clarissa Valim*

Case study authors: *André Brunoni and Felipe Fregni*

In the field of observation, chance favors the prepared mind.
—Louis Pasteur (French scientist, 1822–1895)

It is the theory that decides what can be observed.
—Albert Einstein (Physicist, 1879–1955)

INTRODUCTION

In this chapter, we will introduce you to the major designs of observational studies. With this topic, we now enter the world of epidemiology.

Epidemiology is a field of research that studies "the distribution and determinants of health-related states or events in specified populations" and applies "this study to control [...] health problems" [1]. Its objective is to measure parameters relevant to public health, ranging from birth and death rates to cleanliness of drinking water to disease occurrence. Another main purpose of epidemiological research is to identify risk factors associated with disease. Finally, epidemiologists develop models to predict future disease burden based on current data (e.g., the impact of hypertension on global public health within the next 20 years given unchanged lifestyle). Recommendations on lifestyle factors may be one consequence of such predictions. Importantly, where clinical research assigns interventions to as even study groups as possible, epidemiological research observes unexposed and exposed individuals under "real-life conditions" without intervening itself.

We will provide you with the main tools to assess the quality of an observational study and identify possible threats to the validity of the obtained results. The next chapter discusses covariates and confounders in observational studies and how to account for them (with emphasis on propensity scores).

In observational studies, data are collected through "observations" (interviews, surveys, database queries, etc.), instead of "actively" being generated or altered. Observational studies can be descriptive, when no comparison group is included in the design. They can be applied to describe the frequency of events in a population. Observational studies can also be analytical, when different study groups are compared. Data can then be used for statistical inference, and relationships between exposures (i.e., risk factors) and outcomes (i.e., diseases) can be investigated.

An exposure may be an environmental factor (such as air pollution), a self-chosen habit (such as smoking), or an intervention that a patient receives independently of the study. To make a comparison with randomized controlled trial (RCT), an "exposure" in an RCT would be the intervention, which is manipulated in RCT, while it is not in observational trials. Due to the non-randomized nature of observational studies, bias and confounding can largely influence study outcomes and must be carefully controlled. Consequently, the study protocol should provide detailed information on the study sample, exposure and outcome variables, sources of data and methods of assessment, sources of bias, and statistical analysis [2].

CLASSIC MEASURES IN EPIDEMIOLOGY

Epidemiology has its own language, and in order to provide you with a better understanding of common statistical measures, we will start by giving a brief overview over several basic terms.

Ratio

A ratio is a division between values, which puts them into relation: $ratio = a/b$ [3]. It can be used to relate different subpopulations to each other, for example the males and females who suffer from the same disease.

Proportion

A proportion relates a sub-entity to an entity. In its simplest form, it can be expressed as proportion = $a/(a+b)$ where the nominator (a) is a part of the denominator $(a+b)$ [3]. Different than ratios, proportions can only take values between 0.0 (if (a) equals zero or is infinitely low) and 1.0 (if (b) equals zero or is infinitely low).

Chance can alternatively be expressed in terms of *odds*. Odds represent the number of times that a favorable event will likely occur [4].

In epidemiology, a specially defined type of proportion is *prevalence*, which is the proportion of those individuals who develop a condition at a specified time within a population at risk. Disease prevalence can be determined as follows [4,5]:

$$Disease\ prevalence = \frac{number\ of\ individuals\ with\ disease}{number\ of\ all\ individuals\ at\ risk\ for\ the\ disease}$$

Rate

Disease frequency can be determined over a specified time period and, in that case, a measure of time needs to be included in the ratio. Rate is a measure of how frequently an event occurs in a population at risk within a given time period. Demographic rates, such as birth or death rate, usually refer to a time period of one year, and the population at risk at the midpoint of the year is commonly used as the reference population. Irrespective of the size of the study population, rates are often expressed per 1,000 or 100,000 population (by using a multiplier). The basic formula to determine rates is the following [3]:

$$Rate = \frac{number\ of\ events\ in\ a\ time\ period}{population\ at\ risk\ in\ the\ same\ time\ period} \times multiplier$$

Box 16.1 General Use of Contingency (2 x 2) Tables

Contingency tables are used to represent data from observational studies in a visually plausible way. They consist of two columns, which show disease status (D), and two rows, which show exposure status (E). Absolute frequencies are displayed in each cell. Cell *a* represents the number of individuals who have the disease and have been exposed to a putative risk factor (E+/D+). Cell *b* contains the number of individuals without the disease who have been exposed to the risk factor (E+/D−). Cell *c* represents the number of individuals who have the disease but were not exposed to the risk factor (E−/D+). Cell *d* contains the number of individuals without the disease and any exposure to the risk factor (E−/D−). Consequently, a+c represents all individuals with the disease (D+), a+b represents all individuals with positive exposure status (E+), and so on. We will later show how to calculate important statistical parameters for each study design.

	D+	D−
E+	a	b
E−	c	d

For example, if 428,077 individuals die in 2012 in a country in which the mid-year population comprised 61,153,780 individuals, the death rate is 700 in 100,000.

The terms ratio, proportion, and rate are the basis for the specific statistical parameters that will be introduced in the context of study designs. Contingency tables (see Box 16.1) can be helpful to calculate these parameters and the adequate formulas will be provided throughout the text.

CLASSIC DESIGNS OF OBSERVATIONAL STUDIES

We will discuss in this section simple designs, such as case report and case series, as well as more classical study designs, such as cross-sectional, case-control, and cohort studies. The reader needs also to be aware that mixed designs are possible—also called *nested designs* (in other words, a small study within a large study). For instance, suppose someone is following a cohort with 1,000 subjects. It is possible to get 100 cases of this cohort and run a nested case-control study. It is beyond the scope of this chapter to discuss nested designs in depth.

Case Report and Case Series

A case report is a descriptive study in which clinical data of an individual patient is presented to the public. It usually includes a detailed description of disease history, clinical presentation, diagnostic approach, and response to given treatment. Certainly, it is not useful to elaborate on typical presentations of a clinical syndrome that is widely known from textbooks. Instead, case reports focus on the description of rare clinical symptoms, unusual combinations of symptoms, unexpected presentations of known diseases, or individual off-label treatments. Furthermore, case reports are an established way to report adverse drug events [6,7]. A case series is a quantitative and qualitative extension of the case report in that it summarizes a number of cases under a clearly defined research question. It thus adds value to the clinical findings and may even be used to build hypotheses on associations. Large case series, which for example analyze data from disease registries, may comprise up to several hundred patients [8].

Statistical Analysis

A very limited amount of statistical analysis can be done in case series. One main parameter is *symptom prevalence*, which is the proportion of cases that have a certain symptom, relative to the total number of cases [9].

$$Symptom\ prevalence = \frac{number\ of\ cases\ with\ symptom\ x}{total\ number\ of\ cases}$$

For example, in a case series on symptoms associated malignant wounds, 21 out of 67 patients reported pain. Thus, symptom prevalence of pain was $21/67 = 31.3\%$ [9].

Advantages

Case reports and case series detect novelty by describing yet unknown clinical presentations or novel treatments [8,10]. When evidence accumulates from several case reports or case series with similar findings, hypotheses on disease mechanisms, associations with risk factors, or treatment effectiveness can be generated. Larger studies with the potential for meaningful statistical analysis (e.g., case-control or cohort studies) may then be initiated to test these hypotheses. In this way, a case report may be the first step to the discovery of a new disease. Similarly, a series of cases with severe adverse events due to a drug may initiate the retraction of that drug from the market [7]. Clinical education can be another positive aspect of case studies, as rare diseases or rare manifestations of a common disease may hardly be seen in clinical daily routine, yet should be recognized once they present.

Disadvantages

The major disadvantage of case reports and case series is the lack of a comparison group. Therefore, they cannot be used to demonstrate the efficacy or safety of a treatment. Also, there is a good chance that a found association is falsely positive. Consequently, associations that are based on data from case series should be treated very carefully. They can only be used to generate hypotheses, which must further be tested in a robust study design with a comparison group, for example a case-control study [11].

Another disadvantage of case reports and case series is their proneness to *publication bias* (see the section "Bias" later in this chapter) [6]. As mentioned earlier, case reports and case serious favor the unusual, and this may lead to an overrepresentation of certain rare cases in the literature.

These arguments explain why case reports and case series are considered to provide a rather low level of evidence. They alone usually do not change medical practice.

Example from the literature
A case series from 1981 described the unusual presentation of Kaposi's sarcoma in eight young homosexual men in New York [12]. In these patients, skin lesions were generalized, whereas classical Kaposi's sarcoma rather affects the lower limbs. Patients were about 30 years younger than usual (in their forties rather than seventies). They all suffered from sexually transmitted diseases, including CMV and hepatitis B infection. Importantly, survival time was markedly reduced (20 months rather than 8–13 years). This case series was among the first descriptions of acquired immunodeficiency syndrome (AIDS). The search for the underlying pathogen of Kaposi's sarcoma, as well as Pneumocystis carinii pneumonia with high lethality in unusually young patients, ultimately led to the isolation of the human immunodeficiency virus (HIV) in 1983.

Cross-Sectional Studies

A cross-sectional study investigates the characteristics of a population sample at a specific time point (Figure 16.1). Subjects are randomly sampled from a target population, and exposure and disease status are measured once and at a specific point of time for each subject. The sampling process itself can take an extended period of time (up to several years), depending on how narrow the study population and how large the required sample size is. Data can be obtained from questionnaires or interviews (13).

Statistical Analysis

On a descriptive level, cross-sectional studies can be used to determine odds and prevalence of the *disease*. On an analytical level, odds ratio and prevalence ratio can be calculated to measure the association of exposure and disease.

We will show here how to calculate these parameters using a contingency table. Let us examine the occurrence of type II diabetes mellitus (D) on a very small Pacific island and investigate the potential association with a body-mass-index (BMI) >35 (E).

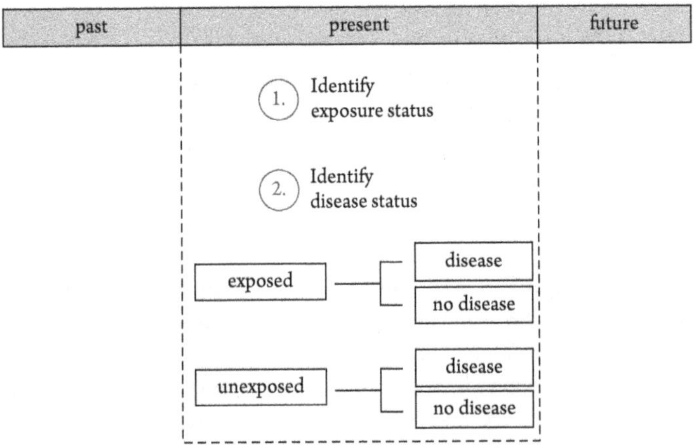

Figure 16.1. Study design of cross-sectional studies.

	D+	D–
E+	125	350
E–	55	850

To determine *disease prevalence*, we divide the number of individuals with diabetes by the number of all individuals (in this case, all of them are at risk for acquiring diabetes) (see section "Classic Measures in Epidemiology" earlier in this chapter). Using the contingency table, we calculate prevalence = $(a+c)/(a+b+c+d)$. The overall prevalence for diabetes in the Pacific island population is $(125+55)/(125+350+55+850) = 0.13 = 13\%$.

To determine the *odds of disease*, we divide the probability of having the disease by the probability of not having the disease. We can calculate this from the 2 x 2 table: odds of disease in exposed subjects = a/b, and odds of disease in unexposed subjects = c/d. In the Pacific island example, the odds for diabetes are $125/350 = 0.36$ in the exposed and $55/850 = 0.06$ in the unexposed.

Prevalence ratio is a statistical parameter that is used to determine associations between exposure and disease in cross-sectional studies. It is the prevalence of disease among exposed subjects compared to unexposed subjects [14]:

$$\text{Prevalence ratio} = \frac{\text{disease prevalence among exposed subjects}}{\text{disease prevalence among unexposed subjects}}$$

One can calculate prevalence ratio from the 2 x 2 table: Prevalence ratio = $(a/(a+b))/(c/(c+d))$. The resulting value is a measure of strength of association. Values >1.0 indicate an increased risk for the disease due to exposure, whereas values of 1.0 or lower indicate no associated risk or a protective effect of the exposure, respectively. In our example, prevalence ratio is $(125/(125+350))/(55/55+850)) = 4.33$, which means that the individuals with BMI >35 have 4.33 times the probability to have type II diabetes mellitus than individuals with BMI of 35 or lower.

Alternatively, associations between exposure and disease can be determined from odds by calculating *prevalence odds ratio (POR)*, which is the *odds ratio of disease*. It can be defined as the odds of disease among exposed compared to unexposed subjects:

$$POR = \frac{\text{odds of disease among exposed subjects}}{\text{odds of disease among unexposed subjects}}$$

We can calculate POR from the 2 x 2 table: POR = $(a/b)/(c/d) = (axd)/(bxc)$. In the Pacific island example, the prevalence odds ratio for type II diabetes mellitus given a BMI >35 is $(125x850)/(350x55) = 5.5$. In other words, the odds for diabetes mellitus in an individual with BMI >35 is 5.5 times the odds for type II diabetes mellitus in an individual with a lower BMI. Note that, due to the particular definition of odds, this cannot be translated into a 5.5-fold higher chance to develop the disease due to exposure.

In order to estimate the impact of confounding variables, logistic regression can be used. This is a multivariate regression method in which we estimate the probability (or odds) to develop an outcome (disease) instead of another outcome (no disease) depending on one or more dichotomous variable (e.g., gender or presence/absence of hypercholesterinemia). Coefficients in this regression model represent odds ratios [15].

Advantages

Cross-sectional studies are an efficient way to gather comprehensive data on common health conditions like diabetes or cardiovascular diseases and are hence used for national surveys [15]. They are used to determine disease and exposure prevalence and measure associations between exposures and diseases. They can in principal be relatively fast and cheap to perform, but this is highly dependent on the sampling process and method of data acquisition, as stated earlier. Cross-sectional studies can easily be integrated into cohort studies to measure the characteristics of the study cohorts at baseline or any other defined time point. Another major advantage is no need for follow-up [4].

Disadvantages

Cross-sectional studies in a general population are not suited to study rare diseases. For rare diseases, a case series can be an alternative to measure exposure prevalence in a subset of diseased patients [13].

The measurement of prevalence in cross-sectional studies can lead to an underrepresentation of cases, when a disease is of short duration, or to an overrepresentation of cases, when a disease has a long duration (*prevalence-incidence bias*; see section "Bias" for further explanation). In this situation, prevalence may not be a good estimate for disease occurrence [15].

Since subjects are assessed at a single point in time, no temporality of an association can be determined. Therefore, it is extremely difficult to establish causality with cross-sectional data [15]. Cross-sectional studies can, however, be used to build hypotheses about causal relationships, which are tested in a case-control or cohort design in a second step.

Example from the literature

A large cross-sectional study on 3,090 patients with Parkinson's disease determined the prevalence of impulse control disorders (ICDs) in Parkinson's disease [16]. Patients with Parkinson's disease were recruited from movement disorder centers in the United States and Canada and were assessed in semi-structured interviews. Problem or pathological gambling occurred with a prevalence of 5%, whereas compulsive buying was a habit for 3.5% of the patients; 5.7% displayed compulsive sexual behavior and 4.3% were affected by binge eating. ICDs were unequally distributed between male and female patients (men were more likely to have compulsive sexual behavior (OR 11.98), but less likely to have compulsive buying (OR 0.55) and binge-eating disorder (0.57). Furthermore, an association of dopamine replacement therapies with ICDs was established. The likelihood of developing an ICD under therapy with dopamine agonists was higher than under therapy with levodopa (OR 2.6). This study (together with others) increased the awareness for ICDs in Parkinson's patients and led to a change in prescription practice.

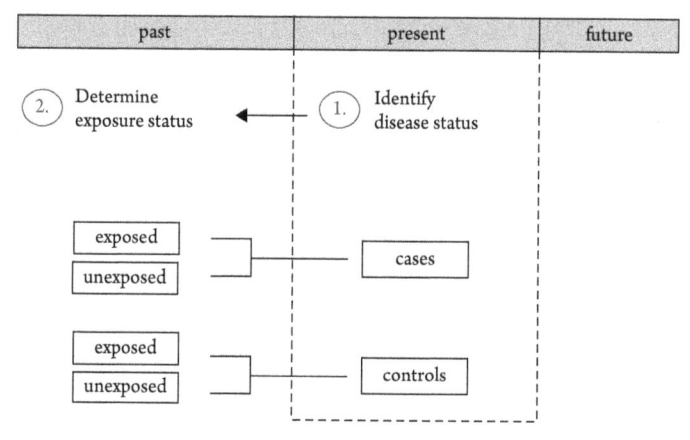

Figure 16.2. Study design of case-control studies.

Case-Control Studies

Case-control studies (Figure 16.2) are studies in which individuals are selected from a defined population based on outcome (i.e., disease) [17]. Individuals that have the outcome are selected as "cases." From the same population, individuals free of the outcome are selected and serve as "controls." Investigators then look back in time to identify possible risk factors (exposure) for developing the disease. Information on previous exposures is gathered directly from subjects (e.g., personal interviews, telephone interviews, paper-based questionnaires) or from preexisting records (e.g., medical charts) [14]. Usually, only one outcome (the one used for the selection of cases) is investigated per study [18,19].

Statistical Analysis

Since the number of cases and controls is fixed by design, case-control studies do not allow the estimation of disease occurrence. Instead, odds ratio can be calculated [4].

To further understand these parameters, let us analyze a fictive example of foodborne disease after eating in a restaurant famous for seafood. We want to find out whether eating seafood was a risk factor for developing food-borne disease in this specific example. Therefore, both cases and controls are drawn from a population of visitors to this restaurant. Exposed subjects had consumed seafood, whereas unexposed subjects had not.

	D+ = cases	D− = controls
E+	49	37
E−	31	43

Similarly to the odds ratio of disease, which we calculated in cross-sectional studies, we can calculate the *odds ratio of exposure* in case-control studies. The odds ratio of exposure is the odds of exposure among the diseased relative to the odds of exposure among the disease-free [15]:

$$\text{Odds ratio of exposure} = \frac{\text{Odds of exposure among diseased subjects}}{\text{Odds of exposure among disease-free subjects}}$$

Using the 2x2 table, we can calculate OR = (a/c)/(b/d) = (a x d)/(b x c) [4]. The odds ratio of exposure in our example is (49/31)/(37/43) = (49 x 43)/(37 x 31) = 1.8. This means that the likelihood of having eaten seafood as a case was 1.8-fold higher than as a control. Seeing the high exposure prevalence of seafood, we can suspect that other risk factors for food-borne disease exist in this restaurant.

Further parameters can be calculated when cases and controls are sampled from a cohort, because only incident cases within the observation time are included [20]. In a case-cohort study, the probability that an initially disease-free subject develops the outcome during the time of follow-up equals the *incidence risk*, or *cumulative incidence*. Building a ratio between the exposed and unexposed group will result in *relative risk*, or *cumulative incidence ratio*. Because controls are longitudinally sampled from the population still at risk in nested case-controls, one can calculate incidence rates for the exposed and unexposed cohort and build a ratio between them, the *incidence rate ratio*, or *relative rate* (see section "Cohort Studies" for further explanation).

In order to control for confounders in the analysis, two main strategies exist: stratification through cross-tabulation methods and regression modelling (see subsection "Control of Confounding" for more details). Among the regression models, logistic regression is commonly used for case-control designs because it is based on odds ratios.

Advantages

Case-control studies present a time- and cost-efficient way to examine a large number of risk factors. Relatively smaller sample sizes are needed to investigate associations in case-control studies than in cohort studies [4]. Case-control studies provide an optimal design to investigate rare diseases and diseases with long latency, since cases are enriched in the sample compared to the population the sample is drawn from. Moreover, they are useful to investigate disease outbreaks [4]. Nested case-control studies and case-cohort studies are well suited to conduct expensive and more elaborate analysis on a subset of a cohort, while benefiting from the prospective design of the cohort (especially the lack of recall bias and the sampling of cases and controls from the same population) [19].

Disadvantages

Selection of cases and controls is a major challenge in case-control studies [17]. Clear diagnostic criteria must be provided to define cases. Controls should be drawn from the same population as cases, as they should have an equal risk of becoming a case. It is also crucial to select cases and controls independently of their exposure history in order to prevent selection bias. Furthermore, if a disease affects survival, those cases that already have died cannot be included in the study [15]. Exclusion of such cases might lead to a serious imbalance in the exposure status of cases and controls.

Case-control studies are not suited to study rare exposures since, even in a very large sample, none of the cases or controls might have experienced the exposure [17].

As exposure histories are obtained retrospectively in the case-control design (from self-questionnaires, chart records, registries, etc.), incorrect or incomplete information can lead to serious bias (*recall bias*; see section "Bias" for further explanation).

Example from the literature

In 1950, when the harmful effects of tobacco smoking were not yet widely known, Doll and Hill published a case-control study on smoking habits in carcinoma patients [21]. They interviewed 2,475 inpatients from 20 hospitals in London, out of which 709 were diagnosed with lung cancer, 709 had non-malignant diseases and served as controls, and the remaining ones had malignant disease other than lung cancer. Subjects were matched according to sex, age, hospital, and the time point of interview. While the majority of subjects had been smokers for at least some time of their lives, the proportion of smokers among patients with lung carcinoma (99.7%) was significantly higher than the proportion of smokers in the control group (95.8%). Moreover, the most recent amount of cigarettes and the total amount ever smoked were positively associated with lung cancer.

This case-control study was the first large study that established an association between smoking and lung cancer. It was followed by the British male doctors study, a large cohort study by Doll and Hill, which, during its 50 years of follow-up, gave valuable insights into mortality in relation to smoking [22].

Cohort Studies

Cohort studies are to epidemiologists what the RCT is to the biostatisticians. They sample subjects based on exposure status and follow them up to an outcome. The term *cohort* originates from the military, where it stands for a group of warriors marching forward in time. Typically, exposed and non-exposed subjects are followed in two parallel groups. Depending on the time of data acquisition, cohort studies can be *prospective* or *retrospective* (Figure 16.3) [23]. Prospective cohort studies examine past and present exposures in a disease-free sample and follow subjects up in pre-defined intervals until the main endpoint occurs or the subject becomes censored (due to study end, loss to follow-up, or death). Retrospective, or historical, cohort studies use existing data (e.g., from past medical records or cohorts that have been studied for other reasons). While often both the exposures and outcomes lie in the past, the chronology of having documented an exposure that is later followed by an outcome is maintained.

Statistical Analysis

Disease risk and rates are primary statistical measures in a cohort study. We will exemplify the calculation of these parameters in a fictive cohort study that examines the effect of air pollution on the development of asthma in children. Children who live in an urban environment and are exposed to particulate matter <10 μm, which reaches the respiratory tract, were considered exposed. Children from an urban environment without exposure to particulate matter <10 μm were considered unexposed and served as controls. The diagnosis of asthma was a primary outcome; 4,003 subjects

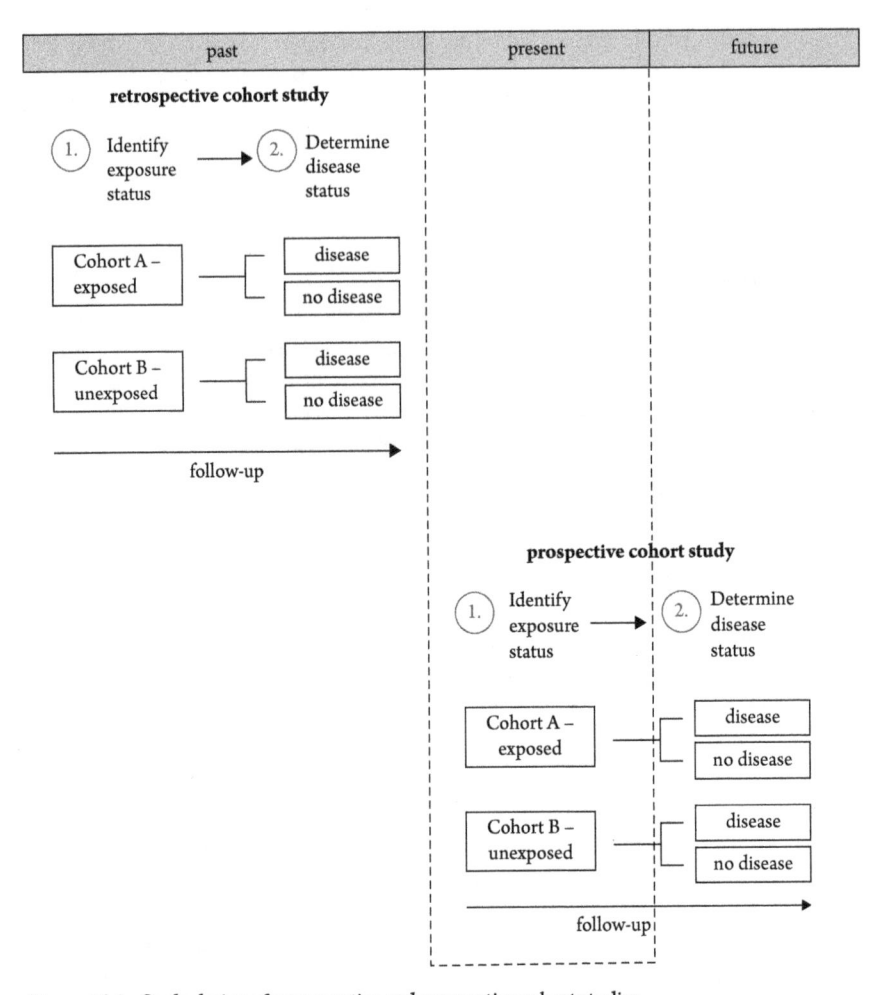

Figure 16.3. Study design of retrospective and prospective cohort studies.

participated in the study and were followed up over five years. For simplicity, we consider person-time in the study as 4,003 x 5 = 20,015.

	D+	D−
E+ = exposed cohort	36	1967
E− = unexposed cohort	28	1972

If the sample is representative of a general population in an urban environment, we can calculate the *incidence* of asthma. Incidence represents the number of individuals newly diagnosed with the outcome within a given time period in a population at risk.

It can be expressed as a proportion or a rate. Incidence as a proportion is called *risk* and can be calculated as follows [15]:

$$Risk = \frac{\text{Number of new cases in a population at risk within a given time period}}{\text{Number of disease-free individuals in the same population at the beginning of the time period}}$$

Since all individuals in a cohort study are free of the outcome at the beginning of the study, those individuals who develop the disease throughout the study will be equivalent to "new cases." Risk must be described in the context of time of follow-up (e.g., 5-year risk). Risk can be calculated from the 2 × 2 table:

Risk among exposed subjects: $\frac{a}{(a+b)}$

Risk among unexposed subjects: $\frac{c}{(c+d)}$

In our example, five-year risk for asthma among children exposed to particulate matter is $36/(36 + 1967) = 0.018 = 1.8\%$. Five-year risk for asthma among non-exposed children is $28/(28 + 1972) = 0.014 = 1.4\%$.

Other than risk, *incidence rate* includes the duration, how long an individual is "at risk" for a disease within the study period. This can largely vary among subjects, depending on the time point of entry into the study, dropout, or occurrence of the outcome (after which a subject is not any more "at risk"). In order to express incidence rate in person-years, we multiply the number of participating subjects by the length of follow-up period (= population at risk during study period). A multiplier is included in the calculation to adjust the result to an easily comprehensible population size (e.g., 100,000 individuals). Hence, the definition of incidence is the following [3]:

$$\text{Incidence rate} = \frac{\text{number of new cases in a time period}}{\text{population at risk for the disease in the same time period} \times \text{multiplier}}$$

In the example of the asthma study, the incidence rate for asthma in children that are exposed to particles <10 μm is $36/20{,}015 \times 10{,}000 = 18$ per 10,000 person-years. The incidence rate for asthma in unexposed children is $28/20{,}015 \times 10{,}000 = 14$ per 10,000 person-years.

In order to measure strength of association, we can calculate the odds ratio of disease from cohort studies, which is analogous to the calculation of odds ratio in cross-sectional studies. However, be aware that outcomes are incident in cohort studies while they are prevalent in cross-sectional studies.

The most important parameter to measure associations in cohort studies is *relative risk (RR)*, or *risk ratio*. It can only be derived from this study type because it is based on incident outcomes. RR is the risk of an exposed individual to develop a disease, relative to the risk of an unexposed individual to acquire the same disease [15]:

$$RR = \frac{\text{risk for disease among exposed subjects}}{\text{risk for disease among unexposed subjects}}$$

Box 16.2 Confidence Intervals

Confidence intervals are a measure of *how precise the estimate of a population parameter is* (sampling distribution). Precision is a measure of exactness. If a sample is repeatedly measured with high precision, the true population mean can be found within a narrow confidence interval at a pre-specified significance level. A 95% confidence interval would contain the true value with 95% probability. Conversely, the true value would lie outside of a 95% confidence interval with a probability of 5%. Confidence levels of 90%–99% are commonly chosen, depending on the degree of imprecision that researchers are willing to accept.

The 95% confidence interval can be calculated by

Sample estimate $\pm 1.96 \times$ SE (sample estimate),

in which SE represents standard error [15].

Confidence interval width is influenced by sample size, dispersion and confidence level [57]. A large sample size increases precision and, therefore, the confidence interval becomes narrower. High standard deviation or standard error results in a wider confidence interval. And, by definition, a 99% confidence interval is wider than a 95% confidence interval.

Statistical significance can be inferred from confidence intervals [57,58]. If the value that represents the null hypothesis lies within the confidence interval (e.g., "0" in case of a mean difference, or "1" in case of odds ratio or relative risk), the null hypothesis is true and the result is considered statistically not significant. If the entire confidence interval lies above this value, in the example of a cohort study, it could be concluded that exposure to a certain factor leads to a higher risk to develop a disease (or to a lower risk if the entire confidence interval lies below this value). Thus, the direction of an effect can be determined, which may also be meaningful in case of a statistically not significant result.

While *p*-value allows conclusions on the statistical significance within a sample, confidence intervals provides an estimation of the true mean value within the entire population of which the sample has been taken [58]. In conclusion, confidence intervals enable us to assess the clinical relevance of study outcomes.

It can be derived from the 2 x 2 table as RR = $(a/(a+b))/(c/(c+d))$.

If an exposure does not present any risk for developing the outcome, RR equals 1. An RR >1 translates into an increased risk that is associated with an exposure, while an RR<1 implies a protective effect that is associated with the exposure. RR should always be interpreted in connection with confidence intervals in order to determine statistical and clinical relevance (see Box 16.2).

In the asthma study example, relative risk is $0.018/0.014 = 1.285$. This means that children exposed to particulate matter <10 μm have 1.3 times the risk of developing asthma compared to non-exposed children.

To learn about the relation between relative risk and odds ratio, see Box 16.3.

A third way to measure associations in cohort studies is based on incidence rates. The *incidence rate ratio (IRR)* sets the incidence rate of the exposed cohort into relation with the incidence rate of the unexposed cohort [14]:

$$IRR = \frac{\text{incidence rate}_{exposed\ group}}{\text{incidence rate}_{unexposed\ group}}$$

Box 16.3 Odds Ratio or Relative Risk?

Odds ratio can be derived from both prevalent and incident data and can provide a useful measure of association in cross-sectional, case-control, and cohort studies. In contrast, relative risk is based on incidence and can only be determined from cohort studies. Relative risk is a more intuitive measure of association than odds ratio. If, hypothetically, the probability to develop a disease outcome is 0.2 in a population, it is easy to grasp that, statistically, every fifth subject randomly sampled from this population will develop the disease. At the same time, this would mean that the odds to develop the disease, 1/5, relative to the odds not to develop the disease, 4/5, equals 1/4, or 0.25. This number is much harder to understand. The same scenario will occur when we build ratios between probabilities (RR) versus ratios between odds (OR). OR is sometimes incorrectly interpreted as RR, resulting in wrong conclusions that are drawn from study results [25].

In some cases, odds ratio will approximate relative risk. If a disease occurs with low probability, which reflects in low numbers for a and c, the denominators of OR and RR will almost be similar: RR = (a/a+b)/(c/c+d) ≈ OR = (a/b)/(c/d) [26]. However, if a disease is more common, the denominator of OR will become smaller than the denominator of relative risk, with the consequence that OR will overestimate the relative risk. This problem is likely to occur when the event probability of a disease outcome is larger than 10% [25].

In the asthma study example, IRR is 18/14 = 1.285.

Risk difference = risk for disease$_{exposed\ group}$ − risk for disease$_{unexposed\ group}$

Rate difference = incidence rate$_{exposed\ group}$ − incidence rate$_{unexposed\ group}$

When we attempt to describe the results of a cohort study, we can interpret relative risk as "times the risk" and incidence rate ratio as "times the rate." A more intuitive and sometimes more meaningful way of expressing the same findings is the excess risk that is associated with the exposure. It is an absolute measure and can be calculated as *risk difference* or *rate difference* by subtracting the risk or incidence rate in the unexposed group from the risk or incidence rate in the exposed group, respectively [15]:

Risk difference in the asthma study is 0.018 − 0.014 = 0.004 = 4/1000. This means that children exposed to particulate matter <10 μm had 4 additional cases of asthma per 1,000 children during the five-year observation period compared to unexposed children. Rate difference is 18 per 10,000 person-years − 14 per 10,000 person-years = 4 per 10,000 person-years. Hence, children exposed to particulate matter <10 μm had 4 additional cases of asthma per 10,000 person-years compared to unexposed children.

Advantages

A major advantage of cohort studies is that the temporal sequence between an exposure and the development of a disease can be directly observed [24]. It can be useful to characterize the natural history of a disease. Furthermore, temporality is the best way to infer causality from an association, as long as investigators efficiently control for bias and confounding variables. Measuring exposures before the outcome occurs has the benefit of reducing information bias. The particular strength of prospective cohort studies is that well-matched cohorts can be assembled, which reduces selection bias. Instead, retrospective cohort studies are usually more time- and resource-efficient. In both designs, multiple outcomes can be studied simultaneously [15].

Disadvantages

Among the observational study designs, cohort studies are the most expensive. Depending on the research question, study duration usually lasts several years, in exceptional cases even decades (see the following Example from the literature). In order to handle large cohorts, an enormous effort of personnel resources and logistics, as well as monetary expenditure, can be required. Loss to follow-up is an important issue in cohort studies, especially if it occurs unequally among cohorts (see the section "Bias"). Furthermore, exposure status of a subject can change while the study is running [24], for example, when a worker with an occupational exposure leaves his working environment. Cohort studies are not useful for studying rare outcomes, since the subjects enrolled in the study may never experience the outcome [13].

Example from the literature

The Framingham study was the first long-term cohort study and, until today, is the largest of its kind. It started in 1948 with a cohort of 5,209 residents of the town Framingham in Massachussetts, United States, and was designed to study the pathomechanisms of heart disease. The Framingham study continued with the offspring in 1971 and the third generation in 2002, and has included more than 14,000 participants since its initiation [27].

One of its major contributions to the field of cardiovascular diseases has been the finding that chronic atrial fibrillation is associated with an increased risk for stroke [28]. A total of 5,184 subjects at the age of 30–62 years and without a prior history of stroke were followed up over 24 years by biennial routine examinations and additional neurological evaluation in the case of suspected stroke. The incidence rate of stroke in subjects with chronic atrial fibrillation was 41.48/1,000 person-years and showed to be 5.6-fold higher than in subjects without atrial fibrillation after adjustment for age, sex, and hypertension. Importantly, stroke outcomes positively correlated with duration of atrial fibrillation, with a median duration of 39.5 months prior to stroke. The authors concluded that treatment with anticoagulants might reduce the incidence of stroke in patients with atrial fibrillation, which has become standard care since the 1990s.

BIAS AND CONFOUNDING

As we have learned in previous chapters in this book, association can be attributed to four different factors: chance, bias, confounding, and cause. If an association between a risk factor and a disease is found in an observational study, investigators will primarily be interested in identifying the extent of causal relationship. For this reason, they will investigate to which extent chance, bias, and/or confounding have skewed the results.

Bias

Bias is a systematic error that leads to an over- or underestimation of the true association between an exposure and an outcome. It can present a serious threat to the internal validity of a study. Importantly, it is independent of sample size [29]. Two main types of bias are relevant in observational studies: selection bias and information bias.

Selection Bias

Selection of subjects for observational studies can be very difficult, as randomization is not feasible. Selection bias is present when selected subjects differ in relevant characteristics among study groups, and these factors have an influence on the associations that are investigated. Case-control studies are especially prone to selection bias, because they require careful considerations regarding which population (and based on which criteria controls) should be selected in order to resemble cases as much as possible [15].

Several types of selection bias can be distinguished:

Attrition bias arises when subjects lost to follow-up substantially differ in certain baseline characteristics from those subjects who remain in the study. Although initial subject selection may have been unbiased, missing observation is the critical point that leads to imbalances among groups in this type of bias. This can especially occur in cohort studies that require long-term follow-up, but is not an issue in cross-sectional studies [30].

Admission-rate bias (or Berkson bias) is present when hospital admission rates differ between the case and control groups. Admission-rate bias becomes relevant when the sample population is recruited from hospitalized patients. Some patients may be more likely admitted for a disease when they had a certain exposure, for example when they are carrying medical devices, which can be better handled by a specialist. If these patients are compared to a control group recruited from the same hospital, a relationship between exposure and disease may show in the measurements where none exists [31,32].

If a study sample is recruited from volunteers, *volunteer bias* is likely to occur, as volunteers tend to be healthier and less exposed to risk factors. Similarly, one should be aware of *non-respondent bias*, for example in surveys from households, where non-responders often have different demographic characteristics than responders [31,33].

If a disease leads to death or recovery within a short time, this may result in *survivor bias*. Incidence and prevalence may differ significantly for such diseases. For example, cases of an aortic aneurysm rupture may not be representative of the occurrence of the disease, as many patients die quickly. This type of bias is also called *incidence-prevalence bias*, or *Neyman bias* [29,34].

Publication bias is a systematic error that occurs when publication is directly related to the direction and significance of the results. In other words, publication bias is present when some results (mostly positive ones) are more likely to get published than others (mostly negative results). The origin of this type of bias has essentially been a lack of consensus of what should be published. It is introduced by investigators, editors, and even by funding sources, and its extent is difficult to assess [35].

Information Bias

Data collection is another process during epidemiological research where bias can occur. Information bias arises if data on exposures or outcomes are acquired in a systematically different manner from study groups. It may be introduced by the subject who provides information to the interviewer, by the interviewer him- or herself, or by the instruments used to measure or diagnose exposures and diseases, respectively. Knowledge of exposure or disease status increases the likelihood that information bias is present [15].

In the following, we will describe different types of information bias:

Recall bias (or reporting bias) is important to consider in case-control studies where disease status is known and data on exposures are acquired retrospectively. The problem here is that cases are more likely to remember exposures. For example, women with breast cancer may be more attentive to their personal history of contraceptives use, substance use, menstruation, or family history than women without breast cancer. This may lead to an overestimation of certain risk factors for breast cancer [36].

Interviewer bias can occur when an investigator who obtains data on exposures is aware of a subject's disease status. An interviewer may be more careful in reviewing personal history, may pay attention to even rare exposures, and may explain questions differently if a patient is suffering from cancer. Similarly, determination of the disease status may be influenced by knowledge of the exposure status in a prospective cohort study [29].

Lead-time bias becomes relevant when a disease is diagnosed in two different stages. Suppose a formerly asymptomatic patient suddenly dies from hypertrophic cardiomyopathy. In a screening, another family member is diagnosed with hypertrophic cardiomyopathy in an asymptomatic stage and thereafter receives treatment. He dies five years later from congestive heart failure. One may perceive this as a clue that treatment is beneficial. An alternative explanation could be that the patient was diagnosed five years before clinical presentation of the disease (this interval would be the lead time) and the treatment had no real effect on the course of the disease [29].

Misdiagnosis of cases or controls can produce serious *misclassification bias*, if it affects case and control groups unequally. If a control is mistaken as a case, the association between exposure and disease may be overestimated, and vice versa [4].

Performance bias occurs when subjects receive different care or treatment apart from the treatment under investigation. This may be the case in an observational study that compares two surgical procedures when operating surgeons have different levels of skills to perform these procedures [37]. Another example may be different levels of additional intensive care treatment in a multi-center study.

Detection bias is caused by uneven diagnostic procedures between study groups. If exposure counts as a diagnostic criterion for a disease, its presence will lead to the initiation of certain diagnostic procedures and, subsequently, a higher likelihood to discover the disease (*diagnostic suspicion bias*) [31,38]. In a case-control study, the exposure status of cases will therefore be biased by selection. Similarly, exposure can lead to a symptom that will direct the diagnostic process toward detection of a disease. This type of bias is called *unmasking (signal detection) bias* [31,38].

Assessment and Control of Bias

The fundamental basis to any assessment of bias is a thorough report of how a study was conducted. With this information at hand, magnitude and direction of bias can be determined based on judgment. A number of assessment tools have been proposed for observational studies, in the form of scales and checklists [39]. One challenge in observational studies is their diversity and different susceptibility to bias in different study designs. Generally, a suitable tool to assess bias should cover all relevant domains of bias. Use of scales is not advisable because resulting scores usually represent arbitrary numbers that do not allow any conclusions about the real impact of different types of bias. To provide an example, the Cochrane Collaboration's tool for assessing risk of bias analyzes six domains: selection bias (in this case: allocation to study groups), performance bias, detection bias, attrition bias, reporting bias, and any other type of bias [39]. Authors are required to provide detailed information on how subjects were allocated to study groups, whether and how participants and researchers were blinded, how outcomes were assessed, how attrition within study groups has been, and how outcomes were reported. Additionally, the estimated direction and magnitude of bias should be described for each domain. Suggested terms for magnitude of bias are "low risk" (no bias identified, or bias that is unlikely to seriously affect results), "high risk" (results may be seriously altered), or "unclear risk" (bias that raises some doubt about the internal validity of results). Although it was originally developed for systematic reviews of randomized trials, the general structure of the tool can be similarly useful for observational studies [40].

Control of bias is not an easy task, as bias is in many cases difficult to assess. It is most important to anticipate potential bias and account for it while designing a study because it cannot be corrected in the analysis [11].

We will further discuss how to control certain types of bias:

Control of selection bias is an important issue in observational studies because randomization is not possible. Investigators should carefully choose a representative sample of the target population, as a means to minimize selection bias. Based on a clearly defined study question, they need to define inclusion and exclusion criteria and decide how to obtain a sample that best represents the target population. This is especially challenging in case-control studies because both the exposure and the disease have already occurred at the time of inclusion in the study and *controls* need to be drawn from the *same population as cases*. This means that they should be at risk to develop the outcome and resemble cases in potential confounding variables [11,17]. Cases can be recruited in the hospital setting or from a defined population (e.g., a registry). A *hospital-based sample* may be preferred as patients can be more easily recruited, particularly those with rare diseases who attend specialty clinics. Controls can be recruited from the same hospital so that they are ideally derived from the same subpopulation that is commonly referred to this particular hospital. Also, they might resemble cases in their willingness to participate and ability to remember relevant aspects of their own history [15]. However, bias can potentially be induced by hospital-based controls, if the disease they are admitted for is associated with the exposure under investigation [4,15].

If cases are drawn from a registry, *population-based controls* should be chosen. These ideally represent the general population, if the registry is comprehensive. If doubt exists about how appropriate controls are, more than one control group can be defined [4].

In prospective cohort studies, special attention needs to be paid to subjects' adherence and all possible measures should be taken to minimize loss to follow-up (see Chapter 7).

An attempt to reduce publication bias has been made by the International Council of Medical Journal Editors that, since September 2004, requires *registration* of any new clinical trial in a publicly accessible registry in order to be considered later for publication [41]. Furthermore, publishers and journal editors have increasingly become aware that the reporting of negative results needs to be stimulated and have started to open negative results sections, and even have created new journals that focus on negative trial results [42,43].

Two fundamental principles should be followed in order to minimize information bias. First, data collection instruments should be as precise and objective as possible; and second, the administration of these instruments (e.g. by interviewers, examining physicians, or radiologists) should be consequently blinded. Both principles serve the goal of leaving as little room for judgment as possible [11].

Interviewer bias can be controlled by both *consequent blinding* and use of standardized interviews [29]. If the interviewer is a blinded rater who is not informed about the disease status, he or she will more likely interview cases and controls in a uniform way, and will not be more thorough with case subjects. Interviewers should receive extensive training before they first start to evaluate subjects, so that inter-rater reliability can be ensured [4].

In order to control for recall bias, *standardized questionnaires* or protocols with specifically phrased, closed-ended, and preferably objective questions should be used. Medical records or existing databases may be useful to gather more objective data. Nevertheless, one should be aware that prior documentation itself might be incomplete or misleading. Subjects should be blinded and can be kept unaware of the exact study hypothesis, if feasible and ethically acceptable [11]. In order to conceal risk factors under investigation, "dummy" risk factors can be included in questionnaires [4]. Another way to control recall bias is to include controls who suffer from a disease that is different from the disease under investigation in cases. Compared to healthy controls, such control subjects will be more likely to remember any relevant exposure [29].

Strict criteria for diagnoses and exposures should be used in order to avoid misclassification. Clinical diagnoses should be complemented by standard *diagnostic tests*, including laboratory tests, imaging, electrophysiological tests, and, if appropriate, even invasive diagnostics. Use of multiple sources (e.g., records from both hospitals and primary care physicians) can help to verify diagnoses or exposure to risk factors [11].

Performance bias can be minimized by stratification of subjects by country, center, or surgeon in a surgical study [37].

Confounding

Confounding leads to the assumption that a risk factor is correlated with an outcome, while the actual effect is influenced by a third, independent factor. A confounder is both related to exposure and a risk factor for the outcome [15,44]. For example, in a study that investigates the risk of coffee consumption for myocardial infarction, smoking is a confounder, as smoking is positively correlated with coffee drinking and is a known risk factor for myocardial infarction [4]. If a confounder is positively correlated with the exposure and the outcome, this may lead to an overestimation of the studied association. If it is negatively correlated to either the exposure or the outcome, this may lead to an underestimation. Note that a confounder is also predictive of the outcome in unexposed subjects. However, since it is related to exposure, it is more likely to be present in the exposure group and thereby introduces bias [44].

Despite its relationship with the exposure and outcome, a confounder does not lie on the causal pathway between them. Instead, a variable that positively or negatively regulates existing associations in subgroups of a population, and is therefore causally linked to the outcome, is called an *effect modifier* [4]. This results in different magnitudes of effects among subgroups. For example, hypercholesterolemia is a link between diet and coronary artery disease and in part explains how a wrong diet can lead to increased risk for coronary artery disease. Therefore, hypercholesterolemia is in this case not a confounder but an effect modifier. The different relationships of confounders and effect modifiers to exposure and outcome variables are visualized in Figure 16.4.

One special type of confounding is called *confounding by indication*. It reflects the fact that certain treatments (e.g., a surgical procedure or escalation treatment with a medication that is very potent but may cause serious side effects) will more likely be indicated in a carefully pre-selected subgroup (e.g., patients with a more severe disease course). Outcomes, such as increased mortality, may be mistakenly attributed to treatment, although they are in reality causally linked to disease severity [4,38]. One example is a prospective cohort study that assessed the risk of cardiovascular disease in patients with rheumatoid arthritis exposed to glucocorticoids [45]. While it seemed that glucocorticoids were associated with a higher incidence of cardiovascular disease, this finding could not be confirmed after adjusting for disease activity and severity. Rather, use of glucocorticoids was associated with higher disease activity, which by its own seemed to be associated with higher risk for cardiovascular disease.

Confounders need to be anticipated in any observational study in order to allow proper data interpretation. This is especially important in extreme cases of confounding, such as Simpson's paradox (see Box 16.4), in which the true direction of the association becomes reversed. P-values alone are not suited to identify

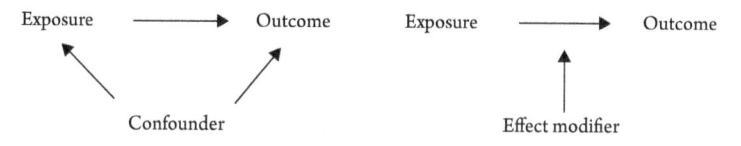

Figure 16.4. Relationship of confounders and effect modifiers to exposures and outcomes.

Box 16.4 Simpson's Paradox

Simpson's paradox is a special situation in which the association between two variables changes its direction due to the presence of a predictor [50]. This may occur if the size of treatment arms is largely unbalanced with respect to this predictor. Simpson's paradox has been exemplified by Baker and Kramer using hypothetical data [51]: In a clinical trial that compares treatment A and B, treatment A results in better survival than treatment B in both men (60% vs. 50%) and women (95% vs. 85%; see Figure 16.5). However, when data for women and men are aggregated into one dataset, treatment A seems to be associated with worse survival than treatment B (72% vs. 80%). This happens because two conditions are true: (1) women survive better than men in both treatment groups, and (2) a higher fraction of women than men is subjected to treatment B.

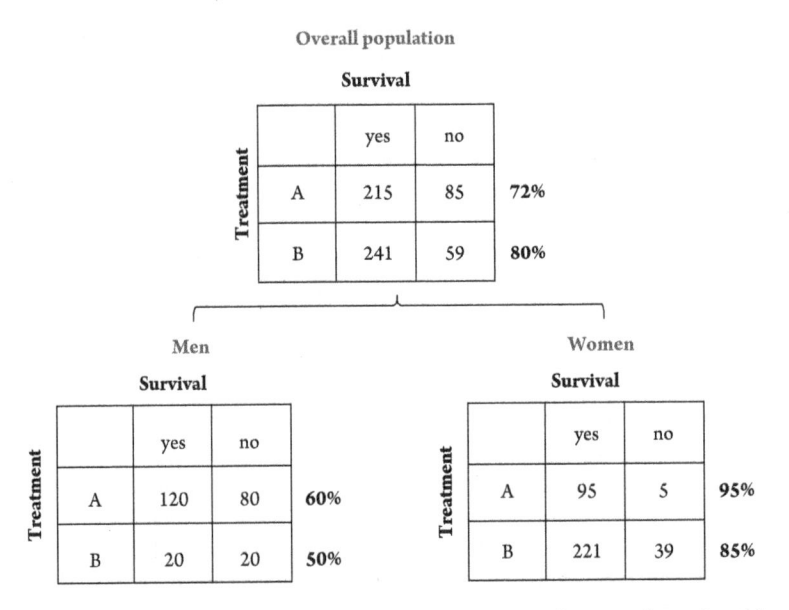

Overall population

Treatment	Survival		
	yes	no	
A	215	85	72%
B	241	59	80%

Men

Treatment	Survival		
	yes	no	
A	120	80	60%
B	20	20	50%

Women

Treatment	Survival		
	yes	no	
A	95	5	95%
B	221	39	85%

Figure 16.5. Contingency tables exemplifying Simpson's paradox using hypothetical data from [51].

There is no statistic criterion that is able to guide the decision whether conclusions drawn from the overall analysis versus conclusions from stratified data are the correct ones. Instead, only the understanding of causal interactions between variables will help to determine clinical meaning from data [52].

confounders because effect sizes may be minor, although they are statistically significant, and not necessarily clinically meaningful [15].

Control of Confounding

Confounding can be adjusted in the phases of study design (restriction, matching) and data analysis (stratification, statistical modelling) [29,46]. To complete the picture, randomization would be an additional way to control confounding; nevertheless, it is not applicable in observational studies. Potential confounders should be identified beforehand and measured rigorously.

Restriction

Inclusion criteria can be restricted to exclude the confounding variable from the study population [4,46]. For example, if tobacco use is expected to be a confounder, all smokers will be excluded. This consequently reduces generalizability with respect to the subpopulation in which the confounder is present. Additionally, it may become difficult to recruit subjects, if the excluded confounder is highly prevalent in the study population (e.g., smoking in patients with psychiatric diseases).

Matching

Matching is a sampling strategy that is most commonly used in case-control studies [4]. It assures that potential confounding variables are equally distributed among study groups. Cases and controls are sampled in a way that they have similar values of potential confounders. For example, if age and sex are considered confounding variables, one will include a 60-year-old female control subject when a 60-year-old female case subject has been recruited. Matching is commonly done for constitutional factors, such as age and gender. Especially when matching is done for too many variables, it can be an expensive process in terms of costs and effort, and may even lead to an exclusion of cases if no corresponding control can be found [4]. It is important to *avoid overmatching*, which occurs when controls and cases become too similar with respect to exposure [15]. It arises when (1) the variable used for matching is in reality part of the causal pathway between exposure and disease, and (2) the variable is associated with exposure (but not linked to the disease). Overmatching leads to a reduced power to detect statistically relevant differences [4].

Stratification

Stratification involves the separate analysis of data according to different levels of a variable, which represent homogenous categories called *strata* [15]. Strata can be built for both dichotomous (e.g., smoking) and continuous (e.g., age) variables. In the latter case, strata size should be selected as to what is considered clinically meaningful, while keeping levels of the confounding variable homogenous so that data within the stratum can be considered unconfounded. Stratified variables and strata per variable are generally limited to a low number; otherwise, there is danger that some strata may remain empty or contain extremely sparse data, and a much larger sample size will be required to prevent this.

Other than in regression-based methods, statistical analysis of stratified data is not based on any hypothetical model of the nature of association and is therefore less dependent on assumptions [47]. Estimates can be calculated separately for each stratum, and these stratum-specific estimates may be pooled to obtain an adjusted estimate that is weighted by strata size. This is commonly achieved by using *Mantel-Haenszel odds ratios* or *risk ratios*. Information on the strength of confounding can be derived by comparing crude and adjusted estimates; if the difference is large, substantial confounding by the stratified variable is present, and adjusted estimates better reflect the true association [15].

Statistical Modeling

Regression analysis uses a hypothetical model to estimate the relationship between an outcome and several explanatory variables, one of which is the exposure. A main advantage is that this procedure can be used to control for many variables simultaneously. For example, in a study that investigates the risk of hyperlipidemia for myocardial infarction, a multiple logistic regression model may be employed to adjust for age, sex, tobacco use, hypertension, diabetes, and family history of cardiovascular events. Similarly, a Cox's proportional hazards model could be used to adjust for the all these factors when investigating time-to-event ("survival") [15].

In regression analysis, one can take advantage of the full information provided by continuous variables in the analysis, while categorizing into strata usually reduces its content [48]. Importantly, control of confounding by regression modeling strongly depends on how well the model reflects the reality. If the model is based on incorrect assumptions, confounding will remain, at least as a residuum [14,45]. Additionally, results from regression modeling cannot be intuitively understood because complex relationships are condensed to few numbers, and therefore the choices made during regression modeling should be well explained in any publication.

Propensity scores are used to estimate the probability of receiving treatment for each subject based on covariates, and to balance treatment groups to obtain less biased estimates [46,48,49]. Matching, stratification, weighting, or regression modeling can all be implemented in propensity score models. Additionally, confounding by indication can be addressed by this method. (More detailed information on propensity scores is provided in Chapter 17.)

SAMPLE SIZE DETERMINATION IN OBSERVATIONAL STUDIES

Sample size determination is used in observational studies to estimate the required population size for a valid inference. Associations between exposure (risk factors) and outcomes may be missed due to a lack of power if the study sample is too small. On the other hand, while there is no threat of exposing subjects to unnecessary risks in observational studies, overestimation of sample size may still result in a waste of valuable resources.

As we have learned in Chapter 11, the required parameters for sample size determination are (1) significance level (α); (2) desired power ($1 - \beta$); (3) measure of variation of the outcome variable (σ); (4) anticipated treatment/exposure effect. In terms of these basic principles, observational studies are essentially not different from RCTs. However, since randomization is not feasible in observational studies, one cannot exclude the presence of confounders. Therefore, sample size determination is rather *estimation* in these types of studies.

If an important confounder is anticipated and will be investigated in the statistical analysis, it should as well be included in the sample size estimation [4]. This can be achieved by multivariate methods, such as linear and logistic regression. *Adjustment for confounders* usually results in considerably larger sample sizes, which depends, among other factors, on the prevalence of the confounder and the strengths of association between exposure or outcome with the confounder [4,53,54].

Another issue in sample size estimation is loss to follow-up of subjects during the study. Its extent should be estimated a priori and incorporated into the sample size calculation [55].

If required, sample size can be minimized by using continuous rather than dichotomous variables, using paired measurements, choosing more precise variables or employing unequal group sizes [4,56].

Sample size calculation for observational studies can be achieved with two main approaches: either it is based on power (when the analysis will be based on statistical testing) or on precision (when the analysis will be based on confidence intervals) [15].

To calculate *sample size for means based on power*, the following formula can be used [56,59]:

$$n = \frac{(Z_\beta + Z_{\alpha/2})^2 \sigma^2}{(\mu_2 - \mu_1)^2},$$

where n is sample size, Z_β is the Z statistic for the desired power, $Z_{\alpha/2}$ is the Z statistic for the desired significance level, σ is the assumed standard deviation, and μ1 and μ2 are the two estimated means.

Sample size for proportions based on power can be derived using the formula [55,59]:

$$n = \frac{(Z_\beta + Z_{\alpha/2})^2 \left[p_1(1-p_1) + p_2(1-p_2)\right]}{(p_2 - p_1)^2},$$

where n is sample size, Z_β is the Z statistic for the desired power, $Z_{\alpha/2}$ is the Z statistic for the desired significance level, and p_1 and p_2 are the two estimated proportions.

To calculate *sample size for means based on precision*, the following formula can be used [56,60]:

$$n = \frac{Z^2_{\alpha/2} \sigma^2}{d^2},$$

where n is sample size, $Z_{\alpha/2}$ is the Z value for the corresponding significance level (Z = 1.96 for the commonly used significance level of 0.05), σ is the assumed standard deviation, and d is precision (i.e., total width of the confidence interval).

Sample size for proportions based on precision can be calculated with the following formula [56,60]:

$$n = \frac{Z^2_{\alpha/2} \, p(1-p)}{d^2},$$

where n is sample size, $Z_{a/2}$ is the Z value for the corresponding significance level (Z = 1.96 for the commonly used significance level of 0.05), p is the estimated population proportion, and d is precision (i.e., total width of the confidence interval).

Special Considerations for Sample Size Determination in Different Study Designs

Descriptive studies analyze characteristics in a single group (i.e., in case reports, case series, and surveys) based on precision [4]. For sample size calculation, researchers need to specify (1) the assumed standard deviation of the variable of interest (for continuous variables) or expected proportions of this variable in the population (for dichotomous variables), (2) desired precision, and (3) confidence level.

Cross-sectional studies compare characteristics between two study groups at a single time point, and therefore sample size estimation should be based on power. The parameters p_1 and p_2 represent the estimated prevalence of the outcome of interest in the two study populations [60].

Case-control studies retrospectively compare a disease and a control group regarding their exposure to risk factors. Sample size estimation should be based on power, and parameters p_1 and p_2 represent the odds of exposure, that is, the estimated proportion of exposed subjects among controls and the proportions of exposed subjects among cases [15,60]. Cases and controls are usually selected in a 1:1 ratio; however, when costs for selecting cases are especially high or cases are extremely rare, the control-to-case ratio can be changed to up to 4:1 [14]. In this case, a correction term must be implemented into the sample size calculation.

Cohort studies prospectively investigate a disease outcome in two groups of unexposed and exposed subjects. Sample size estimation should be based on power, and parameters p_1 and p_2 represent the risk of developing an outcome either of the groups [60]. Cohort studies typically require larger sample sizes than case-control studies due to the low rate of outcome in a population (compared to the prevalence of exposure).

OBSERVATIONAL STUDIES IN SURGERY

Surgical research is a topic that deserves a special place in clinical research because of the particular considerations that have to be made. To date, surgical research is mainly conducted using observational studies, such as retrospective case-control studies or prospective registry-based cohort studies. RCTs are difficult to perform for several reasons [61–64]: (1) randomization is often not feasible as patients prefer a certain procedure; (2) it may be difficult to recruit a sufficient number of patients, especially for rare conditions; (3) surgeries are difficult to standardize as procedures tend to be modified and refined with time, and skill levels vary among performing surgeons; (4) blinding of surgeons, nurses, and patients is very difficult; (5) surgical intervention itself is typically complex and cannot be evaluated separately from pre- and postoperative medical care, anesthesia, or rehabilitation [64].

The use of placebo in surgical research is a matter of controversy. Opponents of sham surgery criticize that sham surgery cannot be compared to placebos in medication trials because, unlike a placebo pill, sham surgery may cause serious harm to subjects due to surgery-related complications, use of antibiotics, wound-healing issues, and the need for general anesthesia in case of some procedures [65]. They argue that the principle of minimizing harm for subjects in clinical studies would be violated. Other researchers proclaim that it may even be unethical and a "double standard" not to perform a rigorous RCT to answer important clinical questions in surgery, as long as equipoise principle is met and informed consent is carefully obtained [66,67]. Sham surgery would make blinding of patients possible and therefore abolish one important source of bias. However, these authors stress that the decision to choose sham surgery as a control condition should be made individually for any study. Evaluation of scientific value, methodological rationale for sham control, risk-benefit assessment, informed consent, and the consequences of not performing a sham-controlled trial are suggested criteria to guide this decision [66].

Where Does Surgical Research Begin?

In contrast to drug research, surgery is not subject to FDA regulations, and new surgical procedures can be performed without prior approval [62,68]. While surgical techniques are constantly modified and improved by operating surgeons, innovation is further promoted by special clinical problems encountered during surgery and the development of new instruments. Furthermore, the reduction of complication rates is a perpetual goal, which, for example, leads to the development of minimally invasive techniques. In practice, a new surgical procedure is introduced by a single or few innovators, usually very skilled surgeons, and slowly spreads by the training of other surgeons within the same and other clinics to eventually become adopted by the community [68].

The right timing of scientific assessment in a clinical study is difficult to determine: a too early timepoint, when surgeons are at the beginning of the learning curve and the procedure is still refined, might introduce bias. Conversely, it may become too late to introduce a study based on the equipoise principle once surgeons and patients have accepted a procedure. An expert group of methodologists and clinicians, the IDEAL network, has recently developed a framework to describe stages of surgical innovation and has provided recommendations for clinical research in surgery [64,68,69]. They propose a stepwise use of different study designs related to the stage of innovation, which range from (1) reporting any new procedure in a register available to all surgeons to (2) retrospective and prospective observational designs at the stages of development and evaluation and (3) RCTs at the stage of assessment where the procedure has been refined and dispersed to a larger network of performing surgeons, and (4) registries for long-term surveillance.

Interpreting Data from Surgical Studies

In interpreting data from surgical studies, several issues need to be given special consideration:

1. Selection of subjects: Subjects with certain comorbidities may not be eligible to get surgery. Also, patients in late disease stages may be precluded from surgical intervention because of the elevated peri-operative risks. This may lead to indication bias [37,62]. It can later become difficult to distinguish whether better outcome in

patients assigned to the new treatment group was causally linked to the procedure itself or to an initially better prognosis of this study group.
2. Blinding is difficult to achieve in surgical studies, and loss of blinding may result in significant bias. Apart from the non-blinded operating surgeon and assisting staff, study investigators and patients may guess group allocation due to the location or dimension of the scar, different postoperative care, or clues from diagnostics, such as radiographs [70]. Certainly, it should be a general rule to blind as many individuals as possible: definitely the statisticians, and possibly the outcome raters, any staff providing patient care that do not need to know treatment allocation (the anesthesiology team, ward nurses, physiotherapists, pharmacists, etc.), and the patient. For example, scars can be concealed and, more creatively, radiographs can be digitally altered, as long as this does not preclude proper assessment of the outcome [71]. Finally, bias can be reduced by choosing "hard" outcome measures, such as death or recurrence of a disease [62].
3. Skills of the performing surgeons can influence outcomes and introduce performance bias, if they are unbalanced in the study groups [37]. This can even occur if the same surgeon performs both surgical interventions in a study that compares two surgical techniques, as the surgeon may be more used to performing one of the procedures. This problem can be addressed, for example, by allocating study groups by surgeons [37,61]. If only highly specialized surgeons perform a procedure within a study, resulting data may not be generalizable. One solution to this issue can be a multi-center study in which surgeons of different skill levels perform the intervention [64].

When Does a New Surgical Procedure Become Accepted?

Adoption of a new surgical technique is not necessarily a rational process, as scientific evidence usually comes into play after a certain dispersion of the procedure has already occurred. Some critical factors for adoption are (1) the effort a surgeon has to undertake to learn and perform the procedure, (2) patients' demands, (3) promotion of new technologies by manufacturers, and (4) perceived benefit over alternative treatment options [71]. More than any other intervention, a surgical procedure needs to be feasible. If only a few highly trained surgeons in the world can do it, it will most likely not become common practice. Furthermore, the opinion of leading surgeons may facilitate or constrain the widespread implementation of a surgical procedure [69]. Yet, even widely accepted procedures have been rapidly abandoned in the past after randomized control trials have shown no benefit [71], (see the following Example from the literature).

Example from the literature

The Carotid Occlusion Surgery Study (COSS), an open-label RCT conducted from 2002 to 2010, was designed to investigate whether patients with atherosclerotic internal carotid artery occlusion and hemodynamic cerebral ischemia benefit from extracranial-intracranial (EC-IC) bypass surgery with regard to subsequent to ipsilateral ischemic stroke [72]. The procedure had previously been performed for about 20 years and small case series had been published on potentially beneficial effects. A second interim analysis of the COSS study analyzed completed outcomes of 194 participants (out of an estimated sampe size of 372 patients) for futility. The primary end point was "the combination of (1) all stroke and death from surgery through 30 days after surgery and (2) ipsilateral ischemic stroke within 2 years of randomization" [72]. The two-year rates of reoccurrence of ipsilateral stroke were 21.0% for the surgical group and 22.7% for the non-surgical group. The confidence interval for the detected difference of 1.7% included the null hypothesis (95% CI, −10.4% to 13.8%). Within 30 days after surgery, 14.4% subjects in the surgical group and 2.0% subjects in the control group had an ipsilateral ischemic stroke, which made a difference of 12.4% between groups (95% CI, 4.9% to 19.9%). The trial was prematurely terminated in 2010 based on these results. The decision was further explained by the authors in the discussion of the original publication: "The DSMB considered redesigning the trial to detect a smaller absolute difference of 10% in favor of surgery. This would have required increasing the overall sample size from 372 to 986 to achieve 80% power. The DSMB recommended stopping the trial, citing that (1) the prespecified statistical boundary for declaring futility had been crossed using the design effect size and, (2) given the unexpected relatively low rate of observed primary end points in the nonsurgical group, a clinically meaningful difference in favor of surgery would not be detectable without a substantial increase in sample size, which was not feasible" [73].

CASE STUDY: OBSERVATIONAL STUDY—PURSUING A BETTER UNDERSTANDING OF PSYCHOTIC DISORDERS

André Brunoni and Felipe Fregni

Stockholm—Sao Paulo

Professor Mauro Tufo was glad. Dr. Fernando Martins was excited. Dr. Frida Abba was apprehensive.[1]

The three of them would meet in a couple of days. Everything started 15 years ago when Professor Tufo did his postdoctoral fellowship in the Department of Public Health at the University of Stockholm in Sweden just after finishing his PhD in Clinical Epidemiology at the University of Sao Paulo in Brazil. At that time, he was already a brilliant psychiatrist with a solid foundation in social psychiatry, interested in continuing his studies in the Swedish Cohort of Mental Health. When he moved back to Brazil, he carried with him the dream of making a similar study in his home country. Many years passed, and finally after settling down with all the necessary support, he was able to establish the Sao Paulo Mental Health Cohort (SP-MH) five years ago. Since then, Prof. Tufo has published several excellent papers and has earned the respect of the local and international community in the field of psychiatry.

Six months back, he felt that a cycle was complete when he received an email from his former mentor, Bjørn Andersson: "Hi, Mauro. Great to meet you in California last week. I have been thinking and believe that I have the perfect postdoctoral fellow to help us in Brazil. My best student is Frida, whom you met in the conference. She was delighted with the perspective of doing her postdoc with you in Brazil. She is really brilliant. Initially I was reluctant to let her go but I finally agreed when I realized she would certainly learn a lot with you and this would strengthen our relationship. Let me know your thoughts. Best, Bjørn."

After extensive email exchanges, Mauro Tufo, Frida Abba, and Bjørn Andersson decided that Dr. Abba would spend two years with Prof. Tufo in the SP-MH cohort. The summer was nearly ending. Dr. Abba would arrive in two days. Prof. Tufo asked his doctorate student, Dr. Fernando Martins, to meet her at the airport and help her out in the first few weeks in Sao Paulo. Fernando delightfully agreed to receive Frida at the airport.

Frida arrived tired after a 24-hour journey, flying from Stockholm to Sao Paulo with a flight connection in Barcelona. The time zone difference was six hours. She was frightened, too—"Two years abroad! What can I expect? Should I have stayed in Stockholm? Should I have done my postdoc in Europe, or the United States? Well, let's try not to think about this now. Prof. Tufo said a student of his would meet me here in the airport."

---

[1] Dr. Brunoni and Professor Fregni prepared this case. Course cases are developed solely as the basis for class discussion. Although cases might be based on past episodes, the situation in this case is fictional. Cases are not intended to serve as endorsements or sources of primary data. All rights reserved to the author of this case. Reproduction and distribution without permission is not allowed.

It was not difficult for Fernando to find Frida. After a brief introduction, they connected well and both realized that the project could gain momentum extraordinarily quickly with a sense of excitement in the air. The challenge of working in a real observational study is the dream of an epidemiologist, and Frida was not an exception to this rule.

Observational Studies

Observational studies offer a worthwhile alternative for clinical researchers when ethical or feasibility issues preclude the performance of a randomized placebo-controlled clinical trial. It is a robust design that can provide reliable results if carefully planned and executed. Although there are key issues with observational studies, such as lack of blinding and poor control for unmeasured confounding, results from well-designed observational studies might be similar to placebo-controlled clinical trials. A recent review published in the *New England Journal of Medicine*, in which authors searched for meta-analyses of randomized controlled trials and meta-analyses of either cohort or case-control studies published in five leading medical journals, showed that well-designed observational studies do not overestimate the magnitude of the effects of treatment when compared to results of randomized controlled trials on the same topic.[2]

Finally, well-designed observational studies can provide data on long-term drug effectiveness and safety. The main types of observational studies are (1) prevalence survey or cross-sectional study; (2) case-control study; and (3) cohort study, which can be either prospective or retrospective.

Cohort Studies

It was 2:30 p.m. when Frida arrived at the University Hospital. Prof. Tufo was tremendously relieved to see her. She said, "I had to get a taxi! I tried to get the subway but I could not find the yellow line that goes under Avenida Reboucas." Fernando smiled and said, "That's because the yellow line does not exist yet. Did you not see in your map that the line is dashed? That means it is under construction." Everyone laughed and started working on the Sao Paulo cohort study.

Frida Abba was genuinely impressed with the Sao Paulo Mental Cohort Study. They were doing state-of-the-art research in psychiatry. For example, in one ancillary study—the PSYCHOSP (Psychosis in Sao Paulo)—they had been following all patients at risk of developing psychosis since 2005. The patients had neuroimaging studies and blood tests repeated every year, as well as complete neuropsychological batteries and follow-up with mental health professionals. As previously decided, Frida would work on the PSYCHOSP project.

"As I told you before, Dr. Abba," Prof. Tufo said, " PSYCHOSP is our main project. We have already 2,150 patients being followed up. Our cohort has completed five years

---

[2] Concato J, Shah N, Horwitz RI. Randomized, controlled trials, observational studies, and the hierarchy of research designs. *N Engl J Med.* 2000 Jun 22; 342(25): 1887–1892.

now and we are starting to see the initial results." After a short pause, he concluded, "Well, as you know this is the main caveat of cohort studies—they are very costly and they demand a long time for follow-up. In this case, we are interested in observing the natural history of psychosis. What is the prevalence in our population? What is the one-year incidence in our city? And naturally, we have the fundamental question in psychiatry, a question unresolved since the first studies of Kurt Schneider: how many patients go on to develop schizophrenia? Therefore, the main goal of PSYCHOSP is to increase our understanding of psychotic disorders."

"Yes, Prof. Tufo, that is the main advantage of a cohort study," Frida said, "We start observing patients free of the disease—in this case, we are observing patients with a high risk of developing psychosis. I imagine you use the common risk factors, such as familial history of schizophrenia, cannabis use, social withdrawal—is that right?" As he agreed, she continued, "So, after that, we start the follow-up of these patients... and we wait. It can take 5, 10, or even 15 years until the data can tell us anything." "That is right, Dr. Abba. And the data are already talking—we have almost one thousand cases now, and we are comparing these cases with those patients who have not developed the disease. So, that is the main strength: we can infer causality—i.e., that the risk factors developed before the disease—thereby we can distinguish cause from effects."

"Indeed, Prof. Tufo, the level of clinical evidence of cohort studies is particularly strong and even comparable to, if not better than, randomized clinical trials. Some studies have shown that, for the same disease, cohort studies and randomized trials provide the same results—but overall the confidence interval observed in cohort studies is narrower, meaning that the results are more precise. But then, tell me—how do you handle the dropouts? Because the studies are time-consuming, follow-up is a serious issue in almost all cohort studies. Another question is about subject selection—how is it done? That is a potential source of bias in this type of study. For instance, you are following subjects at high risk of developing psychosis. How can you be sure that these subjects do not have the disease at time zero? This would be a serious bias. But, do not get me wrong, I think cohort studies are one of the best types of observational studies; however, they are expensive and have their limitations. This is the reason why I think we should consider other options." Frida and Prof. Tufo kept talking and sharing ideas until evening. Prof. Tufo then invited Frida and Fernando for a dinner in a charming Thai restaurant nearby. As a competent psychiatrist—and also an experienced observer—Prof. Tufo could observe some sparks between his two students. Both were young, smart, and charismatic—but they also had some narcissistic traits, outbursts of irritation, and some passive-aggressive behaviors. At least they could enjoy a pleasant evening without talking about epidemiology.

Cross-sectional versus Case-Control Studies

A few weeks later, Frida presented her study plan in a lecture—a cross-sectional study based on the PSYCHOSP project. She started her lecture with confidence, "My idea is to do a cross-sectional study to determine the prevalence of psychotic disorders in our PSYCHOSP sample. As you know, a cross-sectional study is the best way to determine prevalence. Besides being relatively quick, we can also study multiple outcomes—for instance, in our study we can determine the prevalence of several psychotic disorders simultaneously. In addition, we could extend the original score of PSYCHOSP to make sure we truly have a population-based survey and therefore we would avoid the issue of case selection as we usually see with convenience samples."

"I am sorry to interrupt you, Dr. Abba," Fernando said, "But I personally don't like cross-sectional studies. This type of study does not allow us to differentiate between cause and effects or the sequence of events. It is just like taking a snapshot—we freeze a specific moment of time and infer causality. Although it is quick, it does not have the beauty like other types of observational studies—don't you think, Frida?"

She quickly replied, "Well Dr. Martins, beauty is in the eye of the beholder. But talking about study designs, I do agree that cross-sectional studies have significant limitations. On the other hand, they can show us something new and provide evidence for further studies. I want to suggest something new here. As you know, I work with neuroimaging. And talking with Prof. Tufo, we thought that it would be interesting to assess the neuroimaging studies in this sample and then try to correlate our findings with the diseases. And then, if we find something interesting, we can do very beautiful studies with the results in hand, Dr. Martins!"

He smiled and continued the emotional argument with her, "Naturally the idea of doing beautiful studies is worthwhile. But again—I think your design is missing the point. How would you know if the changes in the brain scans were not a cause, but a consequence of the disease? It seems to me a waste of time and energy in analyzing the neuroimaging of the entire sample to get stuck in an egg-chicken situation."

Prof. Tufo was restless and wanted to stop this endless debate. "OK, Fernando, so what is your point?"

He quickly replied, "I want to propose something new. Cohort study might take a long time and be too costly to produce results, plus the cross-sectional study is too superficial. I suggest running a case-control study. It is also simple to organize and relatively quick. We can compare the cases of our cohort with controls. A critical issue in this type of design (case-control) is to identify the proper controls. That is why we match the controls for age, gender, and several other variables. Then, this source of bias can be controlled. So, by selecting the right controls we can compare their brain scans with the cases. And we can also infer causality via calculation of an odds ratio."

"Wait!" Frida said—she was just waiting for a moment to shatter Fernando's ideas—"Are you saying odds ratio can infer causality? I do not agree with you, Fernando. Causality can only be inferred through cohort studies and relative risk. You criticized my design on the basis that it cannot differentiate cause and effects—but case-control studies are just slightly better on this topic. You should also not forget that choosing controls is a really difficult task! Also, there is the important problem of recall bias. When you ask someone if she or he was exposed to toxic fumes, it is much more likely that someone with lung cancer recalls this exposure as compared to a healthy subject. Therefore, I do not agree when you say 'this source of bias is controlled'—I think it is not quite like that."

Prof. Tufo intervened, trying to select the best words to calm down the situation, "OK, let me explain something here. This is a common confusion even for experienced researchers. Relative risk is the test used in cohort designs, while the similar test for case-control studies is the odds ratio. Relative risk—as the name says—is the possibility of developing a condition due to the exposure to a risk factor. It is a ratio, that is, the two probabilities are divided: the ratio of subjects with the disease exposed to the risk factor divided by the ratio of subjects with the disease not exposed to the risk factor. Therefore, the risk of developing the disease due to the exposure is determined. Odds ratio is different. First, odds are the opposite of probability. So, if the probability of developing a disease is 10%, then the odds of developing the disease are 1 to 9 and the odds of not developing the disease are 9 to 1. The odds ratio is, therefore, the ratio of the odds between two groups; for instance, let's take the classical example of lung cancer. Suppose that 100 patients with lung cancer are compared to 100 patients without lung cancer. Ninety patients who had lung cancer smoked, while only 10 patients without lung cancer smoked. So the odds of smoking in cancer patients are 90 to 10; while the odds smoking in non-cancer patients are 10 to 90. Dividing one by another, we have the odds ratio of 81—that is, the odds of being a smoker in lung cancer is 81 times as compared to subjects with no lung cancer—an extraordinarily strong association. But this can only be transposed to a risk ratio of developing cancer if the disease is rare (<1%). If it is not, then the association of the disease with the risk factor is overestimated—as probably other risk factors are also contributing to cause the disease—and then we need a cohort study."

Prof. Tufo realized that he had accomplished enough for that meeting and decided to end it. He returned to his office to check his emails. Bjørn, Frida's mentor in Stockholm, had just sent one, "Hello, Mauro! How are you? Any news from my student? I am concerned. She did not answer my last emails! Is there something wrong there? Best, Bjørn."

Prof. Tufo replied, "Hello, Bjørn! Everything is fine here. I think Frida is so involved in our projects that she does not have enough time to check her personal emails!" Prof. Tufo looked through the window to the room of postdoctoral students and saw the students interacting. He continued his email, "By the way, do you remember Dr. Fernando Martins? He is a brilliant student and I was thinking—perhaps he could continue his postdoc with you, Bjørn? Let me know your thoughts. Best, Mauro

CASE DISCUSSION

This case deals with a very interesting situation: we are introduced to an already running, long-term observational study and are asked to plan a new observational study on the same disease background in parallel. Let us take a closer look: On the one hand, we have Prof. Tufo's PSYCHOSP study, which has been running over the last five years. It has been designed to analyze the natural history of psychosis, determine risk factors, measure prevalence, and observe the development of schizophrenia as a consequence of psychosis. More than 2,000 patients have so far been followed up, while the study is still continuing.

On the other hand, Dr. Frida Abba, the new postdoc from Sweden, plans her own study. She has two ideas, which are (1) to determine prevalence in the PSYCHOSP or an extended, population-based sample, and (2) to compare neuroimaging in healthy and psychotic as well as diagnosed schizophrenic subjects. Her postdoc is, according to the current plan, limited to two years. Dr. Abba's task is now to choose the best design for her study.

First, she could do a cross-sectional study. The advantage is that prevalence can be well assessed in this study design. The time frame and expenses will depend on whether she uses the PSYCHOSP sample or a population-based sample. However, she will not be able to address causality between risk factors or neuroradiologic findings and psychosis. Misclassification bias is a major threat in this study design because psychotic symptoms are, among others, one hallmark of schizophrenia, and therefore a thorough diagnosis of schizophrenic patients is crucial.

Second, Dr. Abba could develop a case-control study. A major advantage is that the number of cases is enriched due to the study design and rare diseases can be studied well. As almost 1,000 cases have already been identified in the PSYCHOSP cohort, Dr. Abba could perform a case-control study within this cohort. Depending on her study question, she would have to decide between the designs of a nested case-control study or a case-cohort study. This would also require a thorough reflection on the sampling of controls. Misclassification of cases can lead to serious bias in this design. While she cannot study disease prevalence in a case-control study, she would deal with incident data from the cohort, which will allow her to address other interesting questions (e.g., how high the incident risk associated with an exposure is). Recall bias would be an important issue if Dr. Abba recruited a sample independently of the PSYCHOSP study. However, within the PSYCHOSP cohort, exposures have been identified at the beginning of the cohort study so that recall bias will not be a concern.

Third, Dr. Abba could directly use data from the PSYCHOSP cohort study or design her own cohort study. A cohort study is best suited to assess temporal association and thus causality. This might be of importance if Dr. Abba wanted to show a causal association between distinct neuroradiological findings and the development of psychotic disorders. However, cohort studies are generally very expensive. Moreover, psychotic disorders may take years to develop after exposure to a risk factor. Anyway, if Dr. Abba wanted to start her own cohort apart from the PSYCHOSP study, she would need convincing reasons to do so.

All in all, Dr. Abba's decision is largely dependent on her exact research question, a realistic time frame and cost estimation, and the potential limitations of the study design that she is willing to accept.

CASE QUESTIONS FOR REFLECTION

1. What are the main issues in this case for choosing the optimal study design?
2. What are their main concerns?
3. What should the group consider in making the decision?

FURTHER READING

Books

dos Santos Silva I. *Cancer epidemiology: principles and methods*. Lyon: International Agency for Research on Cancer; 1999.

Hulley SB, et al.,*Designing clinical research*, 4th ed. Philadelphia: Lippincott Williams & Wilkins; 2013.

Journal Articles

Beral V, et al. Ovarian cancer and hormone replacement therapy in the Million Women Study. *Lancet (London, England)*. 2007; 369(9574): 1703–1710.

Danforth KN, et al. A prospective study of postmenopausal hormone use and ovarian cancer risk. *Br J Cancer*. 2007; 96(1): 151–156. Available at: http://www.ncbi.nlm.nih.gov/pubmed/17179984\nhttp://www.nature.com/bjc/journal/v96/n1/pdf/6603527a.pdf.

Freemantle N, et al. 2013. Making inferences on treatment effects from real world data: propensity scores, confounding by indication, and other perils for the unwary in observational research. *BMJ*. 2013; 347: f6409. doi:10.1136/bmj.f6409

Higgins JPT, et al. The Cochrane Collaboration's tool for assessing risk of bias in randomised trials. *BMJ (Clinical research ed.)*. 2011; 343: d5928. doi:10.1136/bmj.d5928

van der Woude FJ, et al. Analgesics use and ESRD in younger age: a case-control study. *BMC Nephrology*. 2007; 8: 15.

Odds Ratio and Relative Risk

Katz K. The (relative) risks of using odds ratios. *Arch Dermatol*. 2006; 142(6): 761–764.

Bias

Delgado-Rodriguez M, Llorca J. Bias. *J Epidemiol Comm Health*. 2004; 58(8): 635–41.

Confounding

McNamee R. Confounding and confounders. *Occup Environ Med*. 2003; 60(3): 227–234.

Simpson's Paradox

Bickel PJ, Hammel EA, O'Connell JW. Sex bias in graduate admissions: data from Berkeley. *Science (New York, N.Y.)*. 1975; 187(4175): 398–404.

Surgical Research

McCulloch P, et al. No surgical innovation without evaluation: the IDEAL recommendations. *Lancet*. 2009; 374(9695): 1105–12.

REFERENCES

1. Last J. *A dictionary of epidemiology*, 4th ed. New York: Oxford University Press; 2000.
2. von Elm E, et al. The strengthening the reporting of observational studies in epidemiology (STROBE) statement: guidelines for reporting observational studies. *J Clin Epidemiol*. 2008; 61(4): 344–349.
3. Friis RH, Sellers T. *Epidemiology for public health practice*, 5th ed. Burlington, MA: Jones & Bartlett; 2013.
4. Hulley SB, et al. *Designing clinical research*, 4th ed. Philadelphia: Lippincott Williams & Wilkins; 2013.
5. Szklo M, Nieto J. *Epidemiology: beyond the basics*, 3rd ed. Burlington, MA: Jones & Bartlett; 2012.
6. Rao A, Ramam M. The case for case reports. *Indian Dermatol Online J*. 2014; 5(4): 413–415.
7. Vandenbroucke JP. In defense of case reports. *Ann Intern Med*. 2001; 134(4): 330–4.

8. Carey TS, Boden SD. A critical guide to case series reports. *Spine.* 2003; 28(15): 1631–1634.
9. Maida V, et al. Symptoms associated with malignant wounds: a prospective case series. *J Pain Symptom Manage.* 2009; 37(2), pp.206–11.
10. Rao A, Ramam M. The case for case reports. *Indian Dermatol Online J* [serial online] 2014; 5: 413–415.
11. Buring JE. *Epidemiology in medicine,* Vol. 515, 1st ed. Philadephia: Lippincott Williams & Wilkins; 1987.
12. Hymes K, et al. Kaposi's sarcoma in homosexual men: a report of eight cases. *Lancet,* 1981; 2(8247): 598–600.
13. Mann C. Observational research methods. Research design II: cohort, cross sectional, and case-control studies. *Emerg Med J.* 2003; 20(1): 54–60.
14. Zocchetti C, Consonni D, Bertazzi PA. Relationship between prevalence rate ratios and odds ratios in cross-sectional studies. *Int J Epidemiol.* 2997; 26(1): 220–223.
15. dos Santos Silva I. *Cancer epidemiology: principles and methods.* Lyon: International Agency for Research on Cancer; 1999.
16. Weintraub D, et al. Impulse control disorders in Parkinson disease: a cross-sectional study of 3090 patients. *Arch Neurol.* 2010; 67(5): 589–595.
17. Schulz KF, Grimes DA. Case-control studies: research in reverse. *Lancet.* 2002; 359(9304): 431–434.
18. Vandenbroucke JP, Pearce N. Case-control studies: Basic concepts. *Int J Epidemiol.* 2012; 41(5): 1480–1489.
19. Szklo M, Nieto J. *Epidemiology: beyond the basics,* 3rd ed. Burlington, MA: Jones & Bartlett; 2012.
20. Rodrigues L, Kirkwood BR. Case-control designs in the study of common diseases: updates on the demise of the rare disease assumption and the choice of sampling scheme for controls. *Int J Epidemiol.* 1990; 19(1): 205–213.
21. Doll R, Hill AB. Smoking and carcinoma of the lung: preliminary report. *Bull WHO.* 1999; 77(1): 84–93.
22. Doll R, et al. Mortality in relation to smoking: 50 years' observations on male British doctors. *BMJ (Clinical Research Ed.).* 2004; 328(7455): 1519.
23. Grimes DA, Schulz KF. Cohort studies: marching towards outcomes. *Lancet,* 2002; 359(9303): 341–345.
24. Grimes DA, Schulz KF. Bias and causal associations in observational research. *Lancet.* 2002; 359(9302): 248–252.
25. Katz K. The (relative) risks of using odds ratios. *Archives Dermatol.* 2006; 142(6): 761–764.
26. Schmidt CO, Kohlmann T. When to use the odds ratio or the relative risk? *Int J Public Health,* 2008; 53(3): 165–167.
27. Mahmood SS, et al. The Framingham Heart Study and the epidemiology of cardiovascular disease: a historical perspective. *Lancet,* 2014; 383(9921): 999–1008. Available at: http://dx.doi.org/10.1016/S0140-6736(13)61752-3.
28. Wolf PA, et al. Epidemiologic assessment of chronic atrial fibrillation and risk of stroke: the Framingham study. *Neurology.* 1978; 28(10): 973–977.
29. Tripepi G, et al. Bias in clinical research. *Kidney Int.* 2008; 73(2): 148–153.
30. Krishnan E, et al. Attrition bias in rheumatoid arthritis databanks: a case study of 6346 patients in 11 databanks and 65,649 administrations of the Health Assessment Questionnaire. *J Rheumatol.* 2004; 31(7): 1320–1326.

31. Sackett DL. Bias in analytic research. *J Chronic Dis.* 1979; 32(1–2): 51–63.
32. Berkson J. Limitations of the application of fourfold table analysis to hospital data. *Int J Epidemiol.* 2014; 43(2): 511–515.
33. Criqui MH, Barrett-Connor E, Austin M. Differences between respondents and non-respondents in a population-based cardiovascular disease study. *Am J Epidemiol.* 1978; 108(5): 367–372.
34. Neyman J. Statistics: servant of all sciences. *Science (New York, N.Y.).* 1955; 122(3166): 401–406.
35. Dickersin K. The existence of publication bias and risk factors for its occurrence. *JAMA.* 1990; 263(10): 1385–1389.
36. Skegg DCG. Potential for bias in case-control studies of oral contraceptives and breast cancer. *Am J Epidemiol.* 1988; 127(2): 205–212.
37. Paradis C. Bias in surgical research. *Annals Surgery.* 2008; 248(2): 180–188.
38. Delgado-Rodriguez M, Llorca J. Bias. *J Epidemiol Comm Health.* 2004; 58(8); 635–641.
39. Higgins J, et al. Chapter 8: Assessing risk of bias in included studies. In: Higgins J, Green S, eds. *Cochrane handbook for systematic reviews of interventions.* 2011. The Cochrane Collaboration. Available at: www.handbook.cochrane.org
40. Reeves B, et al. Chapter 13: Including non-randomized studies. In: Higgins J, Green S, eds. *Cochrane handbook for systematic reviews of interventions.* 2011. The Cochrane Collaboration. Available at: www.handbook.cochrane.org.
41. Abaid LN, Grimes DA, Schulz KF. Reducing publication bias through trial registration. *Obstet Gynecol.* 2007; 109(6): 1434–1437.
42. Dirnagl U, Lauritzen M. Fighting publication bias: introducing the Negative Results section. *J Cereb Blood Flow Metab.* 2010; 30(7): 1263–1264.
43. Goodchild van Hilten L. Why it's time to publish research "failures." 2015. Available at: https://www.elsevier.com/connect/scientists-we-want-your-negative-results-too [Accessed September 10, 2016].
44. McNamee R. Regression modelling and other methods to control confounding. *Occup Environ Med.* 2005; 62(7): 500–506
45. Sijl AM Van, et al. Confounding by indication probably distorts the relationship between steroid use and cardiovascular disease in rheumatoid arthritis: results from a prospective cohort study. *PLoS One.* 2014; 9(1): e87965. doi:10.1371/journal.pone.0087965.
46. Jepsen P, et al. Interpretation of observational studies. *Heart.* 2004; 90(8): 956–960.
47. McNamee R. Confounding and confounders. *Occup Environ Med.* 2003; 60(3): 227–234.
48. Freeman TB, et al. Use of placebo surgery in controlled trials of a cellular-based therapy for Parkinson's disease. *N Engl J Med.* 1999; 341(13): 988–991.
49. Okoli GN, Sanders RD, Myles P. Demystifying propensity scores. *Br J Anaesth.* 2014; 112(1): 13–15.
50. Simpson EH. The interpretation of interaction in contigency tables. *J Roy Stat Soc. Series B (Methodological).* 1951; 13(2): 238–241.
51. Baker SG, Kramer BS. Good for women, good for men, bad for people: Simpson's paradox and the importance of sex-specific analysis in observational studies. *J Womens Health Gend Based Med.* 2001; 10(9): 867–872.
52. Pearl J. Simpson's paradox, confounding and collapsibility. In *Causality.* Cambridge: Cambridge University Press; pp. 269–274, 2009.
53. Drescher K, Timm J, Jöckel KH. The design of case-control studies: the effect of confounding on sample size requirements. *Stat Med.* 1990; 9(7): 765–766.

54. Lui, K-J. Sample size determination for case-control studies: the influence of the joint distribution of exposure and confounder. *Stat Med.* 1990; 9(12): 1485–1493.
55. Whitley E, Ball J. Statistics review 4: sample size calculations. *Critical Care (London).* 2002; 6(4): 335–341.
56. Eng J. Sample size estimation: how many individuals should be studied? *Radiology.* 2003; 227(2): 309–313.
57. du Prel J-B, et al. Confidence interval or p-value?: part 4 of a series on evaluation of scientific publications. *Deutsches Ärzteblatt Int.* 2009; 106(19): 335–339.
58. Akobeng AK. Confidence intervals and p-values in clinical decision making. *Acta Paediatrica.* 2008; 97(8): 1004–1007.
59. Chow S-C. Sample size calculations for clinical trials. *Wiley Interdisc Rev: Comp Stat.* 2011; 3(5): 414–427.
60. Hajian-Tilaki K. Sample size estimation in epidemiologic studies. *Caspian J Int Med.* 2011; 2(4): 289–298.
61. Lilford R, et al. Trials in surgery. *Br J Surgery.* 2004; 91(1): 6–16.
62. McLeod RS. Issues in surgical randomized controlled trials. *World J Surgery.* 1999; 23(12): 1210–1214.
63. Cook JA. The challenges faced in the design, conduct and analysis of surgical randomised controlled trials. *Trials.* 2009; 10: 9. doi:10.1186/1745–6215-10-9.
64. Ergina PL, et al. Challenges in evaluating surgical innovation. *Lancet.* 2009; 374(9695): 1097–1104.
65. Macklin R. The ethical problems with sham surgery in clinical research. *N Engl J Med.* 1998; 341(13): 992–996.
66. Miller FG. Sham surgery. *Surgery.* 2003; 3(4): 41–48.
67. Freeman TB, et al. Use of placebo surgery in controlled trials of a cellular-based therapy for Parkinson's disease. *N Engl J Med.* 1999 Sep 23; 341(13): 988–992.
68. Barkun JS, et al. Evaluation and stages of surgical innovations. *Lancet.* 2009; 374(9695): 1089–1096.
69. McCulloch P, et al. No surgical innovation without evaluation: the IDEAL recommendations. *Lancet.* 2009; 374(9695): 1105–1112.
70. Demange MK, Fregni F. Limits to clinical trials in surgical areas. *Clinics (Sao Paulo).* 2011; 66(1): 159–161.
71. Karanicolas PJ, Farrokhyar F, Bhandari M. Blinding: who, what, when, why, how? *Can J Surgery.* 2010; 53(5): 345–348.
72. Wilson CB. Adoption of new surgical technology. *BMJ (Clinical Research Ed.).* 2006; 332(7533): 112–114.
73. Powers WJ, et al. Extracranial-intracranial bypass surgery for stroke prevention in hemodynamic cerebral ischemia: the Carotid Occlusion Surgery Study randomized trial. *JAMA.* 2011; 306(18): 1983–1992.

17

CONFOUNDERS AND USING THE METHOD OF PROPENSITY SCORES

Author: *Chin Lin*

Case study authors: *Rui Imamura and Felipe Fregni*

It is the mark of an educated mind to rest satisfied with the degree of precision which the nature of the subject admits and not to seek exactness where only an approximation is possible.
—Aristotle

INTRODUCTION

In Unit III, you have been presented with several aspects of observational studies and their basic designs. Important concepts concerning bias and confounders, as well as methods to address them, were explored in Chapter 16.

One of the key aspects of an observational study is the fact that researchers have no control over treatment assignment [1, 2]. In practice, large differences on observed covariates may exist between treated and non-treated (control) groups. These differences can lead to biased estimates of treatment effects: a relationship effect could be established when actually there is none, or a true effect will remain hidden instead of being observed [2, 3]. In contrast, randomizing patients to treatment allocation, as is done in experimental studies, is a very efficient method to reduce bias and potential confounding by balancing groups with regard to known and unknown variables, and thus reduce their influence on the interpretation of results.

In order to decrease the influence of confounding variables, when planning an observational study it is highly recommended to list the potential characteristics of patients that may impact outcome, attempt to record them, and propose a method to control the bias resulting from them [3].

In this chapter, we will discuss one of the most robust methods to reduce the impact of bias generated by group imbalance, which therefore increases greatly the validity of observational studies: the propensity score.

DEFINITIONS

Propensity Score

In the historical article by Rosenbaum and Rubin [4], the authors provided this definition: "The propensity score is the conditional probability of assignment to a particular treatment given a vector of observed covariates" (p. 41). Intuitively, it works as a balancing score and measures the tendency of a subject being in the "treated" group (or more generally, in the group with exposure of interest) considering his or her observed background (pre-treatment) covariates. This score is frequently estimated by logistic regression where the treatment variable is the outcome and the covariates are the predictor variables in the model [5]. The propensity score tries to mimic some aspects of randomized trials by balancing patients' characteristics, and the distribution of baseline covariates between groups will be dependent on conditional probability.

Confounding and Confounder

Confounding (as a causal effect) is the distortion in the estimate attributed to a given factor in causing or contributing to the outcome [6]. Usually there is some confusion about the terms *confounder* and *covariate*. A covariate is a variable that is highly predictive of the outcome, and sometimes is referred to as a *patient variable* (i.e., baseline characteristics).

A *confounder* is a covariate that is related to both the exposure and the outcome, and either partially or completely accounts for the effect of the exposure on the outcome. Once controlled for, the relationship between exposure and outcome can either be diminished or disappear [6,7]. In the presence of a confounder, systematic error (bias) may be induced to measurement of the data and interpretation of the results.

To qualify as confounder, the variable must be a risk factor, the cause or surrogate of the disease; positively (overestimation) or negatively (underestimation) correlated with the exposure—if the population is divided by exposure (or not) to it, the prevalence in both groups is different; not an intermediate factor in the pathway between exposure and outcome; and not affected by the exposure [6,8].

Some epidemiologists consider confounding indistinctly as a type of systematic bias, but there is an important difference. In principle, it is possible to measure a confounder, and its effect can be eliminated by adjustment. By contrast, once any random or systematic bias is present in any study, its effect cannot be eliminated [9].

Bias

Bias is the systematic deviation (or error) of measurements or inferences/conclusions that are different from the truth. In a clinical study, bias may be introduced during: (1) conception and design of the study; (2) data handling, collection, analysis, interpretation, reporting, or review processes [10].

METHODS TO CONTROL FOR CONFOUNDERS

As discussed previously, confounders play an important role in the non-experimental studies, especially in those concerned with causality. Patients with certain characteristics tend to be related to certain exposures. The aim of an observational study is to examine the effects of the exposure, but sometimes the apparent effect of the exposure is actually the effect of another covariate that is associated with the exposure and with the outcome [11].

Several methods have been proposed as an attempt to control for the effects of patients' characteristics on treatment outcomes in observational studies. Basically, there are two principal ways to achieve this goal: prevention in the planning phase by *restriction* or *matching*; and statistical analysis adjustment in data handling by *stratification* or *multivariate regression modeling* [4].

Restriction

In this method, also known as specification, *the study population is restricted to those subjects with a specific value of the confounding variable*. We can perform the restriction by determining specific exclusion criteria for the study; thus the potential confounders are eliminated. A disadvantage of this method is that findings cannot be generalized to those subjects left out by the restriction.

Matching

The matching process *constrains subjects in different exposure groups to have the same value of potential confounders*. The samples are conditionally drawn from the populations ensuring that characteristics are similarly distributed across samples, based on the propensity scores. It is commonly used in case-control studies, but can also be used in cohort studies. With increasing number of matching variables, the identification of matched subjects becomes progressively demanding, and matching does not reduce confounding by factors other than the covariates used for the matching.

Stratification

Stratification is also known as *sub-classification*. The basic idea is *to divide study subjects—treated and non-treated—into a number of subgroups (or strata) within the covariate*, so that subjects within a stratum will share the same characteristics. Stratification is important because it provides a simple means to display data, to measure an unconfounded estimate of the effect of interest, and to examine the presence of effect modification.

Within each stratum, a simple comparative statistic is calculated, and the results for both groups are compared. If there are many potential covariates at one point, this method will not be practical, due to the overwhelming number of required strata, which may also impact the number of subjects within each stratum, as this method requires that the resultant strata must be large enough to yield conclusive results [7].

For both matching and stratification, there is an additional disadvantage when dealing with continuous variables, as these variables have to be recoded into categories, which may lead to the use of arbitrary criteria during the process.

Multivariate Regression Modeling

This method *uses the regression model* and usually *expresses the risk of the outcome as a function of the exposure (treatment) of interest and the effects of potential confounders*, especially when there is a large number of covariates.

Multivariate analysis enables the simultaneous adjustment/control of several variables to estimate each one's effect independently. Usually in this model, the patient's exposure (or type of treatment) is assessed as the independent variable of interest and patient's outcome is described as the dependent variable. Other variables can be included as prognostic factors and potential covariates. The effect of the exposure on the outcome is estimated, based on the similarity of the covariates between the exposed and reference patients. Frequently used methods are the Cox proportional hazard model (survival analysis), and the logistic and linear regression models [12].

An important disadvantage of these methods is the risk of extrapolation when too many covariates are included into the analysis. It may result in errors in the estimation of the effects of the treatment of interest. In the literature, a ratio of 10–15 subjects or event per independent variable in the model is desired [12].

METHOD OF PROPENSITY SCORES
Theoretical Background

There are two basic steps to perform a propensity score (PS) analysis. First, a model to predict the exposure is built (treatment model); then a model including propensity score information is constructed (outcome model) to evaluate the association between exposure and outcome [13]. From this model, a summary of each study subject's pre-treatment covariates is replaced by a single index. This "new covariate," or the expected probability, is the person's propensity score. In theory, it is expected that with increasing sample size the pre-treatment covariates are balanced between study subjects from the two exposure groups who have nearly identical PS [14].

Consider the formula

$$e(X) = \text{prob}(Z = 1/X)$$

where X is the observed pre-treatment covariates; Z is an indicator of treatment allocation (Z = 1, for treatment; Z = 0, for control). The X for one subject might entail several pretreatment covariates which describe that particular subject's characteristics. *The propensity score, e (X), will be the probability of a person with X covariates to be exposed to treatment (Z).*

In a simple randomized trial comparing two interventions, subjects are assigned to treatment or control, so $e(X) = \text{prob}(Z = 1/X) = 1/2$ for every X, which means that subjects will have the same chance of receiving the treatment, and the potential effects of baseline characteristic on the outcome are minimized due to the process of randomization.

But, in an observational study, some subjects are more likely than others to receive the treatment, so $e(X) \neq \frac{1}{2}$, and thus the X covariates patterns often help to predict which treatment a particular subject will receive.

By having this conditional probability, subjects in treatment and control groups with equal (or nearly equal) propensity scores will tend to have similar distributions in terms of the baseline characteristics (i.e., covariates). Therefore, these adjustments made using the propensity score aim to remove imbalance across baseline characteristics. The bias-removing adjustments can then be performed using the propensity scores, instead of adjusting for all the covariates individually [5].

Most Common Techniques to Adjust Using Propensity Scores

The propensity score complements model-based procedures and is not a substitute for them. Once the propensity score is computed, there are four different ways or techniques to adjust for the uncontrolled assignment of treatment: (1) as a matching variable, (2) as a stratification variable, (3) as a continuous variable in a regression model (covariance adjustment), and (4) as a coefficient for adjustment (weighting).

Matching

Matching is a technique used to select control subjects who are similar to the treated subjects. This similarity across groups is achieved by controlling several baseline characteristics that are thought to have an potential impact on the outcome. It is useful in situations when there is a limited number of patients in the treated group and a larger (often much larger) number of control patients [5].

It is often difficult to find subjects who are perfectly similar (i.e., that can be matched) on all important covariates, even if there are only a few background covariates of interest. Propensity score matching will then be a method that allows an investigator to control simultaneously for many background covariates by matching on a single scalar variable.

There are several matching techniques that can be performed. Mahalanobis metric matching [15] is a common one. It is performed by first randomly ordering the subjects, and then the distance between the first treated subject and all controls is calculated. The distance between a treated subject (i) and a control subject (j) is defined by the Mahalanobis distance: $d(i, j) = (u - v)^T C^{-1} (u - v)$ where (u) and (v) are matching variables values for treated (i) and control subjects (j), respectively, and C is the sample covariance matrix of the matching variables from the full set of control subjects. The control subject (j) with the minimum distance $d(i, j)$ is chosen as the match for treated subject (i), and both of them are removed from the pool. This process is repeated until matches are found for all treated subjects.

The major disadvantage of this technique is the difficulty of finding close matches when there are many covariates included in the model. As the number of covariates increases, the average distance between observations increases as well.

There are three techniques proposed by Rosenbaum and Rubin for constructing a matched sample using the propensity scores:

a) *Nearest variable matching on the estimated propensity score*

This method consists of first randomly ordering the subjects in the treated and non-treated groups. Then the first treated subject is matched to a subject with the closest propensity score from the non-treated group. After this, both subjects are removed from the pool, and the next patient from the treated group is selected.

b) *Mahalanobis metric matching including the propensity score*

This technique is performed exactly as described earlier for Mahalanobis metric matching, with an additional covariate—the logit of the estimated propensity score ($\^q(X)$) which is included in the covariates for the calculation of the Mahalanobis distance.

c) *Nearest available Mahalanobis metric matching within calipers defined by propensity score*

This method is a hybrid of the previous two techniques; first, subjects in the treated group are randomly ordered, and then a subset of potential non-treated subjects whose propensity scores are near to the ones on the treated group ("within calipers") is determined. The subject from the non-treated group is selected from this subset by using nearest available Mahalanobis metric matching. The caliper size is determined by the investigator, and the recommendation is to keep the size of the caliper to 1/4 of the standard deviation of the logit of the propensity score.

Rosenbaum and Rubin suggested that the nearest variable matching on the estimated propensity score is the easiest technique, and the nearest available Mahalanobis metric matching within calipers defined by propensity score is the best technique for producing the best balance between the covariates in the treated and control group [7].

Stratification

Stratification or subclassification consists of *ordering subjects into subgroups (strata) defined by certain background covariates. After the definition of the strata, treated and control subjects who are in the same stratum can be compared directly.*

According to Cochran [16], 90% of the bias can be removed by creating five strata. However, there is a natural problem related to subclassification [17], because the number of strata grows exponentially with increases in the number of covariates [18]. The propensity score is a scalar summary of all the observed background covariates; therefore, the stratification method can balance the distributions of the covariates in the treated and control groups without the undesirable increase in number of strata. Ideally, the perfect stratification based on the propensity score will produce strata where the average *treatment* assignment is an unbiased estimate of the truth treatment effect. Usually in order to perform this stratification, the propensity score is estimated by logistic regression for binary outcomes or discriminant analysis. The investigator then must determine the cut-off point for the boundaries for different strata, and also whether this will be based on the values of the propensity score for the combination between groups or in the treated group alone. A suggestion is to use the quintiles or deciles of the propensity score of treatment and control groups combined.

Regression (Covariance) Adjustment

The propensity score can also be used in regression (covariance) adjustment. Consider the formula for the treatment effect, τ, is estimated as $\tau = (Y_t - Y_c) - \beta (X_t - X_c)$.

The (t) indicates treatment group and (c) the control group. By subtracting out the second term on the right hand of the equation, the effects of the covariates are adjusted. The β coefficient is an estimate of the regression of the responses for the treated and control groups on the background covariates. By using this method for both the treated and the control group, it is possible to adjust the final estimate to reflect better the treatment effect.

Another possibility is to use a large set of covariates to estimate the propensity score, and then use a subset from the covariates in the regression adjustment. This method is also similar to performing Mahalanobis metric matching within calipers using a subset of the covariates including the propensity score.

Weight by the Inverse of Propensity Score

The inverse of the propensity score is used to weight each subject in the treated group, and one minus the inverse of the propensity score (that is, the propensity of not being in the treated group) in the controls. This way, weighing is a process that includes all the data, and does not depend on random sampling. It was shown that weighting based on the inverse of the propensity score produces unbiased estimates of the treatment effects [19].

Propensity Score Weights

There are several weighting methods that use the propensity score. We will present the weighting by odds to estimate the average treatment effect. Subjects in the treated group receive a weight of 1, and subjects in the untreated one receive a weight of pi (1/pi), where pi refers to an individual probability to receive the treatment (which is the individual propensity score).

The control subjects who are different from the treated group will have a pi near zero and a weight near zero, while the control subjects who are more similar to the treatment group will have a larger pi, and thus a larger weight.

The propensity score weights are then incorporated as weights into a standard outcome linear regression model, which has no covariates and only the treatment as a predictor of variable [20].

CASE STUDY: USING THE METHOD OF PROPENSITY SCORES: A TASK FORCE TO COMPARE APPLES AND ORANGES

Rui Imamura and Felipe Fregni

A Life-Threatening Experience

Professor Minoru has recently returned to work after a three-month medical leave to treat his prostate cancer. He underwent prostatectomy surgery that did not go well because he developed a local infection that progressed to septicemia. He was in the ICU (intensive care unit) for almost a month. Although he had a good recovery and now is able to go back to work, he was uncomfortable with the ICU management as he felt that procedures there did not follow evidence-based medicine. Professor Minoru has dedicated his entire life to offer treatments with the best evidence to his patients, and he was not comfortable with the treatment offered to him in the ICU.

Prof. Minoru is a calm and methodical physician—he is frequently described as a cold person. He makes decisions and takes action wholly on the basis of logic. Evidence-based medicine was therefore for him the foundation of medicine. Prof. Minoru is a well-known professor of internal medicine in Osaka, Japan. He leads a large team of physicians in the largest and busiest hospital in Osaka.

He decided to propose to the Japanese Ministry of Health the idea of a Task Force aiming to determine the value of medical procedures in ICU based on evidence-based medicine. His goal is to produce a document that could serve as recommendations for medical care in ICUs throughout Japan. In fact, the government was interested and helped gather first-class specialists from the entire country to join this Task Force.

Swan-Ganz Catheterization: Should We Be Using It?

For this task force, Prof. Minoru's first assignment was to determine the efficacy of right heart catheterization (RHC) to improve overall mortality rates in emergency care units. He decided then to recruit his colleague from medical school, Dr. Tanabe—who is one of the leading experts in this topic. Dr. Tanabe has the opposite personality of Prof. Minoru—he is extremely energetic, seemingly uncontrolled, a bit disorganized, and driven by his feelings.

Although Prof. Minoru was a bit concerned with his work ethic, Dr. Tanabe has published many studies in the field and is recognized worldwide for his expertise in this topic. He would be a great asset to the team. In addition, he has one of the largest databases of RHC in Asia.

RHC (also known as Swan-Ganz catheterization) is a common procedure in critically ill patients. The catheter is guided through the right chambers of the heart into the pulmonary artery, providing vital information about heart functioning and large vessels pressures. Most experts believe that when indicated correctly, it may help to better manage some critically ill patients. However, its use is not devoid of severe complications, such as major bleeding, pneumothorax, arrhythmia, and even rupture of pulmonary artery. So, the physician must balance the pros and cons of its use in each patient in order to decide whether or not to use it.

Prof. Minoru recognizes this opportunity as one of the most important in his career. A positive evaluation by his peers will definitely put him among the medical leaders of his country. On the contrary, a negative one may leave him in the shadows for a long time.

He schedules a meeting with Dr. Tanabe and his research team: one associate professor of cardiology (Professor Shiro Yasuda, a young but experienced clinician) and three of his postdoc students (Drs. Dan Yoshida, Hideki Ueno, and Liang Chen). He has an idea of how to conduct a study to assess the evidence of RHC, but he wants to discuss the problem with his research team and Dr. Tanabe. In addition, Professor Minoru likes to challenge his postdoc fellows.

How to Design a Study to Evaluate RHC

Prof. Minoru schedules the first meeting on Friday morning. He is anxious to get the work done. As usual, he gets to the conference room—a nice room on the 10th floor of the research building—earlier than others, at 6:45 a.m. In preparation for the meeting, he writes on the whiteboard: "How do you design a study to evaluate RHC?"

It is 7:00 a.m. and everyone is there except Dr. Tanabe; but Prof. Minoru decides to start the meeting anyway. He begins with the discussion of logistics issues and deadlines. At 7:19 a.m., Dr. Tanabe opens the door and goes to his seat trying to catch his breath. He gets immediate disapproval from the group and especially from Prof. Minoru who thinks to himself, "This will not be easy." But they continue the meeting.

Prof. Minoru continues, "As I explained briefly in my email scheduling this meeting, I need help to design a study to estimate the efficacy of RHC. I would like to hear your comments and suggestions."

Dr. Ueno, the newest research fellow, wants to start, "Scientifically speaking, the best design to access efficacy would be an RCT. I am just concerned with the endpoint you mentioned, mortality, because it would imply long-term follow-up and relatively large sample size."

Prof. Yasuda then quickly intervenes, "We might have an ethical problem with this design, though. As you know, RHC may provide vital information on critical care patients, but on the other hand, it may cause serious complications. The indication of its use is dictated by the physician's experience and must be considered on a case-by-case basis. If in the particular case he or she believes RHC would be necessary, then how do you deny the right to use it? Randomization would do just that. Would it be ethical to run such a study? Also here we are speaking of extremely severe conditions."

Dr. Yoshida, the most productive fellow, comments, "I agree with you. Besides, Dr. Tanabe has a large and detailed database on such patients and it would be much more cost-effective if we could use it through a retrospective study, for example. Furthermore, one of the strengths of observational studies, as they do not have the artificial environment of RCTs, is the ability to estimate treatment effectiveness in real-life conditions."

Dr. Ueno, feeling the pressure of being a new fellow, is afraid to disagree, but he decides to defend his position, "I understand that there are ethical concerns involved, but as you know, observational studies lack scientific rigor that might lead to biased results. How do you guarantee comparability of the groups at baseline without randomization? We might have strong selection bias. It's like comparing apples to oranges. I believe we are in the crossroads between ethics and science. Which road should we take?"

Prof. Yasuda, a more experienced clinical researcher, then proceeds with a more detailed explanation:

> You got to the point. If not interpreted carefully, observational studies may lead to biased results and history has shown that faulty conclusions and recommendations for medical and public-health policy can follow. A typical example in the literature regards the use of estrogen in hormone replacement therapy in post-menopausal women. In 1985, the observational Nurse's Health Study reported that women taking estrogen had only a third as many heart attacks as women who did not. For the next several years, HRT became one of the most popular drug treatments in America. By the end of the last century and beginning of this one, two clinical trials (HERS and WHI) concluded that, on the contrary, HRT constituted a potential risk for postmenopausal women, with increased risks of heart disease and stroke. The question of how many women may have died prematurely or suffered heart attacks or strokes because they were taking HRT, which is supposed to protect them against heart disease, is unknown. Maybe tens of thousands would be a reasonable estimate. Why did conclusions in these studies differ so much? We have to consider the influence of confounders biasing the results in order to understand it. In continuation, our main task, if we decide to keep with the retrospective cohort design, will be how to control for confounders.

Confounding in Observational Studies

A confounder is a covariate that is associated with the exposure and also determinant of the outcome. It is not part of the causal pathway from the exposure to the outcome. Suppose, for example, that you run an observational study on the relationship of drinking coffee and lung cancer. So, you follow two cohorts of subjects, one that drinks coffee and another that does not, and you look for the incidence of lung cancer in each group. You may find significant differences in the comparison groups. Would that mean that coffee causes lung cancer? Not necessarily. What may be happening is that drinking coffee is just a "marker" of other habits, let us say smoking, which is related to lung cancer. Smoking here is a confounder because it is associated with the exposure under consideration (drinking coffee) and the outcome (developing lung cancer). If the investigators do not adjust results for this confounder, biased conclusions will result. In RCTs, on the other hand, the investigator is protected against confounders as they are theoretically balanced in the two groups. If an association is detected in the presence of a confounder, it reflects the combined effect of the exposure and the effect of the confounder. Actually, the exposure may have no effect on the outcome, and the reported association may be due only to the effect of the confounder.

In the Nurses' Health Study, the main issue was that nurses who spontaneously adopted HRT were those with conscious healthy habits, thus less prone to cardiac events. This is known as the healthy-user bias. Although the possibility of confounding was raised by the authors, as the magnitude of the effect between groups was large, the outcome (less cardiac events) was considered related to exposure (HRT). Results of this study may have motivated disseminated use of HRT aiming at the protection to cardiac diseases. This is in fact an important issue, especially for physicians who do not know what confounding is and how it may affect results of a given trial.

Propensity Scores or a Multivariate Outcome Regression Model?

After this productive discussion, Dr. Tanabe stops responding to emails from his Blackberry. Although he seems careless when he speaks, he does so with passion:

> Thank you Shiro! Those were really helpful considerations. I agree with you: we may keep the retrospective cohort design, but we will have to control for confounders. Although other methods are available, outcome models and propensity score analysis are the most commonly used methods to achieve this goal. Briefly, outcome modeling is the way most statisticians address the issue. It allows one to calculate the coefficient to each identified risk factor, which represent the effect of that factor on the outcome, adjusting for other factors in the model. Propensity score (PS) analysis, on the other hand, creates a model that reflects risk factors' effects on the EXPOSURE (in our case RHC would be the exposure). Propensity score becomes a single summary variable that predicts the probability of receiving the intervention as a function of the confounders. By the way, we have advanced quite a lot this morning. Can we take a break and return in the afternoon to continue this discussion?

Prof. Minoru was not happy with this interruption; but he decided to agree, "OK, I would like that you, postdoc students, remind us of the methodology of propensity scores, and the pros and cons of outcome regression versus propensity scores. Is that OK for everybody? Let us meet after lunch."

During the extra time, Drs. Ueno, Yoshida, and Chen went to their offices and started looking on the Internet to get the information they needed. In the afternoon, they were ready and eager to show their progress on the topic. Dr. Yoshida starts after waiting 10 minutes for Dr. Tanabe to arrive:

> As Dr. Tanabe introduced, propensity scores is a method that creates a model that reflects risk factor effects on the exposure, but not on the outcome. The exposure in our case is the use or not of the intervention (RHC). As the exposure is binary, the most suitable model to predict is logistic regression. We could include in the model many covariates that we believe would act as confounders in our study and calculate, for each patient, the chance (or propensity) of exposure (using RHC) according to the model. In other words, with PS, we try to resume factors that influence the choice of a given procedure (exposure). It is important to note that patients with similar propensity scores present similar distribution of confounders, therefore

becoming comparable. So, after defining propensity scores for each study subject we may:
1. Match on propensity scores: with some algorithm (greedy or optimal match);
2. Stratify on propensity scores;
3. Control for propensity scores in an outcome model; and
4. Weight by propensity scores.

Prof. Minoru quickly gave positive feedback to Dr. Yoshida. "Great summary, Dr. Yoshida. What about advantages and disadvantages of each method? Could you tell us something about it, Dr. Chen?"

Dr. Chen, always concerned about speaking in public, goes ahead:

With the propensity scores method, advantages include: first, it is an easier method to explain to a nontechnical audience as groups with similar baseline characteristics (covariates) are created and compared; second, the diagnostics for the efficacy of propensity scores modeling requires just checking for balance of covariates in both comparison groups. It is much more straightforward than regression and allows determination of the range over which comparisons can be made; third, it is objective, as PS modeling and adjustment can be completed without looking at the outcome variables. That allows complete separation of modeling and outcome analysis and protects against deliberate choice of covariates during modeling that could bias the results; fourth, propensity scores may be less sensitive to incorrect model assumptions; lastly, propensity scores may be better when the number of outcome events/number of confounders is less than 7.

Dr. Ueno was itching to reply and he finally had the chance to do so: "On the other hand, propensity scores obscure identification of interactions between treatment and confounders. Furthermore, if matching by propensity scores is the method chosen, we do not use all patients in analysis, only those who could be matched in both groups. That means we will lose power in the analysis. Advantages of outcome regression models include allowing to estimate the effect size of each confounder and also to identify interaction effects between treatment and confounders."

Dr. Yoshida decides to go with Dr. Chen's position and completes,

That is true. However, there are some drawbacks of outcome regression models, as well. Diagnostics for regression (residual plots, measures of influence, etc.) are not so straightforward as for propensity scores (i.e., just checking for balance in baseline characteristics between comparison groups). Also, outcome regression models do not allow separation of modeling and outcome analysis as propensity scores do. Also, modeling may influence the choice of covariates in the model and how they are used (squares, interaction, etc.). Manipulating covariates, in turn, may change the strength or even the direction of the intervention on the outcome. Furthermore, it is not so straightforward to explain to a nontechnical audience how regression controls for confounders.

Dr. Chen, happy with the support, makes a final brief comment, "Finally, I would like to add that there are limitations for both methods since neither is able to adjust for unmeasured confounders (hidden bias)."

Prof. Minoru, who does not usually show enthusiasm in public, makes an exception, "Great job, folks! I believe we are much more prepared to decide which method we will use to analyze the role of RHC." At the end of the day, Prof. Minoru was feeling that his painful experience in the ICU could result in a great contribution to medicine. He felt some comfort with that thought as he had dedicated all of his life to medicine.

CASE DISCUSSION

Professor Minoru plans to determine the efficacy of right heart catheterization (RHC) to improve overall mortality rates in emergency care units. This is an example of a condition in which the use of a RCT can be problematic.

Alternatively, observational studies are considered to be not as controlled as RCTs and therefore if not carefully interpreted, conclusions derived from them can be misleading. One famous example is the Nurses' Health Study, a large cohort study, in which only a third of the women taking estrogen had as many heart attacks as women who did not (for more details about this study, see Stampfer et al., 1991) [21]. This had a tremendous impact in health policy. But between the exposure to estrogen and the outcome there was also one factor that was not on the causal pathway. In this study, nurses who were taking estrogen were also the ones having conscious healthy habits—this is known as the healthy user bias.

This healthy user bias is a clear example of a confounder, a covariate associated with the exposure and the outcome, but not part of the causal relationship between them. Confounders can lead to unrealistic estimations of treatment effects, and they need to be addressed in order for accurate conclusions are to be drawn. This can be performed by using statistical modeling. Outcome modeling calculates a coefficient for each identified risk factor influence on the outcome, adjusting for other factors in the model. But it is based on the outcome, and for instance the choice of covariates or the way they will be used may change the strength and/or direction of the association between intervention and outcome. Propensity scores follow a different assumption, and attempt to summarize in a single variable the probability of receiving an intervention based on a set of confounders. One major advantage of this method is that it is not necessary to take the outcome into consideration, which allows for a separation between the modeling and the outcome analysis, ultimately preventing a deliberate choice of covariates that can bias the results. But at the same time, they can obscure the relationship between exposure and outcome (by not looking at the outcome), and will reduce the sample size if only matched patients are used.

Considering the strengths and limitations of both methods, now Prof. Minoru and his research team have to decide which method they will use to analyze the role of RHC.

CASE QUESTIONS FOR REFLECTION

1. What are the issues involved in this case that should be considered in order to design this study? What are the concerns here?
2. Have you seen similar studies to the one discussed in the case?

FURTHER READING

Rosenbaum PR, Rubin DB. The central role of the propensity score in observational studies for causal effects. *Biometrika*. 1983; 70; 41–55.

Rosenbaum PR, Rubin DB. Reducing bias in observational studies using subclassification on the propensity score. *JASA*. 1984; 79; 516–524.

Rosenbaum PR, Rubin DB. Constructing a control group using multivariate matched sampling methods that incorporate the propensity score. *Am Statistician*. 1985; 39; 33–38.

These are historical articles related to the conceiving process of the propensity score; the first contains the authors' introduction of the theoretical and mathematical basis for the propensity score. The others are the method application by using the stratification and the matching techniques.

D'Agostino RB Jr. Propensity score methods for bias reduction in the comparison of a treatment to a non-randomized control group. *Stat Med*. 1998; 17: 2265–2281.

It is a comprehensive and illustrative review of the propensity score.

Cook EF, Goldman L. Performance of tests of significance based on stratification by a multivariate confounder score or by a propensity score. *J Clin Epidemiol*. 1989; 42; 317–324.

Here the authors compare the performance and the efficiency of methods for confounder control based on stratification, multivariate confounder score, and propensity score.

Winkelmayer WC, Kurth T. Propensity scores: help or hype? *Nephrol Dial Transplant*. 2004; 19; 1671–1673.

This editorial comment brings us a critical review of the propensity score and also discusses briefly the issue of confounding.

Miettinen O, Cook F. Confounding: essence and detection. *Am J Epidemiol*. 1981; 114; 593–603.

In this interesting article, the authors discuss the confounding issue in different studies—follow-up and case-control, illustrated by several examples.

REFERENCES

1. Mann CJ. Observational research methods. Research design II: cohort, cross sectional, and case-control studies. *EMJ*. 2003; 20(1): 54–60.
2. Joffe MM, Rosenbaum PR. Invited commentary: propensity scores. *Am J Epidemiol*. 1999; 150(4): 327–333.
3. Cochran WG, and Rubin DB. Controlling bias in observational studies: a review. *Sankhyā: The Indian Journal of Statistics, Series A (1961–2002)*. 1973; 3(4): 417–446. www.jstor.org/stable/25049893.
4. Rosenbaum PR, Rubin DB. The central role of the propensity score in observational studies for causal effects. *Biometrika*. 1983; 70(1): 41–55.
5. D'Agostino RB Jr. Propensity scores in cardiovascular research. *Circulation*. 2007; 115(17): 2340–2343.
6. Rothman KJ. A pictorial representation of confounding in epidemiologic studies. *J Chron Dis*. 1975; 28(2): 101–108.
7. Rosenbaum PR, Rubin DB. Constructing a control group using multivariate matched sampling methods that incorporate the propensity score. *Am Statistic*. 1985; 39(1): 33–38.
8. McNamee R. Confounding and confounders. *Occup Environ Med*. 2003; 60(3): 227–234.

9. Porta M. *A dictionary of epidemiology*. Oxford: Oxford University Press; 2008.
10. Francis CE, Goldman L. Performance of tests of significance based on stratification by a multivariate confounder score or by a propensity score. *J Clin Epidemiol*. 1989; 42(4): 317–324.
11. Jepsen P, Johnsen SP, Gillman MW, Sørensen HT. Interpretation of observational studies. *Heart*. 2004; 90(8): 956–960.
12. Klungel OH, Martens EP, Psaty BM, Grobbee DE, Sullivan SD, Stricker BH, et al. Methods to assess intended effects of drug treatment in observational studies are reviewed. *J Clin Epidemiol*. 2004; 57(12): 1223–1231.
13. Winkelmayer WC, Kurth T. Propensity scores: help or hype? *Nephrol Dial Transplant*. 2004; 19(7): 1671–1673.
14. McNamee R. Regression modelling and other methods to control confounding. *Occup Environ Med*. 2005; 62(7): 500–506, 472.
15. D'Agostino RB Jr. Propensity score methods for bias reduction in the comparison of a treatment to a non-randomized control group. *Stat Med*. 1998; 17(19): 2265–2281.
16. Cochran WG. The effectiveness of adjustment by subclassification in removing bias in observational studies. *Biometrics*. 1968; 24(2): 295–313.
17. Austin PC. A tutorial and case study in propensity score analysis: an application to estimating the effect of in-hospital smoking cessation counseling on mortality. *Multivar Behav Res*. 2011; 46(1): 119–151.
18. Cochran, WG, and Chambers SP. The planning of observational studies of human populations. *J R Stat Soc Series B Stat Methodol*. 1965; 128(2): 234–266. www.jstor.org/stable/2344179.
19. Posner MA, Ash AS. *Comparing weighting methods in propensity score analysis*. 2015. Available at http://www.stat.columbia.edu/~gelman/stuff_for_blog/posner.pdf
20. Lee BK, Lessler J, Stuart EA. Weight trimming and propensity score weighting. *PLoS One*. 2011; 6(3): e18174.
21. Stampfer MJ, Colditz GA, Willett WC, Manson JE, Rosner B, Speizer FE, et al. Postmenopausal estrogen therapy and cardiovascular disease. *N Engl J Med*. 1991; 325(11): 756–762.

18

ADAPTIVE TRIALS AND INTERIM ANALYSIS

Authors: *Priscila Caldeira Andrade, Nazem Atassi, and Laura Castillo-Saavedra*

Case study authors: *André Brunoni and Felipe Fregni*

Failure to prepare is preparing to fail.
—Benjamin Franklin

INTRODUCTION

Other chapters in this Unit have discussed special cases of randomized clinical trials (non-inferiority trials, for instance). This chapter discusses the reasons and methods to perform interim analysis, adaptive design (used during clinical trials to modify trial design or statistical procedures based on preliminary results from interim analysis), and the particularities of clinical trials with medical devices.

INTERIM ANALYSIS: STARTING AS A LARGE TRIAL AND FINISHING AS A SMALL TRIAL

Interim analysis of randomized clinical trials enables investigators to make more efficient use of limited research resources and to satisfy ethical requirements that a regimen is discontinued as soon as it has been established to have an inferior efficacy/toxicity profile [1].

The idea of interim analysis is examining results as the data accumulate, preferably by an independent data monitoring committee and with a clear plan, thus avoiding that investigators look at data and decide to stop as soon as the result is significant, considering that multiple looks will make type I error much higher than previously established. For example, if the accumulating data from a trial are examined at five interim analyses that use a P value of 0.05, the overall false positive rate is nearer to 19% than to the nominal 5%.

Interim analysis involves many ethical aspects and statistical warnings and must be planned in advance, including clear rules for early termination. The committee, responsible for appropriate monitoring, assesses if the ongoing study can answer the primary question, inclusion rate of patients is as expected, unexpected life-threatening adverse events, poor adherence, fraud, importance of collected information, and finally, if the results of the interim analysis present statistical significance between the treatments. The committee, based on their observations, can recommend the early termination of a clinical trial [2].

Interim analysis can be planned in the middle of the trial (i.e., one-year duration study) or according to the enrollment (after the enrollment of 50% of the patients), depending on the study, outcome, and disease characteristics. The analysis can be planned to look for the following:

1. *Safety*: assess whether the treatment is associated with severe adverse events. In this moment, the committee can recommend stopping the trial for ethical reasons, exposing fewer patients to unnecessary risks.
2. *Efficacy*: if the treatment demonstrated superiority over placebo. In positive case, the trial should be stopped, offering the active treatment to the control patients.
3. *Futility*: if the new treatment has not shown any benefit over the control arm and will not likely change over time, the new treatment may be considered futile and thus efforts should not be spent.

The reasons to stop a trial earlier based on interim analysis results can result in advantages, as earlier publication diminish costs and resources utilization and expose fewer patients to unnecessary risk. However, the balance between clinical and statistical significance should be observed.

Statistical significance may be reached, but not the clinical significance, leading to criticism from the scientific community that the results are not robust enough. In fact, one of the main issues is perception of results from a small trial that may not validate the results clinically. Even demonstrating important clinical significance, an early termination may impact the statistical significance of the trial and may limit the power to look at secondary outcomes.

To preserve the overall significance level, there are specific methods to statistical stopping rule, which must be pre-established in the analysis plan.

The Alpha Spending Function

Repeatedly interim analysis can increase type I error if not handled appropriately. Assuming that the probability of type I error was set at 5%, this 5% has to be shared—not necessarily equally—among all analyses. The alpha spending function implement boundaries that control the type I error rate over the interim analysis. Otherwise, if you assume 5% for the interim analysis and 5% for the final analysis, then at the end you will have a 10% chance of type I error.

The O'Brien Fleming Approach

The O'Brien Fleming approach is widely adopted because the stopping criteria are more conservative at earlier stages, because the boundaries of the test are very large—it uses a very small *p*-value at the earlier stages. Thus, the results should be extreme to cross the boundaries, leading to trial termination. At the more advanced stages of a trial, then the boundaries become quite close to the first statistical value and the penalty for conducting interim analysis is not too high [3].

The Haybittle-Peto Rule

In this approach, the trial is stopped when there is overwhelming evidence to stop the trial. This threshold has been considered at $p < 0.001$ [4,5].

The Pocock Approach

The Pocock approach is a fixed nominal level approach. This means that it sets the same value (threshold) for each interim analysis (divides the p-value equally). However, the number of interim analysis must be fixed during planning the study, and it is not possible to change the number of analysis. Another disadvantage is that it is difficult to report the results [6].

> **Example:** From Schulz KF, Grimes DA, Multiplicity in randomised trials II: subgroup and interim analyses. *Lancet*.
>
> In a given study, a data monitoring committee does an interim analysis every 6 months for 5 years. At 18 months, the analysis slips under $p < 0.05$, but never again attains significance at that level. An early decision by the committee to stop the trial based on this result might have led to an incorrect conclusion about the effectiveness of the intervention.
>
> On the basis of the number of interim analyses planned, the methods define p-values for considering trial stoppage at an interim look while preserving the overall type I error (α; Table 18.1).
>
> O'Brien-Fleming and Peto methods were selected. Both adopt stringent criteria (low nominal p values) during the interim analyses (Table 18.1). If the trial continues until the planned sample size, then all analyses proceed as if basically no interim analyses had taken place. The procedures preserve not only the intended α level but also the power. As a general rule, investigators gain little by doing more than four or five interim analyses during a trial.
>
> **Table 18.1** Interim Stopping Levels for Different Numbers of Planned Interim Analyses by Group Sequential Design
>
> | Number of planned interim analyses | Interim analysis | Pocock | Peto | O'Brien-Fleming |
> |---|---|---|---|---|
> | 2 | 1 | 0.029 | 0.001 | 0.005 |
> | | 2 (final) | 0.029 | 0.05 | 0.048 |
> | 3 | 1 | 0.022 | 0.001 | 0.0005 |
> | | 2 | CC22 | 0.001 | 0.014 |
> | | 3 (final) | 0.022 | 005 | 0.045 |
>
> *(continued)*

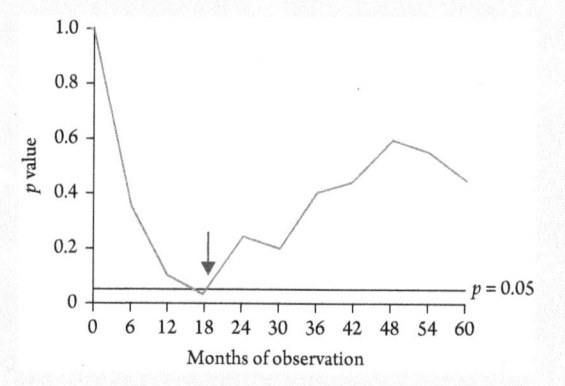

Table 18.1 Continued

Number of planned interim analyses	Interim analysis	Pocock	Peto	O'Brien-Fleming
4	1	0.018	0.001	0.0001
	2	0.018	0.001	0.004
	3	0.018	0.001	0019
	4 (final)	0.018	0.05	0.043
5	1	0.016	0.001	0.00001
	2	0.016	0.001	0.0013
	3	0.016	0.001	0008
	4	0.016	0.001	0.023
	5 (final)	0.016	0.05	0.041

Overall $\alpha = 0.05$.

The Peto (or Haybittle-Peto) approach is simpler to understand, implement, and describe. It uses constant but stringent stopping levels until the final analysis (Table 18.1). For some trials, however, investigators believe that early termination of a trial is too difficult with Peto [7].

Additional Reading

Fossá and Skovlund reported in a very elegant way the penalties for the investigators in not following the planned interim analysis [8]:

[...] The article by Negrier et al (2000 – Journal of Clinical Oncology) gives an example of misconduct of a clinical trial in this respect as the investigators disregarded their own study design and the role of the predefined interim analysis. Based on favorable though preliminary phase II trial results with selected chemoimmunotherapy in metastatic renal cell carcinoma, the combination of subcutaneous interleukin-2 (IL-2), interferon alfa (IFN), and fluorouracil was compared with the combination of IL-2 and IFN. This comparative study was planned before the final phase II results were known, which proved the chosen chemoimmunotherapy to be ineffective in this malignancy. When the phase III trial was designed, it was evident from the medical literature that only few patients with metastatic renal cell carcinoma would benefit from immunotherapy: those with a good performance status and minimal metastatic disease, preferably in lung and lymph nodes. Oncologists treating these patients knew that the majority of the patients would experience significant constitutional toxicity from IL-2/IFN–based immunotherapy without tumor response or prolongation of life. Because of this uncertainty, the principal investigators wisely planned a randomized phase II design with 21 patients in each arm and a subsequent interim analysis. The protocol contained clear stopping rules to be based on the results of the interim analysis: if a ≤10% response rate was obtained in either trial arm and a difference in response rates of greater than 15% between the two alternatives were observed, then the trial would be discontinued. [...] Despite their clearly defined stopping rules, Negrier et al. did not follow their own design: patient

> inclusion was continued during the period of interim analysis until the trialists themselves required the premature end of the trial because of an unexpectedly low response rate. At that time, 131 of the 182 planned patients had been entered, whereas the results of the interim analysis would have led to closure of the trial after 42 patients. The continuation of the trial is even more unexplainable, as the disappointing results of the preceding phase II trial should have been suspected at the time when the interim analysis was due. Proper interim analysis after 42 patients and the results of their own previous phase II study would also have led to the consideration of another problem with the study by Negrier et al: because of the very rapid inclusion rate in this phase III study, despite its being a multicenter effort, the principal investigators should have suspected an inadequate selection of patients. In their final report, the authors correctly discuss this fact as a reason for the low response rate. This problem could, however, have been largely avoided by a proper interim analysis and discussion of inclusion rate with the trialists during an investigator meeting. [...]

DATA SAFETY MONITORING BOARD

The history of data safety monitoring boards (DSMB) dates back to the "Greenberg Report," presented in 1967 by the National Institutes of Health (NIH), as a result of a sponsored expert task force, directed by Dr. Bernard Greenberg. Initially, DSMBs acted as policy advisory boards, and over time they evolved into a committee in charge of monitoring the safety and efficacy of ongoing clinical trials, with a main focus on oversight of interim data of clinical trials, and a main responsibility of ensuring safety of participants. The relevance and procedural extent of DSMBs has grown considerably over the years, so much that the NIH now requires most clinical trials to have a DSMB.

When Are DSMBs Needed?

As part of a research protocol and before the initiation of patient recruitment, researchers must submit a detailed monitoring plan to the local institutional review board (IRB) and the NIH. It is important to emphasize that the functions of a DSMB in monitoring safety of a clinical trial go beyond those of the local IRB. The establishment of a DSMB is required for every multi-site clinical trial, most phase III trials, and any protocol that involves interventions that may entail risk to participants. Smaller trials, such as phase II and I clinical trials, are required to include an appropriate monitoring plan, but DSMBs are not a requisite. The following parameters established by the National Heart Lung and Blood Institute (NHLBI) can be used as general guidelines for understanding the requirements for a DSMB:

- Phase III clinical trials: require a DSMB, which can be formed by the funding agency or by the local IRB, according to the level of risk entailed by the trial.
- Phase II clinical trials: a DSMB is not a requirement, but may be convened by the funded institution according to the characteristics of the trial.

- Phase I clinical trials: a DMSB is not required, unless the trial entails the study of a new and potentially risky intervention. In most cases, thorough monitoring by the principal investigator and local IRB are sufficient.
- Observational studies: the need for a DSMB is determined on a case-by-case basis, according to the size and complexity of the study.

When trying to determine if a specific study requires the conformation of a DSMB, investigators should analyze each case based on the size of the study, number of participating sites, potential risks of the intervention, and outcomes, especially when they include morbidity and/or mortality. Thus, some of the parameters that should be taken into account when making this decision are the following:

- Do any of the outcomes include mortality as an endpoint?
- Does the study require a large patient population?
- Will the study be conducted in several study sites?
- Is the trial designed to determine safety or efficacy of a new intervention?
- Does the trial entail a high risk of toxicity?
- Can the trial be stopped early?

How Do DSMBs Operate?

Every DSMB should include a charter, which is a document outlining and defining the responsibilities, roles, and procedures of the DSMB, with the primary purpose of guaranteeing that its main responsibility is to ensure patient safety. Charters should include a specific data safety monitoring plan, also known as a manual of operations, which includes specifics about the function, frequency, and content of meetings, reporting guidelines, need of blinding of the board, and statistical guidelines for decision-making. Another critical function of any DSMB is to protect study quality, as well as to ensure that an appropriate number of participants are enrolled in the study, which will allow an adequate analysis of outcomes.

In general, the DSMB is in charge of ensuring that the progress of the trial is adequate and in accordance to the initial estimates, so that it can determine if the path followed by the study should be modified or not. This function is accomplished mainly by ongoing protocol monitoring, regular face-to-face meetings, and availability for unexpected crises (see Box 18.1).

Box 18.1 Specific Functions of a DSMB

Ensure patient safety
Ensure the integrity and credibility of the study
Make sure that initial assumptions and results are valid
Determine if enrollment rates are too low
Determine if ineligibility rates are too high
Determine if dropout rates are too high
Determine if rates of adverse events are too high
Determine if any violations to the protocol have been committed
Determine need for early termination of the trial

Member selection is another crucial component of the adequate functioning of DSMBs; members should be experts in an area pertinent to the study, have no identifiable conflicts of interest, be accepted by the sponsor, but hold no affiliation with them, and have no direct involvement in the conduction of the trial.

Early Termination of a Trial

The main role of the DSMB is to continuously monitor adverse events occurring in a trial, and determining the specific relationship of such events to the intervention being evaluated. As a result of their ongoing review of study quality and safety, DSMBs are expected to make recommendations to the funding agency, which will then make a decision to whether accept, reject, or modify such recommendation.

The decision of terminating a study early is a critical one, and it can be based on different termination parameters, some easier to identify than others. The main early termination triggers are based on the safety and efficacy of the study. If there is clear evidence of harm resulting from the intervention, or if it is evident that the intervention is leading to clear benefits, then the study should be stopped early, as continuing it would be inappropriate. The DSMB can also recommend that a study be terminated early if it is clear that even if the study is continued no benefit will be obtained, or if any external force justifies the early discontinuation; for example, another technique has recently been proven to be life saving for the same condition being studied.

Nonetheless, more frequently than not, the decision to terminate a study early is not always straightforward and a careful benefit versus risk analysis should be made. This judgment should take into account the possible impact that such decision may have on other ongoing trials and on operational costs of the study. It should also carefully consider whether or not data are both convincing and sufficient to terminate a trial; for example, is the trend observed on either efficacy or safety just due to lack of sufficient observations, or is it a final direction? So, if the trial were allowed to continue, would investigators identify that the initial lack of efficacy was only due to a low number of subjects? Or, would they identify that the initial high number of adverse events was just a partial observation that is no longer evident or relevant by the end of the trial?

In general, the decision to discontinue a trial should be made based on a careful analysis and thoroughly reasoned consideration of all available data and information, rather than solely on a statistical observation.

ADAPTIVE (FLEXIBLE) DESIGN

Adaptive design methods have become very popular in clinical research, mainly in industry studies due to their flexibility and efficiency. Adaptive designs are used to modify the trial design or statistical procedures based on preliminary results from interim analysis without minimizing the validity and integrity of the trial. However, advantages of adaptive designs do not come without a cost. Adaptive designs can induce some methodological shortcomings in the trial that invalidate the results.

A common selection rule is to pick the most promising treatment, for example, the treatment with the numerically highest mean response, at the interim stage. However, there is a concern regarding the overall type I error after the adaptations, which result from possible deviation from the original target population.

The main goal is to increase the success of clinical development, making the studies more efficient and more likely to demonstrate the effect of a treatment.

The range of possible study design modifications must be planned in the written protocol. It has been used to change the following:

- study eligibility criteria
- randomization procedure
- treatment regimens of the different study groups (e.g., dose level, schedule, duration)
- total sample size of the study (including early termination)
- concomitant treatments used
- study endpoints
- hypotheses
- analytic methods to evaluate the endpoints (e.g., covariates of final analysis, statistical methodology, type I error control)
- assessment of clinical responses.

The following are examples of adaptive designs:
1. Adaptive randomization design (described in Chapter 6): Patients are randomized according to the outcome of the previous patient);Disadvantages of adaptive randomization:
    - Adaptive randomization is more difficult to execute then static randomization.
    - There are several sources of error.
    - Results of errors are poorly understood.
    - Using Adaptive randomization adds costs and risk to running a trial.
2. Sample size re-estimation design: Starting out the study with a small initial commitment of patients but is willing to factor in the possibility that the sample size might need to be increased during the course of the trial. Usual in vaccines and HIV studies [10].

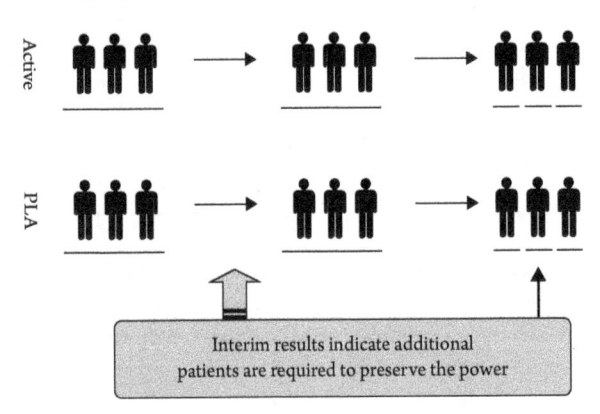

(Chow 2008)

- Nuisance parameter adaptive methods: Accurate estimation of a nuisance parameter is crucial for proper sample size determination. (Ex: If SD is 20% larger than initially proposed, the sample size must be increased 44% to maintain 90% power).

- Re-estimation and resizing a trial for a clinically insignificant difference in treatment effect in not desirable.
3. Drop-the-loser design: This design allows dropping the inferior treatment groups, very useful in phase II trials (dose level adjust). Usually has two phases. Only the "winners" proceed to the second phase. The loser group plays a very important role, provide information about dose response. Dropping the non-promising treatments at an early stage helps to save the resources and expedite the trial.
4. Adaptive dose finding (escalation): This design is used to identify the minimum effective dose (MED) and/or the maximum tolerable dose (MTD), which is used to determine the dose level for the next phase clinical trials.
5. Hypothesis-adaptive design: This design allows modifications or changes in hypotheses based on interim analysis results. It is possible to switch from superiority to a non-inferiority hypothesis.
6. Multiple adaptive design. Combine several adaptive designs:
group sequential design
drop-the-losers design
adaptive seamless trial design
adaptive dose-escalation design
adaptive randomization design.

There is potential to increase the chance of erroneous conclusions in adaptive designs:

- Study results can be difficult to interpret
- Chance to introduce bias (through modification) that increases the chance of a false conclusion that the treatment is effective (a type I error)
- Bias associated with the multiplicity of options
- Difficulty in interpreting results when a treatment effect is shown
- Operational bias.

Therefore, although adaptive designs are attractive as they seem to increase the efficiency of a given trial, they should be carefully considered, as there is an important chance of adding bias when using these designs and therefore invaliding the results. Adaptive designs in fact should be used only in special situations and when there is a good rationale for its use [8]. It is not the goal of this chapter to discuss in depth each type of adaptive design, but rather to give the reader a general overview of different types of adaptive designs. There are some references given at the end of this chapter discussing each type of design and the uses and potential biases associated with them.

OTHER TYPES OF DESIGNS: DESIGN WITH MEDICAL DEVICES

Drugs versus Medical Devices Trials: Are They Different?

In 1970, Dr. Theodore Cooper (at that time the director of the National Heart, Lung, and Blood Institute) submitted a report on the regulations of medical devices. He wrote in the report: "medical devices are unlike pharmaceuticals in significant ways, and as such, direct application of the drug-model is not desirable or feasible."

What are the differences between drugs and medical devices (for instance, pacemakers, stents, deep brain stimulators) for clinical trial design?

Medical device differs from drug in several aspects, including indication—drugs are used to treat patients in specific clinically indicated populations, whereas devices are used to treat wide indications and populations, user effects that are expressive in the case of medical devices, influencing outcomes, whereas drugs are not or minimally affected by user effects.

Available evidence and evidence generation differs between medical devices and drugs. The design and analysis of clinical studies of devices can be more challenging than comparable studies of drugs, owing to ongoing device modifications, user "learning curves," and difficulties associated with blinding, randomization, and sample size definition.

On the other hand, the current demand for clinical evidence in medical devices has been increasing, leading to specific solutions to answer this need. Actually, the interest in effectiveness grew over efficacy, the same for health-care value, real-time data analysis, longitudinal follow-up, comparative effectiveness research (CER), patient-centered outcomes research (PCOR), and clinical registries.

Alternatives to RCTs are usually observational studies—case reports, case series, cross-sectional, case-control, and cohort studies—that avoid sham procedure, which may raise ethical concerns. Non-randomized clinical studies play an important role in this scenario. In addition, non-randomized clinical studies offer the possibility of comparing two groups, using data collected. However, it is the need to avoid bias (temporal and selection) and confounding, which is very easy to be present in surgical studies. It is needed to balance the distribution of patient characteristics and the risk factors and assess the quality of historical data. The interpretation of the results needs to take into account bias, confounding, chance, and causality.

Despite these factors that are discussed in many papers, evidence regarding the safety and effectiveness of medical devices still is considered as drug evidence—the gold standard remains in randomized controlled trials, with adequate blinding and a control arm, usually placebo. The issues start appearing exactly at blinding and placebo control (or sham) point, since it is very difficult and many times impossible to perform this type of design for medical devices.

In the following we describe some exclusive features and issues of clinical trials with medical devices and why they have to be differentiated of drug clinical trials [11].

Rationale for RCT

The best evidence based-medicine level originates from RCTs, once observational studies may be confounded. However, clinical trials with medical devices are especially vulnerable due to operative covariates (user effect, learning curve) and the placebo effect.

Placebo Effect

Placebo effect is a consequence of cognitive dissonance, while medical devices are more invasive. In addition, it is very difficult and usually impossible to blind the study and to develop a perfect "placebo device." Yet, although it is easy to develop a sugar pill that serves as placebo for drug studies, adverse effects of drugs may serve as potential unblinding factors.

Primary Endpoint Considerations

Drugs usually are measured by systemic metrics as effect of chemotherapy on overall survival, or effect of cholesterol lowering on coronary heart disease. Although the final goal of medical devices is to have a clinical impact, medical devices usually also measure more frequently surrogate outcomes given their more focal effects in most of the cases.

Sample Size Considerations

Sample size is an important consideration for medical devices, as usually the large phase III trials for medical devices are not as large as drug trials. The reasoning for smaller sample sizes are based on costs and feasibility. Usually, medical device treatments cost more than drug treatments and also are developed for more restricted population. Thus recruitment may be a challenge in a good number of them. However, an adequately powered phase III trial needs to be developed, and thus the investigator should find methods to consider power optimization.

CASE STUDY: INTERIM ANALYSIS: TROJAN'S HORSE IN THE SERENIUM TRIAL? PLANNING AN INTERIM ANALYSIS

André Brunoni and Felipe Fregni

An International Call

It was a warm night in Paris. The summer had just begun. Dr. Jean-Luc Richelieu was in a pleasant dream but was obligated to wake up due to the annoying ring of his mobile (he wishes he had not chosen the Beethoven's Ninth Symphony to alert incoming calls).[1]

"Bon soir ... What time is it?" Jean-Luc said with a very sluggish voice.

"Good afternoon, Dr. Richelieu. This is John Williams, research assistant of Professor Gregor Briggs. Prof. Briggs wants to talk with you right now about your email to which he just replied. Is it possible?"

"Oh—hummm—of course, Mr. Williams! I was not doing anything important." Jean-Luc quickly ran to his computer and opened his mailbox. It was 3 a.m. in Paris.

"Good afternoon, Jean-Luc!" Prof. Briggs said, "I mean, good afternoon here. What time is it there?"

"Oh, not to worry. I was looking forward to talking with you again! I read your email and was responding," said Jean-Luc, trying to open the file. ("Saved in docx, it does not open!")

"My apologies for disturbing you—I do not want to rush you. In fact, I am calling about something I had forgotten to address in the email—a crucial aspect in the project we forgot to discuss last month when I was in Paris—we should plan an interim analysis!"

Jean-Luc panicked. He planned the trial so carefully—but he had completely forgotten this topic!

"Interim analysis. Yes, how did we forget? But do you think it is necessary? I mean, we are studying insomnia ... "

"I know what you are going to say, Jean-Luc. We are studying insomnia, so it is not necessary to do an interim analysis due to ethical issues. But as the PI, I need to wear the physician's hat, too. And although insomnia is not a life-threatening condition, I do think it is an important condition. We are testing against placebo and the trial has four-week duration. I do not think it is ethical to let people not sleep for four weeks. But I know this is a delicate matter. I would like to set up a meeting. But this time in Los Angeles. What do you think?"

As Jean-Luc agreed, Prof. Briggs continued, "But—in order to move quickly with this study—if you can board tomorrow, it would be great. How about tomorrow at 6 p.m. Pacific Time—is that OK?"

---

[1] Dr. Brunoni and Professor Fregni prepared this case. Course cases are developed solely as the basis for class discussion. Although cases might be based on past episodes, the situation in this case is fictional. Cases are not intended to serve as endorsements or sources of primary data. All rights reserved to the author of this case. Reproduction and distribution without permission are not allowed.

It was a tight schedule, but Jean-Luc knew that this project would be his pathway to his greatest success—or his worst failure. At least, Prof. Briggs was right—having insomnia is awful. Jean-Luc was now too excited to fall asleep again.

The Successful Negotiation of Serenium Trial

A mid-size pharmaceutical company from France, Psychotics™, is sponsoring the Serenium trial. This young company has aggressive plans to become the market leader. This company is now developing a new antipsychotic drug called *Serenium* to be used as a treatment for insomnia. Its pharmacists have been working with the first antipsychotic drug—Chlorpromazine. They changed its molecular structure in order to enhance its sedative effects while diminishing its extrapyramidal side effects—they plan to re-launch the drug in the market after the confirmatory clinical trials.

Jean-Luc had taken the job of medical director of Psychotics™. But he has been feeling the pressure of this new job—if he fails now, he will need to be looking for another job.

The project has been going well so far. After a tense but successful negotiation with Prof. Briggs—a renowned psychiatrist and clinical researcher from the United States—who is now the PI of this study, the initial study steps have been uneventful. But now this call from Los Angeles from Prof. Briggs has raised an important and potentially problematic issue for this study: the issue of interim analysis. Interim analysis is an important and ethical issue that needs to be addressed. The use of interim analysis could also bring methodological problems to the study.

Boarding to LA: Advantages and Disadvantages of Interim Analysis

The next morning, Jean-Luc and his research assistant, Dr. Helen Curie, took a flight to LA.

Dr. Richelieu was taking two pills. "Melatonin—do you want? We are traveling to the west and we need to avoid jet lag. We have a meeting today!"

Dr. Curie thought, "Psychiatrists and their psychiatric pills—a delicate issue!" She said, "No, I still prefer caffeine. Dr. Richelieu, I am curious. Why should we be so worried about doing an interim analysis?"

"Well, Helen, first of all, the idea of interim analysis is to analyze the results before the trial finishes. If it were planned to have a two-year duration and an enrollment of 100 patients, then an interim analysis would be done, for instance, after half of the trial was conducted, after the enrollment of 50 patients. Or if a trial planned to enroll 300 patients, interim analyses could be done after 100 and 200 patients. In this case, the interim analysis can unmask some issues: (1) safety issues—we can detect, for instance, that the active treatment is associated with an increased risk of an adverse event and thus should be stopped earlier; in this case, an interim analysis is a good chance to see if "things are going just fine"; (2) efficacy issues—we can detect whether our drug reached statistical significance over placebo and that would allow us—in fact, obligate us—to stop the trial at this point as the principle of equipoise would be violated and therefore patients should be offered the active treatment. Finally, in trials that compare an experimental treatment against the standard treatment (a drug-drug trial), the interim analysis can also reveal that new drug is worse than the standard drug (at a statistically significant level) and thus that would be another reason to terminate the trial."

Helen said, "Dr. Richelieu, I am confused. Interim analysis sounds like an excellent idea! I mean, stopping the trial earlier is good, isn't it? It is almost impossible that our drug performs worse than placebo, so that is not something to worry about. Our pilot trials showed that Serenium is not associated with important adverse events. We planned a sample size calculation not only for statistical significance but also for clinical significance! So it is very possible that if we stop the trial at half the sample size, then we will have a statistically significant result. So that means we can publish sooner, we can expend fewer resources in this current economical crisis—and most important, we can expose fewer patients to unnecessary risks. What is the catch here?"

"Yes, Helen, interim analysis is certainly a very good idea with important advantages, but as you know in clinical research, almost everything you do has a cost. One point is the variability of results during a clinical trial. For instance, results might favor treatment A after 50 patients, then change to treatment B after 100 patients, and so on. In addition, you may reach the statistical significance level during the interim analysis but not the clinical significance level. This is a result of less stability of data with smaller samples. As a result, academics, and editors of medical journals can argue that the results are not robust enough. Let me give you an example: suppose a trial that tests a new anticoagulant agent versus warfarin for stroke prophylaxis in patients with chronic atrial fibrillation. Such a trial would need to enroll a large number of patients, for instance, 2,000 patients. Let me give you two scenarios then: with 1,000 patients, the new drug is significantly better than warfarin ($p = 0.01$) to avoid ischemic stroke: 8% versus 6% (incidence of stroke). What is the number needed to treat (NNT) in this case?"

Helen quickly calculated the NNT, a measure that she knows is very important to address the clinical utility of a given treatment. "The absolute risk reduction is 8−6 = 2%. NNT is 1/ 2%. Fifty?"

"Yes, NNT is 50. And, also if the drug is very expensive and is associated with an increased risk of an adverse event (e.g., hemorrhagic stroke), then its utility will certainly be jeopardized since the NNT is very high—that means a physician would have to treat 50 patients with the new drug (and not warfarin) to avoid one ischemic stroke. Now, let me give another scenario: suppose that the trial ends when it was planned and it still shows statistical significance and now the risks are: 16% of stroke in the warfarin group and 4% in the new drug group—with more patients and time, the differences of the drugs are clearer. In this scenario, the NNT is 7. What can you conclude?"

"I understand. With this new NNT, the new drug is obviously better than warfarin and should be chosen, even if it is more expensive. So you are saying that interim analysis might also hurt a study?"

Jean-Luc opens a smile before responding, "Yes—exactly—that is the *catch*! Another issue here is that even if you show an important clinical difference between the two treatments with the interim analysis, the impact of your trial might be less

significant as you are presenting a trial with a sample size of n/2 (or n/3, n/4, ...)."
After a brief pause, he continues, "There are other issues: first, studies are planned to address one primary hypothesis. In our study, we planned to enroll 300 patients. We calculated our alpha level and beta level for this sample size, not less. We will not have full statistical power with fewer subjects. And there is more: we have some secondary hypotheses—that are very prone to fail, as secondary hypotheses are naturally not as powerful as the primary hypothesis. And then the argument of exposing fewer subjects to unnecessary risks turns the side: I can argue that it is better to resolve all the issues in one trial than in two. Suppose that a study with an interim analysis has a small impact, and then a subsequent study will be necessary. And that is also true when looking at the economic aspect: we are already prepared to do this trial now, but we might not be in one year. So, I agree that an interim analysis can save costs but only in the short term. In the long run, doing two trials instead of one will certainly be more expensive and challenging. Helen, in fact, stopping a trial due to early efficacy is usually not well accepted by aca xxx it is difficult to define that a given risk is unacceptable—this might be subjective and depends on a given patient, as you know medicine is a risk-benefit analysis."

Jean-Luc stopped for a moment and then concluded, "So, Helen, I personally think that interim analysis is a Trojan's horse. It is a beautiful idea and, so you bring it to your trial, but it might end up destroying the trial!"

Helen replied, "I understand, Dr. Richelieu. But I still think that the advantages of the interim analysis cannot be underestimated."

"I know, Helen, I know." He sighed, "I did not make up my mind yet. Let's hear the opinion of Prof. Briggs. He is a brilliant researcher and I want to discuss this matter very carefully with him. This project is very important and it is critical to analyze all the options carefully."

The Sun Still Shines: Statistical Aspects of Interim Analysis

Helen Curie was exhausted. The flight time (Paris—LA) is 11 hours, but the time zone difference is 9 hours. So, they left Paris at 1 p.m. and arrived in LA at 3 p.m. The sensation was of a terrible hangover.

"I cannot believe it, Dr. Richelieu," she said, "We traveled for 11 hours, and the sun still shines!"

She also noticed that Jean Luc was feeling much better than she was. Perhaps it was due to the melatonin pills?

"Well, look on the bright side, Helen! The sun still shines! That is a good augury! But if you wish you can stay in the hotel and sleep a little before the meeting."

"No, if I sleep I will only wake up tomorrow! Let's go to UCLA!"

"Ok, but first let me get you a coffee. You need lots of caffeine—you will have a strong double espresso!"

They went to the hotel just to leave the bags and then they headed to UCLA. Professor Briggs was waiting for them and they quickly started their meeting. The first topic was the conversation Helen and Jean-Luc had in the plane.

"OK, very good!" he said, "Just let me clarify some statistical issues first. One important thing is that each time we do an interim analysis, there is a 'penalty' for that so as to avoid increasing type I error. Let me explain: assume that the probability of type I error was set at 5%, as most trials do. This 5% has to be shared—not necessarily equally—among all analyses. Otherwise, if you assume 5% for the interim analysis and 5% for the final analysis, then at the end you will have a 10% chance of type I error. Therefore, the sum has to be 5%. So suppose that a trial is planned with one interim analysis. If we calculate the results with a p of 2.5%, then the final p also has to be 2.5%. If we calculate the interim analysis with a p of 1%, then the final p would be 4%. That is just an example for your understanding. The calculation is not simple arithmetic, using some statistical calculations that demand a statistician, but it is the logic of 'alpha spending.'"

"Prof. Briggs," Helen said, "should we distribute the p-value equally or unequally, as you gave the example of 1% / 4%?"

"Well, Helen, it depends. If you believe that the study results will be accepted with a smaller sample, then you can divide the p-value equally—that increases your chances of getting a significant p-value at earlier stages. So, if we are going to do an interim analysis, we should also decide which type of analysis is more recommended, or in statistical terms, the most appropriated 'alpha spending function.'" He continued, "The O'Brien Fleming approach is more conservative at earlier stages, because the 'boundaries' of the test are very large—it uses a very small p-value at the earlier stages. Thus, the results should be extreme to cross the boundaries, leading to trial termination. At the more advanced stages of a trial, then the boundaries become quite close to the first statistical value and the penalty for conducting interim analysis is not too high. The Pocock approach sets the same value for each interim analysis performed (divides the p-value equally). Also, there is the option of conducting the interim analysis for safety only."

"So, I think we have several options here," Jean-Luc said, "(1) do nothing; (2) do an interim analysis for safety only (not looking at the efficacy and therefore not paying the p-value penalty; (3) do an interim analysis for safety and efficacy. Right? Also, if we go for safety and efficacy, we will also have to decide which method to use for alpha spending—Pocock or O'Brien Fleming."

Helen Curie looked at the wall clock. It was still 6:30 p.m. She was tired, thinking about how odd it was to have a day with 33 hours! But then she thought that when she goes back to Paris her day would only have 15 hours! "There is no free lunch—an interim analysis implies a type I penalty—gaining time today implies losing time tomorrow. We now need to decide whether interim analysis here will be our Trojan's horse."

CASE DISCUSSION

For the case discussion, the reader should consider the advantages and disadvantages of having interim analysis.

Advantages:

- Reduce the duration of the trial, reducing costs and patients exposure to potential risks.
- Treatment safety is an important concern—assess unexpected life-threatening adverse events related to the treatment.
- Anticipate efficacy issues, providing important information to continue or to stop the trial.

Disadvantages:

- Statistical significance level could be reached, but not clinical significance (easily criticized by publishers).
- Sample size planned at the beginning could be reduced, then losing power.
- NNT issue: clinical results in favor of the treatment can differ if the analysis is made in the middle or in the end of the trial.
- Statistical issues: increase type I and II errors due to underpowered analysis, and further studies may be needed, which increase unnecessary costs.
- Secondary hypothesis are prone to fail.

Statistical Power and Interim Analysis

Another important issue for this case is the p-value penalty for doing interim analysis. This penalty might influence the power of the study. There are different ways to address this, such as the O'Brien-Fleming procedure (most of the p-value is considered at the end of the study) or the Pocock procedure (in which p-value is divided evenly for the interim analysis).

CASE QUESTIONS FOR REFLECTION

1. What is the reason for performing an analysis in the middle of the trial, and what should you do with the results?
2. What are the advantages and disadvantages for running interim analyses?
3. When should a trial be terminated early? What are reasonable stopping rules?
4. What penalties does the investigator need to pay when doing the interim analysis?
5. Which method do you think is more appropriate?
6. Also one issue here is abstracts for conferences; do you pay the statistical penalty when you analyze your results to write an abstract?

FURTHER READING

Papers

Observational Studies• Avorn J. In defense of pharmacoepidemiology. Embracing the yin and yang of drug research. *N Engl J Med*. 2007 Nov 29; 357(22): 2219–2221. PMID: 18046025.

Interim Analysis• Snapinn S et al. Assessment of futility in clinical trials. *Pharm Stat*. 2006 Oct–Dec; 5(4): 273–281. PMID: 17128426.

Adaptive Designs• Chow SC, Chang M. Adaptive design methods in clinical trials: a review. *Orphanet J Rare Dis*. 2008 May 2; 3: 11. PMID: 18454853.

- Gallo P, Chuang-Stein C, Dragalin V, Gaydos B, Krams M, Pinheiro J, PhRMA Working Group. Adaptive designs in clinical drug development: an executive summary of the PhRMA Working Group. *J Biopharm Stat*. 2006 May; 16(3): 275–283; discussion 285–291, 293–298, 311–312.

Medical Devices• Bonangelino P, et al. Bayesian approaches in medical device clinical trials: a discussion with examples in the regulatory setting. *J Biopharm Stat*. 2011 Sep; 21(5):938–953. PMID: 21830924.

- Li H, Yue LQ. Statistical and regulatory issues in nonrandomized medical device clinical studies. *J Biopharm Stat.* 2008; 18(1): 20–30. PMID: 18161539.

Online: Interim Analysis
- http://www.consort-statement.org/consort-statement/3-12---methods/item7b_interim-analyses-and-stopping-guidelines/ç

Data Safety Monitoring Boards (DSMBs)• He P., Leung Lai, T., Su Z. Design of clinical trials with failure-time endpoints and interim analyses: An update after fifteen years. Contemporary Clinical Trials. 2015.
- Chalmers I, Altman DG, McHaffie H, Owens N, Cooke RW. Data sharing among data monitoring committees and responsibilities to patients and science. *Trials.* 2013; 14: 102.
- Sartor O, Halabi S. Independent data monitoring committees: an update and overview. *Urologic Oncol.* 2015; 33: 145–148.

Books

- Kirkwood BR, Sterne JC. *Essential medical statistics.* Malden, MA: Blackwell Science; 2003.
- Portney LG, Watkins MP. *Foundations of clinical research: applications to practice.* 3rd ed. Upper Saddle River, NJ: Pearson Prentice Hall; 2015.
- Rothman KJ. *Epidemiology: an introduction.* 2nd ed. Oxford: Oxford University Press;
- Williams OD. Data Safety and Monitoring Boards (DSMBs). In: Glasser SP, ed. *Essentials of clinical research.* 2nd ed. Heidelberg: Springer; 2014.

REFERENCES

1. Fleming TR, DeMets DL. Monitoring of clinical trials: issues and recommendations. *Controlled Clin Trials.* 1993; 14(3): 183–197.
2. Su HC, Sammel MD. Interim analysis in clinical trials. *Fertil Steril.* 2012; 97(3): e9. PMID: 22285749.
3. O'Brien PC, Fleming TR. A multiple testing procedure for clinical trials. *Biometrics.* 1979; 35: 549–556.
4. Haybittle JL. Repeated assessments of results in clinical trials of cancer treatment. *Brit J Radiol.* 1971; 44(526): 793–797.
5. Peto R, Pike MC, Armitage P, et al. Design and analysis of randomized clinical trials requiring prolonged observation of each patient. I. Introduction and design. *Brit J Cancer.* 1976; 34(6): 585–612.
6. Pocock SJ. Group sequential methods in the design and analysis of clinical trials. *Biometrika.* 1977; 64(2): 191–199.
7. Schulz KF, Grimes DA. Multiplicity in randomised trials II: subgroup and interim analyses. *Lancet.* 2005; 365(9471): 1657–1661. PMID: 15885299.
8. Fosså SD, Skovlund E. Interim analyses in clinical trials: why do we plan them? *J Clin Oncol.* 2000; 18(24): 4007–4008. PMID: 11118460.
9. Chow SC, Chang M. Adaptive design methods in clinical trials: a review. *Orphanet J Rare Dis.* 2008; 3: 11. PMID: 18454853.
10. Chuang-Stein C, et al. Sample size reestimation: a review and recommendations. *Drug Inform J.* 2006; 40: 475–484.
11. Li H, Yue LQ. Statistical and regulatory issues in nonrandomized medical device clinical studies. *J Biopharm Stat.* 2008; 18(1): 20–30. PMID: 18161539.

UNIT IV
Study Designs

19

INTEGRITY IN RESEARCH
AUTHORSHIP AND ETHICS

Authors: *Sandra Carvalho and Gustavo Rivara*

Case study authors: *André Brunoni and Felipe Fregni*

The right thing to do is often hard but seldom surprising.
—Adam Gopnik (2012)

INTRODUCTION

So far in this book we have had chapters focusing on research methodology, statistical analysis, and trial design, among others. In this chapter we will focus on another important concept: integrity in research. Integrity in research refers to the active commitment to ethical principles, norms, regulations, and guidelines governing the responsible conduct of research. Research integrity requires that the research process is governed by honesty, objectivity, and verifiable methods, rather than preconceived ideas and expectations.

Although practices of responsible conduct of research may vary from country to country or even from one institution to another, there are some shared values, which include, but are not restricted to, the following: honesty, accuracy, efficiency, objectivity, confidentiality, and responsible publication of research findings [1]. These shared values ensure the accuracy and replicability of study findings, reinforcing the commitment to good practices in research among professionals. Integrity in research governs all the stages of a research process—planning, implementation/execution, interpretation of results, and report writing and publication. Therefore, before starting any research process, all research members involved must be aware of professional codes, government legislations, and institutional policies governing research with human subjects and animals, research misconduct, and conflicts of interest.

In this chapter we will focus on several aspects of integrity in research: authorship, conflict of interest, and ethics.

AUTHORSHIP

Publication of the research findings in scholarly journals is one of the most important stages of the research process and a career in academia. Research findings must be disseminated to readers and peers in a standard form, language, and style [2]. Publication must be done in the most accurate and honest way possible, so research methodologies and research findings can be replicated, and can support future scientific advances. It constitutes an ethical obligation for an investigator to make research findings accessible, in a timely manner, and with sufficiently detail so that other investigators could replicate the study [3]. The ultimate objective of any research is to make research findings available to the community, and any publication must give the appropriate credit and accountability to all authors who contributed to the scientific work.

Authorship credit is attributed to persons who have substantially and intellectually contributed to the study and to the scientific report. According to the International Committee of Medical Journal Editors (ICMJE), authorship provides credit for an individual's contributions to a research study, has important academic, social, and financial implications, and carries accountability and responsibility [4]. Since there is no universally accepted standards governing authorship assignment, researchers should be aware of specific practices, guidelines, or recommendations within their own institution. Because authorship order may be governed by different guidelines, some research journals require authors to state for each author the specific contribution to the scientific report. This practice has the advantage of removing some ambiguity surrounding contributions, acknowledging each specific contribution. However, this does not resolve the problem of quantity and quality when assigning authorship.

The ICMJE developed guidelines with specific criteria for authorship. Authors should be accountable for their contribution, and also should be able to identify the contribution and responsibility of co-authors listed in the scientific report. This definition of authorship acknowledges an author's accountability for his or her own work, as well as co-authors' contributions. Therefore, according to ICMJE, in order to be considered an author, the individual must meet the following criteria:

1. Considerable contribution the research process, including study design and main concept; or data acquisition, data analysis, or interpretation of the research findings; *and*
2. Substantial work on drafting or reviewing the scientific report, with important intellectual contributions; *and*
3. Provide final approval of the version to be published; *and*
4. Be responsible and accountable for all the aspects related to the accuracy or integrity of the published work.

Thus, every investigator who meets these four criteria should be listed as an author, and those who do not meet the four criteria should be acknowledged (in the acknowledgment section of the manuscript) for their contribution to the study. It is important to stress that if the first criterion is met, individuals should be given the opportunity to work on the report, including drafting, revising, and approving the final version of the scientific report. This is the collective responsibility of the authors listed in the manuscript, and it is not a responsibility of the journal where the work is going to be published. Some journals require details about authorship (i.e., a list of each specific author's contribution) and some even require authors to sign a statement on authorship responsibility, conflict of interests (COI) and funding, and copyright transfer/publishing agreement. If an agreement among authors on authorship cannot be reached, the institutions where the work was conducted should be requested to investigate and find an appropriate solution. After the manuscript submission or publication, any change in authorship—order, additions, deletions, contributions being attributed differently—should be justified, and journal editors should require a signed statement of agreement from the requested change from all listed authors, including those being added or removed.

According to the American Psychological Association (APA) [5], people who provided mentorship, or funding or any resources to the project, but did not participate in the final report, should not necessarily qualify for authorship. Despite these efforts from ICMJE and APA, among others, in providing guidelines governing scientific publication, several institutions do not follow them. For instance, in some institutions it is a common practice that heads of the department are listed as authors even though they have never been directly involved in the research process or contributed to the final publication. These are the so-called guest authors or gift authors (including authors who did not contribute significantly to the report) (Table 19.1), and this practice is not endorsed or allowed by many of the most important peer-reviewed journals.

Table 19.1 Different Types of Authorship, with Different Ethical Concerns

Different Forms of Authorship

First authorship	The main researcher and the main writer of the article. This person is usually responsible for writing the first draft of the paper and is also the corresponding author.
Last authorship	An author who contributed with expertise and guidance. This person is usually a senior researcher, who critically revises the manuscript, assuring that the good quality standards of research and publication have been met. Typically, this person represents the institution in which most of the actual research was performed (if the study is not a multicenter trial). The last author can also be listed as corresponding author.
Corresponding author	The corresponding author is the person who submits the paper to a journal and has the responsibility to review and answer reviewers' questions, as well as all the correspondence related to the published paper (i.e., reprint requests or any contact with the research group). This person is listed in the manuscript with detailed contact information. This is not only an administrative role, but also a sign of seniority.
Gift or honorary authorship	Listed authors who did not contribute substantially to the manuscript and the research project. Example: award authorship credit to someone who has power and prestige rather than for intellectual and substantial contribution to the work. This is not endorsed by most medical journals or ICMJE.
Ghost authorship	Failure to list as author someone who meets the criteria for authorship. Example: a company (or a busy researcher) hires someone to write the paper.

(continued)

Table 19.1 Continued

Different Forms of Authorship	
Coercion authorship	Authorship is demanded or imposed rather than voluntarily awarded. Examples: a chair of the department who demands authorship in all manuscripts; a senior researcher forcing a junior researcher to include a gift or guest author in the manuscript; or a researcher forcing a specific authorship order (for instance, first or last position) when his or her work does not justify that position.
Group authorship (corporate, organization or collective)	For publications with very large number of authors, a name for the group may be created and every author who contributed to the published work is listed in the article text. The group name in this case represents a specific consortium, or committee or a study group. If necessary, more than one group name can be created for the citation, or both group name and author names can appear in the citation. Example: An organization that take full responsibility for the creation of the scientific work; can be an alternative to long author lists in multi-authored manuscripts.
Mutual support/admiration authorship	Authors agree to list each other's names on their own manuscripts despite minimal or no participation in the research project and manuscript. Examples: friends or colleagues who want to rapidly increase their number of publications agree to list each other's names in their own publications. Authors agree to share the main authorship positions in the paper (first and senior positions), though their work does not fulfill the criteria for that position.

(based on (6, 7)).

"Ghost authorship" happens when someone that significantly contributed to the scientific work and has no authorship position assigned in the manuscript (Table 19.1). It is also a practice of some companies (such as pharmaceutical companies) to hire "ghost" writers for clinical studies and to use others names as authors in the manuscript. Other examples of gift or guest authors is when busy investigators hire someone to write their own manuscripts, or when someone is invited to participate in the manuscript due to prestige or as a way of "returning a favor." One of the problems with ghost writers is that they may not fully understand the underlying experiments, and may not be able add any intellectual contribution to the final report, or to explain the experiment and findings to other scientists (Table 19.1).

Authorship Order

According to the ICMJE guidelines, authorship order should always be the co-authors' joint decision. Authors should be informed of authorship order, as well as the reasons

First author
- ✓ Fulfills ICMJE authorship criteria.
- ✓ Performs bulk of the experimental work.
- ✓ Able to describe the procedures and the results described in the paper.
- ✓ Has the major contribution to the manuscript writing.

Last author
- ✓ Fulfills ICMJE authorship criteria.
- ✓ Directs and supervises the work.
- ✓ Takes responsibility for the scientific accuracy of the research findings, data integrity, and research methods used.
- ✓ Able to explain all the results described in the paper.

Middle author
- ✓ Fulfills ICMJE authorship criteria.
- ✓ Does not fulfill the criteria to be the first or the last author.
- ✓ Order of the middle author (relative to other listed authors) reflects his/her contribution to the paper.

Corresponding author
- ✓ Fulfills ICMJE authorship criteria.
- ✓ Communicates with editors and readers of the published paper.
- ✓ Ensures that submission of the manuscript is done properly and that all co-authors have the opportunity to review and approve the final proof.

Acknowledgments
- ✓ Does not fulfill ICMJE authorship criteria.
- ✓ No significant contribution to the manuscript writing:
    - ✓ Participated in data collection.
    - ✓ Proofread and language edited the manuscript.

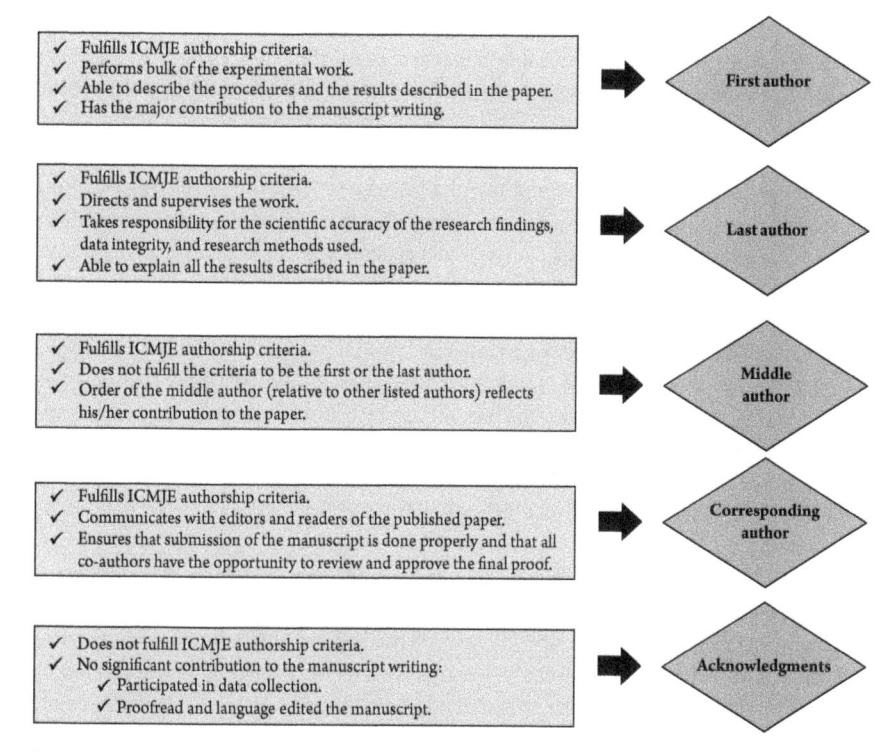

Figure 19.1. Decision diagram for authorship order [adapted from 9].

for that particular order. In some cases, authors are listed alphabetically, with the justification that all authors made equal contributions to the study and to the publication. Whenever this happens, it is important to make that clear in the manuscript, by adding a note in the manuscript.

A general recommendation to a young researcher who has made substantially intellectual contributions and may have drafted the manuscript is to be the first author in a paper and/or the corresponding author. For someone in career progress, being the last author or the corresponding author usually means that this person is a senior author in the field or was the main person responsible for the contents of the manuscript/and the study [8].

The following are some descriptive guideposts on authorship order to help in deciding the sequence of authorship (based on [10]):

1. Authors sequence should be determined by their relative overall contribution to the study and the manuscript. Equal contributors should be highlighted in the manuscript.
2. Typically, the first author is the one that takes responsibility for writing the first draft of the manuscript. However, in certain cases, especially when the first author is a research student without experience in manuscript writing, the senior author may take responsibility for drafting the manuscript, or, supervisors/senior researchers give the student a fixed period of time (for instance, 3 months)

to write the first draft of the manuscript. If the student does not deliver or if he or she completely fails to complete the first draft, the supervisor may then take full responsibility for writing the manuscript (and therefore, will put his or her name first).

3. The first author should be the person who contributed most to the work, including manuscript writing. This person may be associated with the development of the basic concept of the study, the main hypothesis, study design, data collection, (and/or) data analysis. This person was certainly one of the major contributors to the main data interpretation and discussion in the manuscript. It is also worth noting here the possibility of co-first authorship, where two or more individuals who equally contributed to the manuscript have the opportunity to share the primary credit. In this case, it is recommended that co-first authors be listed in alphabetical order. In cases of co-first authorship, and if this is made clear in the manuscript, being listed as second or third or even fourth should not be seen with prejudice. First authors, along with senior/last/corresponding authors, also typically assume primary responsibility and accountability of the reported results and conclusions.

4. The last author is typically the one who plays a mentoring/stewardship role for the overall conduction of the study, supervising and providing overall guidance for the research project. He or she is typically the head of the laboratory that hosted most of the research. The last author is usually an established and senior researcher in the field for that particular work. Similarly to all authors, the last author should meet all criteria for authorship in order to be listed as author in the manuscript.

5. For the middle authors there is less clarity around the significance of authors' contributions. Order may quantify contribution, meaning that authors are listed according to their overall contribution to the manuscript. In some research fields, the second author is listed as the second person, following the first author, who contributed more to the research project and manuscript writing. And, the second-to-last author is also a senior author in the research field who has made substantial contributions to the manuscript.

One curious and interesting aspect is that in other fields of science, authorship order has other criteria compared to those just discussed that are used in health sciences. In fact, promotion committees should pay more attention to the real authors' contribution as cited at the end of the articles, as requested by some journals; this may decrease, at least at some extent, some of the authorship disputes.

Authorship Disputes

In theory, assigning the appropriate credit for intellectual contributions in a scientific work is a straightforward process. However, authorships disputes regarding authorship position are somewhat frequent. In most of the cases, these disputes happen because it may not be easy to define whether someone's contribution was substantial or not [6].

In order to minimize the likelihood of authorship disputes, it is generally recommended that all potential authors in a research project discuss authorship with the principal investigator (PI) when the study in still being planned [4]. It is the responsibility of both co-investigators and the PI to prioritize this conversation. If necessary, researchers can use a signed agreement, in the format of a contract regarding publication intent. In this case, researchers agree about their responsibilities/roles in the project and also about authorship order. The agreements can also specify that authorship order can be renegotiated if researcher's responsibilities change substantially, or if a researcher fails to perform his or her role as previously agreed. Winston (1985) [11] suggested a procedure for determining authorship order in any research publication. The basic concept of this authorship instrument is that potential authors should complete it in a collaborative way, with discussion that includes all contributors. This checklist helps facilitate the organization and delegation of responsibilities in the research project, and provides the opportunity to discuss and negotiate authorship and authorship order in a collaborative way.

Even though authorship should be discussed or negotiated in advance, this good practice does not always prevent authorship conflicts. At the time of manuscript writing, authorship has to be reassessed. Therefore, it is important to ask the following type of questions: Have all investigators fulfilled their contributions according to what they agreed upon initially? Has the scope of the project changed during its course and therefore the contribution of the participating research study members [12]?

In order to prevent authorship disputes, it is important to follow four basic principles:

1. Create and reinforce a culture of ethical authorship (be informed about the institution policies on authorship, or propose one if there is not, and discuss that with your PI and research team);
2. Start discussing authorship when planning the research study (when it is possible, discuss that in a face-to-face meeting, so all authors will be aware of authorship decisions);
3. Reassess authorship during the course of the study (if there are any substantial changes in the roles of any author, authorship may be discussed as the project evolves); and
4. Decide authorship before manuscript writing (discuss expectations and responsibilities on manuscript writing, revision and submission to a journal) [6].

Summary of Authorship

Everyone who makes substantial intellectual contribution to a research project is a potential candidate for authorship. In addition to the contributions to the researcher project, the researcher needs to make substantial intellectual contributions to the manuscript in order to be listed as author. All persons who substantially contributed to the research project, or who are listed as authors in the manuscript, should have the opportunity to participate in the manuscript writing and to approve the final version to be published. It is ultimate responsibility of the lead investigator(s) to manage authorship credits and authorship order with integrity and honesty, and to promote and facilitate discussions within the research team whenever authorship disputes occur.

Finally, authorship has a great impact on the scientific career, because it means credit and recognition for the work performed. However, it also involves responsibility and accountability for the published work.

ETHICS IN RESEARCH

Scientific research is built on a foundation of trust and credibility. Both society and the scientific community expect that every scientist is devoted to describing the world in the most accurate and unbiased way. This trust in research conduct and research findings has led to unparalleled scientific investments and productivity in the last centuries. Nevertheless, it is important to stress also that the history of science includes examples of research misconduct or unethical procedures. Despite the negative consequences of these research trials, it is important to stress that they also impacted the quality of research, by promoting the need to create guidelines and rules governing research conduct. One famous example of this is the case of the Tuskegee syphilis study.

The Case of the Tuskegee Syphilis Study

In 1932, the US Public Health Service, working with the Tuskegee Institute, began a study of the effects of syphilis on the human body. The study took place in Macon County, Alabama. The true objective of this study was to study the natural course of syphilis in black men. This study was called the "Tuskegee Study of Untreated Syphilis in the Negro Male." When this study was designed, there were no proven available treatments for syphilis, and no knowledge about the natural course of the disease. Initially, researchers enrolled a total of 600 African American males, 399 with untreated syphilis (experimental group) and 201 without the disease (control group). The recruitment was performed by government officials and participants were told that they would be compensated for their participation in the study with "free medical care," free examinations, and free meals on the days of the examination, and burial insurance. The recruited men were mostly sharecroppers from Macon County, in Alabama, due to a high rate of syphilis cases in that region. These men had difficult lives and very limited access to health-care services. They were never told by the research team that they had syphilis, but solely that they were being treated for "bad blood"—a vague term used at that time to describe several types of diseases. They were never told also that autopsies would eventually be required in order to get the final data necessary to complete the study. In fact, they never signed any consent form or received details about the experimental procedures, or the potential benefits and risks related to their participation in the trial. Since the objective of this study was to evaluate the effects of untreated syphilis, the 399 syphilitic subjects did not receive the "treatment that they were assigned to," and were never told that the "treatment" that they were receiving was placebo (i.e., without any medical properties). The objective of the researchers was solely observing the natural progress of untreated syphilis. In addition, the study, which was previously projected to last 6 months, went on for about 40 years. And in order to prevent possible dropouts from the participants, researchers used specific promotional campaigns with suggestive titles such as "Last Chance for Special Free Treatment."

The experiment continued in spite of the Henderson Act in 1943 (a public health law requiring testing and treatment for venereal disease) and also in spite of the World Health Organization's Helsinki Declaration in 1964 (see details about the Helsinki Declaration later in this chapter and in [13–15]). In fact, even when penicillin was introduced as a possible cure for syphilis in 1947, none of the subjects participating in this study had access to this treatment or was informed about this possible available treatment. In 1972, when this study was exposed, a total of 28 men had died of syphilis and 100 men were dead due to complications related to the disease. In addition, about 40 wives have been infected, and 19 children contracted the disease at birth.

The study was ended on July 25, 1972, when Jean Heller of the Associated Press broke the story, both in New York and Washington. (For more details about this study, see Brandt et al. [16].)

The Belmont Report: Three Principles for Ethical Research

The Belmont Report summarizes the basic ethical principles identified by the National Commission for the Protection of Human Subjects of Biomedical and Behavioral Research. It provides ethical principles and guidelines for the protection of human subjects of research.

This report was prompted in reaction to previous violations involving human subjects. Examples of these violations include the Tuskegee syphilis study and the Nuremberg trials on human experimentation, among others. The report resulted from an intensive four-day period of discussions that were held in February 1976 at the Smithsonian Institution's Belmont Conference Center. The Belmont Report was published in the Federal Register and was made available to scientists, institutional review boards, and federal employees in order to rapidly and easily change boundaries between research and practice in the United States.

The Belmont Report resulted in two important definitions: (1) the boundaries between research and practice, and (2) basic principles governing research with human subjects. Practice is defined as any intervention that aims to solely enhance or improve the well-being of any individual. Research is defined as any activity designed to test hypotheses, generate conclusions, and add knowledge to the existing theories and practices.

The three basic principles are (1) respect for persons, (2) beneficence, and (3) Justice (Figure 19.2).

Ethical Principles	Requirement
• Respect for Persons	• Informed Consent
• Beneficence	• Risk/Benefit Ratio
• Justice	• Subject Selection

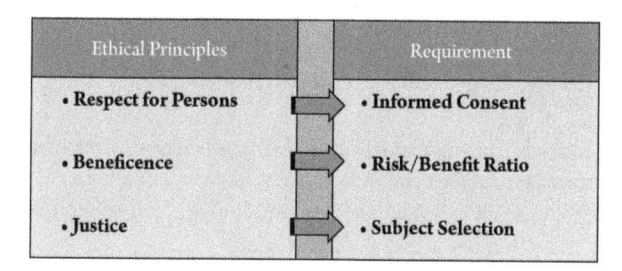

Figure 19.2. According to the Belmont Report (1979), ethics in human research should be based on three interrelated basic principles: respect for persons, beneficence, and justice.

Respect for persons in research refers to the basic ethical principle that participants involved in the research study are volunteers and have the right to be informed about the research goals (such as the objective of the study, benefits, risks, etc.). This basic principle involves two important ethical considerations. The first one is that the participant should be treated as an autonomous being (i.e., a person who has the right to make decisions or deliberations about her or his personal goals and desires). The second one is that persons who are not able to make decisions for themselves (any vulnerable populations, such as children, prisoners, people with some mental disorders or impairments) should be protected from any type of coercion from others or any activity that can cause any harm to them.

Beneficence refers to the obligation of maximizing possible benefits and minimizing possible harm to the participants involved in the study. In this sense, investigators and institutions have to plan to maximize benefits and minimize risks to the participants, following the best judgment possible, with the available knowledge. By following the principle of beneficence, investigators will use the available knowledge to decide whether there is another way to obtain the data/knowledge but with lower risks to participants, and therefore, benefits should outweigh the risks.

The principle of justice refers to the distribution of benefits and burdens related to the experimentation, so that there is fairness and study participants are treated equitably. The principle of justice will guide, for instance, the selection of participants, preventing that some populations that are easily available or vulnerable or easy to manipulate are systematically recruited, rather than participants being chosen for reasons directly related to the research problem being studied.

Applications of the Belmont Report

Informed Consent

The informed consent process is an important and mandatory component of respecting human participants. Voluntary participation in any study should always be preceded by the informed consent and should protect the privacy of all volunteers. The informed consent form is a written summary of information about the study. It should be written in a way that participants will be able to understand the objective of the study, all the procedures involved in the study, and all the direct benefits and risks associated with his/her participation in the study. And, therefore, it should enable people to voluntarily decide whether they want to participate as research subjects. There are several rules governing the informed consent process, and some of them may vary according to the specific research protocol and also specific institutional guidelines. In general, the consent form process requires that

1. Informed consent is always prospectively obtained from participants or their legally authorized representatives;
2. Both parties (research team, participant and/or legal representative) have access to a signed and dated copy of the consent form;
3. All information should be conveyed in understandable and adequate language (avoiding excessive use of scientific terms);

4. Participants are given sufficient time to read, understand, and decide whether they want to participant in the study;
5. Any type of coercions or influence must be avoided when performing the informed consent process;
6. Participants must not be made to give up legal rights or any treatment in order to be involved in the study.

Assessment of Risks and Benefits

The careful assessment of potential benefits and risks to participants before starting any study derives directly from the basic principle of beneficence. The basic principle of beneficence is that it is the ultimate responsibility of the research team and all the institutions involved in research to assess all potential risks and benefits before starting any research protocol. All procedures must be performed with the least risk possible to participants, and risks must be reasonable in relation to benefits. Research must be performed in a way that does not cause any harm to participants, and confidentiality should always be maintained.

Selection of Subjects

According to the principle of justice, there must be fair procedures and outcomes in the selection of research participants. Therefore, researchers must avoid exploitation of vulnerable populations and avoid providing benefits only to populations that they favor.

When confronting an ethical dilemma in research, the first option is always to carefully examine the situation and keep these three ethical principles in mind. This may help in clarifying some issues and making appropriate decisions. The example presented in the preceding—the Tuskegge syphilis study—is an example of a clinical trial in which researchers violated all three of these principles, as participants were lied to about their condition, about the "treatment" they were receiving during their participation in the trial, and about the objectives of the study. Additionally, participants were selected based on race, gender, and economic class.

Research Misconduct

Research misconduct occurs when standard codes, regulations, and ethical behavior that governs scholarly conduct research are violated [17]. The main purposes of research misconduct policies and guidelines are to provide clear definitions of research misconduct, to provide protection for those accused of research misconduct, and to outline standard procedures of reporting and investigation of any research misconduct [1]. According to the Singapore Statement on Research Integrity, drafted in 2010 at the Second World Conference on Research Integrity in Singapore, and with 51 countries represented, there are four common principles of research integrity:

1. Honesty in all research stages;
2. Accountability in the conduct of research;
3. Professional courtesy and fairness in working with others; and

4. Good stewardship of research on behalf of others [18].

In order to be considered research misconduct, three criteria should be fulfilled:

1. The behavior represents a clear and significant deviation from accepted practices, policies, and guidelines governing research; and
2. These evidences can be proven; and
3. There are clear evidences that the behavior was committed intentionally, and with negligence. The primary author and other authors whose results are found culpable are accountable.

When there is any suspicion of research misconduct, all researchers who are involved in the specific data and publication are investigated. In order for a formal investigation to occur, an investigative committee is appointed by the associate provost. This committee has the responsibility to determine whether research misconduct has occurred or not, and to determine possible disciplinary sanctions to those involved in research misconduct. When federal funding is involved, that particular funding agency must be informed that a formal investigation of possible research misconduct has been initiated. The formal investigation can take several days and usually requires the examination of several research documents related to the subject being investigated, correspondence, and interviews. When the formal investigation is completed, the chair of the investigation prepares a detailed report to be sent and discussed with the associate provost. The disciplinary procedure may vary dependent on the status of the researcher (i.e., if he or she is a faculty member, a research assistant, a student, etc.).

Examples of misconduct in research include data fabrication or falsification, plagiarism (both plagiarism-fabrication and self-plagiarism), ghost writing, data manipulation, and breaches of confidentiality (Box 19.1). Honest mistakes or divergent opinions are not considered research misconduct, and therefore should be approached in a different manner. Research misconduct needs to be proven by sufficient evidence, and the behavior must be committed intentionally.

In 2008, the Office of Research Integrity from the US Department of Health and Human Services carried out a study to examine scientists' reports on suspected misconduct in biomedical research. In their final report, a total of 192 scientists have reported 265 incidents of research misconduct, which were coded and evaluated based on the federal definition of research misconduct. Overall, 64 descriptions (24% of the total) did not meet the criteria of the federal research misconduct. The remaining 201 reports were related to fabrication or falsification (60%) and plagiarism only

---

Box 19.1 Common Lapses in Research Integrity in Human Subjects Research

Falsification of data on scientific reports
Data fabrication
Failure to report all adverse events/reactions or serious adverse events/reactions related to the study
Failure to report all data [19].

(36%) [20]. However, in general it seems that researchers fail to report 37%–42% of suspected research misconduct findings. The reasons for that may be due to lack of protection for the whistleblowers, lack of knowledge on the research misconduct, and the need of a system with clear policies and guidelines for reporting these allegations in an anonymous way. And the researchers who are more likely to observe and report research misconduct are the ones who are more familiar with the institutional misconduct policy.

CASE STUDY: MUCH ADO ABOUT NOTHING— A DISPUTE FOR A PLACE IN HEAVEN

André Brunoni and Felipe Fregni

A long dispute means both parties are wrong.
—Voltaire (French Philosopher 1694–1778)[1]

The Vendetta—A Surprise during the Argentinian Summer

The past months have been really difficult for Juan Guevara—a postdoctoral fellow in the neurobiology department at Macondo Institute of Mental Health in Buenos Aires, Argentina. He has been in an authorship dispute with his PhD mentor, Prof. Isabel del Carpio, that could have a significant impact on his career. He has been exhausted by this situation. Stressed and sleep-deprived, he feels that no solution would address all the problems. He is at a crossroads and has to decide whether to fight for what he believes is fair, or to accept a compromise solution to protect his future career.[2]

The main reason for this dispute is the authorship of a study Juan Guevara has been working on for years—transplantation of neuronal cells to robotic devices—that would certainly gain publication and an editorial in a top scientific journal with a huge impact factor such as *Nature*.

Juan remembers in detail the day that everything started. It was the warmest day of the year in Buenos Aires, between Christmas and New Year's Eve. The city was virtually empty; besides some loyal tourists who could be seen in local restaurants, it seemed that everybody had left town—including his family, who was in Florianopolis (Brazil) enjoying the summer on the marvelous beaches. Juan Guevara, though, had stayed at Macondo Institute with his research. He thought he was alone when Prof. del Carpio arrived. He knew that there was something wrong, as she usually did not go to the institute during holidays.

"Hi Juan! I am glad to see you here!"

"Hi Isabel!" he replied "I am using the holiday break to prepare my oral presentation for the next Congress and to start writing our *Nature* paper."

"Yes—about that . . . we need to talk, Juan," she said, changing her expression. "Prof. Carlos Ferrucci [head of the neuroscience department of Macondo Institute] and I talked yesterday, and although we are glad to have you as first author in the abstracts—you will not be the first author of this paper, Juan. I am sorry, but I hope you understand."

"What? How is that so, Isabel?" He was starting to lose control of his emotions. "I have been leading this research for years—and we talked about this in the beginning

---

[1] Bornstein NM, Norris JW. The unstable carotid plaque. *Stroke*. 1989 Aug 1; 20(8): 1104–1106.

[2] Professor Felipe Fregni and Dr. Brunoni prepared this case. Course cases are developed solely as the basis for class discussion. The situation in this case is fictional. Cases are not intended to serve as endorsements or sources of primary data. All rights reserved to the author of this case. Reproduction and distribution without permission are not allowed.

and it was implicit that I would be the first author of this study; otherwise, I would have gone to another lab."

"Juan, things change and science is a dynamic process. Also we are a team of 12 researchers! *We* have been leading this research! I have also put a lot of work into this project. And also thanks to Prof. Ferrucci, who earned a huge grant of the Ministerio de Salud, we were able to pay the scholarships of four postdoctoral fellows—including *you*, Juan—and to import equipment from overseas, to avoid the premature termination of the project. I am sure *you* remember this, Juan. In a nutshell, you are the arms of our study, but Prof. Ferrucci is the soul of our great, collective work. In addition, he had the idea for our work and he helped significantly with the design of this study; that's why he will be the first author. Besides, Juan, you should see the big picture here: you are at the beginning of your career and you will have lots of opportunities to get your first author paper. We really need to think here on what is best for our group and the institution."

Juan Guevara was furious. "But I did more than him—this project *is* my life. I dedicated so many years to it—this is really unfair! And I suppose you are the last author, *aren't you*?", Juan replied, becoming increasingly more aggressive.

"Naturally, Juan, I am the mentor of this work," she said. "That's it, you are the arms, I am the head, and Prof. Ferrucci is the soul. You can be the second author—but I have good news, we also talked about writing an invited review on the topic for an Argentinian science journal. You can write it, we will help you, and you will be the first author for this one. You are young and one day you will understand. If you work with us, we will help your career."

Juan was perplexed. He could not recognize the person in front of him. He had always admired Isabel del Carpio as for him she was the role model of a scientist—someone who stayed in Latin America and had been able to, despite all the challenges, change knowledge in her field of research. But he would not accept that. "Sorry, Isabel. I don't agree with you. I deserve to be the first author. You know it. This question is still unsettled."

"Juan Guevara, you are such an idealist. You should focus more on science instead of *politics*. Please do not become a rebel here; we are trying to accommodate everyone in this situation; besides, a second authorship in a paper such as *Nature* is a great breakthrough for you.

"Again, you are very smart, and also very young. I am sure you are going to publish many papers in the future," she continued, but her expression then became harsh. "Besides, you don't want to go against Prof. Ferrucci and me. You do not want to ruin your career for a paper, do you?"

The Issue of Authorship

Authorship of a paper is a more complex matter than it seems to be: in fact, in academic settings, the overall number of articles published and the number of first-authored publications heavily influence how colleagues view the researcher. Therefore, authorship is not a trivial matter and it is recommended that it should be discussed before the trial/study starts. Failure to do so might lead to authorship disputes that can waste a significant amount of time and energy of the involved authors and result in significant damage to one's career. One important issue is that either small or large collaborations can lead to authorship disputes if not well planned.

The importance of authorship is not only to acknowledge someone's work; it is the critical piece for appointments in medical centers, promotion, grant support, and participation in society committees. Therefore, it is crucial for academic life. In the traditional authorship model, authorship order is of vital importance, and usually the first and last author get most of the credit for the work performed.

There are other forces playing into authorship disputes, such as scientists' self-esteem. Currently when a paper is cited, it is cited usually as the first author's name followed by "et al."—for instance, "Guevara et al. presented remarkable findings . . .." Though this is never noted as an official reason in debates, this certainly plays an important role. Scientists are in a sense very similar to artists, and some are known for having an over-inflated ego.

One important issue of authorship is that only researchers who have contributed *intellectually* to the work should be included in the list of authors. The manuscript should be seen as the intellectual product of the research. So, for instance, the clinician who refers patients to the study or the technician who only does the laboratory experiments do not qualify for authorship according to medical journals and the ICMJE. The problem here is how then to acknowledge a clinician who has dedicated time referring and finding patients to the study, as this person might have been critical for a clinical study to happen. That is one of the problems of clinical research—lack of extrinsic motivators.

Radical Solutions

Juan was really stressed by this situation. He stopped all of his work and could not function well—he spent hours on the Internet looking for similar cases. This project was his life—something he had worked very hard for, and he could not let go of this issue, even knowing that it could have detrimental consequences for his career.

While thinking about how to act on this issue, he was considering a more dramatic approach, such as filing a lawsuit. In fact, he knew about a recent dispute between two microbiologists at the University of Gottingen that ended up in court. Juan knew that it was a similar case to his. In this story reported in *Nature*,[3] the team leader removed the name of the postdoctoral fellow at the last minute and the postdoctoral fellow decided to take legal action. In the end, the court ruled in favor of the postdoctoral fellow, based on the original verbal agreement that both researchers had agreed to in the 14 months before the submission. According to the court, "this understanding constituted an implicit contract." He was prepared to go in that direction if needed; however, he knew that this would have devastating consequences, as the

---

[3] Dispute over first authorship lands researchers in dock, *Nature*. 2002; 419 (p. 4).

academic world is a very small one and he could be labeled as a "difficult researcher" and no one might agree to work with him in the future. But on the other hand, he kept remembering a famous Argentinian saying, "Hay que endurecerse" (in English: "have to become stronger").

Another radical solution would be to send an email to the editor of the journal expressing his disagreement with the authorship order. Usually, editors do not want to publish papers in which there is a dispute on authorship. This could persuade his mentor to go back and agree with him about being the first author. However, he knew that this option would also bring much grievance and impact his career negatively. Also he knew he needed a letter from his mentor to get a permanent academic position. He was feeling like a hostage to this situation. He decided then to try to cool off and wait some weeks before doing anything radical.

Diplomatic Solutions

Summer had long finished in Buenos Aires and things were not going well for Juan Guevara. He had tried to schedule a meeting several times with Prof. Feruccci but he always refused, rescheduled, or simply missed the appointment. Finally, when Juan sent him a firm email, Prof. Feruccci agreed to meet, but they failed to settle the question. In fact, he was very rude, threatening Juan with losing his position and career if he continued to stand with his "rebel point of view."

Juan, then, decided to act. He sent an email to Dean Catarina Mendez, Dean of Research Integrity for Malcondo Institute. A few days later, during a long, tense meeting, Juan explained to Prof. Mendez what was going on in the Neurobiology Department. She listened carefully. One point that was not clear to her was the implicit agreement they had made. In Guevara's own words, "Dean Mendez, this is what every PhD student expects: that he or she would be first author in his or her main PhD project—if this was not the case this should have been communicated to me before." After a pause, Dean Mendez commented, "Well, Juan, I understand, but again this is a gray area that may be interpreted in different manners. But let me see what I can do." Later, after she had listened to Prof. Feruccci and Prof. del Carpio, she realized she had a time bomb in her hands and she would need to address the situation very carefully. In fact, she realized the problem was too important for her to judge alone. She did not want Juan or the others to get into a personal war. One option here would be to set up a committee. There are two committee options:

1. To create an internal, advisory committee—this committee would listen to both sides and would try to provide a fresh set of eyes for the problem, suggesting an ethical, professional, and fair solution to the quarrel. This option would be less aggressive and would aim to provide a "gentleman's" solution. This committee would not, therefore, impose anything; it would only provide a recommendation. However, she also thought things had gone too far in this matter, and that neither side could be reasonable anymore.
2. To create a mandatory committee—in this case, the committee would listen to both sides, but ultimately support one of them. Also, such a committee would

have the power to institute disciplinary actions if authorship abuse were seen. The advantage would be to provide a clear, final solution on the matter. The disadvantage is that it would be an authoritarian solution that goes against the principles of academia. Also, such a committee would not obviously have "force of law"—that is, someone could get very angry with the solution and tell the media about what is going on—possibly ruining the institution's reputation, or could leave the institution with some of the data, burying the paper's publication.

Time for a Decision

Juan had another conversation with Dean Mendez and she explained that this was a difficult situation. She also mentioned that she understands that he could make a radical decision as he explained to her initially (such as filing a lawsuit); but she advised him to consider it carefully and that a diplomatic solution could be worthwhile (such as setting up this review committee). Juan was relieved to talk with Dean Mendez; he felt that she was ethical and fair. But he did not make up his mind yet and also did not know if Prof. Feruccci and Prof. del Carpio would support such a committee. It was like playing chess—the next play would be decisive.

Juan listed the options in his head: (1) do nothing; (2) file a lawsuit; (3) complain to the editor-in-chief; (4) try to convince the dean to set up an advisory committee or a mandatory committee). Since the first conversation with Prof. Carpio, 6 months had passed and it was mid-July in Buenos Aires, and a light snowfall was expected for that evening—the first in 90 years! He was freezing. He knew that authorship conflicts happen all over the world. He got on the bus and, for just this day, the slow traffic near the La Plata River did not bother him as he had too much to think.

CASE DISCUSSION

This case discusses an authorship dispute between a postdoctoral researcher—Juan Guevara—and his PhD mentor—Prof. Isabel del Carpio. Juan has to decide whether to fight for what he believes is fair (i.e., being the first author), or to accept a compromise solution with his mentor and, therefore, be the second author. This decision is rather difficult, and both have pros and cons. First authorship position is very important to both Juan and del Carpio—it has an important career impact and represents recognition for their hard work and contribution to the final work.

Cases like Juan Guevara's remind us that ethical ideals and integrity in research often bend to the reality of ego, power, and self-interest in the real world. Regardless of how one thinks this case should ethically be resolved, we must acknowledge that many times in practice, we fail to live up to the normative expectations we set for ourselves. There are important open issues from this case to allow for disagreement about assignment of authorship. For example, if it were true that Carlos was the main idea generator for the research and was the key study designer, and that Juan executed Carlos's ideas while intellectually contributing less as results came to be known, it might make sense to assign co-first authorship to both. The point is, the only way we can ethically "solve" this dispute is for each party to honestly detail precisely what and how he or she contributed to the study. Of course, each party will infuse his or her own contribution with as much substantive importance as possible and this is where leadership from an *impartial* judge proves vital to maintaining procedural integrity. Whether Dean Mendez or her faculty colleagues or others can fill this role is context specific, but it should be clear that Isabel is no longer a "neutral" party. This case also reveals the importance of "anticipatory authorship ethics." When so much is at stake, it behooves all junior investigators who have made a commitment to a career in scientific investigation to proactively engage their mentors/senior project advisors on the issue of how authorship is assigned on work coming out of the lab. Unfortunately, we can no longer rely on "understanding" and "expectation" from customary practices. Ideally, junior investigators should choose labs and mentors only after they have a clear understanding of how their "boss" approaches authorship assignment. At a minimum, junior investigators should have a clear understanding of how their "boss" will manage specific potential authorship disputes.

This case is important therefore to make the reader consider what he or she would do it in this case, also what would be the scenario if Juan were right or vice versa? This exercise can help to resolve and perhaps prevent future authorship disputes.

CASE QUESTIONS FOR REFLECTION

1. What are the issues in this case that resulted in the dispute?
2. What are the authors' concerns? And the institution's?
3. What should the authors consider in making the decision?
4. Have you experienced a similar situation?

FURTHER READING

Gopnik A. Facing history. *New Yorker*. April 9, 2012.

REFERENCES

1. Steneck NH. ORI: Introduction to the responsible conduct of research. Washington, DC: Government Printing Office; 2007.
2. Derntl M. Basics of research paper writing and publishing. *Int J Tech Enhanc Learn*. 2014; 6(2): 105–123.
3. Graf C, Wager E, Bowman A, Fiack S, Scott-Lichter D, Robinson A. Best practice guidelines on publication ethics: a publisher's perspective. *Int J Clin Practic*. 2007; Supplement (152): 1–26.
4. Editors ICoMJ. International Committee of Medical Journal Editors (ICMJE): uniform requirements for manuscripts submitted to biomedical journals: writing and editing for biomedical publication. *Haematologica*. 2004; 89(3): 264.
5. Association AP. Publication practices & responsible authorship. Retrieved from http://www.apa.org/research/responsible/publication/
6. Albert T, Wager E. How to handle authorship disputes: a guide for new researchers. The COPE Report 2003; 32–34.
7. Babor TF, McGovern T. Coin of the realm: practical procedures for determining authorship. In: Babor TF, Stenius K, Savva S, eds. *Publishing addiction science: a guide for the perplexed*. 2nd ed. London: Multi-Science Publishing Company; 2004: 110–123.

8. Bhattacharya S. Authorship issue explained. *Ind J Plast Surg*. 2010; 43(2): 233–234.
9. Strange K. Authorship: why not just toss a coin? *Am J Physiol-Cell Physiol*. 2008; 295(3): C567–C575.
10. Riesenberg D, Lundberg GD. The order of authorship: who's on first? *JAMA*. 1990; 264(14): 1857.
11. Winston RB. A suggested procedure for determining order of authorship in research publications. *J Counsel Devel*. 1985; 63(8): 515–518.
12. Liesegang TJ, Schachat AP, Albert DM. Defining authorship for group studies. *Arch Ophthalmol (Chicago, Ill: 1960)*. 2010; 128(8): 1071–1072.
13. World Medical Association. World Medical Association Declaration of Helsinki: Ethical principles for medical research involving human subjects. *JAMA*. 2013; 310(20): 2191–2194.
14. Rickham P. Human experimentation: code of ethics of the world medical association: Declaration of Helsinki. *BMJ*. 1964; 2(5402): 177.
15. World Medical Association. World Medical Association Declaration of Helsinki: Ethical principles for medical research involving human subjects. *Bull WHO*. 2001; 79(4): 373.
16. Brandt AM. Racism and research: the case of the Tuskegee Syphilis Study. *The Hastings Center Report*. 1978; 8(6): 21–29.
17. Nylenna M, Andersen D, Dahlquist G, Sarvas M, Aakvaag A. Handling of scientific dishonesty in the Nordic countries. National Committees on Scientific Dishonesty in the Nordic Countries. *Lancet (London, England)*. 1999; 354(9172): 57–61.
18. Resnik DB, Shamoo AE. The Singapore statement on research integrity. *Account Res*. 2011; 18(2): 71–75.
19. Titus S, Bosch X. Tie funding to research integrity. *Nature*. 2010; 466(7305): 436–437.
20. Titus SL, Wells JA, Rhoades LJ. Repairing research integrity. *Nature*. 2008; 453(7198): 980–982.
21. Misconduct OFPoR. 2005. Available from: http://www.ostp.gov/html/001207_3.html.

20

THE BUSINESS OF CLINICAL RESEARCH

Authors: *Lívia Caroline Mariano Compte, and Jorge Leite*

Case study authors: *André Brunoni and Felipe Fregni*

Money won't buy happiness, but it will pay the salaries of a large research staff to study the problem.
—Bill Vaughan (1915–1977)

INTRODUCTION

In previous chapters you have learned the main aspects of designing, planning, and conducting a clinical study. By now it should be clear that clinical research is an activity that requires careful planning, right methodology, and good execution. In order to accomplish that, several requirements need to be met, including a budget that will allow the proper execution of the study. Thus, even if clinical research is mainly based on academia, at its core it is still a business and should be approached and managed as such.

In this business model, potential sources of funding (i.e., sponsors) need to be identified and research funds secured prior to the execution of the research plan. The *budget* therefore is a pivotal object for financing a research project and, depending on the sponsor, may require not only extensive justification, but also some complex negotiations.

Most researchers are not aware of the extent to which the *source of funding* can impact research. For instance, in the United States a researcher seeking funding from the government for research activities can be awarded a grant or a contract. If the researcher is awarded a grant, this means that research will be developed for public good; if instead research is funded as a contract, this will be a means of procuring a service that will benefit the contractor (in this case the government).

In the previous example, the distinction was between grants and contracts provided by the government. This distinction would even be more significant for clinical research funded by corporate interests.

THE PARTNERSHIP BETWEEN ACADEMIA AND INDUSTRY

In the aftermath of World War I, partnerships between industry and academia became increasingly popular. Pharmaceutical companies created the infrastructure to conduct their own independent research, and sought scientific expertise in academia [1].

But in 1930, the National Institutes of Health (NIH) was created in the United States, and in less than 20 years the NIH became the leading source of funding for biomedical research in academia. However, with the advent of large federal funding, there was one caveat: the ownership of discoveries and inventions made with taxpayers' money. At that point, everything that was a product of research that was funded by federal funds was "owned" by the government. This was a major limitation to the involvement of the industry in clinical research. But the plummet of research funds from the NIH in the 1970s, mainly due to the oil crisis, stock market crash, and inflation, led academic researchers to look for industry sponsorship in order to conduct their research.

But it was not until 1980, with the Bayh-Dole Act, that the relationship between industry and academia changed. This act was intended to be a competiveness and economic revitalization initiative; it followed three controversial cases in which the government asserted ownership of products from research that it had funded (Gatorade, 5-fluorouracil, and the phenylketonuria test). Probably the most interesting one was the flourouracil, an anti-neoplastic" or "cytotoxic" chemotherapy drug. The US government claimed the title of the patent because US$120 on reagents was erroneously charged from a federal grant, instead of the US$500,000 industry-sponsored grant from Roche.

This government effort of stimulating the relationship between academia and industry followed a simple premise, that in order to improve health care, the shared knowledge derived from academia research could also be applicable to industry. Thus the university becomes a unit of entrepreneurship, capitalizing on the knowledge generated by its members [2]. This change was so successful that the estimates are that around 68% of US and Canadian universities have a partnership with industry.

This has also meant that sponsors from industry are more willing to invest in research. For instance, in the United States, the NIH is probably the most well-known source of funding, but industry, as in the case of pharmaceutical and biotech companies or venture funds, are the largest investors in clinical research. In fact, data from 2007 suggests that industry was sponsoring 58% of ongoing biomedical research, comparing to 33% from NIH and other federal agencies [3]. Academia and industry can develop various forms of partnership, such as material transfer, clinical trial agreements, consortia, joint ventures, consulting, equipment loans/rentals, and spinoff companies, or by procuring a service by means of a contract.

One of the major motivations for industry-sponsored trials is that Food and Drug Administration (FDA) marketing approval requires clinical phase III trials demonstrating efficacy of the agent/device combined with reasonable safety in humans. In order to achieve this, sponsors from industry reach out to clinical researchers at academic research organizations (AROs) in order for clinical trials to be conducted. The process of approval of a new drug or device is very long, and requires multiple clinical trials until the new intervention translates "from the bench to the bedside." An Investigational New Drug/Device (IND) needs to be requested 30 days prior to the start of the first clinical trial. If in that period, or at any time point during the clinical trial execution, the FDA finds a problem with the IND, it can put it on "clinical hold" or actually interrupt the trial if it is an ongoing one. Only after several trials in which there is enough evidence of safety and efficacy on the new drug/device that matches FDA requirements for marketing approval, then a New Drug/Device Application (NDA) can be submitted. Taken into consideration all the required steps for an NDA, it is not surprising that sponsors from industry strive to protect their investments with patents or other sort of intellectual property (IP) agreements. Therefore, depending on the agreement specificity and on the institution, the ownership of data can be considered as a part of the sponsoring company's IP. Very often the sponsor claims the responsibility for data analysis and eventual publication rights. This sometimes leads to some complex negotiations between the sponsor and the ARO, as some academic institutions require having data ownership and no role of sponsor in study design, data analysis, or publication.

This has led to a blooming of specialized private businesses—contract research organizations (CROs)—in order to manage clinical trials. CROs usually promise lower costs and speedy completion of the study by breaking the study into several steps, while emphasizing the speedy completion of each step [3]. But these lower costs are achieved with some workforce qualification problems that ARO usually are not affected. Moreover, some sponsors still prefer the use of academic centers, due to their reputation, as well as the lead scientist's prestige in the scientific community.

There are mutual benefits from this academia-industry relationship. For the academy, such partnership allows the translation to clinical applications of discoveries made on the basic science field. The patents obtained during academic research can also provide a valuable source of funding for other research activities. And conducting quality clinical research is also an important training aspect for educating medical students and future researchers. For the industry, the clinical research benefits from increased credibility; reduced costs since the workforce and the laboratories are already implemented; stimulation and strengthening of the activities of R&D (research and development); competitive advantage due to access to cutting-edge technology and research; and tax credits for sponsoring academic centers (Table 20.1).

Sources of Conflicts Between Academia and Industry

However, even in the presence of mutual advantages, there is also potential for conflicts. This was showed in a survey about academy-industry agreements published by the *New England Journal of Medicine*, in which industry-academia disputes are relatively frequent, most of them involving payments (75%), followed by intellectual property (30%), and control of or access to data (17%) disagreements [4].

Such conflicts are inevitable, because there are distinct interests between the two institutions. While academia strives for excellence in research, minimizing or eliminating potential conflicts of interest, industry is motived by different senses of urgency, tighter deadlines, and trade secrecy.

These potential sources of conflict between industry and academia can be daunting for researchers, especially if they are in the middle of a tense negotiation between academic institutions and industry. In order to prevent any potential issues toward the research team, offices responsible for research in the host academic center usually lead the negotiation process with the industry sponsor, ensuring that the research team will focus on the research aspects.

Table 20.1 Academia and Industry

Academia		Industry	
Advantages	Disadvantages	Advantages	Disadvantages
Allows basic research to be applied in the interest of society	Ownership issues	Stimulate and strengthen internal R&D	Ownership issues
Potential financial rewards of patents/licenses provide a means for continued academic funding	Publication disagreements over timing and/or details of methodology	Outsourcing to CROs and AROs	Publication disagreements over timing and/or details of methodology
Training of students and future employment opportunities	Potential ethical and conflict of interest issues	Enhances credibility of research	Threatens trade secrets gained during collaboration
	Threatens freedom to pursue research topics not in interest of industry	Access to cutting-edge research provides a competitive advantage	Different senses of urgency
	May not have access to all the data generated	Can provide more inexpensive lab space Enhance research personnel	

Despite the challenges, this synergy might be beneficial for both sides, but careful and thoughtful consideration must be given when planning the agreement.

> In 2000 the University of California suffered a $7 million legal action from a biopharmaceutical company. The reason? Researchers refused to include in the manuscript the company's statistical analysis. This was an attempt to prevent negative results from being published.

Reasons for Partnership Between Academia and Industry

This case is an example of how important agreements between industry and academia are. Agreements lay the foundations for the success of the ongoing collaboration, or they will be the cornerstone that will be used to solve disputes. If in some institutions industry-sponsored clinical trials can represent up to 79% of the ongoing trials [3], the acceptability of restrictive contract provisions can be daunting. Policies regarding what is an acceptable or unacceptable demand from an industry sponsor vary across institutions. Usually, not allowing researchers to alter study design or allowing the sponsor to review the manuscript for a period of time before publication are provisions that research offices are willing to accept in industry-sponsored trials. But reviewing a manuscript written by the investigators for more than proprietary information or decisions that results should not be published are considered to be highly inadmissible by academic research offices [4,5]. Interestingly enough, academic research centers are less restrictive to practices of inserting sponsor data analysis in the manuscript (only 47% of AROs prohibit it) or sponsor manuscript draft (40% of AROs prohibit it, while 50% accept it) [4].

So the resolution of a case such as the one that opposed the University of California at San Francisco and a sponsor can only be resolved based on specific clauses of the pre-established clinical trial agreement.

CLINICAL TRIAL AGREEMENT

The International Committee of Medical Journal Editors (ICJME) requires that the author responsible for a study (see Chapter 19 for more information about authorship) state in writing that he or she was fully responsible for conducting the trial, had access to the data, and controlled the decision to publish [4]. But with an industry-estimated investment of $10.4 billion in 2004 [6], a 2002 survey of the 122 members of the American Association of Medical Colleges showed limited adherence to these recommendations [7].

Despite the fact that there are no guidelines for clinical trial agreements, universities usually use topic checklists, lists of specific and unacceptable provisions, institutional statements of principles, and often employ legal advice in these negotiations with industry [4]. Box 20.1 shows an example of topics that constitute a clinical trial agreement between academia and Industry.

Box 20.1 Structure of a Clinical Trial Agreement Between Industry and Academia

Introduction
- Scope of Work
- Performance Period

Term
Cost and Payment
Responsibilities
Confidential Information
Proprietary Rights
Publications
Indemnification
Study Drug/Device and Materials
General
Amendments
Counterparts
Assignment
Compliance with Law
Arbitration
Insurance
Limitation of Liability
Parties' Relationship
Term and Termination of Agreement
Notice
Disputes

COST AND PAYMENTS

Clinical research is expensive. Data from oncology trials in Ontario, Canada, suggests that the in 2005, the cost per patient for an industry-sponsored trial could be as high as $11,304 [7]. These costs include not only the cost of the drugs and compensation to subjects, but also to the research team and labs, among others.

When sponsoring academia research, industry usually supports several direct and indirect costs. These costs vary across institutions and countries, with great influence on the costs of conducting research. The direct costs are those related directly to the proposed project, namely personnel, consumables, laboratory costs, equipment, services to be acquired, travel, and publication charges. On the other hand, indirect costs are those that are not directly related to the project, but are incurred by the ARO during the project, namely accounting, payroll, building maintenance, utilities, and department and institutional costs, among others. These indirect costs can impact the overall costs of research, as usually they reflect a fixed percentage of the direct costs. For instance, if a research budget for a five-year study is US$1 million in direct costs and the research office of the university has negotiated a 59% rate for indirect costs (also known as overhead), the total cost to be included in the budget will be US$1.59 million. Table 20.2 summarizes the costs that usually need to be included in the contract.

Table 20.2 Budget Costs Definitions

Type of Expense	
IRB/Ethics Committee	IRB/Ethics Committee is usually required prior to the initiation for a drug/device trial. The process of submission, amendments, and reporting of serious adverse events is very time-consuming. Also some IRBs have fees associated with the approval of a protocol. It is the responsibility of the research team to include in the budget the costs of the IRB process.
Overhead/Indirect Costs	Varies from institution to institution, and usually has a negotiated rate with the sponsor. Usually these costs include the rent, building maintenance, utilities, equipment depreciation, and department/institutional costs.
Staff Labor/Training	Usually represents the largest portion of a clinical trial budget. In a clinical trial this can include researchers, nurse coordinators, research assistants, administrative staff, and consultants (e.g., biostatistician). The actual level of the expense will be determined by the sample size, the trial design (e.g., single-blinded design requires less staff than a double-blinded design), the intervention and assessments (whether they can be performed by a research assistant, or only by a medical doctor).
Patient Recruitment/Participation	Costs of advertisement and the enrollment of potential patients, as well as incentives for adherence and participation, should also be in the budget.

Table 20.2 Continued

Type of Expense	
Laboratory Costs	A clinical trial can use several surrogate markers in order to validate the effects of the intervention. The clinical trial can require blood, urine, or other type of biological/genetic samples, and thus it is important to include theses costs in the budget.
Pharmacy Costs	An investigational drug can have several pharmacy costs, such as preparation, storage, dispensation, and accounting. Pharmacy quotes detailing all the costs and staff training (if required) should be included in the budget.
Equipment/Supply Costs	The required equipment to conduct research that is not already available at the institution. If the equipment is already available, then its depreciation should be included. The supplies include reagents and any other type of consumables that are required to perform the clinical trial.
Travel/Missions	Include the required travel between sites, to present in conferences or field work if required.
Publication Expenses	In the budget any fee associated with language editing or open access publication should be included.
Patient Follow-up	Assessing outcomes and serious adverse events has it costs and should also be in the budget.

This process of budgeting ends with the execution of the study contract. This study contract should weight the number of patients to be enrolled, and the level of effort of the research team, as well as any fiscal obligations that may occur during the trial. Also, there should be a payment schedule. The payment could be made based upon the achievement of agreed-upon milestones, or at regular intervals. Also, will there be start-up money to initiate the study before the first patient enrollment? For instance, if training is required for the research team, or if advertisement is required before the first patient is enrolled, are there funds to start the protocol? Also, there should be a provision for screen fails, as even if they are not enrolled in the study, there are costs associated with their eligibility evaluation. Finally, if it is a multi-year protocol (the most common one in clinical research), the costs should be corrected for inflation.

GOVERNMENT FUNDING MECHANISMS FOR INDUSTRY

So far in this chapter we have been focusing on the contract agreement between industry and academia, in which industry supports monetarily the development of a trial by an ARO or a CRO. But in some situations it may be possible that centers from industry (especially small businesses) apply for government-provided R&D funds. For instance, in the United States, small businesses can apply to the Small Business Innovation Research (SBIR) program, in order to develop a product that has a potential for commercialization. Similarly, in the Small Business Technology

Transfer (STTR) program, academia and small businesses develop joint applications in order to help translate science from "the bench to the bedside."

CONTRACT PROVISIONS

Although budget is essential in a clinical trial agreement, there will also be a series of provisions that can be the source of conflicts between academic institutions and industry sponsors. Typically, these contract provisions include intellectual property, publication rights, medical care in case of adverse events, and indemnification.

Intellectual Property

One of the main missions of academia revolves around the dissemination of new knowledge from R&D and training. In the majority of agreements, the industry sponsor retains the IP right for what is specified in the protocol or investigator brochure (Box 20.2). So, new IP that may be developed during a study is not necessarily property of the industry sponsor, if not otherwise specified in the contract. In the cases where new IP is not specified clearly in the contract, general patent law applies, and thus the patent title holder will be the one that developed the new IP. As a gesture of good faith, the industry sponsor of a trial in which new IP was developed may be given the first option to enter into negotiations for the ownership of the new IP, even in the absence of a provision clearly specifying that. Other options could be to give the sponsor a limited period to license the new IP, otherwise it will have forfeited any rights to it; or even to reach an agreement to have a fair license agreement in which the relative contribution of each partner is assured.

The industry has a different position on this matter, as its main goal is to commercialize inventions, and thus if an invention during a trial is related to the study drug/device, then the company should own all the rights related to it. Also industry sponsors generally believe that if they fail to license the product during the option period, the company should nonetheless retain the right to match a third party's license offer. This assumption is in line with the company's "vision" that without access to the IND, the research team will not be able to make that discovery, and thus it should retain the rights to at least match a license offer from a third party.

A contract should state
Scope of the definition of inventions
Disclosure of inventions/discoveries/improvements
Ownership of inventions/discoveries/improvements in the scope of the project
Ownership of inventions/discoveries/improvements not in the scope of the project (e.g., outside the protocol, serendipitous in the course of following the protocol)
Allowed time to exercise option for licensure/match offer from a third party
Type of licensure (e.g., exclusive)
Who will be responsible for the patent costs
Statement about what is not covered by the contract

Publications

Publishing the results of a trial is how in science the dissemination of research is performed. So the general agreement is that if the industry sponsor has more than a certain amount of control over the content and decision to publish, then the article will not be accepted by high-impact peer-reviewed journals. So in academia the dominant vision is that the sponsor from industry should not restrict publication in any way. If accepted, these restrictions would prevent the academic institution from reaching its goal: public dissemination of knowledge.

Thus the principal investigator (PI) in the academic institution should have full access to the data, and will be held responsible for the integrity of the data, any analysis performed, as well as the conclusions from the trial. But academic institutions cannot willingly or knowingly jeopardize any IP property from the sponsor if that is stated in the confidentiality agreement. Thus, the sponsor's objections to the contents of a manuscript should be related to what has been marked as "confidential information" or that may affect the sponsor's IP property or ability to protect any patents.

In the advent of a sponsor objecting to data publication, the academic institution will undertake serious efforts to revert that objection. The ARO can try to find a mediator for the dispute, with a pre-specified time for resolution (usually brief); can decide to go ahead with the publication; or can try to mobilize a publication committee, in which one of the members will be an industry representative, but the majority of the committee will be constituted by independent representatives.

Industry generally is interested in the timely communication of important results. It also has responsibilities in the study design, as well as the integrity of the data. Also, industry owns the database from large multi-center trials that it has sponsored. So usually the industry shares this interest with academia, with the possible exception of basic science trials or even exploratory trials with the primary purpose of generating trials for future research, in which results are not immediately available except for those that can potentially have significant medical importance.

A contract should state

PI/academic institution's right to publish/present or otherwise disseminate the knowledge obtained from the trial
Definition of "confidential information"
If a multi-site study, PI/academic institution's access to data from other sites
Authorship in multi-center trials
Specific requirements for single-site publication in a multi-site trial
Early publication for reasons of public health, safety, or public welfare
Sponsor's right to manuscript review/allowed comments/allowed time for review
Sponsor's time to withhold publication

Indemnification

Indemnification is the term for designating that one party will be responsible for the costs incurred for losses by a second one. In research this second party can be the research subjects in case something harmful happens to them while they are being tested for the IND. The general agreement is that when testing an IND, AROs indemnify and hold the sponsor harmless for any misconduct, negligence, or any intentional acts from their own employees/agents. On the other hand, the industry sponsor will be willingly to indemnify the ARO for protocol-related injuries to patients.

> **A contract should state**
> List of indemnitees: whom the sponsor indemnifies and holds harmless
> Conditions for indemnification (such as claims)
> Exceptions to indemnification per non-compliance
> Scope of indemnification, insurance requirements, survival of obligation to indemnify
> Who will control the defense in the advent of a lawsuit, who pays and in which conditions

Medical Care in the Case of an Adverse Event

Another important topic is who should be accountable if during a clinical trial, medical attention is required for a patient due to an adverse event. The main debate is how much the sponsor should be responsible for—the full amount, or only the portion that is not covered by subject's insurance (or by the government). In some cases, private insurers could even not allow certain procedures from being performed based on the subscribed health-care plan or could forbid any type of billing from non-covered procedures. In those cases, it may happen that the industry sponsor ended up without covering any health-care costs directly related to the IND. This would be unethical and, for some academic institutions, completely inadmissible. Also there should not be any cap for the sponsor's liability in terms of health-care costs, nor unthoughtful claims of patient negligence from the sponsor. "Patient negligence" could indeed signal an (un)expected adverse event of the IND. Patient negligence should only be claimed when there is enough proof that the patient willfully failed to comply with the study protocol. This should be clear in the contract, as well as in the informed consent. Moreover, if the IRB gives the sponsor an exemption from this policy, this needs to be clearly defined in the informed consent to be signed by patients.

Another important issue for the industry sponsor in the case of chronic conditions is how long the sponsor should provide the IND to patients, if the IND has proven to be efficacious for that specific chronic condition. In some countries, industry sponsors are obligated to provide the drug free of charge for the entire life of the subjects. In others, like the United States, usually the obligation ends as soon as the FDA approves the new drug/device.

> **A contract should state**
> As per FDA [8] requirements, serious adverse events should be reported as soon as possible and not exceeding 15 days after PI's awareness. IRB and sponsor should also be notified.
> FDA Investigational New Drug Application (IND), 2017
> Scope of medical expenses that will or will not be covered
> The extent to which subject's insurance coverage may or may not be used to pay for study-related health-care expenses
> Sponsor's agreement about what to do in the advent of a study-related adverse event
> Circumstances under which sponsor will decline any payment/costs.
> Sponsor's obligation to provide ongoing care for efficacious drugs in chronic disorders.

CASE STUDY: THE BUSINESS OF CLINICAL RESEARCH—A STANDOFF IN THE CITY OF LIGHTS

André Brunoni and Felipe Fregni

Goethe's *Faust*

Jean-Luc would be a brilliant scientist if he had decided to stay in academia, but he was more interested in having a "rich future"—that was the opinion of Dr. Jean-Luc Richelieu's colleagues just after he finished his postdoctoral fellowship in Munich. Indeed, his CV was impressive: medical school at the Faculté de Médecine Paris Descartes, residence in neuropsychiatry at the King's College (London), doctorate in neuroscience from MIT (Boston), besides the postdoctoral fellowship in Munich. However, to accept the job proposal from a medium-size pharmaceutical company Psychotics™ to become medical director was beyond doubt for Dr. Richelieu: living in Paris, his beloved city, in a big house, with a big salary and a lot of glamour. But Dr. Richelieu soon realized there is no free lunch—three weeks after being hired, the CEO of Psychotics™ invited him for a business talk, "Jean-Luc, I have big plans for you. You know we hired you because you are brilliant, studied in top-notch universities, have a good influence in academic circles and can speak fluently French, English, and German. I will make you the golden boy of Psychotics™."

"As you know, the aim of our pharmaceutical company is to increase our market share of psychiatric drugs in France. We are developing a new antipsychotic drug called Serenium to be used as a treatment for insomnia. Our pharmacists have been working with the first antipsychotic drug—Chlorpromazine —which as you know was first tested in the Parisian hospitals. They changed its molecular structure in order to enhance its sedative effects while diminishing its extrapiramidal side effects—we plan to re-launch the drug in the market after the confirmatory clinical trials."

"Wait—" Jean-Luc interrupted, "Chlorpromazine was synthesized by the Rhone-Poulenc laboratories which is now Sanofi-Aventis (a huge pharmaceutical industry). Can we use their drug? Are we not violating intellectual properties?"

The CEO answered gently, managing his anger, "Yes, it was synthesized by Rhone-Poulenc—60 years ago! As you know, drug patents are valid for only a few years. In fact, drug patents grant 20 years of protection on average, and given that they are applied for before clinical trials start, the effective life of a drug patent tends to be shorter than that: between 7 and 12 years. So we are all set and it is OK to use—in addition, by changing the molecular structure of this drug we will gain a new patent. Besides, as the new compound is similar to the old compounds, we also can use some of the safety and efficacy data from the old drug that were confirmed by our recent phase I and II trials. Now we need to go straight ahead to a big, multi-center, phase III trial—which you, Jean-Luc, are going to lead! Congratulations! This is a big opportunity to show us what you are able to do."

Those words remained in Jean-Luc's head for a while: "show us what you are able to do." He knew this was the major test of his reputation as the company was depending on the success of this trial in order to remain alive and healthy. He thought aloud, "four to five years from now, if this does not work, I may be doing the second mortgage of my house and selling my car to pay the bills."

The Other Side: Academia

Since the meeting with the CEO, Jean-Luc knew that the clock was ticking and he was constantly planning the next steps. After some thought, he had drafted the main plan, which consisted of having a main academic center oversee this multi-center trial. The other centers then would be coordinated by this main academic center. He chose UCLA as the main academic center and Prof. Gregor Briggs—a renowned psychiatrist who has led many large clinical trials—as coordinator. Jean-Luc did not waste one

---

Box 20.2 Intellectual Property

Intellectual property (IP) is a legal form of establishing that creations of the human mind in its industrial, artistic, and scientific activities are kept as physical objects. In each country, a number of laws allow that inventors limit the use of their ideas.

The need for protection laws that ensure the IP is based on two main goals: to give statutory expression to these creations and promote their economic and social applicability [8].

Intellectual property is usually divided into two major areas: copyright and industrial property. While copyright refers mainly to artistic and scientific productions, industrial property refers to inventions, industrial designs, trademarks, and trade names.

In the area of clinical research, the most common objects of intellectual property protection are categorized as patents, copyrights, and trademarks.

1. Patent: a document issued by an official and specialized government agency that describes an invention and ensures that it is exploited only with the prior permission of the patent holder. This right of ownership has a limited time that can range, but is usually 20 years. To qualify for a patent some characteristics must be fulfilled by the invention: applicability and utility, novelty, non-obvious, and of major importance.
2. Copyright: aims to protect the expression of ideas and not the ideas themselves. It Controls reproduction, public performance, translation, and adaptation of a work. It is assigned for a period of time, which in most countries it starts in the moment of creation to a limited time after the author's death. It is also important to remember that copyright is limited to the geographic extent of the country in which it is registered, although the existence of some international agreements may facilitate the maintenance of these rights. Each country has its own measures to restrain any infringement of those rights, which can range from civil reparations to penal actions that result in imprisonment.
3. Trademarks: signals that allow the distinction of origin of a product. Most countries limit the record to graphical representations, although there is a system of international registration of marks.

Although each country has its laws and departments for the policies of intellectual property protection, the application process begins through a request form that will be examined by the patent office and once under the previous provisions will be registered by the organ responsible.

more minute and contacted Prof. Briggs immediately, who was favorable to the idea initially but wanted to meet to talk about details.

This agreement could be favorable to Prof. Briggs as he had a recent meeting with the dean of medicine—James Tarsy—in which the main topic was how to increase collaboration between academia and industry. In this meeting, the dean mentioned, "As you know, Greg, our university has a long history of collaboration with industry that generated many products to the open market that have improved the quality of life of our citizens. And in fact, this is how I see the role of university: to give back as much as possible to society. But in order to do that, we need to increase our collaboration with industry. That will be one of the flags of my tenure at UCLA. In addition we are losing good faculty to industry, and this can be avoided. On the other hand, we need to defend our interests and guarantee that the agreements we make with industry are good for us as well." Thus, Prof. Briggs saw the recent conversation with Jean-Luc as a great opportunity, but he knew he would need to be careful in this interaction.

The Negotiation Table

One month later, Psychotics™ sponsored a one-week symposium (Serenity, Serendipity, Serenium—because your patient can sleep tight) in a five-star hotel in Paris. Jean-Luc hosted the guests, who were among the most influential names in psychiatry. Before their arrival in Paris, Dr. Richelieu spoke to his staff, "This should be done perfectly as we are hoping to invite our guests to participate in a multi-center randomized trial to test Serenium versus standard therapy. But before doing so, we need to have a detailed conversation with Prof. Briggs, as the main agreement will be decided with him. Let us reserve a nice conference room in the hotel to decide on the main aspects of this agreement. Let us do this the day before the conference, after Prof. Briggs's arrival."

As planned, Prof. Briggs arrived from a long flight from the West Coast to Europe. Unfortunately there were no direct flights, and the connections spoiled the chance of Prof. Briggs to rest during the flights; adding the jet lag, he was not at his best, but he was looking forward to the first round of negotiations.

The next morning, everyone was waiting anxiously for Prof. Briggs. When he arrived, Jean-Luc gave him a warm greeting, "My dear colleague, it is a pleasure to have you here. I hope everything is going well." And not waiting much longer, he continued, "As you know we have a tight schedule, let us go directly to business." After the initial words of Prof. Briggs, Jean-Luc started with a summary of the project, "We aim to perform a large phase-III multi-center trial comparing Serenium versus standard therapy. We are prepared to pay all the study-related costs, including personnel, patient fees, quality assurance, and training. We are going to train all researchers of participating centers here in Paris to guarantee internal validity of our study. We also expect to sponsor the researchers to present the results in international symposiums and local seminaries. The role of the centers will involve recruitment and selection of the sample, and to set a working research center. The idea is to start data collection in 9 months and conclude in 18 months. As you know, we need to launch this drug to the market as soon as possible."

After this initial introduction, Prof. Briggs then spoke, "Thank you Jean-Luc, we have a very good opportunity here. This might be clearly a win-win situation, and we are looking forward to working with your company. But we need to discuss in detail four important topics: (1) intellectual property; (2) rights to the data and publication; (3) payments; (4) performance period, time to complete the study. I know these are delicate topics but we need to discuss them very carefully."

He then continued, "Let us start with intellectual property. As you know, in the United States the Bayh-Dole Act grants universities permission to retain intellectual property rights to inventions resulting from federally supported research—and even to license these inventions to private industry for commercialization. As you know, the idea of the Bayh-Dole Act is to motivate researchers to continue investigating new compounds. Although your company may cover the expenses of this trial, most of the researchers involved will also have federal grants, and some of our equipment (for instance, computers and software) was bought with taxpayers' money. Finally, I would like to help with the design, indication, and dosage of this drug, as treatment of insomnia with antipsychotics is the main line of my research; therefore, I think it would be fair if we share the intellectual property of this trial." This comment created a level of discomfort in the room. Jean-Luc was afraid that he was starting to lose control of the situation and quickly replied, "I think this is a good point. The main issue here is that our company created this compound and made the initial testing; so it would not be adequate to share the intellectual property given that all the creation was done in our company. But I would suggest that we should move to the next point: rights to the data and publication."

Jean-Luc then decided to use a technique of negotiation: when a topic is not progressing well, quickly move to the next topic so as to avoid an increase in tension. He then proceeded, "Regarding the data, because we are sponsoring the trial, all data should be immediately disclosed to us and, as you know, we want the data to be published, but we will write the manuscript and give the academic centers the opportunity to review the manuscripts in a period of 60 days. We will not allow independent publication in order to avoid the disclosure of any confidential information." It seemed that the mood in the room had not improved, as Prof. Briggs also quickly replied, "I understand your position, Jean. But this is not what we are used to, nor is it what we like to do. We usually do the opposite: we have the right to write and publish the results of the study, and prior to the submission of the publication we will send the manuscript to you for your review, and we also would like to have the right to publish a small subset of the data if we want to do so." It seemed that the negotiation was not going well as they had reached another roadblock. Jean-Luc was then betting that the remaining topics would improve the situation.

Jean-Luc then, feeling a bit frustrated, started, "Well, Greg, let us then see if we agree on payments and deadlines! I think this will be an easy one as we are willing to cover all the study-related costs. The protocol used by our company is that we pay one-quarter of the budget after IRB approval and then pay the second quarter after 50% enrollment, the 3rd quarter after 80% enrollment, and the last allotment after the final enrollment and transfer of the data. We would need to have the enrollment done in 9 months and we would withhold part of the budget if there are delays." Judging by Prof. Biggs's expression, this seemed to have not gone well either. He then replied, "We may have a problem here, too. I think 9 months is not enough for us and even considering that we will have other centers. You know that it is becoming increasingly difficult to have patients participating in trials, and in addition our ethics committee might delay the start of the project. If we make the budget dependent on enrollment, then we will have a problem with the fixed costs of the trials—such as salary for the personnel involved in the trial, like the co-investigators and research coordinators. Indeed, if the budget decreases with a delay of the trial, then we will have a big problem with salaries in our institution. We also need to review this."

After this initial round of conversation, both of them were emotionally drained.

The situation had not gone as planned by Jean-Luc. He felt discouraged but decided to end this meeting and take Professor Briggs on a nice tour in Paris—that was his last ace in the hole—perhaps Paris, the city of lights, would improve the chances of reaching an agreement for both sides.

CASE DISCUSSION

Jean-Luc had the potential to become a gifted scientist, but chose instead to become an executive in a pharmaceutical company. His first challenge, in his new role, is to lead a trial to test a new drug named Serenium. This new drug is a modification of Chlorpromazine, the first antipsychotic drug that was developed more than 60 years ago. Previous phase I and II trials have already shown its efficacy and safety for insomnia, and thus the company thinks that now is the time to sponsor a large phase III, multi-center, randomized clinical trial for regulatory approval.

To conduct this study, Jean-Luc invites Prof. Briggs, a world-renowned psychiatrist, with a vast experience in clinical trials. This could be a win-win situation for both parties: academia and industry. Industry benefits from the expertise of Prof. Briggs, while academia will benefit from the resources of the industry to conduct a clinical trial. Despite the advantageous situation, there are four key elements that distinguish industry from academia: (1) intellectual property (IP); (2) rights to the data and publication; (3) payments; (4) performance period.

As already mentioned in this chapter, IP is an important matter for both parties. Industry thinks that it needs to protect its IP and that new IP developed during the course of an ongoing research should also belong to its IP portfolio. For academia, new IP developed during the clinical trial does not necessarily belong to the sponsor, even if the sponsor is the federal government (cf., Bayh-Dole act). So the question here is what to do with new IP that can arise from this trial.

The second point in which industry and academia see themselves on different trenches is in the publication rights. Who has the right to publish? Usually the sponsor owns the database of the trial that it sponsored. But that does not necessarily mean that it owns the data that arise from research. As we discussed previously, some industry sponsors want to keep control of publications that arise from sponsored trials, as these will be determinant for the future commercialization of their product. But the general vision in academia is that, apart from "confidential information" that could jeopardize the sponsor's IP, all the decisions about the manuscript should belong to the ARO. The sponsor could be given a period to review the manuscript, but should limit its comments to topics that could limit its ability to commercialize the product.

The budget and the payment plan can be another source of potential conflict between industry and academia, simply because of different goals and timings. Industry is concerned with commercialization of the drug/device, so wants to disseminate the results as soon as possible. In order to achieve that, sponsors from industry attempt to impose payment milestones for academia, in order to achieve their goal. So payments by objectives, or payment withholds, are common tactics that industry employs over the sponsored academic research centers. But, again, the focus of academia is not to commercialize products, but instead to train people and create and disseminate knowledge. That means that getting paid by objectives will limit academia's ability to keep staff, especially if enrollment goes below the one anticipated. This is interconnected with the last point: the performance period. The sponsor from industry plans a duration of the trial, which very often is not realistic for the ARO. And there are many possible reasons for that: the academic research center is focused on different trials; the IRB/ethics committee may delay the start of the trial, even if amendments to the original protocol are not required. For instance, if there is no agreement in place between IRBs from different institutions, it may be possible that each performance site involved in a multi-center trial may be required to secure an independent IRB approval. If that is the case, any modification required by one of the IRBs needs to be accepted by all of them. This can be time-consuming, and thus can actively endanger a study performance period.

CASE QUESTIONS FOR REFLECTION

1. What are the issues involved in this case that should be considered by both parties in order to make an agreement?
2. What are the concerns for the university? And for the company?
3. Should both walk away or try to negotiate?
4. Do you think it is possible to establish a "win-win" relationship among the company and the university?
5. Have you seen or been in a similar situation?

FURTHER READING

Papers

To deepen the movement of translational research obtaining historical data, financing models, and career building:

- Translational research: getting the message across. *Nature.* 2008; 453(7197): 839. doi:10.1038/453839a
- Nathan DG. Careers in translational clinical research—historical perspectives, future challenges. *JAMA.* 2002 May 8; 287(18): 2424–2427.

Porter P, Longmire B, Abrol A. Negotiating clinical trial agreements: bridging the gap between institutions and companies." *J Health Life Sci Law.* April 2009; 121.

Mello M, Claridge B, Studdert D. Academic medical centers' standards for clinical trial agreements with industry. *N Engl J Med.* 2005 May 26; 352: 2202–2210.

Online Information

- http://hms.harvard.edu/content/hmshsdm-fcoi-policy-sponsored-research—Example from Harvard Medical School about policy on the relationship between industry and academia.

- http://www.wipo.int/about-ip/en—A world intellectual property organization, where you can found more information about this topic.
- http://www.mrc.ac.uk/Ourresearch/MRCIndustry/index.htm—UK organization whose goal is to improve human health through research. The site has interesting information on policy, training, and opportunities in partnership with industry.
- http://www.bostonreview.net/BR35.3/angell.php—Dr. Angell, former *New England Journal of Medicine* editor-in-chief and now senior lecturer in social medicine at Harvard Medical School, comments on the partnership of academia and industry.
- http://www.newyorker.com/reporting/2009/06/01/090601fa_fact_lepore?currentPage=all—The Parrot Fever Pandemic of 1930 and the "Hygienic Laboratory."
- www.dcri.duke.edu/ccge/contracts—Example of a Clinical Trial Agreement.

Books

- In: Gallin JI, Ognibene F. *Principles and practice of clinical research*, 2nd ed. New York: Elsevier; 2007: 341–350.

REFERENCES

1. Swann JP. *Academic scientists and the pharmaceutical industry cooperative research in twentieth-century America*. Baltimore, MD: Johns Hopkins University Press; 1988.
2. Dorsey E, de Roulet J, Thompson JP, et al. Funding of us biomedical research, 2003–2008. *JAMA*. 2010; 303(2): 137–143.
3. Shuchman M. Commercializing clinical trials—risks and benefits of the CRO boom. *N Engl J Med*. 2007; 357(14): 1365–1368.
4. Mello MM, Clarridge BR, Studdert DM. Academic medical centers' standards for clinical-trial agreements with industry. *N Engl J Med*. 2005; 352(21): 2202–2210.
5. Steinbrook R. Gag clauses in clinical-trial agreements. *N Engl J Med*. 2005; 352(21): 2160–2162.
6. Wright JR, Roche K, Smuck B, Cormier J, Cecchetto S, Akow M, et al. Estimating per patient funding for cancer clinical trials: an Ontario based survey. *Contemp Clinical Trials*. 2005; 26(4): 421–429.
7. WIPO Intellectual Property Handbook. Word Intellectual Property Organization. Second Edition. ISBN 978-92-805-1291-5
8. FDA Investigational New Drug Application (IND), 21 CFR § 312.32 (2017).

21

DESIGN AND ANALYSIS OF SURVEYS

Authors: *Ana R. Martins and Inês C. R. Henriques*[1]

Case study authors: *André Brunoni and Felipe Fregni*

Quand on ne sait pas ce que l'on cherche, on ne voit pas ce que l'on trouve.
[If you do not know what you are looking for, you do not see what you have found.]
—Claude Bernard (French physiologist, 1813–1878)

INTRODUCTION

Surveys are often used in clinical research. A survey could be defined as a method where information is obtained from a sample of individuals through a series of questions. This definition already contains the key elements of a survey: the goal of a survey is to gain knowledge on a certain topic; a sample is defined and selected as a representative part of a target population; data are collected through a number of questions using interviews or questionnaires.

In medical research, surveys are used in descriptive, exploratory, and experimental studies to assess parameters such as quality of life, pain levels, and mental health. While measurements in experimental and observational studies yield objective data with explanatory weight, information collected through surveys is subjective and mostly descriptive. This might be one reason why surveys are not given the credit and attention they deserve. Another reason might be that researchers tend to assume that design and analysis of a survey is rather trivial. A further problem is the lack of reporting guidelines of survey research [1], which makes it difficult to assess the quality of a survey and the true implications of its findings

In fact, survey research involves many methodological challenges, which may strongly influence the quality of the survey results. Nevertheless, survey data can generate many interesting new questions and provide new insights, consequently leading to new hypotheses and further research studies.

In this chapter, we discuss the most important aspects of designing, administrating, and analyzing surveys in clinical research and highlight important points to consider. We provide a general overview of each of the following main stages of survey research:

1. Design and planning phase
   - Defining the aim(s) of the survey study

---

[1] Both authors contributed equally to the work presented in this chapter.

- Sample design
2. Instrument design
   - Method for survey administration, data collection, and data capture
3. Data analysis

We also discuss problems and pitfalls, as well as legal and ethical issues when conducting survey research. Since this chapter cannot replace an entire book about survey research, we refer to external sources to complement this chapter. We hope that at the end of the chapter you will be able to better interpret published surveys, will have higher appreciation of the information provided in surveys, and will be better prepared for conducting your own survey research. Although very few investigators will design a survey throughout their research career, most of the clinical researchers will use a survey in their research; thus learning the methodology of surveys will help the investigators to use this instrument adequately.

DESIGN

Defining the Aim(s) of the Survey Study

As discussed in Chapter 2, you should start your research project by defining your research question. What are your aims? What are the specific objectives? What is the purpose of your study? Do you have a hypothesis? Do you want to explore a relationship, or do you just want to describe a condition or trend? Defining the aims is necessary in order to select the appropriate primary outcome, the target population, and a suitable survey design. A common mistake is that researchers instead start with the instrument design based on the topic of interest, and then try to make the other parts of the survey design fit to it.

An example for an experimental use of a survey is a study by Schron et al. where a questionnaire was used to compare the quality of life (QoL) of patients on antiarrhythmic drug (ADD) therapy versus patients with implantable cardioverter defibrillator (ICD). While the survival benefit of ICDs is unquestionable, this study tried to answer what impact each treatment has on patients' QoL [2].

A recent study in the *New England Journal of Medicine* surveyed residency program directors regarding the effect of the new Accreditation Council for Graduate Medical Education (ACGME) rules one year after implementation [3]. This is an example of an exploratory study. The purpose of this study was to evaluate if there is a relationship between implementation of the new ACGME rules and changes (good or bad) perceived by the residency program directors in regard to patient care, resident education, and quality of life.

As discussed in the previous chapter, the investigator designing a survey must have a clear idea of the objectives of that survey: *What is it measuring? How is it going to be used? In what population is the survey going to be used?* Based on the goals, the investigator can design an appropriate survey.

Instrument Design

Stage 1: Planning and Development

Through surveys, data are collected in a systematic way, generally based on a standardized assessment instrument [4]. This instrument is either an interview or a self-completion questionnaire. The conception of the instrument requires careful planning and design, as the format and order of the questions may influence the respondent's answer and thus produce biased results.

Before starting to design the survey instrument, you should collect some background data of your research topic and consult the literature, searching for instruments used in previous studies. You should then decide whether they can be applied or adapted to your survey. If there are instruments that can be applied, it is necessary to consider and make adjustments according to the differences of the target population and the specific objectives of your survey. Even if no suitable instrument exists, examples from the literature may raise thoughtful insights into the development of a new instrument.

Questions

A well-designed survey instrument consists of questions that are

- Brief, direct, and clear: Avoid complex questions that may be misunderstood and questions that allow for more than one specific answer. Use neutral language and avoid unclear definitions or use of uncommon terms.
- Unambiguous: Avoid double-barreled questions, which may lead to misunderstanding and incorrect answers (e.g., "Do you have problems with climbing stairs or do you have chest pain?" A person might give the desired answer when she has congestive heart failure, but if the person has sprained her leg, you will receive an answer that will lead you to a wrong conclusion).
- Directed to address the main research question: Non-specific questions lead to lack of interest and influence the instrument validity.
- Valid and reliable: Measure what is intended to measure (internal validity).
- Attention and interest catching: Questions should be following a sequence from neutral and general items to more specific and sensitive questions, respecting a logical and congruent sequence.

Questions should be written so that responses given will help answer the research question. If the aim of the study is to test or confirm a specific hypothesis, attention has to be paid not to bias answers by providing an answer choice that is more likely to be chosen since it suggests what the study's hypothesis is. Similarly, leading questions that skew answer choices should be rephrased as unbiased questions by removing leading phrases (*doctors believe* that acupuncture . . .) or judgmental wording (*should, ought to, bad, wonderful*, etc.).

Validity and Reliability

Validity reflects the degree to which a question can truly assess the desired information. For example, asking age in years will provide answers with very high validity. On the other hand, how can you assess or measure QoL? How happy a person declares himself? How much money she makes? Each answer alone might not have high validity to reflect QoL, which is the reason that multiple questions are asked to increase the overall validity.

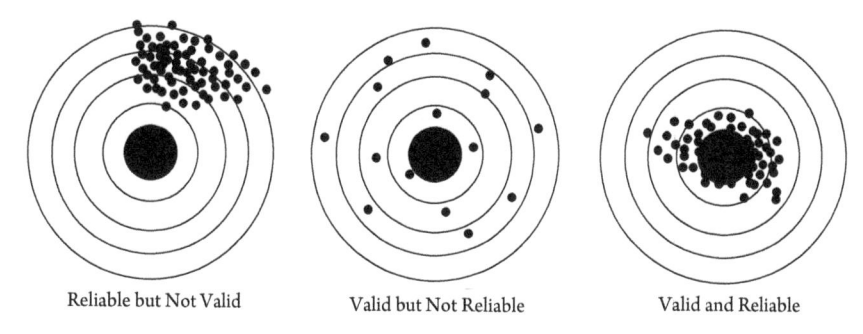

Reliable but Not Valid   Valid but Not Reliable   Valid and Reliable

Figure 21.1. Reliability versus validity.
Source: http://ccnmtl.columbia.edu/projects/qmss/measurement/validity_and_reliability.html

Reliability reflects the degree of how likely a question would be answered in the same way if repeated. It is a measure of consistency and precision. A clearly asked question will yield a higher reliability. But a question that is ambiguous or asks something not well known will cause a participant to guess, introducing random error and therefore reducing reproducibility. High reliability, however, does not automatically mean high validity (Figure 21.1). A question can generate reliable answers that have no validity (e.g., asking kindergarten children if they prefer chocolate milk or regular milk as a question to assess what drinks should be provided in the cafeteria).

The length of the instrument also deserves careful consideration, as very lengthy and time-consuming questionnaires or interviews are less likely to raise interest and motivation, leading to imprecise, wrong, or random answers, or even no responses at all. In this context, short instruments can actually be more valid than longer instruments.

Question and Answer Types

Open-Ended Questions Open-ended questions allow subjects to answer in their own words. The major advantage of using this type of questions is the amount of information that can be extracted. Answer choices can bring up topics that were not anticipated, with the potential to stimulate new ideas, but that might also be irrelevant to the research questions. Additionally, due to the broad range of possible answers, analysis and interpretation are more difficult (and time-consuming), Open-ended questions are typically used in unstructured interviews.

Closed-Ended questions More commonly used are closed-ended questions, in which the respondents choose from a set of defined answer choices. Data derived from closed-ended questions are easier to quantify and analyze. However, closed-ended questions by their nature limit answer choices, and the recorded answer therefore might not correctly reflect what the participant really thinks if an important answer choice is not anticipated and therefore not included. This would diminish the validity of a question, but can be alleviated by including an "other" response choice or "not available/applicable." Closed-ended questions are preferred when designing structured instruments [5].

Answer Types Nominal answers can be either categorical (e.g., race) or multiple choice (e.g., past medical diseases).

Ordinal answers reflect a rank order (e.g., rank the following items from 1 to 7 as how important they are for your happiness, with 1 being the most important and 7 the least important item to you: money, child(ren), reputation, education, health, spouse, food).

Interval answers reflect an order and are evenly spaced (e.g., age: 16–25, 26–35, 36–45).

Numerical answers are continuous variables that have a meaningful zero and are usually open-ended (e.g., what is your height in centimeters?).

Response scales (e.g., Likert scales—scales with several rating options of agreement or disagreement) are usually used to record attitudes or values in a series of questions that ask for favorable and unfavorable characteristics [6].

When constructing the survey, consider who your target population is. Do you think language might be a problem for them? Should you translate the survey or use pictograms instead or in addition to words? It is also important to match the layout/graphical presentation to your target population. The graphical design should motivate participants to complete the survey and improve clarity and easiness to answer (e.g., how many questions are presented on one page, do you arrange answer choices in a grid, maybe a slider is helpful, maybe a progress bar, etc.).

Structure

A brief introduction should summarize the purpose of the survey and include a confidentiality statement. An estimate of the time required to complete the survey should be provided (in electronic questionnaires a progress bar would be useful).

Following is the main body of the survey with the set of questions, best grouped into subsets.

The order of questions is important. Demographic questions should be asked at the end, taking into consideration that the participant may be exhausted after a long survey and therefore less challenging questions can be more easily answered toward the end. Asking demographics might be felt personal or intrusive and may make participants defensive and therefore alter the answer pattern of the survey. On the other hand, if demographic information is important for the analysis (e.g., subgroup analysis, adjusting for gender), the questions might be put at the beginning, to make sure that those questions are answered, in case there is a chance of not finishing a survey.

The end of the survey can conclude with a short summary of how the answers will be used and a thank you statement. If deemed useful, permission to re-contact can be asked for.

Stage 2: Pre-test and Validation

Once you have designed your survey instrument, either entirely from scratch or through adaptation, it is mandatory to test it before using it in your final study. Also, if established instruments are used, it may be warranted to perform a pre-test. The questionnaire or interview is applied to a small pre-test sample drawn from the target population (5–10 subjects), following the same procedures, which are defined for the main survey. In a pre-test you will be able to identify existing flaws, thus identifying in advance potential pitfalls of the main survey. These can be problems with your instrument (e.g., wording, answer choices, length) but also with your study design (e.g.. mode of administration, response rate) [3].

A common strategy used for the development of an adequate instrument includes using open-ended questions in the pilot phase to identify the most important answer choices for inclusion and then design closed-ended questions in the finalized survey instrument. In summary, the pilot study's utmost purpose is to allow refining the quality and validity of the data collection instrument and improve the overall study design. Thus, despite the fact that a pilot study is time-consuming and increases the cost of the research project, it deserves serious consideration.

There are some methods to validate a survey. As this is beyond the scope of this chapter we will only briefly cite the methods used for validation. They can be divided into two categories: (1) based on judgment, in which other methods are used to validate the survey; (2) based on checks against the data, in which the investigator compares the data against data that are considered valid.

The methods to validate a survey using judgment are the following: (1) face validity (or logical validity) where the investigator assesses whether the measurement is logically consistent—for instance, assessing age by the birth certificate seems logical and accurate; (2) content validity, which indicates that all aspects that are aimed to be investigated are being assessed in the survey (e.g., if a survey aims to assess quality of life, the investigator needs to ensure that all aspects of quality of life are being measured); and (3) consensual validity, which occurs when experts in the field agree that the instrument is valid.

The methods to validate surveys using data include the following: (1) Criterion validity, in which the survey is checked against another survey or similar instrument. For instance, blood pressure measured with sphingomanometer can be measured and checked with direct intra-arterial measurement of blood pressure. (2) Convergent and discriminant validity, in which the new survey is checked against other surveys. The goal is to find other alternative methods that are correlated with other instruments but correlation is not perfect. These are not the best methods due to be need to have both, convergent and discriminant validity in order to achieve (3) construct validity. That is used when novel instruments are checked against a related variable; for instance, an investigator developing a new instrument to measure angina correlates this instrument against imaging exam of coronaries. The last two methods are (4) predictive validity (measured against a future event, for instance mortality in the future) and (5) responsiveness (when the new instrument is assessed in different conditions to measure if it can change).

Stage 3: Final Survey Design and Planning

Before fielding the survey, review and if necessary revise the sampling plan, the survey instrument, and the operations plan (administration strategies, data collection, and capture). In fact, a very important point for surveys is the sampling method.

Sample Design

Sample design is actually one of the greatest challenges of survey research. You have to define the target population, determine the accessible population, and finally, obtain a representative sample from the accessible population. *Which subjects should be included? To what degree are they accessible and how can they be accessed? To what extent do we want our results to be generalizable?*

The population of interest is predetermined by the research question, but time is well spent to clearly define it. While in other forms of research, inclusion and exclusion criteria are critically considered and published, survey research is not that transparent. Nevertheless, it is advisable to characterize the target population as exactly as possible, so that you can define the criteria by which you select your sample. Similarly to the sampling process in experimental research, a non-biased sample must be selected from an accessible portion of the target population (see Chapter 3 for more about study sample). In survey research especially, much thought has to be spent on the degree of accessibility of the target population given the mode of survey administration (e.g., if you choose to do a telephone survey, will you be able to equally reach senior people, who often still have landlines, and younger people, who are mostly cellphone users and therefore not registered in a phone book). Your ability to select a random and representative sample will be essential to determine the generalizability of your findings.

Types of Sample Design: Probability and Non-Probability Sampling

In order to ensure the representativeness of the sample, a probability sampling method is usually recommended [5]. These sampling methods are based on the principles that, in random selection or chance, every subject of the target population has the same chance to be included in the sample. They increase the generalizability of the results, thus allowing the researcher to make inferences on the target population. Still, we need to be aware of potential sampling bias, and the influence this will pose on the generalizability of the results. Random sampling is usually chosen when quantitative methods are used for data collection [3].

Simple random sampling selects members completely at random, with each member having the same probability to be chosen. Systematic sampling is another approach to obtain a representative sample. Here individuals are drawn at fixed intervals (e.g., every 10th person). If the research question supports stratified sampling, the target population is divided into strata, and a proportional sample is drawn from each stratum.

Cluster sampling is usually used when practical reasons permit and support sampling from one geographical location (e.g., schools).

However, sometimes practical reasons dictate to use non-probability sampling.

Purposive sampling selects individuals to enter the sample based on a certain characteristic. Purposive sampling is done based on certain characteristics and when the research question does not require the sample to reflect a certain proportion (e.g., Asian people between the age of 20 and 40 to survey if they had a history of gastritis and whether they sought treatment). The advantage is that the required sample size can be reached quickly.

Convenience sampling is recruitment based on "first come, first served" (e.g., recruiting patients from a neurology outpatient clinic).

Snowball sampling is done when participants are asked to recruit others who they know might meet the criteria for the survey. This is helpful if the target population is very difficult to access (e.g., people with agoraphobia).

If non-probability sampling is used, the degree to which our results are generalizable will always remain unclear.

When selecting the sample strategy, you have to balance several factors (e.g., cost vs. precision, time vs. seasonality) and consider how to accommodate/exploit the structure of the population, language differences, and geographical restrictions.

Method for Survey Administration, Data Collection, and Data Capture

The two major distinct survey methods are interviews and questionnaires. The differences inherent to each approach make both very useful for different situations. Interviews allow gathering important data on respondents' behavior and attitudes toward the survey topic. They allow for a more complex assessment of the participants and their answers and therefore are preferred in qualitative studies. Questionnaires are more useful to assess phenomena that can be reported through "self-observation," such as values and attitudes [5]. They are limited to the questions asked and the provided answer choices and are more useful in quantitative studies.

Based on the selected method of conducting the survey, it is possible to use several modes of administering the survey instrument, as face-to-face interviews, telephone interviews, postal and email self-completion questionnaires. But how can we choose which method is the better for our survey?

The selection of the method for survey administration is a very important step in the survey design process. Validity and representativeness of the collected data will strongly depend on how the survey has been administered to the sample. Table 21.1 presents an overview of the main methods, including reference to the main advantages and disadvantages of each. The decision of which administration approach to choose depends on several factors, including the time and available resources (budget, staff, etc.), the expected response rate, the characteristics of the sample, the accessibility of survey subjects (e.g., older people have less access to email and Internet or are less willing to complete electronic surveys), privacy issues, and also the nature of the topic being explored (e.g., if it is a delicate or controversial issue).

Sometimes, it is possible to combine administration methods—for instance, if you mail a self-report questionnaire and follow up by telephone interviews. Alternatively, you could give individuals the choice of which format they would like to use to complete the survey. The ultimate goal of combining such strategies is to reduce the number of non-responders and enhance the overall response rate. As discussed in the sample design section, several strategies exist to increase the response rates. Data analysis, on the other hand, will be more complex.

Table 21.1 Methods of Survey Administration

Method	Advantages	Disadvantages	Response Rate
Face-to-face interview	Interaction between the interviewer and responder Helps to interpret concepts and clarify doubts Can clarify misunderstandings Reduces non-responses Interviewers may reinforce confidentiality	Costly Time-consuming Requires training of the interviewers May produce interviewer-induced bias and social desirability bias	Higher comparing with other methods
Telephone interview	Limited interaction between the interviewer and responder Can help interpret concepts and clarify doubts Can clarify misunderstandings Reduces non-responses Effective in terms of time	Less expensive than face-to-face interviews Less time-consuming compared to face-to-face interviews High rate of non-responses Administration more difficult due to cell phone use	Higher than postal mail method
Postal questionnaire	Reduced cost compared to face-to-face interviews (but still higher than telephone and email) Bias can be minimized (e.g., social desirability bias) High level of confidentiality	There is no contact between interviewer and responder May not be time effective; it may take months to receive the surveys Requires a larger sample to address the non-response rate issue	Usually low
Email questionnaire	Low cost Quick and easy administration to a large number of individuals More effective in terms of time Convenient and straight-forward for Internet users Easy data capture	All the responders need to have Internet access Low response rate (spam filters, "survey fatigue") Increased chance of randomly/wrongly answered questions	Usually low

Data Collection and Data Capture

Whether we are using an interview, questionnaire, or both methods, how data is collected is critical. It is important to assure quality during data collection while maintaining confidentiality. Data can be collected manually, but computer-assisted or computer-based data collection methods are being used more and more. There are many data capture methods available that have the benefit that entry problems can be already eliminated or reduced at this stage (e.g., entering weight in pounds instead of kilograms, skipped answers) and that answers will already be coded and can be exported to data analysis programs.

DATA ANALYSIS

After design and administration of the survey, the next step is the analysis of the collected data. This is, indeed, one of the most critical and time-consuming aspects of the whole survey process. As previously stated, it is recommended to have a data analysis plan written up at the beginning of the survey design process. This is recommended because it will prepare you to design the survey in a way that data obtained can be analyzed, and it prevents a data-driven analysis.

Before you can analyze your data you will have to code them (unless you have used a data capture technique that already provides you with coded data). Coding means to convert answers into data that can be handled by a statistics program.

In survey instruments with closed-ended questions, this is a relatively straightforward process, as it is possible to code answers as strings or numerical variables (binary, integers, floating points) for quantitative analysis.

The next step is to edit/clean the data set. This step could be considered quality control, where data entry problems (answers put in the wrong field, wrong units used, etc.) can be detected, as well as outliers and missing data. Missing data can be distinguished as data-missing and case-missing. *Data-missingness* means that some responses are missing, while *case-missingness* occurs when an individual selected for the sample either did not respond or dropped out [7]. Missing data have to be planned and addressed for. (See Chapter 13 for methods of how to address missing data.)

The actual data analysis step depends on the type of analysis we aim to conduct. For a descriptive approach, summary statistics can be easily compiled, for instance central tendency (mean, median, mode), dispersion (ranges), and frequencies. For hypothesis testing, the appropriate statistical test has to be selected based on data type and study design (parametric vs. non-parametric, paired test, chi-square, correlation, etc.).

If the survey was designed with open-ended questions generating qualitative data, the most common approach is to report answer frequencies for each item, generally converted to percentages with other established methods available, such as content analysis [8].

The most often used type of analysis for surveys is the non-parametric approach, given that most of the surveys are based on ordinal scales. However, as discussed in the statistical section of this book, some survey results may be considered parametric and are analyzed using parametric tests such as ANOVA or regression modeling.

BIAS IN SURVEYS

As with any method in clinical research, surveys are also subjected to many types of biases. One important type of biases is the non-response bias. Non-response bias occurs when responders differ from non-responders; therefore results will be biased, as they will reflect the characteristics of responders only. The impact of this bias to surveys results will depend on how different the non-responders are from responders, and how that can affect the main results/main hypothesis.

Sampling bias is also a potential important limitation of surveys. Did sample bias occur? How representative was your sample, and therefore how strong is the external validity?

Recall bias can distort the reported information if the person does not remember correctly or remembers certain (usually negative) experiences better than others. This phenomenon is related to the issue of under- and over-reporting, which can easily become very complex (e.g., a potential BMW buyer might find it more important that he can sync his iPhone with the onboard computer, while a potential Toyota driver might pay more importance to the fuel efficiency of a car).

REPORT OF RESULTS

Similar to the data analysis plan, you should already have drafted a report outline at the design stage of your survey research project. This helps to write a concept-driven report rather than a data-driven report. Reports should be aimed at a specific target audience that you should have already had in mind when formulating your research question. This will increase the chance that your study will have the impact and recognition it deserves.

The final report of your survey should include the aim, instrument used, administration process, data analysis, and results. If you used an established survey instrument, justify the reason for its use in the context of your study. If you have developed a new survey instrument, you have to submit proof of its validity. In both cases you have to validate that the sample size you chose was appropriate. When reporting your results, make sure to include confidence intervals and margin of error. (For additional information regarding manuscript writing and submission, see Chapter 23 of this book.)

ETHICAL AND LEGAL ISSUES

The ethical considerations involved in clinical research, which were explored in Chapter 1, equally apply to survey research. *Is it ethical to provide respondents financial incentives in order to improve response rate? Do respondents always need to sign the informed consent? And what are the main issues involved when breaking confidentiality?* Questions such as these need to be discussed and addressed ahead of administering the survey, so that it is possible to conduct the survey following all rules of Responsible Conduct of Research. The two key aspects to pay special attention to are informed consent and confidentiality.

All surveys conducted at academic institutions have to be approved by the institutional review board (IRB). This is required to ensure HIPAA (Health Insurance Portability and Accountability Act of 1996) compliance to protect the subjects' rights and privacy. Informed consent for face-to-face interview can be obtained before the interview in writing. For telephone interviews, complete survey information can be disclosed before the interview and consent obtained orally. For mail questionnaires, a cover letter explaining the survey or an informed consent form can be included. Return of the questionnaire would imply consent [5]. Return of emailed questionnaires would equally imply consent. For web-based questionnaires, a start page with the survey disclosure can be used with the requirement to click "agree" to the terms of the survey before proceeding.

Preserving confidentiality is not just essential due to legal reasons, but it also increases the chance to obtain complete and honest answers.

CASE STUDY: USING SURVEYS IN CLINICAL RESEARCH—SIGNS OF SMOKE

Adapted from the original by Ana Rita Martins and Inês C. R. Henriques André Brunoni and Felipe Fregni

Economic Crisis and the Department of Social Medicine

"Please, Prof. Marley, have a seat," said Dean Marcondes, pointing to a beautiful leather chair.[2] Even before Prof. Marley could make himself comfortable, the dean started to speak, "As you know, Professor, this economic crisis is hitting the University of California hard. We have lost several funding opportunities and many good projects had to be terminated. As a sign of the severity, we received only one-third of gifts and donations this year as compared to before the crisis, as most of our donors have been affected by the slowdown of the American and global economy. Therefore, in this critical situation we are obligated to . . . review our agenda and our priorities," continued the dean, choosing his words carefully and trying to find any emotion in the pale, blue eyes of the older professor. But his reactions were not easy to read. "Now our priorities are to keep and potentially increase our partnership with the industries of Silicon Valley—that will help our engineering departments. We are also focusing heavily on some agreements with biotech companies—this will keep the medicine departments safe. Unfortunately, Prof. Marley, as you know, there is less interest in funding the health policy and social medicine departments." After a short pause, he then continues, "In fact, our observation is that your department of Social Medicine and Health Policy spends too much vis-à-vis your financial and academic output." The dean took a long breath and gave his final blow, "That's the reason why our board voted to cut your budget by 75% for the upcoming year. I know that this is three-quarters of your budget. So, in this scenario, I see two options, Professor Marley. The first is to look for alternative public or private funding. The second is to *resize* your department."

After some silence, Prof. Robert Marley finally spoke, "Resize—do you mean, fire my professors, staff, reduce the number of postdoctoral fellows and PhD students, and rent some of our space to other rich departments and terminate some of our disciplines—including the courses for medical students?"

"Yes, Bob. As tough as it might sound, that is it," the dean replied.

An Emergency Meeting

Two hours later, Prof. Marley set up an emergency meeting with the faculty and postdocs of the social sciences department. After briefing them on the talk with the dean, Prof. Marley stated strongly that he did not want to "resize" the department; nevertheless, they needed to come up with an alternative to increase the funds of

---

[2] Professor Fregni and Dr. Brunoni prepared this case. Course cases are developed solely as the basis for class discussion. The situation in this case is fictional. Cases are not intended to serve as endorsements or sources of primary data. All rights reserved to the authors of this case. Reproduction and distribution without permission are not allowed.

the department, and his idea was to submit a large research proposal to the National Institutes of Health (NIH) to try to get some funds and also to show the dean that the department is still producing good scientific papers—he concluded his remarks with the phrase, "not only to get papers in high-impact journals, but we also need to get onto the cover of *Times* or *Newsweek*."

As social scientists, they quickly agreed that they would propose a survey study—but on which topic? Professor Ford had an idea: "We are in California. We know a sensitive and difficult topic here and throughout the US is the use of *cannabis*. In fact a recent survey found that the US has the highest level of cocaine and cannabis use.[3] The population of some areas seems to have a sympathetic view toward its use, but we do not know if such populations also represent regular users of the drug, and therefore if the observation is biased. Although there is a debate regarding the use of *cannabis* for medical conditions, the use of *cannabis* is associated with significant mortality and morbidity. It seems that the epidemiological profile of *cannabis* users is different here in California: besides college students, the drug seems also to be utilized by older men and women who were previously married. However, we know nothing for sure, and that is an issue of public interest. We could conduct a very carefully designed survey on *cannabis*."

Prof. Marley and the others agreed—indeed, it is a very urgent, sensitive, and difficult topic, with many medical, social, and legal implications. This will also have a broad impact, especially with this new federal administration that is proposing a radical health reform. "OK! How are we going to do it? How are we going to ask people if they are *cannabis* users?"

First Point: Question Wording

Mary Jane, the postdoctoral fellow, started the discussion with a very important point: question wording. She started paraphrasing Sudman, "Everyone knows that a badly worded questionnaire, like an awkward conversation, can turn an initially pleasant situation into a boring or frustrating experience." After a small pause, she continues, "Well, then the problem begins here. We can use two types of questions: open or closed. For instance, suppose we have the question: 'Who introduced you to *cannabis*?' If it is asked openly, the advantage is, since this is a delicate topic, the subject is given a chance to answer our questions in his or her own way, without feeling morally judged. However, subjects might also give us answers about which we are not interested or that are not the goal of our survey. On the other hand, closed questions—for instance: "() college friends; () girlfriend or boyfriend; () older brother/sister, etc." might make it easier to quantify and analyze the results, but if we do not plan this thoughtfully, we can forget important options—for instance "() high school friends." Also when we use closed questions we should be very careful to not include alternatives that are confusing or overlap each other—in my example, the subject could answer: "It was my

---

[3] Degenhardt L, Chiu W-T, Sampson N, Kessler RC, Anthony JC, Angermeyer M, et al. Toward a global view of alcohol, tobacco, cannabis, and cocaine use: findings from the WHO World Mental Health Surveys. *PLoS Med*. 2008; 5: e141.

boyfriend who was at one time my college friend." There are other problems in doing surveys: simplicity is a key factor, especially if we are going to use mail questionnaires. For instance, if our questions are too wordy or academic or long, then people will get confused or bored and will start to answer anything. We are in a state with many non-native English speakers—should we also build our questionnaire in Spanish? Another issue is using positively versus negatively worded or neutral versus non-neutral questions—as one of the issues is the response set bias in which respondents tend to simply agree with every question—for instance, we can ask: "Have you stopped smoking cannabis in the last year?" or "Have you continued to smoke cannabis in the last year?" There is also the problem of "double-barreled questions"—meaning that "one question to one idea"—for instance, if we ask: "Do you do drugs when you are sad *or* happy"? It is possible that some people use only when they are sad, and others only when they are happy—so it is better to ask two questions. Finally, there is an important issue: should we include "no opinion" or "do not know" alternatives? The issue here is that by including these options, we might give an easy way out for people to respond instead of forcing them to think about the alternative. On the other hand, not including them might create inaccurate responses, and respondents might mark an alternative that is the least inaccurate one—but not the one reflecting his or her opinion. This should be applied to the question: "Under which circumstances should the use of the drug *cannabis* be allowed?" Mary Jane finished her discussion.

"Good, Mary Jane," said Prof. Marley, "So, your observation leads us to a second question—should we do a pilot study first"?

Second Point: The Pilot Study

Professor Marley then continued with his idea for a pilot study: "What about a pilot study with open questions to gather some answers to create a more precise, closed-question survey? In the pilot phase, we should perform an open, unstructured interview with a small number of subjects—in that phase we should try to maximize rapport to gather all the possible answers and detect potential flaws in our survey—we will not be interested in the answers themselves, but in all possible answers that we should use to build a structured questionnaire for the study phase. Another alternative to a small pilot study with a couple of subjects is to conduct a field test with a smaller population in order to test our instrument. However, we might not have enough time, as we need to submit our proposal as soon as possible—we can also try to look for questionnaires in the literature—using already validated questionnaires might also make it easier to apply for grants and to publish our results. So, let's keep that in mind. Next question: How are we going to do our survey?"

Third Point: Administering the Survey

The other postdoctoral fellow, Ursula Heiman, a German physician who has been in the United States for four years, started with this subject: "One of the most important decisions is deciding how the survey is going to be administered." Then she continued, "Basically we need to decide if this is going to be administered by an interviewer or if this is going to be a self-completion survey. Between these two modes, we have some options, like mail, telephone, face-to-face interview, and Internet." As she had the floor to herself, she continued, "I think that use of drugs is a delicate topic. People tend to lie regarding substance use, especially if they do not feel comfortable with the interviewer. In addition, although a face-to-face interview usually yields the best response rate with a good representative sample, it is an expensive method. One less expensive method I like is mailing as a method of survey. We can mail the surveys to the subjects, with a brief cover letter explaining the purpose and importance of our research, and then using a small questionnaire (less than 10 minutes) with simple questions. We can assure the respondents that we will guarantee anonymity and no personal information will be revealed. However, the response rate might be moderate to poor—it might be difficult to get a good response rate with this method. Finally, an intermediate solution would be telephone interview—less expensive than face-to-face, less problematic regarding a delicate topic, and might yield a higher response rate as compared with mailing. Also, we should not forget that because we live in California, a high-technology state, we could use other methods of interview: for instance, electronic mail, Internet websites, text messages to cell phones, and so on. Therefore, we will be able to quickly reach a large number of subjects at a relatively low cost."

Pedro Mendonza, the other assistant professor, said, "Good ideas, Ursula. But I think that *because* the topic is delicate, we cannot rely on some of the methods you mentioned: people who feel comfortable with the use of *cannabis* will be precisely the ones who will not waste their time answering a mail survey. Also, the subjects who do not use *cannabis* will not waste their time either; therefore we might collect inaccurate data using mail—an overestimated and biased sample." Professor Mendonza continued, "I know it is more expensive and more difficult, but my proposal is that we go to the community and ask the questionnaires ourselves. We should train a dozen interviewers—maybe some of our graduate students—to give them skills to show empathy and reassurance and to establish trust in the subjects when they are being asked these tough questions. For instance, it is easier to gain rapport when we validate the behavior—it is useful to start our questions with a statement such as: "In College, students suffer from a lot of pressure from professors, parents, bosses. Sometimes it is difficult to deal with all the pressure, and a common form of relaxation and way to unwind is to use *cannabis*." Finally, they should be trained to assure a good inter-rater reliability."

Fourth Point: Sampling Techniques

"I agree with you both," said Prof. Marley, "When listening to you, I was thinking that we have populations with very different profiles. On one hand, we have the most common profile of *cannabis* users—young people, high school and college students—this group has a relatively low prejudice on talking about this topic (whether or not they use *cannabis*). In this situation, a method of survey that is not specifically focused on establishing trust, validity, and empathy might do the job. On the other hand, we have cannabis users in the general population—and here it is a very mixed population—maybe we have housewives, retired men, veterans of war, multiple substance users, important businessmen, and so on. I think these people have mixed feelings about this topic—some might be comfortable, but many others probably feel ashamed or guilty about using *cannabis* and if we want to survey them—and we do—then the approach should be carefully elaborated. In addition, the method to find these different groups will vary."

Prof. Ford continued, "OK—we discussed the *what* and the *how* of our study. Now the question is *where* are our subjects? Are we going to use a random sample—selecting among all people in California? Are we going to focus only on some cities of the state—therefore performing a cluster sampling to cut costs? Or use a convenience sample if we do not get NIH funding?"

Mary Jane tried to answer, "Of course, the best method is to use a random sample. But it is also the most expensive one. Another method would be to stratify our population in subgroups and then use random techniques in this stratified sample. Using non-random samples is surely the easiest but most biased method, and we might overestimate the number of users."

Final Point: Enhancing Response Rates

Although the meeting was almost over, someone from the back of the room said, "We should not forget that we need to think about methods to enhance response rate." It was Chris Raley, a research assistant from Vermont who was applying to medical school. He then continues, "There are several ways to increase response rate. For instance, making the questionnaire clear and concise—especially having simple questions and clear instructions—might help with our response rate. Another point here is to reduce costs of responding by providing prepaid return envelopes and even gift cards as a monetary incentive. I remember receiving in the past a $10 Starbucks gift card for answering a mail survey. Although the value was small, it was the incentive I needed to do it."

Prof. Marley was very excited about the brainstorm session. He summarized the meeting: "We had a very interesting discussion here. Let's continue in three days—I will assign each of you one topic to elaborate on further and we will resume our discussion this Friday. As you know, the more time we spend discussing and planning this survey, the better results we will get. Also we should not underestimate the amount of work ahead. But we will learn together along the way and enjoy the process. See you all on Friday!"

CASE DISCUSSION

Using Surveys in Clinical Research: Signs of Smoke

In the case study Prof. Marley and his team are faced with a big problem in their department, due to the current economic crisis. In order to face this situation, Prof. Marley sets up an emergency meeting presenting his idea of submitting a large research proposal to the NIH with the goal of trying to get some funds for his department. In fact, every member of the study team agrees that they should propose a survey study about the use of *cannabis* in California, mainly because this is a very urgent, sensitive, and difficult topic, but also because it presents a variety of implications to several fields, such as medical, social, and legal.

It is fundamental to understand the purpose of a survey. Survey research has the main goal of providing information about a specific topic at a specific time, like a "snapshot" of how things are at a certain time in a specific population [5,9]. Surveys are usually descriptive, but they can be explorative as well, to seek for explanation and provide data to test hypothesis [5].

In this specific case Prof. Marley and his team quickly identify five crucial points that are common to all surveys and influence directly the quality and impact of a survey. The issues to discuss are how to word the questions, whether a pilot study should be performed, and the potential methods of survey administration. Additionally, they have to decide what the adequate sampling technique is to obtain a representative sample, which increases generalizability of the results to the target population. Finally, while reaching the target population is very important, the response rate is also a critical parameter that should not be overlooked. Therefore, approaches that can enhance the response rate must be carefully planned for.

The wording of questions is a critical point of the survey design, because if the question is not clear to the participants, they may get confused and frustrated and respond incorrectly or randomly just to continue with the questionnaire. Social desirability bias is another problem that can skew answers and can occur if a sensitive topic is asked and the respondent either answers what he wants to be true (e.g., income) or what he thinks the surveyor wants to hear. Thus, results may be biased. In the case study, the discussion between the team members is centered on the types of questions that should be included in the questionnaire. This particular decision depends heavily on the study question topic. It should be noted that simplicity is the key to design a good questionnaire [6]. There are three types of questions that could be selected to be in the survey instrument: open-ended questions, closed-ended questions without and closed-ended questions with the option "do not know"/"no opinion"/"prefer not to answer." Open-ended questions allow the participant to answer freely and spontaneously, whereas closed-ended questions are stricter and just allow the participant to choose among the options provided. In some cases, a neutral option (like "do not know"/"no opinion"/"prefer not to answer") is provided to the respondents. This, however, can offer the respondent an easy way out instead of forcing him to reflect on the questions and provide an opinion. Furthermore, in some particular questions it is possible that closed-ended questions have an option "other," which provides the opportunity to give a more adequate and informative answer. A questionnaire with closed-ended questions has the advantage that questions are easier to quantify, analyze, and publish. In summary, it is important to weigh all possibilities in designing an instrument, because all of them have advantages and disadvantages. Prof. Marley has to make his choices considering the topic, the target population, the method that will be used to reach the target population, and which strategy will allow them to achieve a sufficiently high response rate.

After the discussion of question wording, one team member suggests performing a pilot study to pre-test the instrument and collect preliminary data. The pilot study is performed before the main study. Its purpose is to test the feasibility of the study and also to search for evidence of possible effects and associations in a small scale [10,11]. Thus, the main goal of a pilot study is to test the methods and procedures that will be later used on a larger scale, and to demonstrate that the methods and procedures are appropriate [10]. Although a pilot study seems to be a good option, it has to be evaluated it in the context of the case study. Options that are theoretically ideal cannot always be considered in practice. In Prof. Marley's case, a pilot study will provide the opportunity to explore a variety of options to refine their own instrument for the evaluation of *cannabis* use. Consequently, this will allow for a more complete data collection, and will yield an instrument that will collect more reliable and valid data from the sample population. Despite all the advantages of performing a pilot study, Prof. Marley and his team must consider the required time for designing and planning the survey, and the necessary budget. In fact, another valid option would be the use of questionnaires that are already validated and published in the literature. With the latter choice, it would be possible to submit the survey proposal more quickly and the survey design and planning process would be shortened. In summary, it is important to consider a pilot study in light of the existing literature, and the amount of time and resources that the study team has.

The next point that is added to the discussion is about how to administer the survey. According to McColl et al. (2001) the mode of administration is one of the first decisions to be made in designing and conducting a survey. Basically the main decision is "between interviewer administration (either face-to-face or by telephone) or self-completion by the respondent (with delivery of the questionnaire either by post or to a 'captive audience')" [12]. These different methods have distinguishing features: if we opt for an interviewer administration, we will have a high response rate and the participant will more likely provide a "truthful" answer. On the other hand, self-completion methods will have lower response rates, which may be due to a lack of interest about the survey topic, perceived lack of time, misunderstanding of questions, or overly long questionnaires. This is why, in Prof. Marley's case, it is important to understand the characteristics of the population the instrument will be applied to. The most expensive method is the face-to-face interview; it is indeed the approach that has the best response rate, due to interpersonal interaction. In contrast, the least expensive approach is mail (with email being even cheaper). It is, however, difficult to reach a good response rate through this technique. The telephone interview is the better balanced method in regard to cost and response rate, because it is less expensive than face-to-face interview, less problematic regarding the mode of application, and may yield a relatively high response rate. The topic "use of *cannabis* in California" chosen by Prof. Marley's team is a sensitive topic, which may make the participants feel judged and, thus, may influence the survey results. Therefore, the mode of survey administration has important implications. Additionally, consider the fact that the target population is very broad. Therefore, a mixed-mode survey administration according to the variety of subgroups in this population might be useful, for instance, email questionnaires to young people, and interviews of parents or business people. Still, we need to be aware of the potential drawbacks of combining administration modes, such as complicated data analysis.

Accordingly to Berten et al. (2012) there are two types of *cannabis* users: the common profile is the young high school or college student, and the second profile is someone from the general population, such as parents, retired men, war veterans, multiple substance users, or important business people [15]. In order to reach both types of *cannabis* users, Prof. Marley's team has to use a sampling method that allows reaching a representative sample of this disperse target population. Before choosing the sampling technique that fits this constellation best, it is fundamental to decide whether the target population is too heterogeneous to apply the sampling technique, or if it is justifiable to sample this mixed population with a single approach. One possibility that Prof. Marley's team considers is the use of a random sampling technique that assures good representativeness of the sample. Using random sampling, every individual belonging to the target population (all subjects who have smoked *cannabis*) will have the same probability to be selected for the survey. Although random sampling is a preferred method, it requires a previous enumeration of all potential subjects, which is an expensive process that may not be feasible to implement [13] unless sampling frames already exist. Another alternative is to opt for cluster sampling, for example using schools as a cluster. This method will reduce expenses if face-to-face interview administration is chosen. On the other hand, it is certainly not free of bias, because people who do not belong to the chosen clusters will be inevitably omitted. If the research team selects schools as clusters and randomly chooses a certain number, students who attend schools that were not selected will be automatically excluded from the sample. Since schools in certain areas might differ greatly in their students' characteristics, complete elimination might skew the survey results. The easiest method to apply, not only to a survey research but also to research in general, is the convenience sample. If Prof. Marley's team chooses this method, they will have to be aware that this is a non-probability sampling method and that participants are not representative of the target population. This is the most biased method of all considered. Since the study has to be conduct in a short period of time, representativeness of the sample will be further decreased. Prof. Marley's team could consider purposive sampling to account for the short time available. They could also consider snowball sampling to accelerate the process of identifying prospective participants. To account for the two distinct groups of cannabis users, stratified sampling could be also a valid option.

And last, but equally important, Prof. Marley's team faces the issue of enhancing the response rates. In the discussion, it was mentioned that creating a concise and simple questionnaire might increase the response rate, owing to less time required for completion, but also to a low level of complexity of the questions. In addition, a team member also proposed providing incentives (vouchers, gifts) to respondents as a reward for the time invested to complete the questionnaire; this is another important suggestion that should be taken into consideration, since evidence suggests that monetary incentives can increase response rates [14]. Due to low response rates reported for surveys, the use of strategies that allow obtaining a good response rate becomes essential. While measures to obtain a higher response rate might increase study costs at the administration phase, they can contribute to decreased time and therefore reduced costs during the data analysis phase.

CASE QUESTIONS FOR REFLECTION

1. What are the main issues involved in designing the methodology of the survey?
2. Which are the implications of using interview or questionnaire as the data collection instrument?
3. Which are the main drawbacks of using open-ended questions versus closed questions?
4. Which are the main advantages of performing a pilot study?

5. How can one choose an adequate sampling technique?
6. How is it possible to enhance the response rate?

FURTHER READINGS AND REFERENCES IN THE CASE DISCUSSION

Papers

- Berten H, Cardoen D, Brondeel R, Vettenburg N. Alcohol and cannabis use among adolescents in Flemish secondary school in Brussels: effects of type of education. *BMC Public Health*, 2012; 12: 215.
- Deasy C, Bray J, Smith K, Harriss L, Bernard S, Cameron P. Functional outcomes and quality of life of young adults who survive out-of-hospital cardiac arrest. *EMJ*. 2012; 30: 532–537
- Edwards P, Cooper R, Roberts I, Frost C. Meta-analysis of randomised trials of monetary incentives and response to mailed questionnaires. *J Epidemiol Comm Health*. 2005; 59(11): 987–999.
- Giles LGF, Muller R. Chronic spinal pain: a randomized clinical trial comparing medication, acupuncture, and spinal manipulation. *Spine*. 2003; 28(14): 1490–1502.
- Kelley K, Clark B, Brown V, Sitzia J. Good practice in the conduct and reporting of survey research. *Int J Qual Health Care*. 2003; 15(3): 261–266.
- Kiezebrink K, Crombie IK, Irvine L, Swanson V, Power K, Wrieden WL, Slane, PW. Strategies for achieving a high response rate in a home interview survey. *BMC Med Res Method*, 2009; 9: 46.
- McColl E, Jacoby A, Thomas L, Soutter J, Bamford C, Steen N, Thomas R, et al. Design and use of questionnaires: a review of best practice applicable to surveys of health service staff and patients. *Health Technol Assess (Winchester, England)*. 2001; 5(31): 1–256.
- Thabane L, Ma J, Chu R, Cheng J, Ismaila A, Rios LP, Robson R, et al. A tutorial on pilot studies: the what, why and how. *BMC Med Res Method*, 2010; 10: 1.

Marston–Non-responder Bias in Estimates of HIV Prevalence

Journals

- *Survey Methodology*
- *Public Opinion Quarterly*
- *Journal of Official Statistics*

Books

- Aday L, Llewellyn JC. *Designing and conducting health surveys: a comprehensive guide*. 3rd ed. San Francisco: Josse-Bass; 2006.
- Andres L. *Designing and doing survey research*. Los Angeles, CA: Sage Publications; 2012.
- Czaja R, Blair J. *Designing surveys: A guide to decisions and procedures*. Thousand Oaks, CA: Pine Forge Press; 2005: Chapters 2, 6, 7, 9.
- Dillman D, Smyth J, Christian LM. *Internet, mail, and mixed-mode surveys: the tailored design method*, 3rd ed. New York, NY: John Wiley & Sons, Inc.; 2008.
- Everitt BS. *Medical statistics from A to Z: a guide for clinicians and medical students*, 2nd ed. Cambridge: Cambridge University Press; 2006.

- Fowler, *Improving survey questions: design and evaluation.* Thousand Oaks, CA: Sage; 1995.
- Fowler FJ Jr. *Survey research methods,* 4th ed. Thousand Oaks, CA: Sage Publications; 2008.
- Friis RH, Sellers TAS. *Epidemiology for public health practice,* 4th ed. Burlington, MA: Jones & Bartlett Learning; 2009.
- Groves RM. *Survey errors and survey costs.* New York: John Wiley & Son; 2005.
- Korn EL, Graubard BI. *Analysis of health surveys, vol. 323.* Hoboken, NJ: John Wiley & Sons; 2011.
- Kraemer HC, Thiemann S. *How many subjects?* Newbury Park, CA: Sage; 1987
- Last JM. *A dictionary of epidemiology.* Oxford: Oxford University Press; 2000.
- Lohr S. *Sampling: design and analysis.* Scarborough, ON: Nelson Education; 2009.
- Lumley T. *Analysis of complex survey samples.* Department of Biostatistics, University of Washington; 2004.
- Portney LG, Watkins MP. *Foundations of clinical research: applications to practice.* Upper Saddle River, NJ: Prentice Hall; 2009. Chapter 15.
- Rea LM, Parker RA. *Designing and conducting survey research: a comprehensive guide.* New York: John Wiley & Sons; 2012.

Webpages/Online Analysis Resources

http://oea.uchc.edu/tips_creating/index.html
http://www.hcp.med.harvard.edu/statistics/survey-soft/
http://www.snapsurveys.com/
http://www.socialresearchmethods.net/kb/survey.php
http://www.statisticssolutions.com/academic-solutions/resources/dissertation-resources/survey-research-and-administration/
http://www.surveymonkey.com
http://www.virginia.edu/processsimplification/resources/survey_design.pdf
http://www.zoomerang.com
https://collaborate.hms.harvard.edu/display/CETHelp/Qualtrics+Survey+Tool
https://whatisasurvey.info/downloads/pamphlet_current.pdf

REFERENCES

1. Bennett C, Khangura S, Brehaut JC, Graham ID, Moher D, Potter BK, Grimshaw JM. Reporting guidelines for survey research: an analysis of published guidance and reporting practices. *PLoS Med.* 2010 Aug; 8(8): e1001069. doi: 10.1371/journal.pmed.1001069.
2. Schron EB, Exner DV, Yao Q, Jenkins LS, Steinberg JS, Cook JR, Kutalek SP, Friedman PL, Bubien RS, Page RL, Powell., the AVID investigators. Quality of life in the antiarrhythmics versus implantable defibrillators trial. *Circulation.* 2002; 105: 589–94.
3. Drolet BC, Khokhar MT, Fischer SA. The 2011 duty-hour requirements--a survey of residency program directors. *N Engl J Med.* 2013 Feb 21; 368(8): 694–697. doi: 10.1056/NEJMp1214483
4. Czaja R, Blair J. *Designing surveys: a guide to decisions and procedures.* Thousand Oaks, CA: Pine Forge Press; 1996.
5. Kelley K, Clark B, Brown V, Sitzia J. Good practice in the conduct and reporting of survey research. *Int J Qual Health Care.* 2003; 15(3): 261–266.

6. Portney LG, Watkins MP. Foundations of clinical research: applications to practice. Upper Saddle River, NJ: Prentice Hall; 2009: Chapter 15.
7. www.epidemiolog.net, © Victor J. Schoenbach 16. Data management and data analysis—540 rev. 10/22/1999, 10/28/1999, 4/9/2000.
8. Morse JM, Field PA. *Nursing research: the application of qualitative approaches.* London: Chapman and Hall; 1996.
9. Rea LM, Parker RA. *Designing and conducting survey research: a comprehensive guide.* New York: John Wiley & Sons; 2012.
10. Last JM. *A dictionary of epidemiology.* Oxford: Oxford University Press; 2000.
11. Thabane L, Ma J, Chu R, Cheng J, Ismaila A, Rios LP, Robson R, et al. A tutorial on pilot studies: the what, why and how. *BMC Med Res Method,* 2010; 10: 1.
12. McColl E, Jacoby A, Thomas L, Soutter J, Bamford C, Steen N, Thomas R, et al. Design and use of questionnaires: a review of best practice applicable to surveys of health service staff and patients. *Health Technol Assess (Winchester, England).* 2001; 5(31): 1–256.
13. Friis RH, Sellers TAS. *Epidemiology for public health practice,* 4th ed. Burlington, MA: Jones & Bartlett Learning; 2009.
14. Edwards P, Cooper R, Roberts I, Frost C. Meta-analysis of randomised trials of monetary incentives and response to mailed questionnaires. *J Epidemiol Comm Health.* 2005; 59(11): 987–999.
15 Berten H, Cardoen D, Brondeel R, Vettenburg N. Alcohol and cannabis use among adolescents in Flemish secondary school in Brussels: effects of type of education. *BMC Public Health,* 2012; 12: 215.

22

ASSESSING RISK AND ADVERSE EVENTS

Authors: *Laura Castillo-Saavedra, Suely Reiko Matsubayashi, Faiza Khawaja, John Ferguson, and Felipe Fregni*

Case study authors: *Rui Imamura and Felipe Fregni*

A man who has committed a mistake and doesn't correct it, is committing another mistake.
—Confucius

INTRODUCTION

This chapter provides an overview of safety assessments in clinical trials, including challenges for designing and reporting safety studies. The previous chapters gave you the methodology to design a clinical trial (Unit I), the best statistical approach to analyze your data for the primary and secondary outcomes (Unit II), how to do an interim analysis, and how to power this analysis in order to stop a trial before its completion (Unit III).

HOW IS THE SAFETY OF A DRUG ASSESSED IN CLINICAL TRIALS?

In all countries, pharmaceutical companies are required by law to perform clinical trials to test new drugs on a selected group of people before the drugs are made generally available. In fact, one of the main goals of clinical trial development is not only to assess efficacy, but also safety. As a matter of fact, the formulation and progression of clinical trial methodology and the need for systematic clinical research have come in part from previous disastrous events as a consequence of the lack of knowledge about drug adverse events, such as the thalidomide disaster (see Chapter 1). The phases of clinical trial development are a perfect explanation for how safety is measured [1]:

- Pre-clinical studies: These studies in animals can provide the first evidence of safety. Invasive testing of test subjects can also help to determine the physiological effects of a drug.
- Phase I trials: These studies aim to assess the maximum tolerable dosage in a small sample of healthy subjects, therefore providing a good background for drug safety.
- Phase II trials: These studies include approximately 20 to 50 subjects with the disease of interest, and drug efficacy is tested. Safety is usually one of the outcomes of interest as well.

- Phase III trials: In these studies a larger and broader sample of subjects is recruited, allowing to test for safety outcomes on a larger scale; thus rarer adverse effects can be assessed.
- Phase IV postmarketing surveillance: In this phase, post-approval reports of adverse effects are monitored and compiled in order to inform about adverse effects that were not identified during the testing phase.

LIMITATIONS TO SAFETY ASSESSMENT IN CLINICAL TRIALS

Although safety assessment is one of the main goals when designing a clinical trial, it is not easy to evaluate this parameter in these types of studies [2]. Although clinical trials, in general, do provide a critical amount of information about how well a drug works and what potential harm it may cause, there are many factors that can affect the results and thus give inaccurate reports regarding the safety of a given procedure. Some of the main challenges are discussed in the following:

- Sample size: Most clinical trials do not have the resources and infrastructure to include large samples sizes; therefore, safety is assessed in small samples, resulting in lack of power to detect rare adverse events.
- Trial duration: Clinical trials usually have short duration due to costs of conducting large clinical trials and also adherence issues; thus adverse events that require a minimum time to develop may not be observed.
- Design: The design is also critical; for instance, cross-over trials may not be adequate to assess safety when adverse events are long lasting or have a long latency.
- Biases: Similarly to efficacy, assessment of safety in clinical trials is vulnerable to biases. For instance, measurement biases (due to lack of proper blinding) can result in adverse events being overestimated in the treatment group and underestimated in the placebo group.
- Sample characteristics: It is important to understand the biological basis of adverse events so as to predict whether specific baseline or clinical characteristics (such as use of other drugs) would accentuate or suppress adverse events.
- External validity: Results of clinical trials in a narrow or homogeneous population may not be applicable to a larger population in terms of adverse events. Therefore when safety is one of the main aims in a given study, the investigator needs to be aware of this limitation.

INSTRUMENTS TO MEASURE ADVERSE EVENTS IN CLINICAL TRIALS

Monitoring safety parameters is a critical component of the process behind drug development; nonetheless, clinical trials are in general developed and powered toward a main endpoint: efficacy. Determination of safety outcomes tends to be relegated to a secondary objective, which leads to most new drugs being marketed on the basis of limited safety information, by the methodology and design of the clinical trials used for this purpose [3].

This monitoring process should be dynamic and evolving, as to encompass all of the stages of the development process and ensure that any important adverse events are discovered and reported in a timely manner. To accomplish this purpose, an investigator should be able to accurately distinguish how to best collect and analyze study data, and what available instruments are most helpful in determining the safety of an intervention. Choosing an adequate study design, and therefore data source, for safety determination is intimately related to the study question and the adverse events that are being evaluated. Each approach to safety assessment, discussed in the following, has advantages and limitations that need to be considered during the design stage of a study, so as to guarantee that they can be properly used and the most benefit is acquired [4].

Spontaneous Reporting Systems

These are based on the voluntary reporting of suspected adverse drug reactions to a coordination center by manufactures, health-care professionals, or researchers. This system allows early identification of signals, which in turn leads to formulation of investigational hypotheses that can convey new information on the drug and its safety profile. This method constitutes the mainstay of pharmacovigilance through post-marketing surveys, representing up to two-thirds of the major regulatory actions taken by the FDA.

This instrument captures a wide range of events, providing safety information throughout the marketed life of a drug. It is a simple and cheap reporting system that has the potential of identifying the signals of events that are rare or that have a low incidence. Another important advantage of this instrument is related to the new and sophisticated techniques that have been developed for the analysis of signal detection, which lead to earlier and more accurate identification of adverse reactions occurrence.

Nonetheless, there are significant disadvantages and limitations to this approach for safety assessment. Given that these are individual reports, there is no control group that can allow for estimation of rates and, therefore, there is no reliable quantification of risk, causality appraisal, and determination of risk factors. The type and amount of information received can vary substantially between reports, and clinical details of each case may be incomplete. Another major limitation is the frequent selective reporting and underreporting. In general, these limitations can be conquered by using the spontaneous reporting system as a base for the development of new hypotheses and clinical trials to assess possible relationships between a drug and a suspected adverse event.

Randomized Clinical Trials (RCT)

These are the mainstay of clinical research for the determination of drug efficacy; nonetheless, they are rarely, if ever, powered to correctly determine possible harmful effects. This is due to either a small sample size or to a study design that does not correctly measure safety outcomes. Another major disadvantage of the use of RCTs for safety determination is the fact that many of them have limited generalizability, given that strict selection criteria are applied to ensure a homogenous study population.

Randomized trials have relevant strengths in safety determination. They are highly convenient for the evaluation of safety outcomes that can be measured early during the execution of the trial, especially if they have a high baseline incidence. These outcomes can be represented using statistical measurements, such as absolute or relative risk increase. In accordance, this type of study design is not helpful in assessing rare or unexpected adverse events [5].

Given that in RCTs the intervention is well defined and it is randomly distributed among study participants, it is possible to draw an unconfounded conclusion by comparing groups. If allocation concealment is adequately guarded, then randomization also offers a significant protection against selectively reporting or diagnosing adverse events. Finally, certain reactions can be prospectively specified so that they can be monitored specifically, in order to avoid ascertainment bias. This can be done by using results from previous studies on adverse events, or by determining possible reactions on the basis of pharmacological mechanisms.

Non-Randomized Studies

This approach to safety determination carries important advantages. First, it assesses "real-world" circumstances, providing data with higher generalizability and longer follow-up periods. This provides an ideal background for the evaluation of rare adverse events that could potentially present after long periods of treatment. For such purpose, study designs should be selected carefully; for example, case control studies allow assessment of adverse events as the primary outcome of the design. Second, it is also possible to obtain relevant information regarding event relationship to the intervention, for example, to dosage, duration of exposure, or risk factors [6].

Some of the major limitations of this type of approach are associated with the lack of randomization, which can lead to higher susceptibility to confounding. The duration and monitoring rigor of the trial will also determine its ability to detect long-term problems and rare events, respectively. Finally, a major disadvantage of non-randomized studies is their inability to accurately specify the exposure, because their determinations are based on history records, rather than on dispensing or actual use.

Meta-Analysis of Controlled Observational Studies and/or Trials

Using a single study design for safety assessment may not reliably measure all possible adverse events; therefore pooling of available information allows for a broader estimate of intervention safety. By rigorously searching available information and assessing its validity and heterogeneity, it is possible to construct a more complete set of information than by analyzing individual trials. It also provides higher power to detect uncommon events, and allows for evaluation of consistency of data [7].

Some of the major limitations of this approach are associated with the constraints of the primary data used, which are highly susceptible to selective outcome reporting and high heterogeneity, therefore limiting the information available for pooling. This is also associated with poor or lack of reporting of data on adverse events.

DESIGNING A SAFETY STUDY

Investigators interested in designing trials to respond to the question of whether the intervention is safe need to follow the same steps as described in Unit I (i.e., formulating a study question, choosing the most appropriate design, selecting the population, and determining other methods such as randomization and blinding). One important point, as explained in Chapter 2 on choosing the research question, is that investigators need to be specific: for instance, a study cannot answer the question of whether a drug is safe, but it can answer the question of whether a certain drug is not associated with an increase in seizures as compared to placebo.

Another important point when designing a study is to determine whether safety is the primary aim of the study and thus the study is powered and designed to answer a safety question, or whether safety is a secondary outcome and thus study will not be confirmatory in terms of the safety questions.

ADVERSE EVENTS CAUSALITY

One of the most important issues in assessing adverse events in clinical trials is to determine the causality relationship with the intervention being used. The best and most reliable way to determine whether a drug is casually related to a specific adverse event is to make a head-to-head comparison of the rate of such event in a group of subjects exposed to the drug in question, and the rate in a group without the exposure. Nonetheless, such comparisons never include a large enough group of subjects, nor last for a long enough period of time to detect rare adverse events. Therefore, post-marketing surveys are still required to detect adverse events that were not caught in the initial trials.

When determining causality in an adverse reaction, it is necessary to consider the following criteria, established by the Surgeon General's Advisory Committee on Smoking and Health (1964). Although they are all important, the following criteria are not all necessary, nor do they all carry the same importance when establishing causality:

- *Consistency*: The drug-adverse event association should be consistent, so that it can be reproduced and lead to the same conclusion if replicated by different investigators, in different scenarios and by different methods.
- *Strength of the association*: The relationship between drug and adverse event should be strong, both in magnitude and in dose-response association.
- *Specificity*: There should be a specific, unique, distinctive association between the intervention and the event, and not a common or spontaneous occurrence, or frequent association with other external conditions.
- *Temporal relation*: The drug or intervention should be temporally related to the event, so that the exposure precedes the initial manifestation of the adverse reaction.
- *Biological plausibility*: There should be a coherent and plausible biological explanation that is in accordance with the natural history of the disease. This is a less robust criterion, and if negative it should not rule out causality.

An association should be considered strong if the evidence is based on the following:

- Human studies conducted that demonstrate an association between the adverse event and the drug by testing a hypothesis determined a priori. In descending order of strength, the following studies can be used to prove such association: RCTs, cohort studies, case-controlled studies, and controlled case-series.
- More than one human study that demonstrates a consistent association between the intervention and adverse event, conducted by different investigators, with different study designs and in different populations.

REGULATORY ISSUES: REPORTING ADVERSE EVENTS

Reporting of adverse events is a critical aspect of the drug development process, specifically, safety determination. The surveillance of this process is highly regulated and its legislation is always evolving, leading to more strict reporting parameters, in order to ensure drug safety. Worldwide, up to 5% of hospital admissions are due to drug-related adverse events; however, only 10% or less of such events are reported to the regulatory authorities or manufactures. This fact highlights the need to understand and clarify the regulations commanding reports of adverse events [8].

Reporting of adverse events is based on its categorization in accordance to three main parameters:

- *Seriousness*: This refers to events that lead to negative outcomes such as death, prolonged hospitalization, persistent or significant disability or incapacity, or congenital anomalies. An event is also considered serious if it leads to the requirement of medical or surgical intervention to prevent one of the previous outcomes, or if it is categorized as life threatening (i.e., the patient was at risk of death at the time the event occurred).
- *Expectedness*: This concept is based on whether the event was or not previously observed or reported in the local product labeling. An event is considered "unexpected" if it was previously unobserved, and its nature and/or severity are inconsistent with documented information. "Expected" events are not typically reported to regulatory authorities on an expedited basis.
- *Relatedness*: This category refers to the likelihood that an event is related or not to the exposure. In order to make such determination, factors like biological plausibility and temporal relationship should be considered. This concept is usually graded according to the possible degree of causality, such as certainly, probably, possibly, or likely related. Nonetheless, there is no standard nomenclature scale. In general, all voluntary reports are considered to carry a casual relationship

In general, once an unexpected serious event is suspected to be reasonably related to a drug, the research sites should report it to the manufacturer or sponsor, given that they are expected to be more efficient at evaluating and reporting such event. In other circumstances, the sites can report adverse events directly to the regulatory commission, but this can lead to lack of knowledge by the manufacturer and/or double reporting of events.

Serious and unexpected events should be reported in an expedited manner. If the manufacturer considers that there is a reasonable association between the event and the product, there is a 15-calendar-day limit for notification. In order to accomplish such a timeline, it is expected that all affiliated sites report serious, unexpected, and possibly related events to the manufacturer or sponsor within a 2-calendar-day limit. If an event does not meet the requirement for expedited reporting, it should be reported through an appropriate safety update (i.e., New Drug Application Annual Report, Period Report, or Safety Update Report).

CASE STUDY: RISK ASSESSMENT AND ADVERSE EVENTS—WHEN TO PULL THE TRIGGER?

Rui Imamura and Felipe Fregni

It's 7 a.m. on Friday and John Sullivan, the chief medical officer of Pharmatec company, drives to work with a funny sensation. He feels that there is something wrong. He received an email the day before from the vice president of research, Terry Morgan, asking for an urgent meeting the next morning. He knows Terry—when there is something urgent, there may be something wrong. He is expecting problems with one of the drugs being developed and he ruminates on the potential crisis: Market production? Fall in sales? Lack of efficacy in phase III trials?[1]

As he enters his office and greets his secretary, he sees Terry seated and waiting for him. Her expression suggests she is anxious. "Good morning, Terry—let's go into my office." After closing doors, Terry goes directly to the point: "John, I have bad news. The results of our recent study on the comparison of MECAR (a novel NSAID that is also a selective inhibitor of COX-2) against the traditional NSAID (that is a COX-1 and COX-2 inhibitor) showed that although MECAR outperformed the traditional NSAID in terms of lower incidence of gastrointestinal events, there was a problem as MECAR had a higher incidence of myocardial events and strokes." John's intuition was correct: this was bad news.

THE DEVELOPMENT OF MECAR

Non-steroidal anti-inflammatory drugs (NSAIDs) are one of the most common medications used for the treatment of pain. Although they are associated with significant benefit for a wide range of pain syndromes, they have one important problem: their association with a gastric ulcer that might induce a life-threatening condition. Because the mechanisms of traditional NSAIDs involve inhibition of COX-1 and COX-2 enzymes that act as catalysts to produce prostaglandins, these drugs can induce important adverse events as COX-1 is responsible for the production of stomach mucus lining. Therefore, traditional NSAIDs can lead to stomach irritation, digestive tract problems, and even intestinal or stomach bleeding.

Therefore, the development of painkillers that inhibit only COX-2 might represent a great advance as it would enhance safety for the gastrointestinal tract compared to traditional NSAIDs, while maintaining its effects on pain. Pharmatec then invested millions of dollars to develop this new compound after several years OF pre-clinical, phase I, II- and III studies. Pharmatec showed that its new drug MECAR has a significant effect to relieve pain and that this drug was associated with less gastrointestinal ulcers as compared to traditional NSAIDs. This gave new energy to Pharmatec, as after that huge investment, Pharmatec had a blockbuster drug on the market. In fact, the launch of MECAR increased Pharmatec's revenue by more than 30% and raised its stocks

---

[1] Professor Fregni and Dr. Imamura prepared this case. Course cases are developed solely as the basis for class discussion. Although cases might be based on past episodes, the situation in this case is fictional. Cases are not intended to serve as endorsements or sources of primary data. All rights reserved to the authors of this case. Reproduction and distribution without permission are not allowed.

by almost 60% in 6 months. John at that point got a raise of $300,000—bringing his salary to $1.3 million—and a bonus of $1.9 million. Everyone seemed to be enjoying the success of MECAR.

THE ISSUE OF ADVERSE EVENTS

A major concern in medical practice is the safety profile of a given treatment. For the patient, drug safety assures minimum risk with application of a drug in a given indication, and for the physician, indication of the appropriate treatment based on a favorable benefit-risk ratio.

Adverse drug reactions (ADR) are common and may be serious. Indeed, ADR is the fourth to sixth largest cause for mortality in the United States and may cost up to $5.6 million each year per hospital, depending on hospital size. Also, 16% of hospital admissions in the United Kingdom are due to ADRs.

ADRs also have great financial impact on pharmaceutical industries, as the life cycle of a medical product is directly influenced by its safety profile. Safety concern is especially important in patient-oriented research. In clinical trials, safety monitoring is of utmost importance for various reasons:

- Allows appropriate modification of study protocols, improvement in study design and procedures to protect safety of subjects in the clinical trials. If necessary, determines termination of subject's involvement or even termination of the trial.
- Improves understanding of the overall safety profile of the product
- Evaluates the benefits and risks of a drug
- Complies with regulatory requirements.

According to the Declaration of Helsinki, the potential benefits, hazards, and discomfort of a new method should be weighed against the advantages of the best current diagnostic and therapeutic methods.

THE AFTERMATH

John knows that this news could be devastating for the company. In fact, the idea of MECAR increasing the risk of vascular accidents is plausible, as prostacyclin acts as a vasodilator and platelet aggregation inhibitor; therefore an increase in the risk of both myocardial infarction and strokes could be theoretically expected. That turned out to be a real dilemma for Dr. Sullivan. After 10 years and hundreds of millions of dollars already invested, the company was recovering its investments with MECAR; in addition, there was no new drug on the pipeline, and a post-market failure of MECAR could even indicate bankruptcy.

The pressure on Dr. Sullivan was quite high at that moment. He knew the issue raised could turn into a major safety concern, and he was pressed by two antagonistic forces. One came from his mind, saying, well, from my experience in research I know that this finding can surely be a false alarm, a false positive. On the other hand, his heart was telling him that there was something wrong and safety issues should always be the main concern of any investigator or physician. In fact, if this drug proves to be unsafe in futures trials, then the company will also likely go bankrupt due to lawsuits.

The situation was not favorable, and he decided then to call an urgent meeting with the company senior executives.

A CLOSED DOORS MEETING

Even within a short period of time, John was able to gather most of the senior-level managers. In his memo he explained the results of these new trials and asked for an urgent meeting to discuss the next steps of the company. The meeting started with a brief exposition from Terry on the results of this recent trial. After she presented many graphs and tables, dissecting the data from different angles, John takes the leading position: "Well, here we have a classic example of a signal that something might be wrong as MECAR was associated with a higher rate of myocardial infarction and stroke as compared with the traditional NSAID. The main question is whether this is a signal that our drug is not safe; as you all know there are many alternative explanations for these results, and although we need to consider safety as the most important parameter, we need to make a decision based on strong theoretical support. Let us then explore different scenarios."

The company CEO, Steve Baylor, is the first to propose one scenario. Steve is a 57-year-old civil engineer with an MBA from Harvard Business School, and he was hired to improve the company's performance. During this tenure he was able to double the stock value and increase by one-third the annual revenue. He spoke with his strong voice: "Well, one radical option is to immediately withdraw the drug from the market even considering that we really do not know whether MECAR is associated with an increased risk of death due to MI or stroke. If we take this pathway, there are two consequences: one is that we will be withholding a drug that might be benefiting a large number of patients without really knowing whether this drug leads to serious detrimental effects; and one important consideration here is the cost-benefit profile as most of the drugs are associated with adverse events—this is an inherent issue to use of drugs. The other consequence is for the company, for if we withdraw MECAR, then we will see an immediate drop in stock values, a huge drop in the company's revenue. In addition, this might affect directly or indirectly the sales of our other drugs such as the second-generation COX-2 selective inhibitor, and most important, we must be prepared for the burden of legal liabilities as lawsuits will be pouring over us. On the other hand, if we do not withdraw MECAR and this drug proves to be associated with a risk of MI and stroke, we will also face legal and economic issues—perhaps even worse. We may not have too many options here!"

The next to speak is Alice Goldstein, a senior scientist and vice president of drug development. "This is certainly a grim scenario for us and we want patients' safety to be our main goal here. But looking at the data that Terry showed us, there is one important issue: Is the difference in the rate of MI and stroke between MECAR and the traditional NSAID due to an increased risk of MECAR, or protective effect of the traditional NSAID? In fact, if we go back to one of the slides that Terry showed us, we can see that this difference was primarily caused by the high rate of myocardial infarction and stroke among the 4% of the study population with the highest risk of a myocardial infarction and stroke, for whom low-dose aspirin is indicated (in fact, the difference in the rates of myocardial infarction and stroke between MECAR and the traditional NSAID was not significant among the patients without indications for aspirin to prevent MI." She then became excited about her finding.

"Because the traditional NSAID used in this study inhibits the production of thromboxane by 95 percent and inhibits platelet aggregation also by almost 90 percent, the use of this drug may be similar to that of aspirin. Therefore, what we are seeing here is a protective effect of the traditional NSAID in high-risk patients." She realized that she got some of the morale back in the room, as this could be good news for everyone in that room. She then continues, "Nevertheless, we would need to run another long-term follow-up trial to assess whether our drug increases the risk of myocardial infarction and stroke. We actually do have a trial that might serve this purpose: our longitudinal trial in which patients are receiving MECAR or placebo for several months for the prevention of adenomatous polyp—in this study we can see then if MECAR increases the risk of MI or stroke as compared to placebo. Therefore, there would be definitive evidence."

The last person to speak is actually Terry Morgan: "This is a good suggestion, Alice. But I would propose a compromise solution between the proposal from Steve to withdraw the drug and the proposal from Alice to run another study. I propose to suggest to the FDA adding a warning label to our product, saying that for patients with high risk of stroke and MI (as defined by a set of criteria), they are at increased risk of another event if they use MECAR. Because this difference in the current study was only on this population, then we would be protecting our patients while not limiting our patients with no risk factors to use MECAR, which I know in some cases is the only drug that is effective and tolerable.

It is almost 7 p.m. on Friday. John decides then to call the meeting off: "Let us then work with these three scenarios and because time is of the essence here as patients will continue to take the drug during the weekend, let us then reflect on these proposals and decide on Monday morning the best option with our complete senior management team—everyone is now aware and some of our colleagues who are out of country were requested to fly back this weekend. Have a good weekend everyone." Monday would be a decisive day for the fate of Pharmatec.

CASE DISCUSSION

Risk Assessment and Adverse Events: When to Pull the Trigger

This case discusses a potential problem that may occur in several studies: how to determine whether adverse events are causally related to the intervention when the trial is not designed for such assessment. In this case, it is important to think how to analyze the data and what are the necessary questions that the investigator needs to make in order to analyze whether the use of the drug needs to be interrupted—that is, if the investigator believes that this is a case of an adverse effect related to the drug. In this case it is important to consider also how to design a trial.

Another interesting topic of discussion for this case is whether this adverse effect of MECAR, if really linked to the drug, is a case of failure to design the trial well, or if it is something that would only be detected in phase IV trials. In fact, the twentieth century is full of cases in which drugs have been put on the market without sufficient safety mechanisms to prevent adverse events or deleterious consequences.

You are encouraged to discuss further historical system failures, other famous cases of pharmacovigilance issues, or recent concerns raised in your specialty/region. You can also discuss if you agree or not (and why) with the last cases of market withdrawal. Besides, are new surgical techniques also monitored? For example, look for papers on LASIK correction at the beginning and compare them to the contemporary limitations of this technique, also the improvement and safety monitory.

CASE QUESTIONS FOR REFLECTION

1. What are the issues involved in this case that should be considered in order to make a decision?
2. What are the concerns? And for the company?
3. What should they consider in order to make the decision?
4. Have you seen a similar situation?

FURTHER READING

Macrae DJ. The Council for International Organizations and Medical Sciences (CIOMS) guidelines on ethics of clinical trials. *Proc Am Thorac Soc* 2007; 4: 176–179.
This article gives an overview of the history of ethics (Nuremberg Code, Helsinki Declaration), international ethical guidelines (Belmont Report, International Conference of Harmonization, Council for International Organizations and Medical Sciences), informed consent, and the study of vulnerable groups.
WHO. Pharmacovigilance: ensuring the safe use of medicines. WHO Policy Perspectives on Medicines, 2004. At: http://who-umc.org/graphics/24753.pdf, accessed December 2012.
This article gives us summary of pharmacovigilance, with definition, aims, monitoring and partners, the international program for drug monitoring, and the increasing of reporting and membership.
Yadav S. Status of adverse drug reaction monitoring and pharmacovigilance in selected countries. *Indian J Pharmacol*. 2008; 40(Suppl 1): S4–9. At: https://www.ncbi.nlm.nih.gov/pmc/articles/PMC3038524/, accessed on November 2016.
This article gives an overview on how the pharmacovigilance of different developing countries (Australia, Brazil, India, Malaysia, Singapore, and South Africa) identify and report adverse drug reactions.
These links are interesting to explore and access the guidelines: safety report, risk management, and so on:
- Council for International Organization of Medical Sciences (CIOMS): http://www.cioms.ch/
- European Medicine Agency (EMA): http://www.emea.europa.eu/ema/
- US Food and Drug Administration (FDA): http://www.emea.europa.eu/ema/

REFERENCES

1. Friedman LM, et al. *Fundamentals of clinical trials*. Vol. 3. New York: Springer; 1998.
2. Leape LL, Berwick DM, Bates DW. What practices will most improve safety?: evidence-based medicine meets patient safety. *JAMA*. 2002; 288(4): 501–507.

3. Terwee CB, et al. Quality criteria were proposed for measurement properties of health status questionnaires. *J Clin Epidemiol.* 2007; 60(1): 34–42.
4. Creswell JW. *Qualitative inquiry and research design: choosing among five approaches.* Thousand Oaks, CA: Sage; 2013.
5. Moher D, Schulz KF, Altman DG. The CONSORT statement: revised recommendations for improving the quality of reports of parallel group randomized trials. *BMC Med Res Methodol.* 2001; 1(1): 1.
6. Li H, Yue LQ. Statistical and regulatory issues in nonrandomized medical device clinical studies. *J Biopharm Stat.* 2008; 18(1); 20–30. PMID: 18161539
7. DerSimonian R, Laird N. Meta-analysis in clinical trials. *Controlled Clin Trials.* 1986; 7(3): 177–188.
8. Nebeker JR, Barach P, Samore MH. Clarifying adverse drug events: a clinician's guide to terminology, documentation, and reporting. *Ann Intern Med.* 2004; 140(10): 795–801.

23

MANUSCRIPT SUBMISSION

Authors: *Alma Tamara Sanchez Jimenez and Felipe Fregni*

Case study author: *Felipe Fregni*

Writers may be classified as meteors, planets, and fixed stars. They belong not to one system, one nation only, but to the universe. And just because they are so very far away, it is usually many years before their light is visible to the inhabitants of this earth.
—Arthur Schopenhauer, *Essays and Aphorisms* (1970)

INTRODUCTION

Manuscript writing and submission can be considered the final steps in a research project. Investigators need to publish their results, not just to inform the scientific world about the work, but to expose their data to scrutiny and have their findings applied to new projects and studies. A track record of published papers is also necessary for career development and is an important criterion for promotions.

However, less than 50% of scientific meeting abstracts actually result in publication, and the proportion of unpublished original work is likely to be even smaller [1]. Challenges to manuscript publication are due to both the writing and submission process. Both require careful consideration and preparation, but the key to success is frequent practice and experience. At the same time, your study does not have to be a randomized clinical trial (RCT) to be considered interesting or publishable. Nor should you give up on publishing your study if the results are negative; it is more important that you have significant statistical power. Furthermore, negative studies play an important role in answering relevant research questions, even if the results are unexpected or controversial.

The basic science argument architecture contains Introduction; (Material and) Methods; Results and Discussion (cum conclusions)—also referred to as IMRaD; this is a standard format for presentation of the data adopted by most medical journals, which is also helpful when comparing information between studies [2].

When drafting your manuscript, be aware that reviewers are asked to check for originality, scientific accuracy, good composition, and interest to the readers. Therefore, important questions to consider as you write include the following: For which audiences are your research question and findings most relevant? How do your findings add information to what we already know? Could your findings change medical practice and, if so, how? What are other likely impacts of your study? The answers to these questions will affect which journals are the best fit for your manuscript, and whether journal editors will ultimately publish or reject it.

Another point to consider is the current publication landscape. On the one hand, the number of publications is increasing at a faster rate than 10 years ago. MEDLINE, the US National Library of Medicine's and primary component of PubMed, started back in 1946 and is the premier bibliographic database, containing over 19 million scientific references. Every day 2,000–4,000 completed citations are added; in 2010, nearly 700,000 citations were added [3]. On the other hand, the number of journals has not increased proportionally, which has made the publication process increasingly competitive and burdensome for all parties involved. The key to successfully publishing a manuscript in a high-impact factor is having high-quality data that demonstrate an important message, clearly presenting this message and its evidence in the manuscript, and choosing the right journal with matching characteristics and requirements. In 2010 the "Authors' Submission Toolkit: A Practical Guide to Getting Your Research Published" was created to increase efficiency in the submission process to accommodate the rising manuscript volume and reduce the resource demands on journals, peer reviewers, and authors [4].

The main focus of this chapter is to prepare you to find the right journal, to understand the quality requirements for reporting your investigation as well as the submission process, to discuss submission strategies and pitfalls and what do to when a paper is rejected. However, we will begin with a short review of the structure of an original research manuscript, providing key aspects that have major consequences on the success or failure of a manuscript submission. Covering the entire manuscript writing process would go beyond the scope of this chapter, but at the end we provide resources that we think will be helpful. We also hope to provide you with some insight into the current state of medical publishing and some of the current issues you need to be aware of.

SCIENTIFIC WRITING: HOW TO PRESENT THE INFORMATION IN YOUR MANUSCRIPT

The scientific method is a fluent organized reasoning process, and therefore a manuscript has to present information in a logical sequence. Research reported by our peers is the source of our knowledge, and we benefit from publications of good quality, produced by trustworthy research that is presented clearly and accurately [5].

Virtually all scientific research is reported using some variant of the IMRAD format (Introduction, [Materials and] Methods, Results, And Discussion). The broad guidelines for presenting medical research can be found at the website for the International Committee of Medical Journal Editors (www.icmje.org). But while guidelines and recommendations are necessary and helpful, writing a manuscript is still a difficult task [6]. Only practice will improve your scientific writing skills, so don't get discouraged by your first efforts. It is helpful to read your peers' work and to learn from them, but it is also a good idea to become a critical reader and reviewer early in your career [7]

In the following paragraphs we will briefly review the format of a manuscript.

Title

The title is the "business card" of your manuscript. This is how you catch the curiosity and interest of your audience. Your title should be an accurate description of your study, expressed in as few words as possible. It is important that the title is in sync with the rest of your manuscript, so that it sends the right signals to editors, reviewers, and readers. While it is important to begin writing your manuscript with a title, this is a working title only—it will not be the final one. It is inevitable that in writing up your research, you will come to a deeper understanding of your work and its significance—and this deepened understanding needs to be reflected in your title. We strongly recommend that at the end of the writing process you re-examine your working title to see whether it is still the best fit for your manuscript. We assume that it won't be. So you will need to change the title, sometimes slightly but other times entirely rewrite it, before you submit your work to the journal. If the title sends the wrong message to an editor, he or she may reject the manuscript out of hand. So craft it to fit the journal's needs and those of its readers. An accurate title will also make it easier for other researchers to find your work in their searches.

Authors

The general consensus is to have the lead scientist who conducted most of the work and drafted the chapter as the first author and the mentor as the senior/last author. Importantly, everyone listed in the manuscript should have contributed intellectually to the manuscript. Data collection only according to the International Committee of Medical Journal Editors (ICMJE) does not qualify for authorship. (See Chapter 19, Integrity in Research: Authorship and Ethics, for more information regarding authorship.)

Keyword List

In addition to the words in the title, your keywords will also be indexed in scientific search engines and databases. This will affect exposure of your paper to your peers and can impact how frequently your paper is cited.

Abstract

The abstract is a short summary of your manuscript with introduction, methods, results and discussion. The abstract is a stand-alone summary of your manuscript that, with the title, is freely accessible, even if the journal itself requires a subscription. Everyone reads the abstract first, and it is your best chance to attract a reader's attention. Even editors and reviewers base their first impression of the manuscript on the abstract. It needs to be very succinct, within the word limit set by the journal, and to highlight the most important aspects of your study.

Introduction

This is your opportunity to win over the reader of your paper (be it a peer scientist, the editor, or the reviewer) and also to explain the motivation for doing that research. The introduction should present important references as a support in your argumentative chain. It should summarize the current state of research and show the knowledge gap that will lead into the importance of your study. The introduction should logically set up your research objective or hypothesis (see Table 23.1 later in this chapter). Remember that the introduction should not be a literature review. Also important journals such as the *New England Journal of Medicine* prefer to have a short introduction with two or three short paragraphs.

Materials and Methods

This section is where you need to demonstrate the scientific validity of your research. It is therefore read very carefully by editors, reviewers, and knowledgeable readers, and errors or lack of clarity here can result in the paper being rejected. You also need to show here that the methods you used were sound and appropriate for addressing your research question. To do so, you should clearly describe all the materials and methods used and ideally allow for the replication of the results of your study. In all this, pay careful attention to whether your readers will likely be familiar with your methods. If, for example, you used very advanced statistical methods that your readers are unlikely to be familiar with, you might put the details of these in an Appendix, while giving an overview in the Methods section. You should also discuss this with the journal editors and follow their recommendations.

Results

Report your findings succinctly using tables and figures. Use words more minimally, mainly to point out main findings, whose details are given in the tables and figures. Establish a logical chronological sequence for reporting your findings, often following the order used in the Methods section. Table 23.1 summarizes the baseline

Table 23.1 How to Choose the Right Journal [10]

Audience/Readers	
General Public	*You must know who you plan to present the information to.*
Physicians	*This is also important during the writing process.*
Health Authorities	*Just stating "There is a new thing" isn't enough.*
Investigators	

(*continued*)

Table 23.1 Continued

Type of journal/Selectivity		
Global (open access journals, WHO publications)		
International (General Journals)		
Peer (Association journals): reject 65%–75%		
Specialized (Highly targeted journals): reject 95%		
Open Access		

Consider timing		
What is the acceptance time lag?		
What are the journal policies for accepting		
and rejecting submitted manuscripts?		

Determine where the paper fits		
What type of study/design did you perform?		Subjects/Approach
Are there similar topics? Does quality match?	Each journal is unique	Requirements
Choose several journals and then narrow down the list.		Time terms
Possible results after a submission	Peer review definition: Unbiased, independent, critical assessment is an intrinsic part of all scholarly work, including the scientific process.	
a) Initial rejection		
b) Rejection after a peer review	Peer review is the critical assessment of manuscripts submitted to journals by experts who are not part	
c) Needs additional experiments	of the editorial staff.	
d) Editors are interested	Peer review can therefore be viewed as an	
e) Editors are very interested	important extension of the scientific process. [11]	

Reasons for rejection
1) Manuscript doesn't fit the journal characteristics
2) Originality; papers are already published containing the information presented
3) Quality

characteristics of your study subjects. Remember what your primary outcome is, because this may be the key figure of your paper and should be given exposure accordingly. Remember that you want to present your findings without any interpretation or subjective assessment; save this for the Discussion.

Discussion

The Discussion is where you interpret you results. What is the meaning of your principal findings in context of what is already known? Only elaborate on what is supported by your results and don't overinterpret their meaning. The common structure of a discussion is a brief summary of the main findings, followed by a comparison of your results with others in the literature, and accounting for differences. This is followed by a description of your study's limitations and a brief reiteration of its strengths. Your Discussion section should end with a conclusion stating the significance of your results and the implications for the field. One of the main critiques of reviewers is "wordiness," and the introduction and discussion sections are most vulnerable to this.

References

It can't be overstated how important a thorough literature search is when writing a manuscript. The aim is not to write up a review paper of the topic, but to include "landmark" papers and relevant contemporary references (about 20 that are not older than 10 years). Keep in mind that the reviewers of your manuscript will most likely have published in your field and will know the literature well. In addition, the formatting of references is unique to each journal, and it is recommended that you use bibliographical software such as EndNote or Reference Manager to accommodate a journal's preferences.

Acknowledgments

Acknowledge funding sources and people who helped with the research work or the manuscript but were not included in the author's list (e.g., media services).

Disclosures

Be sure to disclose any personal or financial conflict of interest (COI) relevant to the work presented in the manuscript. Although the individual journal's definitions and policies differ, most medical journals require disclosure of COI [8].

Non-Native English Speakers

An important challenge for many scientists is how to write in a non-native language. One important aspect of a good scientific manuscript is the logical organization of ideas. Regardless of the native language of a scientist, he or she should know how to organize the ideas logically. As with of any other skill, writing has several components, such as organization of ideas, logical argumentation, correct use of words, grammar, connection of sentences, flow, and elegance. If possible, have a native English speaker read your work. Scientific copyeditors can also be useful, if you have the budget for one.

THE PUBLICATION PROCESS

The Reviewers

Before you start thinking about where to submit your manuscript, you should understand who the reviewers of your manuscript will be. Reviewers of your manuscript are independent scientists and experts in the field who will be selected by the editor of the journal to which you submit your manuscript. They are not being paid for reviewing manuscripts and are not always "real" experts in the topic of your manuscript. Also, sometimes they don't even review the manuscript themselves but instead give it to a postdoc for review. So how can you make these circumstances play in your favor?

Your chances of having your manuscript accepted are certainly higher if the body of your work is at least known to some extent, and in this the importance of networking cannot be underestimated. Present your data at conferences, invite experts to your posters or talks, and interact with your peers, not just to get advice but to make yourself and your work known. Conferences are also an ideal opportunity to learn what is currently "in" and to get a better understanding of the new and innovative research being conducted in your field.

Your goal is to find reviewers who are neutral, who would give you a fair assessment of your work. When you do encounter fair reviewers, you can actually learn a great deal during the review process and usually it is an enjoyable process.

The "X-Factor" of Science

The impact factor in science these days is used as a gauge for how recognized a journal is and in extension how recognized a researcher is. It was, however, initially used by libraries to select which journals should be subscribed to within the limits of their budget. The impact factor is calculated by the *arithmetic mean* of citations the papers in a given journal received in the two preceding years (e.g., the impact factor of 2012 is obtained from the years 2010–2012, but it is published in 2013, since the year 2012 has to be completed before). Factors that influence an impact factor are the discipline and the ratio of original papers and reviews (reviews being cited more frequently).

The impact factor, although its importance is unquestioned, is not without critique. One major critique is that it distorts what is important. "Evaluations of scientists depend on numbers of papers, positions in lists of authors, and journals' impact factors" [9].

Success is measured more by where you publish than by what you have published. It increases competition and adds additional pressure to scientists already struggling with their daily challenges.

Another point here is that more and more academic promotion committees are considering the number of citations of the investigators (summarized by the H-index) as an important metric for promotion criteria. Although it could be argued that publishing in a high-impact journal may increase the chance of being cited, if the manuscript is a strong study with novel results, it can lead to a large number of citations. Thus one strategy researchers are pursuing is to publish in respected open source journals so as to increase the reading of their research.

Where to Submit

Once you have a draft of your manuscript in an advanced stage, you should start thinking about to which journal you plan to submit. This is not an easy decision, and several aspects need to be considered. Please refer to Table 23.1, which depicts the steps that determine a manuscript's fate. Ultimately you have to prioritize what is most important for you, and how you can match this with the submission process. The case discussion that you will find after this section will review the thought and decision process you will go through when preparing your manuscript for submission.

In choosing a journal for your manuscript, go to its website and download its "Instructions to Authors." Follow these guidelines strictly when finalizing your manuscript. Not doing so sends a message to the editors that you cannot be bothered to present the information in the ways that they prefer, which will of course result in your manuscript being rejected. At this stage, you should also review the cost for publication: While charges per page are rarely substantial, consider that color figures can easily increase the cost by more than $1,000 per image.

When submitting your manuscript, you also need to include a cover letter. Briefly state the main findings of your manuscript and why you think it should be published in this journal. If an expert in the field has reviewed your paper before submission, state it here and include the expert's name as a reference. It can also be extremely helpful if you suggest an independent expert as reviewer and, when appropriate, ask that someone be excluded from reviewing it, if you think that person's assessment would likely not be objective.

THE REVIEW RESULTS

The best possible outcome is *acceptance without revisions "as is."* This is, however, a rather rare case. A more common scenario is *possible acceptance after revisions*. The extent of revision requested can vary substantially. If the request is for *minor revisions*, the concerns are mainly in regard to how the manuscript is written. In such a scenario, it is best to revise the manuscript by addressing the reviewer's critique point by point. If you don't agree with a certain comment, explain in detail your reasons for objection. However, if the review response is *possible acceptance after major revisions*, it is usually a request for additional data. In such a case, you have to ask yourself if this is manageable. Can this request be met just by analysis of already existing data, or do you have to conduct new experiments? Do you have the resources and time for these extra experiments? Maybe it would be easier to withdraw your submission and find another journal (see Table 23.1) [12].

WHAT SHOULD YOU DO IF YOUR MANUSCRIPT IS REJECTED?

Average rejection rate of a manuscript can be as high as 95% if you submit to journals such as *Nature* or *Science* [13]. Your manuscript can be administratively rejected, when the editor thinks that the manuscript doesn't fit the journal's content and audience (e.g., submitting a basic research paper to a clinical journal).

If your manuscript is reviewed, but rejected, don't be too disappointed. It is important to control your emotions. Read and evaluate the review and critique and see if you can improve your manuscript for the submission to another journal. Keep in mind that if you submit to rather specialized journals, the chance that your manuscript will end up in the hands of the same reviewer again might be quite high, and you would be well advised to have rectified his concerns in your new submission.

If you think that the journal's decision was unfair, you can try to appeal the decision by contacting the journal, stating what you think was misunderstood, or if you think a certain reviewer was unfairly biased against you. Most appeals, however, are not successful.

The most common reasons for rejection are study-design-related problems (e.g., sample size too small or biased) and problems with the methods section (too brief, incomplete, or inappropriate). Other reasons are "conclusions unsupported by data" and "results unoriginal, predictable, or trivial." Regarding the writing style, the main problem noted is "wordiness" [14,15].

For resubmission you have to again decide what level of journal you should target. Should it be a comparable journal, one with a lower reputation, or even one with a higher reputation? There are arguments for each strategy, and it also depends on the quality of your research and the manuscript writing quality. If a journal is young and not well established, the reputation might be low initially, but it may have good potential to increase significantly over time. Timing might be in your favor, and it might be good opportunity to submit to such a journal.

Also, if your manuscript is rather controversial, it might be indeed a good strategy to try publishing higher by submitting to a journal that might have the scientific magnitude to evaluate and approve such a manuscript.

Finally, take the reviewers' comments seriously. You will certainly get biased comments from reviewers who are not objective and who have another agenda than giving you a fair review; but likely this is a small percentage of reviews. You need then to consider each comment before resubmitting your manuscript and improve as much as possible for the next submission.

Reporting Guidelines

Most reporting guidelines are being endorsed by a growing number of biomedical journals that want to promote transparent reporting, and assess the strengths and weaknesses of studies reported in the medical literature, with the final purpose of improving the quality of the publications and also to help readers to understand what was done or missing during the investigation.

There are several guidelines, CONSORT for RCT, STROBE for observational studies, QUORUM for meta-analyses and systematic reviews of RCT, MOOSE for meta-analyses and systematic reviews of observational studies, STARD for studies of diagnostic accuracy, and STREGA for genetic association studies [16].

CONSORT

CONSORT stands for Consolidated Standards of Reporting Trials and encompasses various initiatives developed by the CONSORT Group to alleviate the problems arising from inadequate reporting of randomized controlled trials. You can find more information at http://www.consort-statement.org/.

Included in the 25-items checklist are the following:

- *Title and abstract.*
- *Introduction*: Background and objectives.
- *Methods*: Trial design, participants, interventions, outcomes, sample size
- *Randomization*: Sequence generation, allocation concealment, mechanism implementation
- *Blinding*: Who was blinded and how
- *Statistical methods*: For each primary and secondary outcome
- *Results*: Participants flow (number, received intended treatment and were analyzed for the primary outcome), recruitment, baseline data, numbers analyzed, outcomes and estimation of effect size and its precision, ancillary analysis and harms
- *Discussion*: Limitations, generalizability, and interpretation
- *Other information*: registration, protocol, and funding.

The site contains a flow chart from assessing eligibility to analysis; it depicts the progress through the phases of a parallel randomized trial of two groups: enrollment, intervention allocation, follow-up, and data analysis [17].

There is also an abstract CONSORT guide.

STROBE

STROBE stands for an international, collaborative initiative of epidemiologists, methodologists, statisticians, researchers, and journal editors involved in the conduct and dissemination of observational studies, with the common aim of *ST*rengthening the Reporting of *OB*servational studies in *E*pidemiology. (32)

The STROBE 22-item checklist for observational studies includes the following:

- *Title and abstract*
- *Introduction*: Background/rationale and objectives
  Methods: Study design, settings (locations, and dates/periods of recruitment, exposure, follow-up, and data collection)
- *Participants*:
  Cohort study: eligibility criteria and methods of selection of participants, and follow-up
  Case/controls study: Reasons for the choice of cases and controls. For matched studies, give matching criteria and number of exposed and unexposed.

- *Variables*: Define all outcomes, exposures, predictors, potential confounders, and effect modifiers.
- *Data sources/measurement*: Assessment of each variable.
- *Bias*: Efforts to address potential sources of bias
- *Study size*
  Quantitative variables: How these were handled in the analyses.
  Statistical methods: All statistical methods, including those used to control for confounding, methods to examine subgroups and interactions, and how missing data were addressed. Describe any sensitivity analysis.
- *Results*: Participants, descriptive data, outcome data, main results, and other analysis.
- *Discussion*: Key results, generalizability, and limitations (potential bias or imprecision), magnitude of any potential bias.

THE PUBLICATION LANDSCAPE

Open Access versus Subscription Journals

The traditional way of scientific publishing is that journals charge a subscription fee for their journal to cover costs. A pool of reviewers is selected and recruited by the journal's editor(s) to review manuscripts without compensation. There is a recent trend toward open access publishing where the article processing charges cover the costs for a journal. This change in the publication landscape has raised concerns that the traditional peer review system might be negatively impacted, risking the quality of scientific publishing. However, more recently an adjusted analysis has shown that scientific impact is comparable between both types of journals [18]. This is not the final word on these competing models, but it will be interesting to see how things will play out.

The Peer Review System

The peer review system is a triangle between authors, editors, and reviewers and can be traced back at least 200 years [19]. The goal of the peer review process is to improve the quality of the publication and to eliminate ambiguity and unsupported conclusions.

Reviewers are experts in the field selected by the journal's editor(s). A reviewer is supposed to be objective and fair. The final review should be constructive and written in a way that if the reviewer were the author of the manuscript, he or she would be satisfied [21].

However, there have been critiques of the system, mainly concerning how to ensure the quality of the review process. Who is reviewing the reviewers? How can bias be avoided during the review process? Should the review process be blinded (removal of the authors' names) [20]?

Another problem is the continued pressure on the author to "publish or perish." What does it matter how well a study was performed, how good the quality of data obtained is, when at the end, political or strategic decisions spoil the final manuscript? An author can decide to exclude controversial data to make the final manuscript's message clearer. The statistical analysis can be changed to accommodate the data and avoid having to publish a negative study. The principal investigator can bend the system and "pull strings" to get a paper into a journal [22].

The system is not perfect, but until it is replaced by a better one, you are advised to understand its flaws to best deal with it and hopefully improve it by not just being a good author but also a good reviewer and eventually a wise editor.

Publication Bias

In this book you have learned the basic principles of how to conduct a research study with methodological rigor and procedural standardization to obtain unbiased and reproducible results. But when it comes to publishing your results and comparing your study to your peer's work, you will soon find out that there are other factors that will determine whether and how research will enter the scientific stage. The current publication landscape reflects a well-documented trend, a bias toward publication of more positive studies than negative ones [23,24]. In case of clinical trials, this phenomenon is accentuated by the fact that positive trials are published faster than results from negative trials [25,26].

In Chapter 4, you've already been introduced to a tool to identify this bias. In Chapter 14 we discussed the funnel plot. Use this tool not just when you write a meta-analysis; also do this for the topic of your research study to get an idea of what the current trend is.

Many reasons can be attributed to the bias of publishing positive studies. A major reason is a lack of incentives for authors, journals, and sponsors to publish negative results. We have also alluded in previous chapters to the role of pharmaceutical and biotech companies and their impact on medical research. Medical ghost writing is one way of how publications from industry-sponsored studies can be skewed, often resulting in an overemphasis of positive results at the expense of reporting possible adverse events [27]. But there are other problems. A recent comment in *Nature* reported that researchers at Amgen were unable to confirm the results of 47 of 53 "landmark studies" in pre-clinical cancer research. The main problem identified was lack of reproducibility, which suggests that most of the findings were false positives [28].

More possible methodological reasons were given in an investigation by Ioannidis: "... a research finding is less likely to be true when the studies conducted in a field are smaller; when effect sizes are smaller; when there is a greater number and lesser preselection of tested relationships; where there is greater flexibility in designs, definitions, outcomes, and analytical modes; when there is greater financial and other interest and prejudice; and when more teams are involved in a scientific field in chase of statistical significance" [29].

Attempts have been made to stir against this trend, for example the *Journal of Negative Results in Biomedicine* (http://www.jnrbm.com/) and *The All Results Journal* (http://www.arjournals.com). Ultimately, however, it is in your hands to contribute to a change in medical research. We hope that with this book, we have given you the ideas and tools to conduct research in a responsible, representative, and reproducible way that will be an inspiration for your peers. Following is one more case and some exercises to complete this chapter. And after that, our best wishes are with you in your endeavor as a clinical scientist.

Search for the truth is the noblest occupation of man; its publication is a duty.
—Madame de Stael (1766–1817)

ACKNOWLEDGMENTS

The authors are grateful to Harvard T. H. Chan School of Public Health writing instructors Donald Halstead and Joyce LaTulippe for their critical review and suggestions in this chapter.

CASE STUDY: MONTEZUMA'S REVENGE OR PRE-SUBMISSION ANXIETY: CHALLENGES FOR MANUSCRIPT SUBMISSION

Felipe Fregni

For the past 45 minutes, Dr. Vengas has been staring at the same laptop screen—it was the final manuscript submission screen for the journal *Circulation* (the journal with the highest impact factor in the field) saying, "Do you confirm that you want to submit this manuscript?" He could not press either "yes" or "no," as he was struggling with his internal thoughts and he was not sure if he had made the right decision for important aspects of the manuscript. And he was not even sure regarding whether it should be submitted to *Circulation*. He was on vacation in his hometown in Cuenca, Ecuador, going over the main issues he had to consider and make decisions about. He was reliving the manuscript writing process in his head. Dr. Vengas knows that this is a critical moment for him: it is the first step that will summarize all the efforts and investments he has made to become an investigator. As Dr. Vengas disclosed to his close friends earlier, "I dream to be able to offer something better to my patients. I dream that I will be able to develop better treatment options that are less invasive for patients with coronary obstructions. I just need the right tools and training to be able to test my ideas and revolutionize cardiology treatments." Although Dr. Vengas has been labeled as a dreamer by some of his colleagues, his passion has given him the fuel to get the initial training, and this important chance of publishing a manuscript may be the first step to change the use of stents in coronary obstruction. But these final moments have not been easy for him, and besides the critical stressful decisions he was facing, an upset stomach has delayed this final moment.

Dr. Andres Vengas is a smart postdoctoral fellow from Cuenca, Ecuador, working in a large cardiovascular laboratory in New York City at Columbia University. He is part of a team investigating the role of a new drug-eluting stent for the treatment of ischemic heart disease. This is considered a hot topic in cardiology, as recent research has shown that drug-eluting stents are associated with an increased risk of thrombotic events when compared with bare-metal stents. Dr. Vengas arrived in New York four years ago after a successful residency in internal medicine/cardiology in the main and largest academic hospital in Cuenca, and some experience in a successful clinical practice where he realized he wanted to be involved with clinical research and decided to train in clinical research in the United States. During these four years, he has been one of the most productive and hard-working fellows in the laboratory. He was usually the first to arrive at 7 a.m. and was still working past midnight. He had very determined goals and also felt responsible to do his best as this fellowship with Prof. Gunpta was being sponsored by the Ecuadorian government—he knew that governmental investment on him was not trivial.

Prof. Ajay Gunpta is one of the world leaders in cardiovascular stent research in the United States. He was born in New Delhi, India, and had received his medical degree from the University of Oxford, England, before moving to the United States for his residency in cardiology at Mount Sinai Hospital and fellowship in interventional cardiology at New York University, where he stayed on as faculty and has now been a full professor at this department for more than 20 years.

Prof. Gunpta is respected worldwide for his contributions to the field of stent research and for his innovative ideas; in fact, he was one of the first to show the long-term potential complications of stent. He had recently been named a Howard Hughes Professor—a prestigious award that is given to the 20 most influential researchers by the Howard Hughes Medical Institute (HHMI) in the United States. These leading researchers are awarded $1 million per year. He was also named one of America's 25 best leaders by *US News & World Report* in 2008. He runs a very successful lab that has two full-time faculty, 15 postdoctoral fellows, six PhD students, and five research assistants (undergraduate level). Dr. Vengas knew that it was a great privilege to be accepted in this laboratory.

The Research Study and Manuscript Draft

Dr. Vengas's project was to conduct a proof of concept trial showing that a new drug-eluting stent is effective to reduce long-term complications associated with drug-eluting stents in patients with coronary obstructions. The idea of this trial was based on recent reports published in *Lancet* and the *New England Journal of Medicine* showing an increased rate of late stent thrombosis with drug-eluting stent (especially with sirolimus-eluting stents). The potential explanation was that drug-eluting stents may delay healing response after implantation and also the synthetic polymers may trigger hypersensitivity reactions. Dr. Gunpta and his team had developed a novel compound that promoted normal healing, and both preliminary preclinical and phase I trials demonstrated that this compound was safe. The next phase was the phase II trial being led by Dr. Vengas. Dr. Vengas was particularly excited about this trial as this supported his belief that current interventions in cardiology were too aggressive and that part of the morbidity was due to the intervention rather than the disease.

In this trial, 140 patients with coronary lesions were randomized to receive the novel drug-eluting stent versus control drug-eluting stent. The main outcome was rate of thrombosis at one year. Two research assistants, two interventional cardiologists, Dr. Vengas, and Dr. Gunpta formed the team conducting this research. Dr. Vengas was leading the project, and thus was named the first author, and Dr. Gunpta was overseeing the project, therefore being the senior author.

After three and a half years of hard work and several difficulties along the way, they finally finished data collection and data analysis. The results were positive, as they showed an overall improvement for the new drug-eluting stent: there was a significant reduction in the rate of thrombosis—zero cases with the new drug-eluting stent compared to seven cases with the control drug-eluting stent. However, to the surprise of Dr. Vengas, the equally challenging part had just started: the manuscript writing.

The first draft done by Dr. Vengas was very poor. He had difficulties writing all the sections in the manuscript from Abstract to Discussion. It was not easy and it took him much longer than he predicted. After several versions, he finally had the courage to send the first draft to Prof. Gunpta for his initial review. He was surprised when what he thought was his masterpiece came back with almost everything changed—he could only see red from the Microsoft Word tracking changes, except for some words such as "and," "however," and names. But these changes were not the final story; this was the beginning of a long iterative process between Dr. Vengas and Prof. Gunpta.

The Art of Manuscript Writing

Papers are one of the most important components in the life of a scientist. It is the tool that the scientist uses to take his or her discoveries to the scientific community and the world. It is also one of the most important outcomes to measure the scientist's productivity and capacity. It is the scientist's most important currency, and is essential for receiving grants and for the promotion process in academia. Although the impact of a paper depends highly on the research idea, methodology, and research design, a poorly written manuscript will certainly not go far and will be rejected by journals with high-impact factor where the competition is so high that editors and reviewers will quickly reject a poorly written paper when other well-written papers are submitted. In addition, the reader now has easy access to a wide range of manuscripts through online access, and therefore will quickly ignore a paper that is difficult to read and understand even if the science is outstanding.

In fact, physicians and other health-care professionals do not usually like writing a paper, mainly due to the fact that they often do not know how to write. Some of them quickly give up as they consider themselves to not have the talent that is essential for the process. Although talent is helpful, good writing, as with any other skill, comes from intensive training. Certainly talent helps, but talent without training is equally useless. In fact, physicians might have additional difficulty as they spend years in medical school and residency without getting formal training in manuscript writing. In addition, non-native English speakers also have language issues that discourage them from writing; however, most of the limitations to writing come not from language but from the overall structure of ideas in the manuscript.

One difficult aspect in the training of manuscript writing is that, unlike other disciplines, there is no recipe for writing. Some fundamental principles need to be followed and can help, but writing needs to be viewed as an art in which creativity, previous knowledge, and a considerable effort are important ingredients in writing an outstanding paper.

There is less room in scientific writing to improvise, as it needs to follow the scientific structure of abstract, introduction, methods, results, and references. In fact, the need to cite other studies sometimes breaks the flow of the paper and makes the writing heavier and less attractive. But there are several options that authors can use to make the text more attractive and easier to understand and read for the readers. Besides being creative, there are several points that should be followed—for instance, extremely long sentences with multiple phrases, parentheses, and numbers are difficult to read and will certainly discourage even the most interested reader.

Flashback in Cuenca, Ecuador

Dr. Vengas has finally finished everything just before boarding for his two-week vacation in Cuenca, Ecuador. He was excited to see his family and friends but was a bit uneasy at not having the manuscript submitted yet. It was constantly coming back to his head as flashbacks of the manuscript writing process. After the arrival in Ecuador he went to have dinner with his friends and had the famous typical dish there—guinea pig (or *cuy* as it is called in Ecuador)—and also the potato soup that he missed very much while in New York. But neither the company of his friends nor the guinea pig could take him away from his thoughts and flashbacks of the discussion with Prof. Gunpta.

The Introduction: The email Discussion

The first episode that has been going through his mind is the introduction. After sending the first draft to Prof. Gunpta at 1:37 a.m., Dr. Vengas received an email back eight minutes later (at 1:45 a.m.) with the following message:

"Glad to receive the first version. We need to finish this ASAP. I skimmed over and the first point that I want to discuss with you is the introduction—it is almost three pages long! The introduction should state the main question, the importance of investigating this topic, and how the main question will be answered. I like to have introductions with two paragraphs only. The first one explains the background and why it is important to conduct the study—it should convince the reader that the study is not a "fishing expedition." The second paragraph is the "therefore" paragraph, as it states clearly the main question hypothesis, and contains one sentence summarizing the study design. In the introduction that you wrote, you explained in detail the findings of studies showing thrombotic events associated with drugs-eluting stents. This can go in the discussion if needed."

After reading it, Dr. Vengas realized that most of the work was actually about to start. He quickly realized that his writing skills needed to be honed. But he responded to Prof. Gunpta that although he would shorten it, he thought it would be impossible to reduce it to two paragraphs. Then another email:

"Yes—I understand. It is challenging. This is also a question of style. Send me the revised version with your shortening and I will review it. But it is important that you learn in this process. I do *not* [he underscored the word not] want to write it for you, as you need to learn! I want to see you leading clinical research in your field in Ecuador or any other place in the world—you have great potential"

The final result, after many reviews by Dr. Vengas and Prof. Gunpta, was an introduction with four paragraphs, as Dr. Vengas insisted that critical information such as the explanation that developing a new drug-eluting stent was necessary as it was associated with increased survival compared to bare-metal stents did not fit in two paragraphs. Now Dr. Vengas was wondering if the introduction was indeed too long and if it should be shortened further.

The next day—the upset stomach—Montezuma's revenge?

The next day, Dr. Vengas woke up sick with stomach cramps and vomiting. He was not sure if that was the guinea pig from the night before or what some people in the Andes use to call "Montezuma's revenge" (it refers to the difficult initial adaption to the high altitudes in the Andes that historically was faced by the Spanish when colonizing this area). Although he was better, he was still a bit weak from being sick during the night. He could not stop thinking about the entire process, and then he remembered the issue on the discussion section.

The Discussion Section and the Title: An Interesting "Discussion"

Two days later, Dr. Vengas arrived even earlier than usual—at 6:30 a.m.—and he encountered some notes from Dr. Gunpta on the whiteboard. He wondered if he wrote them late in the evening or early in the morning. The following was on the whiteboard:

"Andres, Your discussion needs to be rewritten—according to the paper I gave to you, do not forget to add the following points:

(1) Clear statement of what the principal findings were (first paragraph)
(2) Strengths and weaknesses of the study
(3) Comparison of the findings of our study with those of previous studies
(4) Clarification (possible explanations) regarding the similarities and differences (from item 3)
(5) Clear and concise conclusion of the meaning of the study as it relates to clinical practice or future research
(6) Proposal for future research.

Also please no lengthy discussions either!"

After seeing that, Dr. Vengas also remembered something he kept from what Dr. Gupta said before: "Andres, the raw data can be compared to a block of stone—your challenge is to turn this block of stone into a *Pieta*, as Michelangelo did when he was in his twenties—using the raw data you need to learn how it advances science and knowledge and put this in the discussion."

Dr. Vengas then rewrote the discussion, but one point he was not sure about was the limitations. He went to talk to Prof. Gunpta and explained his hesitation, "Prof., I am not sure if we should include the limitations at this stage. I agree that this is important, but let us wait until the reviewers come back to us to then add the limitations of our study. If we add them now, it might decrease the enthusiasm of the editor and reviewers. In addition, our limitations are not major."

Prof. Gunpta quickly responded, "I understand, my dear Andres, but adding it will not make our study worse. You know that regardless of how well the design is thought out in advance and planned, limitations are inherent, as we are studying humans and dealing with practical, ethical issues and resource limitations. So, if you add them, you are showing that you thought carefully about your study. But you know that I want you to decide, as I am less concerned with publications now—I have enough—my goal is rather to help develop young scientists like you. Besides, this is not critical in the first version."

At the end, Dr. Vengas decided not to add the limitations and now he is having second thoughts as well during the submission process.

Also Dr. Vengas was not sure about the title of the manuscript. The initial title was very simple and plain—it was: "Effects of a novel drug-eluting stent on the rate of thrombosis: a sham-controlled, double blind trial." But he also thought about more provocative titles such as "Enhancing post-stent healing to improve outcomes in coronary obstructions."

The Recovery Phase and the Final Decision

After some rest and chicken soup from his grandmother, Dr. Vengas was feeling better and his thoughts were clearer and he could now concentrate on the final submission step; but before, the last flashback came to him: the issue of the impact factor.

The simplest, but also one of the most difficult decisions: where to submit—a high- or low-impact journal?

After reviewing several times and discussing each point with Prof. Gunpta and also getting approval from the other authors, they were ready to submit, but the question now was: where to submit? Both of them discussed it at the end of the laboratory meeting. Prof. Gunpta then summarized his main point:

"So here you mainly have two options: aim high—start with a high-impact journal and then start to go down the list according to the impact factor. The disadvantage of this strategy is that it will delay the publication and also it is a time-consuming process as for each journal you choose, you generally need to reformat the manuscript, change the referencing format—although reference-managing software such as Endnote can help—and write a cover letter. And of course, you need to wait for the formal rejection before submitting to another journal. So, the trade-off is getting the paper in a high-impact journal versus getting the paper published quickly."

Dr. Vengas is not sure—should he change the introduction? The discussion? The title? Submit to another journal? He wonders if he is making the right decision. The stakes are high for him. This final step has been particularly difficult for him—although his grandmother kept saying that his sickness was Montezuma's revenge, he thinks that it is the stress of this final step. The screen is still there and he needs to decide: change some aspects of the manuscript (or even change the journal) or hit "yes."

CASE DISCUSSION

Dr. Andres Vengas, from Cuenca, Ecuador, is part of a team at Columbia University. He has developed a phase II trial to investigate the role of a new drug-eluting stent for the treatment of ischemic heart disease and has proved its effectiveness to reduce long-term complications associated with drug-eluting stents in patients with coronary obstruction.

The study enrolled 140 patients with coronary lesions. The outcome was rate of thrombosis after a one-year period. After three and a half years the study was completed and the results showed a significant reduction in the rate of thrombosis with the new drug-eluting stent compared to control. Dr. Vengas is preparing the manuscript and will be the first author. His mentor, Dr. Gunpta, one of the worldwide leaders in cardiovascular stent research, will be the senior author.

Dr. Vengas has difficulties in writing the manuscript. Dr. Gunpta revised the first draft and found several issues concerning the title, long introduction, long discussion section, and whether discussing the limitations should be included or not. After reading this chapter and the case, think about what you would consider if you were part of this team. Also take this knowledge and apply it to the manuscripts you are working on.

CASE QUESTIONS FOR REFLECTION

1. What are the issues involved in this case that should be considered by Dr. Vengas when deciding whether or not to make changes in the manuscript?
2. What are the mains issues at stake in this case?
3. Have you seen or been in a similar situation?
4. Where should Dr. Vengas submit his article?
5. What appears to be the best submitting strategy when trying to submit to a high-impact journal in his case?

FURTHER READING
Books

Booth WC, Colomb G, Williams J. *The craft of research*, 3rd ed. Chicago: University of Chicago Press; 2008.

Hall GM. Structure of a scientific paper. In: Hall GM, ed. *How to write a paper*, 3rd ed. London: BMJ Books; 2003.

Papers

Bredan A, van Roy F. Writing readable prose: when planning a scientific manuscript, following a few simple rules has a large impact. *EMBO Reports.* 2006; 7(9): 846–849.

Fanelli D. Negative results are disappearing from most disciplines and countries. *Scientometrics.* 2012; 90(3): 891–904.

Jefferson T, Rudin M, Brodney Folse S, Davidoff F. Editorial peer review for improving the quality of reports of biomedical studies: a Cochrane evaluation of the effectiveness of the peer-review system. *Cochrane Database Syst Rev.* 2007 Apr 18; (2): MR000016.

Kallestinova E. How to write your first research paper. *Yale J Biology Med.* 2011; 84: 181–190.

Kern MJ, Bonneau HN. Approach to manuscript preparation and submission: how to get your paper accepted. *Catheter Cardiovasc Interv* 2003; 58: 391–396.

Kliewer MA. Writing it up: a step-by-step guide to publication for beginning investigators. *AJR.* 2005; 185:591–596

Pierson DJ. The top 10 reasons why manuscripts are not accepted for publication. *Respir Care.* 2004; 4 9(10): 1246–1252.

Provenzale JM. Ten principles to improve the likelihood... *AJR.* 2007; 188:1179–1182.

Schulz KF, Altman DG, Moher D, for the CONSORT Group. CONSORT 2010 Statement: updated guidelines for reporting parallel group randomised trials. *BMJ.* 2010; 340: c332. http://www.bmj.com/content/340/bmj.c332

Veness M. Point of view: Strategies to successfully publish your first manuscript. *J Med Imagine Radiat Oncol.* 2010 Aug; 54(4): 395–400.

Von Elm E, Altman DG, Egger M, Pocock SJ, Gøtzsche PC, Vandenbroucke JP; STROBE Initiative. The Strengthening the Reporting of Observational Studies in Epidemiology

(STROBE) statement: guidelines for reporting observational studies. *Ann Intern Med.* 2007 Oct 16; 147(8): 573–577. Erratum in: *Ann Intern Med.* 2008 Jan 15; 148(2): 168. PMID: 17938396.

Wager E. Publishing clinical trial results: the future beckons. *PLoS Clin Trials.* 2006 October; 1(6): e31. PMCID: PMC1626095.

Online Resources

http://www.consort-statement.org

http://www.icmje.org. Look for authorship and manuscript submission and clinical trial registration ICMJE policy.

http://www.strobe-statement.org

[www.ploscollections.org/ghostwriting]

Manuscript Writing

http://www.scidev.net/en/practical-guides/how-do-i-write-a-scientific-paper-.html

Manuscript Submission

http://www.scidev.net/en/practical-guides/how-do-i-submit-a-paper-to-a-scientific-journal-.html

X Factor

http://occamstypewriter.org/scurry/2012/08/13/sick-of-impact-factors/

http://occamstypewriter.org/scurry/2012/08/19/sick-of-impact-factors-coda/

The Publication Landscape

http://articles.mercola.com/sites/articles/archive/2013/02/13/publication-bias.aspx

http://blogs.biomedcentral.com/bmcblog/2012/10/10/no-result-is-worthless-the-value-of-negative-results-in-science/

http://www.theatlantic.com/magazine/archive/2010/11/lies-damned-lies-and-medical-science/308269/?single_page=true

http://www.scilogs.com/the_gene_gym/on-publishing-negative-results/

http://www.ama-assn.org/amednews/2008/02/18/hlsb0218.htm

REFERENCES

1. Scherer RW, Langenberg P, Von Elm E. Full publication of results initially presented in abstracts. *Cochrane Database Syst Rev.* 2007 Apr 18; (2): MR000005.
2. Jenicek M. How to read, understand, and write 'Discussion' sections. *Med Sci Monit.* 2006; 12(6): SR28–SR36.
3. Fact Sheet MEDLINE®, US National Library of Medicine, http://www.nlm.nih.gov/pubs/factsheets/medline.html
4. Authors' submission toolkit: A practical guide to getting your research published. *Curr Med Res Opin.* 2010 Aug; 26(8). Informahealthcare.com/doi/full/10.1185/03007995.2010.499344
5. Booth WC, Colomb G, Williams J. *The craft of research*, 3rd ed. Chicago: University of Chicago Press; 2008.
6. Barron JP. The uniform requirements for manuscripts submitted to biomedical journals recommended by the International Committee of Medical Editors. *Chest.* 2006; 129: 1098–1099.
7. Bourne PE. Ten simple rules for getting published. *PLoS Comput Biol.* 2005; 1(5): e57. doi:10.1371/journal.pcbi.0010057.

8. Blum JA, Freeman K, Dart RC, Cooper RJ. Requirements and definitions in conflict of interest policies of medical journals. *JAMA.* 2009 Nov 25; 302(20): 2230–2234. doi: 10.1001/jama.2009.1669.
9. Lawrence PA. The politics of publication. *Nature.* 2003 Mar 20; 422: 259–261. doi:10.1038/422259a
10. Halstead D. A strategic approach to publishing research. Boston: Writing Program, Harvard School of Public Health; 2011.
11. International Committee of Medical Journal Editors. Uniform requirements for manuscripts submitted to biomedical journals: writing and editing for biomedical publication. Publication ethics: sponsorship, authorship, and accountability. *J Pharmacol Pharmacother.* 2010 Jan–Jun; 1(1): 42–58. https://www.ncbi.nlm.nih.gov/pmc/articles/PMC3142758/ Updated April 2010.
12. Vintzileos AM, Ananth CV. How to write and publish an original research article. *Am J Obstet Gynecol.* 2009; 201: 344.e1–344.e6.
13. Lawrence PA. The politics of publication. *Nature.* 2003 Mar 20; 422: 259–261. doi:10.1038/422259a
14. Byrne DW. Common reasons for rejection manuscripts at medical journals: a survey of editors and peer reviewers. *Science Editor.* 2000 March–April; 23(2).
15. Pierson DJ. The top 10 reasons why manuscripts are not accepted for publication. *Respir Care.* 2004; 49(10): 1246–1252.
16. Brand RA. Editorial: Standards of Reporting: The CONSORT, QUORUM, and STROBE Guidelines. *Clin Orthop Relat Res.* 2009 Jun; 467(6): 1393–1394. doi:10.1007/s11999-009-0786-x
17. Moher D, Schulz KF, Altman DG. The CONSORT statement: revised recommendations for improving the quality of reports of parallel-group randomized trials. *Ann Intern Med.* 2001; 134: 657–662.
18. Björk BC, Solomon D. Open access versus subscription journals: a comparison of scientific impact. *BMC Med.* 2012 Jul 17; 10: 73. doi:10.1186/1741-7015-10-73
19. Kronick DA. Peer-review in 18th-century scientific journalism. *JAMA* 1990; 263: 1321–1322.
20. Jefferson TO, Alderson P, Wager E, Davidoff F. Effects of editorial peer review: a systematic review. *JAMA.* 2002; 287: 2784–2786.
21. Bourne PE, Korngreen A. Ten simple rules for reviewers. *PLoS Comput Biol.* 2006; 2(9): e110. doi:10.1371/journal.pcbi.0020110
22. Lawrence P. The politics of publication. *Nature.* 2003 Mar 20; 422 (6929): 259–261.
23. Chalmers I. Underreporting research is scientific misconduct. *JAMA.* 1990; 263: 1405–1408.
24. Wager E. Publishing clinical trial results: the future beckons. *PLoS Clin Trials.* 2006 Oct; 1(6): e31. PMCID: PMC1626095.
25. Hopewell S, Loudon K, Clarke MJ, Oxman AD, Dickersin K. Publication bias in clinical trials due to statistical significance or direction of trial results. *Cochrane Database Syst Rev.* 2009 Jan 21; (1): MR000006. doi:10.1002/14651858.MR000006.pub3.
26. Fanelli D. "Positive" results increase down the hierarchy of the sciences. *PloS One.* 2010 April 7; 5(4): e10068.
27. The PLoS Medicine Editors. Ghostwriting: the dirty little secret of medical publishing that just got bigger. *PLoS Med.* 2009; 6(9): e1000156.

28. Begley CG, Ellis LM. Drug development: raise standards for preclinical cancer research. Nature. 2012 Mar 29; 483: 531–533. doi:10.1038/483531a
29. Ioannidis JP. Why most published research findings are false. *PLoS Med.* 2005; 2(8): e124. PMID: 16060722.

INDEX

Page numbers followed by b, f and t indicate box, figures and tables, respectively. Numbers followed by n indicate notes.

abstracts, 472
academia-industry partnerships, 417–421
  case study, 427–431
  contract provisions, 424
  further reading, 431–432
  mutual benefits, 419, 420t
  reasons for, 420–421
  sources of conflict, 419–420
academic research organizations (AROs), 418–419
accessible population, 46, 46f
  example, 50, 50f
acknowledgments, 398
active controls, 313
active placebos, 112
acupuncture, 117
adaptive (flexible) design, 383–385
  examples, 383–384
  further reading, 393
  ways to increase erroneous conclusions in, 384–385
adaptive dose finding, 384
adaptive randomization, 92–93, 93t, 383
  case study, 102
  methods of, 101–102
adaptive trials, 77b, 377–393
adherence, 29, 135–138, 138f
  barriers to, 136–137
  definition of, 129, 135–136
  factors that lead to decrease in, 136
  failure issues, 137
  follow-up, 135–136
  further reading, 146–147
  goals of, 138f
  low adherence consequences, 136–137, 138f
  monitoring, 138, 138t
  populations that display difficulty with, 136
  predictors of poor adherence, 136
  problems related to, 136
  regimen, 136
  strategies for enhancing, 137–138, 138t
  techniques to facilitate, 137–138
  techniques to increase, 137
  types of, 135–136
admission-rate bias, 339
adverse drug reactions (ADRs), 465. *See also* adverse events
adverse events, 465
  case study, 464–467, 467–468
  causality of, 461–462
  further reading, 468
  instruments for measurement of, 458–461
  major adverse cardiac events (MACE), 34
  medical care in cases of, 426
  as primary research questions, 37
  reporting, 462–463
advertising for participants, 132–134, 134f
allocation concealment, 88–89, 103
  definition of, 106, 107f
  ensuring adequacy of, 95–96
alpha (α) (significance level), 227–228, 228f
alpha (α) (spending function), 378–379
altruism, 131
Alzheimer's disease trials
  case study, 175–179
  recruitment and retention in, 139

analysis
  of adverse events, 457–469
  in case reports and case series, 327
  in case-control studies, 331–332
  in cohort studies, 333–337
  in cross-sectional studies, 328–330
  of data
    blinding, 116–117
    definition of variables and, 173–174
  of data from surveys, 443
  intention-to-treat (ITT), 260, 261–262, 275, 307, 309
  interim, 313–314, 377–379, 379–380
  meta-analysis, 288, 289–297, 299
    case study, 298–302
    of controlled observational studies and/or trials, 460
  methods of, 301–302
  missing data during, 260–262
  of parallel group designs, 72, 72t
  propensity scores (PS), 365–368
  reporting guidelines for, 479, 480
  risk assessment, 30, 457–469
  sensitivity, 296–297, 296f
  STROBE checklist for, 480
  subgroup, 284–286, 379–380
  for surveys, 443
  survival, 243–256
  of variance. See ANOVA
analysts, 106
ancillary studies, 33, 43
ANCOVA, 272
animal testing, 15
ANOVA (analysis of variance), 184, 184t, 187, 209
  case studies, 202–203, 253
  covariate adjustment for, 272
  one-way
    SPSS commands, 199
    STATA example, 193–196
  summary of how to use, 187
answerability, 30
answers
  interval, 438
  numerical, 438
  ordinal, 438
  types of, 438

ascertainment bias, 51
assay sensitivity, 311, 317
assessment
  of bias, 341–342
  of risk, 30, 457–469
    case study, 464–467, 467–468
    further reading, 468
    for human participants, 407
  risk-benefit, 407
  of safety, 458
assessors, 106
associational questions, 35–36
attending physicians, 106
attrition, 129, 136
attrition bias, 110, 339
"Authors' Submission Toolkit: A Practical Guide to Getting Your Research Published," 471
authorship, 397–404, 411–412
  coercion, 400t
  corresponding authors, 399t
  criteria for, 397, 472
  disputes, 402–403
    case study, 410–414, 414–415
    committee options, 413–414
    diplomatic solutions, 413–414
    further reading, 415
    radical solutions, 412–413
  ethical, 403
  first, 399t, 401–402
  ghost, 398, 399t, 400
  gift or honorary authors, 399, 399t, 400
  group, 400t
  guest, 399
  last, 399t, 402
  manuscript, 472
  mutual support/admiration, 400t
  order of, 400–402
    decision diagram for, 401f
    descriptive guideposts for, 401–402
  principles to prevent disputes, 403
  recommendations for, 421
  requirements for, 421
  summary of, 403–404
  types of, 399, 399t–400t
autonomy, 12
availability of information, 291

average, 162. *See also* mean
awareness campaigns, 133, 144

Bang's blinding index (BI), 115–116
bar charts, 156, 156*f*
baseline carried forward, 266, 279
Bayh-Dole Act, 418, 430
Beck Depression Inventory (BDI), 208–209
Belmont Report (Ethical Principles and Guidelines for the Protection of Human Subjects of Research) (National Commission for the Protection of Human Subjects of Biomedical and Behavioral Research), 12, 405–406, 406–409
beneficence, 12, 405, 405*f*, 406
Berkson bias, 339
best-case scenario carried forward, 266
between-subjects design, 74–75
bias, 338–339, 339–342
  admission-rate, 339
  ascertainment, 51
  assessment of, 341–342
  attrition, 110, 339
  blinding vs, 110
  citation, 290
  vs confounder, 182
  control of, 341–342
  definition of, 110, 363
  detection/observer, 110, 120–121, 340–341
  diagnostic suspicion, 340
  further reading, 358
  incidence-prevalence, 339
  information, 340–341, 342
  interviewer, 340, 342
  language, 290
  lead-time, 340
  misclassification, 340, 342
  multiple publication, 290
  non-respondent, 339
  non-response, 444
  performance, 110, 111*f*, 340, 342
  publication, 297, 339–340, 342, 481–482
  recall, 333, 340, 444
  reporting, 340, 480
  response, 110
  risk assessment for, 341
  and safety assessment, 458
  sampling, 51–52, 110, 111*f*, 444
  selection, 52, 88, 97, 110, 111*f*, 339–340
    control of, 341–342
    in randomized trials, 88–89
  self-report, 110
  sources of, 52
  in surveys, 444
  survivor, 339
  systematic, 51
  with unblinding, 110, 111*f*
  unmasking (signal detection), 341
  volunteer, 339
  ways to minimize, 342
binary variables, 174
biocreep, 313
biomarkers, 39
biomedical research. *See also* clinical research
  industry sponsorship of, 418
  research misconduct in, 408–409
biopharmaceutical industry, 420
biostatistics, 151
biotech industry, 417–421
blinding, 105–128
  in acupuncture, 117
  assessment of, 114–116, 123–124
  Bang's blinding index (BI), 115–116
  vs bias, 110
  candidates for, 106–107
  case study, 119–124, 124–125
  challenging designs for, 117
  in clinical research, 109–110
  consequent, 342
  in COPD trials, 117
  data analysis, 116–117
  definition of, 106, 107*f*
  double-blinding, 107, 109
    case study, 122, 124
  further reading, 125–126
  guidelines for, 116–117
  issues associated with, 120–121
  James's blinding index (BI), 115–116
  open trials with blinded endpoints, 108
  procedure for, 112–114, 113*f*
  quadruple-blind trials, 109
  in rehabilitation trials, 117

blinding (cont.)
  reporting guidelines for, 479
  single-blind trials, 109
    case study, 121, 122, 124
    with third blinded raters, 122, 124
  in surgical studies, 350
  terminology, 107–109, 108f
  triple-blind trials, 109, 123
  unblinding, 110, 111f
block randomization, 90f, 91
  case study, 100
  stratified, 90f, 92
blood pressure, systolic: coefficient of variation for, 168
BMI (body mass index), 154
body fat: ordinal classification of, 154
body mass index (BMI), 154
Bonferroni correction, 286
box plots, 159–160, 160f
budgets and budgeting, 422–423, 422t–423t
business issues, 417–433
  case study, 427–431, 431–432
  further reading, 431–432

carrying forward
  baseline carried forward, 266, 279
  best-case scenario carried forward, 266
  case study, 277
  further reading, 281–282
  last-observation carried forward (LOCF), 265–266, 275, 277
  worst-case scenario carried forward, 266, 278–279
carry-over effects, 74
case reports and case series, 326–327
  advantages of, 327
  disadvantages of, 327
  example from the literature, 328
  statistical analysis in, 327
case-control studies, 331–333, 331f, 353
  advantages of, 332
  vs cross-sectional studies, 354–356
  disadvantages of, 332–333
  example from the literature, 333
  sample size determination in, 348
  statistical analysis in, 331–332
  STROBE checklist for, 479–480

cases, missing, 443
categorical data, 272–273
categorical outcomes, 40, 233
  case study, 178–179
categorical variables, 40, 174
categorization, 34
  case study, 173–179
  of data, 172
catheterization, right heart or Swan-Ganz, 369–370, 370–371
cause-effect relationships, 68–69
CCA (complete-case analysis), 263, 275
censoring, 246, 270
  further reading, 281–282
  interval, 246
  left, 246
  right, 246
  ways to deal with, 247
central limit theorem (CLT), 172, 198–199
  case study, 176–177
central randomization, 103
central tendency: measures of, 162–165
chain sampling, 59
charts and graphs
  bar charts, 156, 156f
  box plots, 159–160, 160f
  forest plots, 292–294, 293f
  frequency polygons, 157, 157f, 158–159, 159f
  funnel plots, 297, 297f
  graphs, 156
  line graphs, 161, 161f
  pie charts, 156–157, 157f
  two-way scatter plots, 160, 160f
Chemie Grunenthal, 8–9
children: recruitment of, 139
chi-square or Fisher's exact test, 184, 184t
citation bias, 290
classification
  of data, 173–174
  sub-classification, 364
  of variables, 221n3
clinical judgment, 312
clinical outcomes, 39
clinical research, 3–7. *See also* human research
  ancillary studies, 33

basics of, 1–148
blinding in, 109–110
business issues, 417–433
core guiding principles, 12
disasters, 7
duration of trials, 458
early termination of trials, 382–383
ethical issues, 30, 404–409
experiments, 4–7
feasibility of, 28, 29–30
history of, 4–7
history of ethics in, 7–15
introduction to, 3–25
with minors, 139
multicenter studies, 29
open-label trials, 108
patient-oriented research, 4
phases of, 457–458
PICOT framework for, 31
practical aspects, 305–393
preliminary studies, 29
recruitment of children in, 139
specific aims, 33
study designs, 68–86
study phases, 15–16, 77–79, 78b
superiority trials, 307–309
surgical research, 349
translational, 17
clinical significance, 34
  case study, 178–179
clinical trial agreements, 421
  example structure, 421b
  further reading, 431–432
clinical trials. See clinical research
clinical variables, 34–35
clinicians, 106
closed or closed-ended questions, 437, 447–448
CLT (central limit theorem), 172, 198–199
clusters, 56–57, 440
Cochrane Collaboration, 341
Cochran-Mantel-Haenszel Test, 222, 222n3
Cochran's Q, 294
coding, 443
coefficient of variation, 168
coercion authorship, 400t

Cohen's d (standardized mean difference), 294
cohort studies, 333–338, 353
  advantages of, 337–338
  case study, 353–354
  disadvantages of, 337–338
  example from the literature, 338
  prospective, 333, 334f
  retrospective, 333, 334f
  sample size determination in, 348
  statistical analysis in, 333–337
  STROBE checklist for, 479–480
co-intervention, 110
cold deck imputation, 265
collective authorship, 400t
commission errors, 136
committee members, 106
Common Technical Document (CTD), 7
comparative trials, 232
comparisons
  group, 35
  paired (within a group), 213–215
  pre-specifying, 287
  subgroup. See subgroup analysis
complete analysis, 263
complete-case analysis (CCA), 263, 275
compliance, 135
composite endpoints, 34, 42–43
concurrent control trials, 75
confidence intervals (CI), 167–168, 296, 336b
confidentiality, 425, 444–445
conflict of interest (COI), 398
confounders, 343, 343f, 362–376
  adustment for, 346–347
  vs bias, 182
  definition of, 363
  methods to control for, 363–365
confounding, 338–339, 343–346
  control of, 344–345
  definition of, 363
  further reading, 358
  by indication, 343
  in observational studies, 371–372
consecutive sampling, 58
consent forms, 406–407

CONSORT (Consolidated Standards of
    Reporting Trials), 478–479
  checklist for publication, 479
  further reading, 489–490
  requirements for reporting missing data,
    257, 258f
constancy assumptions, 311, 317
contingency tables, 115, 115f, 326, 326b
continuous data, 152t, 154
  categorization of, 34
  graphical representation of, 157–161
  summary, 161–162
continuous outcomes not normally
    distributed, 207–208
continuous variables, 40, 154, 171, 173
contract research organizations (CROs), 419
contracts, 424–426
control groups, 122–123
controls, 32. See also randomized controlled
    trials (RCTs)
  active, 32, 313
  adding groups, 122–123
  appropriate, 36–37
  case-control studies, 331–333, 331f
  concurrent control trials, 75
  double-blind controlled trials, 6
  external, 77b
  further reading, 43
  historical, 75, 77b
  observational studies or trials with, 460
  population-based, 342
  selection of, 313
  in surgical studies, 36–37
convenience sampling, 58, 441
COPD (chronic obstructive pulmonary
    disease) trials, 117
copyright, 428b
corporate authorship, 400t
correlation questions, 35–36
corresponding authors, 399t
costs and payments, 422–423, 422t–423t.
    See also financial issues
covariates, 33–34
  adjustment for, 270–273, 367
    advantages of, 271
    case studies, 203, 253–254
    common covariates to adjust, 271–272

  by controlling, 203
  with Cox Proportional Hazards, 248,
    253–254
  further reading, 281–282
  methods of, 272–273
  objectives of, 271
  in observational studies, 272–273
  when to do, 272
  definition of, 363
Cox Proportional Hazards model, 248,
    253–254, 272, 346
cross-over trials, 74–75, 458
  case study, 83
  examples, 78b
  two-group, 77b
cross-sectional studies, 328, 328f, 353
  advantages of, 330
  vs case-control studies, 354–356
  disadvantages of, 330
  example from the literature, 330
  sample size determination in, 348
  statistical analysis in, 328–330
CTD (Common Technical Document), 7
cumulative frequency polygons, 157, 157f,
    158–159, 159f
cumulative incidence, 332
cumulative incidence ratio, 332

data
  categorical, 272–273
  categorization of, 172
    case study, 173–179
  censored, 247, 270
  classification of, 173–174
  continuous, 34, 152t, 154
    categorization of, 34
    graphical representation of, 157–161
    summary, 161–162
  dichotomous, 161
  discrete, 34, 152t, 153–154
    graphical representation of, 157–161
    summary, 161–162
  interval, 152t, 173
  missing, 257–262, 443
  missing at random (MAR), 260, 261t, 275
  missing completely at random (MCAR),
    260, 261t, 275

missing not at random (MNAR), 260, 261t, 275
nominal, 34, 152t, 153
   graphical representation of, 155–157, 156f, 157f
   summary, 161
ordinal, 34, 152t, 153, 206
   graphical representation of, 155–157, 156f, 157f
   summary, 161
ratio, 152t, 173
from surgical studies, 349–350
transformation of, 172
   case study, 177–178
types of, 152–154, 152t
data analysis
   blinding, 116–117
   definition of variables and, 173–174
   in surveys, 443
data analysts, 106
data capture, 443
data collection
   recommendations to minimize missing data during, 259–260
   from surveys, 443
data collectors, 106
data distributions
   assessment of, 171
   for continuous variables, 171
   normal, 51f, 169–172, 170f
   not normal, 172, 207–208
   probability distributions for random variables, 168–169, 169f
   sampling distribution of the mean, 171–172
   standard curve, 170, 170f
   unimodal and left-skewed, 164–165, 164f
   unimodal and right-skewed, 164–165, 164f
   unimodal and symmetric, 164–165, 164f
data handlers/data entry clerks, 106
data imputation. *See* imputation
data retrieval (case study), 299–301
data safety monitoring boards (DSMBs), 107, 380–383
   functions of, 381–382, 382b
   further reading, 393

   guidelines for, 381
   requirements for, 381
data sources, 480
data synthesis, 292
decision making, participant, 131
Declaration of Helsinki (WMA), 6, 11, 15, 405, 465
degenerative mitral valve disease, 251
deletion, listwise, 275
Department of Health and Human Services (HHS), 12
descriptive questions, 36
descriptive statistics, 151–152, 155
descriptive studies, 348
detection bias, 110, 120–121, 340–341
deviation, standard, 166–167
diabetes type I, 141–142
diagnostic accuracy, 479
diagnostic criteria, 342
diagnostic suspicion bias, 340
diagnostic tests, 342
dichotomous data, 161
dichotomous variables, 174
difference questions, 35
diplomacy, 413–414
disasters, 7
   global, 12–15
disclosures, 475
discrete data, 152t, 153–154
   graphical representation of, 157–161
   summary, 161–162
Discussion (manuscript section), 475, 487–488
disease, 68–69
   odds of, 329
   odds ratio of, 329
   prevalence of, 325, 329
dispersion: measures of, 165–168, 165f
distributions of data
   assessment of, 171
   for continuous variables, 171
   normal, 51f, 169–172, 170f
   not normal, 172, 207–208
   probability distributions for random variables, 168–169, 169f
   sampling distribution of the mean, 171–172

distributions of data (*cont.*)
　standard curve, 170, 170*f*
　unimodal and left-skewed, 164–165, 164*f*
　unimodal and right-skewed,
　　164–165, 164*f*
　unimodal and symmetric, 164–165, 164*f*
documentation: consent forms, 406–407
dose finding, adaptive, 384
dose titration, 113, 113*t*
double-blind trials, 109
　case study, 122, 124
　definition of, 107, 108*f*
　example randomized parallels design, 78*b*
　history of, 6
　RCTs, 106
double-dummy design, 112, 113*f*
　case study, 122–123, 124
　example blinding in, 112, 113*f*
　example dose titration in, 113, 113*t*
dropouts, 29
drop-the-loser design, 384
drug development
　investigational new drugs (INDs), 15, 19,
　　418–419, 424
　phases, 15–16
　post-marketing survey, 16
　requirements for, 7
drug safety, 457–458
drug trials
　adverse events in, 458–461
　in Alzheimer's disease, 174–175, 175–179
　case studies, 81–84, 175–179, 316–321,
　　427–432, 464–467
　in dermatology, 81–84
　for Investigational New Drugs/Devices
　　(INDs), 15, 418–419
　large simple trials (LSTs), 79
　vs medical device trials, 385–386
　New Drug/Device Applications
　　(NDAs), 419
　phases of, 19
　preclinical studies, 15
dry eye disease, 48
DSMBs. *See* data safety monitoring boards

early termination of trials, 382–383
effect estimates, 229–230

effect modifiers, 343, 343*f*
effect sizes
　methods for estimation of, 294
　pitfalls, 230
　pooled effect size, 292–294, 293*f*
efficacy, 313–314
　interim analysis for, 378
　measurement of, 39
email questionnaires, 441, 442*t*, 445
endpoints
　clinical, 34–35
　composite, 34, 42–43
　further reading, 42–43
　surrogate, 34–35
enrollment of participants, 135, 143–144
envelope randomization method, 103
enzyme therapy: example study design
　for, 76–77
epidemiology, 324
　classic measures in, 325–326
　further reading, 393
equipment costs, 422, 423*t*
equivalence, 76
equivalence margin (M), 308*f*, 309
equivalence trials, 309, 317
　case study, 316–320, 320–321
　further reading, 323
　vs non-inferiority trials, 307, 308*f*, 308*t*
　vs superiority trials, 307, 308*f*, 308*t*
error rates, 287
errors
　of commission, 136
　of estimation, 52
　in hypothesis testing, 227–228, 227*f*
　of omission, 136
　probability of, 227–228
　statistical, 183–184
　type I errors (false positives), 183,
　　227–228, 227*f*, 286
　type II errors (false negatives), 183–184,
　　227*f*, 228, 286
estimation error, 52
ethical codes, 6
ethical issues, 30, 404–409
　in authorship, 403
　basic principles, 405, 405*f*
　case study, 17–22

further reading, 468
history of, 5–6, 7–15
in research questions, 28–29
in sample size overestimation, 226
in surveys, 444–445
Ethical Principles and Guidelines for the Protection of Human Subjects of Research (Belmont Report) (National Commission for the Protection of Human Subjects of Biomedical and Behavioral Research), 12, 405–406, 406–409
ethics committees, 422, 422t
European Medicine Agency (EMA), 468
European Union (EU), 7
evaluators, 106
exercise after knee surgery, 299
experiments and experimentation
history of, 4–7
human experimentation. See human research
PICOT framework for, 31
quasi-experiments, 69–70, 69f
study designs, 68–70, 69f, 70–75, 70f
exploratory studies, 435
exposure, 68–69
to advertising, 133
criteria for, 342
odds ratio of, 331–332
studies of, 31
extensions, open-label, 108
external historical controls, 77b
external validity, 49–50, 49f, 53f, 62–63, 458

face-to-face interviews, 441, 442t, 445
facilitation, 137–138
factorial designs, 72–73, 73f
case study, 84
examples, 73–74, 78b
for rare diseases, 77b
reasons for, 84
false negatives (type II errors), 183–184, 227f, 228, 286
false positives (type I errors), 183, 227–228, 227f, 286
Faust (Goethe), 427

FCS (Fully Conditional Specification) algorithm, 267
FDA. *See* Food and Drug Administration
FDC (Federal Food, Drug, and Cosmetic) Act, 6, 8
feasibility, 28, 29–30
Federal Food, Drug, and Cosmetic (FDC) Act, 6, 8
financial issues
acknowledgment of funding, 475
case study, 427–431, 431–432
costs and payments, 422–423, 422t–423t
further reading, 431–432
government funding mechanisms, 423–424
indemnification, 425–426
in participants' decision-making, 131
Fischer's Least Significant Difference (Fischer's LSD), 287
Fisher's exact test, 184, 184t
fishing expeditions, 270–271
fixed effects models, 293f, 294–295
fixed margin approach, 312
flexible (adaptive) design, 383–385
flow diagrams, 257, 258f
follow-up adherence, 135–136
follow-up with patients, 29
costs of, 422, 423t
losses to, 230–231
Food and Drug Administration (FDA), 7, 8, 9–10, 18, 265, 468
requirements for marketing approval, 418–419
website, 23
forest plots, 292–294, 293f
Framingham study, 338
frequency
absolute, 155–156
example frequency polygon for, 158–159, 159f
example histogram for, 157–158, 158f, 158t
hypothetical example, 155–156, 156t
cumulative frequency polygons, 157, 157f, 158–159, 159f
relative, 155–156
frequency polygons for, 157, 157f
hypothetical example, 155–156, 156t

frequency polygons, 157, 157f, 158–159, 159f
Friedman test, 184, 184t
Fully Conditional Specification (FCS) algorithm, 267
funding, 29, 423–424
funnel effect, 130–131, 130f
funnel plots, 297, 297f
futility, 314, 378

GCP (Good Clinical Practice) guidelines (ICH), 225
Gehan-Breslow-Wilcoxon method, 246
Gelsinger, Jesse, 18–19, 20
generalizability, 49–50, 53f
genetic association studies, 479
ghost writing, 399, 399t, 400, 481
gift authors, 399, 399t, 400
Good Clinical Practice (GCP) guidelines (ICH), 225
government funding mechanisms, 423–424
graphical representation, 155–161. *See also* charts and graphs
  of continuous data, 157–161
  of discrete data, 157–161
  of nominal data, 155–157, 156f, 157f
  of ordinal data, 155–157, 156f, 157f
Greenberg Report (NIH), 380
group authorship, 400t
group comparisons, 35
  STATA examples, 210–212, 215–218
grouped means, 163–164, 163t
guest authors, 399
guidelines, 30

Hawthorne effect, 120–121
Haybittle-Peto approach, 378, 379, 379t
hazard functions, 245–246, 248
hazards, proportional, 246, 254
  Cox Proportional Hazards model, 248, 253–254, 272, 346
Health Insurance Portability and Accountability Act of 1996 (HIPAA), 444–445
health-care providers, 106
Helsinki Declaration (WMA), 6, 11, 15, 405, 465
Henderson Act, 405

heterogeneity, 294
  quantification of, 295–296
  testing for, 294
H-index, 476–477
HIPAA (Health Insurance Portability and Accountability Act of 1996), 444–445
histograms, 157–158, 158f, 158t
historical control trials, 75, 77b, 78b
history
  of blinding, 106
  of ethics in clinical research, 7–15
  of experimentation, 4–7
History of Clinical trials
  Ancient China, 4
  African Americans: Tuskegee Study of Untreated Syphilis in the Negro Male, 10–12, 404–405, 407
  Cold treatments 6-8
  elderberry oil, 5
  Elixir sulfanilamide, 7–8
  Federal Food, Drug, and Cosmetic (FDC) Act, 6, 8
  Geegs, John, 17–18, 19–20, 21–22
  Germany, Nazi, 12–13
  global disasters, 12–15
  gun wounds, 5
  Kelsey, Frances, 9, 10
  Lenz, Widuking, 14
  Old Testament, 4–5
  Paré, Ambroise, 5
  penicillin, 11
  phocomelia, 15
  Renaissance, 5
  Roman Catholic Church, 11–12
  thalidomide, 8–10, 14–15
  USPHS (United States Public Health Service), 10–12, 404–405
HIV studies
  case study, 17–22
  Marston–Non-responder Bias in Estimates of HIV prevalence study, 454
honorary authorship, 399, 399t, 400
hospital-based samples, 341–342
hot deck imputation, 265
human participants. *See* participants
human research. *See also* clinical research
  assessment of risks and benefits in, 407

basic principles of, 405, 405f
  common lapses in research integrity in, 408b
  costs of participation in, 422, 422t
  critical aspects for, 14
  IRB requirements, 225
  Nazi, 12–13
  recruitment of subjects for. *See* recruitment
  selection of subjects for, 407
hypothesis, 35, 41
  primary, 33
hypothesis testing, 181–199
  errors in, 227–228, 227f
  procedure, 184–185
hypothesis-adaptive design, 384

ICH. *See* International Conference on Harmonization of Technical Requirements for Registration of Pharmaceuticals for Human Use
ICMJE. *See* International Committee of Medical Journal Editors
IDEAL network, 349
impact factors, 476–477, 490
imputation
  cold deck, 265
  hot deck, 265
  mean, 264
  median, 264
  methods of, 277–278
  multiple, 266–268
  regression, 264
  single, 264–266
  stochastic regression, 264–265
IMRaD (Introduction; [Material and] Methods; Results and Discussion [cum conclusions]) format, 470, 471
incidence, 334–335
  cumulative, 332
incidence rate, 335
incidence rate ratio, 332
incidence risk, 332
incidence risk ratio (IRR), 336–337
incidence-prevalence bias, 339
increased random variability method, 265
indemnification, 425–426
independent variables, 31–32
  case study, 202–203

  parallel group designs with one, 71–72, 72t
  parallel group designs with two or more, 72–73, 73–74
INDs. *See* investigational new drugs
industry-academia partnerships, 417–421
  case study, 427–431
  contract provisions, 424
  further reading, 431–432
  government funding mechanisms for industry, 423–424
  mutual benefits, 419, 420t
  reasons for, 420–421
  sources of conflict, 419–420
inferential statistics, 151–152
information
  availability of, 291
  confidential, 425
information bias, 340–341
  ways to minimize, 342
informed consent, 12, 135, 406–407, 445
innovation research, 423–424
institutional review boards (IRBs), 12, 135, 232, 259, 381, 444–445
  costs, 422, 422t
  requirements for human subject research, 225
integrity, 407–408, 408b
intellectual property (IP), 419, 424, 428b
  case study, 427–431, 431–432
  contract provisions, 424
  further reading, 431–432
intention-to-treat (ITT) analysis, 260, 261–262, 275, 307, 309
  further reading, 281–282
  modified (mITT), 260
interaction effects, 73
interim analysis, 313–314, 377–379
  advantages of, 388–390, 391
  case study, 387–391, 391–392
  disadvantages of, 388–390, 391–392
  example, 379–380
  further reading, 393
  planning, 387–391
  statistical aspects of, 390–391
  statistical power and, 392
internal validity, 49, 49f, 53f, 436
  vs external validity, 62–63
  low adherence threats to, 138f

International Committee of Medical Journal
   Editors (ICMJE), 342, 471
  criteria for authorship, 398, 472
  guidelines for authorship order, 400–401
  recommendations for authors, 421
International Conference on Harmonization
   of Technical Requirements for
   Registration of Pharmaceuticals for
   Human Use (ICH), 7
  guidelines for clinical reports, 271
  guidelines for Good Clinical Practice
   (GCP), 225
International Subarachnoid Aneurysm Trial
   (ISAT), 284
interpretation
  of data from surgical studies, 349–350
  of output, 190–191
  of results from statistical software, 188,
   210–217
interquartile range (IQR), 165–166
interval answers, 438
interval censoring, 246
interval data, 173
interventional studies, 69–70
  designs for, 70–76, 70f
  measurement of efficacy in, 39
  testing new interventions, 15–16
interviewer bias, 340, 342
interviews, 30, 441
  face-to-face, 441, 442t, 445
  standardized, 342
  telephone, 441, 442t, 445
investigational new drugs (INDs), 15, 19,
   418–419, 424
investigators, 109
IQR (interquartile range), 165–166
IRBs. *See* institutional review boards
ITT. *See* intention-to-treat

James's blinding index (BI), 115–116
Japan, 7
*Journal of Negative Results in
   Biomedicine*, 481
journals
  impact factors, 476–477
  peer review system, 480–481
  subscription, 480

types of, 474t
where to submit manuscripts to,
   473t–474t, 477
justice, 12, 405, 405f, 406
juvenile diabetes (diabetes type I), 141–142
juvenile patients, 76–77

Kaplan-Meier survival probability estimates,
   245, 254
Kaposi's sarcoma (example case series), 328
Kefauver, Estes, 10
Kefauver-Harris Drug Amendments, 10
keywords, 472
Kolmogorov-Smirnov test, 171
Koop, C. Everett, 129
Kruskal-Wallis test, 184, 184t, 207,
   209, 231t
  SPSS commands, 218
  STATA example, 215–218
kurtosis, 171

labeling, 6
labor costs, 422, 422t
laboratory costs, 422, 423t
language bias, 290
large simple trials (LSTs), 79
Lasagna's Law, 130–131, 130f
last-observation carried forward (LOCF)
   analysis, 265–266, 275
  case study, 277
lead-time bias, 340
left censoring, 246
legal issues. *See also* business issues
  copyright, 428b
  in surveys, 444–445
Likert scales, 438
line graphs, 161, 161f
linear regression, 187–188
  case studies, 203, 253
  multiple, 184, 184t
  SPSS commands, 199
  STATA example, 196–198
  summary of how to use, 188
listwise deletion, 275
literature reviews, 30
  eligibility criteria for, 299–301
  initial search of relevant studies, 289–290

Preferred Reporting Items for Systematic
  Reviews and Meta-Analyses
  (PRISMA) statement, 291
qualitative, 288
quality assessment for, 290–291, 291f
quantitative, 288
studies to include, 289
study selection for, 290–291, 291f
LOCF (last-observation carried forward)
  analysis, 265–266, 275
  case study, 277
log rank test (Mantel-Cox), 245–246
  case study, 253
log transformation, 172
  case study, 177–178
logistic regression, multiple, 184, 184t
logistical support, 131, 138t
longitudinal studies, 74–75, 270

MACE (major adverse cardiac events), 34
Mahalanobis distance, 366
Mahalanobis metric matching, 366–367
mail questionnaires, 441, 442t, 445
main effects, 73
major adverse cardiac events (MACE), 34
Mann-Whitney (Wilcoxon Rank Sum) test,
  184, 184t, 207, 209, 222, 231t
  rationale behind, 212
  SPSS commands, 218
  STATA example, 210–212
Mantel-Cox (log rank) test, 245–246
  case study, 253
Mantel-Haenszel odds ratios or risk
  ratios, 345
manuscript(s), 472–475
  Abstract, 472
  Acknowledgments, 475
  authors, 472
  blinding writers of, 106
  case study, 483–488, 488–489, 489–490
  Discussion section, 475, 487–488
  further reading, 490
  IMRaD (Introduction; [Material and]
    Methods; Results and Discussion
    [cum conclusions]) format, 470, 471
  Introduction, 473, 486–487
  keywords, 472

Materials and Methods section, 473
  by non-native English speakers, 475–476
  presentation, 471–476
  References, 475
  rejection of, 478–479
  Results section, 473
  review results, 477
  submission, 477, 490
  Title, 472, 487–488
  writing, 470–471, 485, 490
MAR (missing at random) data, 260,
  261t, 275
Markov Chain Montecarlo (MCMC)
  algorithm, 267
masking, 108. See also blinding
matching, 345, 363–364
  Mahalanobis metric, 366–367
  nearest available, 366–367
  nearest variable, 366
  with propensity scores, 366–367
  techniques for, 366
Materials and Methods (manuscript
  section), 473
maximum likelihood (ML) techniques, 268
maximum tolerable dose (MTD), 384
MCAR (missing completely at random) data,
  260, 261t, 275
McBride, William, 14
MCMC (Markov Chain Montecarlo)
  algorithm, 267
mean, 162–164
  arithmetic, 476
  based on power, 347
  based on precision, 347
  calculation of, 162
  comparing more than two, 187
    example ANOVA, 193–196
  comparing two, 186–187
    example paired t-test, 191–193
    example unpaired t-test, 188–191
  grouped, 163
    hypothetical example, 163–164, 163t
    mathematical representation, 163
  hypothetical examples, 162, 163
  independent, 199, 232
  mathematical notation, 162
  mathematical representation, 162

mean (*cont.*)
   sampling distribution of, 171–172
   standard error of the mean (SEM), 167
   weighted, 295
mean difference, standardized (Cohen's *d*), 294
mean imputation, 264
mean substitution, 277, 278
measures, numerical summary, 161–168
MED (minimum effective dose), 384
median, 164–165, 164*f*
median imputation, 264
median survival time, 244–245
medical care
   in adverse events, 426
   contract provisions, 426
   and participants' decision-making, 131
   strategies for enhancing adherence, 138*t*
medical device trials, 385–386
   further reading, 393
   observational studies, 385–386
   placebo effects in, 386
   primary endpoint considerations, 386
   sample size considerations, 386
medical devices
   Investigational New Drugs/Devices (INDs), 418–419
   New Drug/Device Applications (NDAs), 419
   regulation of, 385
medical research. *See* clinical research
MEDLINE, 471
Menger, Fred, 151
Merrel, William S., 9
meta-analysis, 288, 289–297
   accuracy of, 288–289
   case study, 298–302
   of controlled observational studies and/or trials, 460
   eligibility criteria for, 299–301
   fixed vs random, 293*f*, 294–295
   initial search of relevant studies, 289–290
   main steps, 299
   methods of analysis in, 301–302
   missing data in, 269–270, 269*t*
   with multiple outcomes, 294
   online resources for, 302

Preferred Reporting Items for Systematic Reviews and Meta-Analyses (PRISMA) statement, 291
   reporting guidelines for, 478–479
   studies to include, 289
   study selection for, 290–291, 291*f*
   technique of, 299
MI. *See* multiple imputation
MICE (Multiple Imputation by Chain Equation), 267
minimization: randomization with, 92–93, 93*t*
   case study, 102
minimum effective dose (MED), 384
minors
   juvenile patients, 76–77
   recommendations for research with, 139
   recruitment of, 139
misclassification bias, 340, 342
misconduct, 407–409
missing cases, 443
missing data, 257–262
   case study, 274–280, 280–281
   further reading, 281–282
   in longitudinal studies, 270
   in meta-analysis, 269–270, 269*t*
   missing at random (MAR), 260, 261*t*, 275
   missing completely at random (MCAR), 260, 261*t*, 275
   missing not at random (MNAR), 260, 261*t*, 275
   in non-inferiority trials, 314
   in observational studies, 269
   recommendations to minimize, 259–260
   reporting, 257, 258*f*
   strategies to deal with, 262–263
   strategies to minimize, 259
   in surveys, 443
   in survival analysis, 270
   types of, 260, 261*t*, 275
missing values, 264
ML. *See* maximum likelihood
MNAR (missing not at random) data, 260, 261*t*, 275
mode, 162, 164–165, 164*f*
models and modeling
   covariate adjustment by, 273

model selection, 188
multivariate regression modeling, 363–364, 364–365
statistical, 346
modified ITT (mITT) analysis, 260
monitoring
  adherence, 138, 138t
  safety, 465
MOOSE, 478–479
MTD (maximum tolerable dose), 384
multi-center trials, 29
  case study, 427–431
  history of, 6
  for rare diseases, 77b
multifactor design, 75
multigroup design, 72
multiple adaptive design, 384
multiple comparisons, 287
multiple imputation (MI), 266–268
Multiple Imputation by Chain Equation (MICE), 267
multiple linear regression, 184, 184t
multiple logistic regression, 184, 184t
multiple publication bias, 290
multiple variables, 34
multistage sampling, 56–57, 440
multivariate analysis
  covariate adjustment by, 273
  regression modeling, 363–364, 364–365, 372–374
murmurs, Austin Flint, 5–6
mutual support/admiration authorship, 400t

National Commission for the Protection of Human Subjects of Biomedical and Behavioral Research, 12, 405–406, 406–409
National Heart, Lung, and Blood Institute (NHLBI), 381
National Institutes of Health (NIH), 17, 232, 380, 418
National Library of Medicine (NLM), 471
National Research Act, 12
Nature, 478, 481
negligence, patient, 426
network sampling, 59

New Drug/Device Applications (NDAs), 419
Neyman bias, 339
NIH (National Institutes of Health), 17, 232, 380, 418
95% confidence intervals, 336b
95%–95% method for estimation of M_2, 313
NLM (National Library of Medicine), 471
N-of-1 studies, 75–76, 78b
nominal data, 152t, 153
  graphical representation of, 155–157, 156f, 157f
  summary, 161
nominal variables, 34
non-compliance, 110
non-equivalent control group design, 75
non-inferiority margin (M), 308f, 309–310, 310f, 312f
  case study, 319–320, 321, 322f
  definition of, 319–320
  selection of, 311–313, 321, 322f
  strategies for estimation of, 312–313, 315f
non-inferiority trials, 76, 309–311, 317
  applying results to patients, 315
  case study, 316–320, 320–321
  vs equivalence trials, 307, 308f, 308t
  further reading, 323
  important issues, 310–311, 317
  interim analysis in, 313–314
  missing data in, 314
  objectives of, 310
  vs superiority trials, 307, 308f, 308t
  switching designs, 314, 315f
non-native English speakers, 475–476
non-parallel design, 74–75
non-parametric tests, 172, 206–224
  case studies, 173–179, 219–223, 280
  examples in the literature, 207–208
  further reading, 224
  vs parametric tests, 188
  summary, 231t
  for survey data, 443
  when to use, 207–209
non-probability sampling, 53, 54f, 57, 440–441
non-random adherence problems, 136
non-random allocations, 75
non-randomized studies, 460

non-response or non-respondent bias, 339, 444, 454
non-steroidal anti-inflammatory drugs (NSAIDs), 464
normal distribution, 51f, 169–172, 170f
NSAIDs (non-steroidal anti-inflammatory drugs), 464
nuisance parameters, 384
null hypothesis, 182
    STATA examples, 212, 215, 217
numerical answers, 438
numerical summary measures, 161–168
Nuremberg Code, 6, 11, 13–14
Nurses' Health Study, 372

O'Brien Fleming approach, 378
observational studies, 31, 68–69, 69f, 324–361
    case study, 352–356, 356–357
    classic designs for, 326–338
    confounding in, 371–372
    controlled, 460
    covariate adjustment in, 272–273
    DSMBs for, 381
    further reading, 357–358, 375, 393
    last observation carried forward, 265–266
    medical device trials, 385–386
    meta-analysis of, 460
    missing data in, 269
    for rare diseases, 77b
    reporting guidelines for, 478–479
    sample size determination in, 346–348
    self-observation, 441
    STROBE checklist for, 479–480
    in surgery, 348–350
    types of, 353
observations, 324
observer bias, 110, 120–121
observers: blinding, 106
odds, 325
odds of disease, 329
odds ratio
    of disease, 329
    of exposure, 331–332
    further reading, 358
    Mantel-Haenszel, 345
    vs relative risk (RR), 337b

omission errors, 136
one-group design, 75
open access, 480
open or open-ended questions, 447–448
open trials with blinded endpoints, 108
open-ended questions, 437
open-label extensions, 108
open-label trials, 108
    parallel design, 78b
    for rare diseases, 77b
order effects, 74
ordinal answers, 438
ordinal data, 152t, 153, 206
    graphical representation of, 155–157, 156f, 157f
    summary, 161
ordinal outcomes, 208–209
ordinal variables, 34, 173–174, 221n3
organization authorship, 400t
Orphan Drug Act, 76
outcome adjudicators, 106
outcome assessors, 106
outcome variables, 231
outcomes, 32
    categorical, 40, 233
    case study, 178–179
    clinical, 39
    definition of, 39
    probability of, 230–233
    robust, 112
    standardization of, 292
    surrogate, 34–35
overhead costs, 422, 422t
overmatching, 345

p values, 182, 212
paired comparisons, 213–215
parallel group designs, 70–73, 70f
    advantages and disadvantages of, 70–71, 71b
    biostatistical plan for analysis of, 72, 72t
    double-blind randomized, 78b
    examples, 78b
    intervention against active agent, 72
    intervention against placebo, 71
    multigroup design, 72
    with one independent variable, 71–72, 72t

open-label, 78b
  with two or more independent variables or two treatments in different formats, 72–73, 73–74
parametric tests, 181–205
  case study, 173–179, 200–203, 204
  further reading, 204
  vs non-parametric tests, 188
  rating scales with, 176
Parkinson's disease studies, 330
participants
  blinding, 106
  decision-making process, 131
  enrollment of, 135, 143–144
  identification of, 131–134
  protection of, 6
  recruitment of. See recruitment
  screening, 135
  selection of, 407
  ways to identify potential participants, 131–132
patents, 418, 419, 428b
patient follow-up costs, 422, 423t
patient negligence, 426
patient variables, 363
patient-oriented research, 4
patients, 29
  participant. See participants
  recruitment of. See recruitment
payments, 422–423
Pearson correlation, 184, 184t
peer review, 480–481
performance bias, 110, 111f, 340
  in surgical studies, 350
  ways to minimize, 342
performance period, 429–431, 431–432
per-protocol (PP) analysis, 260–261, 307, 309
Peto (or Haybittle-Peto) approach, 379, 379t
pharmaceutical industry, 417–421
pharmacovigilance, 468
pharmacy costs, 422, 423t
phase I trials, 19, 457
  DSMBs for, 381
  study designs for, 77, 78b
phase II trials, 16, 19, 457
  DSMBs for, 381

study population for, 47–48
phase III trials, 19, 418–419, 458
  DSMBs for, 381
  study designs for, 77, 78b, 79
  study population for, 48
phase IV trials, 19
  post-marketing survey or surveillance, 16, 458
  study designs for, 77, 78b
phenylketonuria test, 418
physicians, 106
Physicians' Health Study (PHS) I, 73–74
physiotherapy, 299
PICOT (population, intervention, control, outcome, and time) framework, 31–32
pie charts, 156–157, 157f
pilot studies, 29
  case study, 448
  further reading, 43
  history of, 5
  sample size, 231
placebos, 32
  active, 112
  case study, 81–84
  further reading, 43
  history of, 5–6
  loss of, 110
  in medical device trials, 386
  sham procedures, 36, 43
  in surgical research, 348–349
plagiarism, 408
planning, survey, 435–438
Plato, 225
PNAS (Proceedings of the National Academy of Sciences), 20
Pocock approach, 379
polygons
  cumulative frequency, 157, 157f, 158–159, 159f
  relative frequency, 157, 157f
pooled effect size, 292–294, 293f
pooling, 292
population-based controls, 342
postal questionnaires, 441, 442t
post-marketing survey or surveillance, 16, 458

power
  1-β, 227, 228
  alpha level and, 228, 228f
  software programs for calculation of, 240–241
  statistical, 155
  study, 155, 231
PP. *See* per-protocol
practical aspects, 305–393
practice (learning) effects, 74
precision, 52
preclinical studies, 15, 19, 457
Preferred Reporting Items for Systematic Reviews and Meta-Analyses (PRISMA) statement, 291
preliminary studies, 29
pre-randomization screening, 137
prevalence, 325
  symptom, 327
prevalence odds ratio (POR), 329
prevalence ratio, 329
prevalence surveys, 353
primary endpoints, 386
primary hypothesis, 34
primary questions, 31, 32, 33
  adverse events as, 37
  PICOT (population, intervention, control, outcome, and time) acronym for, 31
principal investigators (PIs), 425
PRISMA (Preferred Reporting Items for Systematic Reviews and Meta-Analyses) statement, 291
privacy, 444–445
probability, 168–169
  distributions for random variables, 168–169, 169f
  of errors, 227–228
  of outcome, 230–233
  sampling, 53–54, 54f, 440–441
  of survival, 245, 254
PROBE (prospective randomized open-label blinded endpoint), 108
Proceedings of the National Academy of Sciences (PNAS), 20
prognostic factors, 271–272
propensity scores (PS), 365–368
  case study, 369–374
  covariate adjustment with, 273, 367

definition of, 362–363
further reading, 375
matching with, 366–367
regression adjustment with, 367
stratification with, 367
techniques to adjust with, 365–368
theoretical background, 365
weight by inverse of, 368
weights, 368
property rights. *See* intellectual property (IP)
proportion(s), 325
  based on power, 347
  based on precision, 347–348
proportional hazards, 246, 254
  Cox Proportional Hazards model, 248, 253–254, 272, 346
proportional stratified sampling, 56
prospective randomized open-label blinded endpoint (PROBE), 108
prospective trials, 333–338, 334f
PS. *See* propensity scores
psychiatric research, 140
public awareness campaigns, 133, 144
publication
  "Authors' Submission Toolkit: A Practical Guide to Getting Your Research Published," 471
  further reading, 489–490
  impact factors, 476–477
  manuscripts, 470–492
  open access, 480
  process, 476–477
  review results, 477
  where to submit, 477
publication bias, 297, 339–340, 342, 481–482
publication expenses, 422, 423t
publication rights, 425
  case study, 427–431, 431–432
  contract provisions, 425
PubMed, 471
Pure Food and Drug Act, 6

quadruple-blind trials, 109
quality assessment, 290–291, 291f
quality of life analysis (case study), 253
quality of life scales, 39
quantitative variables, 480

quasi-experimental studies, 69–70, 69f, 75
questionnaires, 30, 441, 442t
  standardized, 342
questions
  closed-ended, 437, 447–448
  double-barreled, 448
  open-ended, 437, 447–448
  statistical (case study), 200–203
  survey, 436, 437–438
  types of, 437–438
  types of answers, 438
  wording, 447–448
QUORUM, 478–479

random adherence problems, 136
random effects models, 293f, 294–295
random sampling, 440
  simple, 54, 440
random variability, increased, 265
randomization, 87–104
  adaptive, 92–93, 93t, 383
    case study, 102
    methods of, 101–102
  block or blocked, 90f, 91
    case study, 100
    stratified, 90f, 92
  case study, 97–102, 102–103
  central, 103
  definition of, 87–88
  effects of lack or failure of, 88
  envelope method, 103
  history of, 6
  main issues associated with, 99–100
  methods of, 89–93, 90f, 98
    checking adequacy of, 95
    implementation, 95–96
    options based on sample
      size and number immportant
      baseline covariates to be
      balanced, 93–95, 94f
  with minimization, 92–93, 93t
    case study, 102
  reporting guidelines for, 479
  simple, 89–91, 90f
    case study, 100
  for small trials, 93–95, 94f
    case study, 97–102
  stratified, 91–92

  with blocks, 90f, 92
    case study, 101
  telephone, 103
  web resources, 103
randomized controlled trials (RCTs), 68–69,
    98, 261, 459–460
  accuracy of, 288–289
  with blinding, 105
  CONSORT checklist for, 479
  covariate adjustment in, 272
  double-blind, 78b, 106
  interim analysis in, 377, 379–380
  key features of, 87
  rationale for, 386
  reporting guidelines for, 478–479
  selection bias in, 88–89
  subgroup analysis in, 379–380
  in surgery, 348
range, 165
  interquartile (IQR), 165–166
rare diseases: study
    designs for, 76–77, 77b
rate(s), 325–326
rate difference, 337
raters, 106
rating scales, 176
ratio, 325
ratio data, 173
R&D (research and development), 419,
    423–424
recall bias, 333, 340, 444
reciprocal transformation, 172
recruitment, 29, 129–130, 138f, 142
  advertising for, 132–133
  in Alzheimer's disease trials, 139
  broad-based, 142–143
  case study, 63–64, 141–144, 145–146
  challenges to, 139–140
  of children, 139
  community-based strategies, 132, 133
  costs of, 422, 422t
  definition of, 129
  effective strategies for, 134–135
  first steps, 130–134
  funnel effect or Lasagna's Law of,
    130–131, 130f
  further reading, 146
  goals of, 138f

recruitment (cont.)
  health-care-provider-based strategies, 132, 133
  human factors, 134–135
  issues that may affect, 139
  methods of, 131–134
  objectives of, 129–130
  obstacles to, 131–134
  in psychiatric research, 140
  public awareness
    campaigns for, 144
  strategies for, 65–66, 138f, 138t
  strategy plans, 134, 134f
  ways to identify potential participants, 131–132
reference population, 45, 46f
References (manuscript section), 475
regimen adherence, 136
regression
  covariate adjustment for, 272, 367
  Cox model, 248
  linear. See linear regression
  to the mean (case study), 62–63
  multivariate modeling, 363–364, 364–365, 372–374
regression analysis, 346
regression imputation, 264–265
regression substitution, 277–278
regulatory issues, 462–463
rehabilitation trials, 117
rejection, 474t, 478–479
relational/correlation questions, 35–36
relative frequency, 155–156, 156t
relative frequency polygons, 157, 157f
relative rate, 332
relative risk (RR), 332, 335–336
  further reading, 358
  vs odds ratio, 337b
reliability, 33, 436–437, 437f
reporting adverse events, 459, 462–463
reporting bias, 340
reporting guidelines, 478–480, 489–490
reporting missing data, 257, 258f
reporting results from surveys, 444
reporting sample size, 226–227
research. See also clinical research
  psychiatric, 140

research and development (R&D), 419, 423–424
research budgets, 422, 422t–423t
research integrity, 407–408, 408b
research misconduct, 407–409
research questions, 26–44
  associational questions, 35–36
  case study, 38–41, 41–42
  considerations for, 28–29
  definition of, 27
  definition of outcomes for, 39
  descriptive, 36
  difference questions, 35
  further reading, 42–43
  key elements needed for, 26
  PICOT framework for, 31–32
  primary questions, 31, 32, 33, 37
  related topics for choosing, 36–37
  secondary questions, 32, 33
  "So What?" test for, 38–39
  statement of, 36
  types of, 35–36
research topics, 28
respect for persons, 12, 405, 405f, 406
response bias, 110
response rates, 130–131, 450
response scales, 438
response to treatment, 48
response variables, 40
restriction, 345, 363–364
results
  application to patients, 315
  reporting, 444
  reporting guidelines, 479
  review, 477
  from statistical software, 188, 210–217
  unexpected, 287–288
Results (manuscript section), 473
retention, 129, 136, 139
retrospective trials
  case study, 249–251, 252–254
  case-control studies, 331–333, 331f
  cohort studies, 333–338, 334f
review results, 477
reviewers, 476
  case study with, 316–320, 320–321
rheumatic fever, 5–6

rheumatic valve disease, 251
right censoring, 246
risk, 335
risk assessment, 30, 457–469
  case study, 464–467, 467–468
  further reading, 468
  for human participants, 407
risk difference, 337
risk factors, 271–272
risk management, 468
risk ratios, 335, 345
risk-benefit assessment, 407
risks and benefits, 30

safety, 314
  drug, 457–458
  measurement of, 457–458
  vs study population, 48
safety assessment
  interim analysis for, 378
  limitations to, 458
  main challenges, 458
  study design for, 461
safety monitoring, 465
Salisbury, 5
sample size
  calculation of, 225–242
    case study, 234–238, 238–240
    for case-control studies, 348
    for cohort studies, 348
    for comparative trials, 232
    for cross-sectional studies, 348
    for descriptive studies, 348
    formula for, 233, 347
    further reading, 240–241
    limitations in literature regarding, 232
    manual, 232–233
    mis-specification problems, 226
    in observational studies, 346–348
    overestimation problems, 226
    probability of errors, 227–228
    re-estimation, 383–384
    required parameters for, 227, 346
    software programs for, 240–241
    steps for, 233
    for two independent means, 232
    underestimation problems, 226

  considerations for, 230–233, 348, 386
  definition of, 225
  in medical device trials, 386
  in meta-analysis, 295
  pilot study, 231
  and recruitment, 130–134
  reporting, 226–227
  and safety assessment, 458
samples and sampling, 45, 46, 46f, 50–59, 130–134
  case study, 449–450
  chain, 59
  cluster, 56–57, 440
  consecutive, 58
  convenience, 58, 441
  definition of, 51
  example, 50, 50f
  hospital-based samples, 341–342
  multistage, 56–57
  network or chain, 59
  non-probability, 53, 54f, 57, 440–441
  probability, 53–54, 54f, 440–441
  proportional stratified, 56
  purposive, 440
  random, 440
  simple, 54, 440
  and safety assessment, 458
  selection scheme, 59, 60f, 441
  snowball, 59, 441
  stratified, 55–56
  for surveys, 440
  systematic, 55
  techniques for, 53–54, 449–450
  voluntary response sample, 52
sampling bias, 51–52, 110, 111f, 444
sampling error(s), 52–53
SBIR (Small Business Innovation Research) program, 423–424
scatter plots, two-way, 160, 160f
scientific writing, 471–476
screening, 135, 137
secondary questions, 32, 33
selection bias, 52, 88, 97, 110, 111f, 339–340
  control of, 341–342
  in randomized trials, 88–89
self-observation, 441

self-report bias, 110
SEM (standard error of the mean), 167
sensitivity analysis, 231–232, 231t, 268–269, 296–297, 296f
SF-36 (Short-Form General Health Survey), 235
sham procedures, 36, 43
Shapiro-Wilk test, 171
Short-Form General Health Survey (SF-36), 235
signal detection (unmasking) bias, 341
significance
    clinical, 34, 178–179
    statistical, 182, 185, 186f
significance level (α), 227–228, 228f
simple random sampling, 54, 440
simple randomization, 89–91, 90f
    case study, 100
Simpson's paradox, 343–344, 344b, 344f, 358
Singapore Statement on Research Integrity, 407–408
single imputation, 264–266
single variables, 34
single-blind trials, 109
    case study, 121, 122, 124
skewness, 171
    left-skewed distributions, 164–165, 164f, 171
    right-skewed distributions, 164–165, 164f, 171
Small Business Innovation Research (SBIR) program, 423–424
Small Business Technology Transfer (STTR) program, 423–424
small trials, 99–100
    case study, 97–102
    randomization for, 93–95, 94f, 97–102
snowball sampling, 59, 441
"So What?" test for research questions (case study), 38–39
social strategies for enhancing adherence, 138t
software. *See also specific programs*
    interpretation of results from, 188, 210–217
    programs for sample size and power calculations, 240–241

Spearman correlation, 184, 184t
spontaneous reporting systems, 459
SPSS software
    commands for Kruskal-Wallis test, 218
    commands for linear regression, 199
    commands for Mann-Whitney/Wilcoxon Rank Sum test, 218
    commands for one-way ANOVA, 199
    commands for paired t-test, 199
    commands for unpaired t-test, 199
    commands for Wilcoxon Sign Rank test, 218
square root transformation, 172
square transformation, 172
Stael, Germaine de, 482
staff and staffing
    costs related to, 422, 422t
    strategies for enhancing adherence, 138t
standard deviation (SD), 166–167, 228–229
standard error of the mean (SEM), 167
Standard of Care Concurrent Control Trials, 72
standardized interviews, 342
standardized mean difference (Cohen's d), 294
standardized outcomes, 292
standardized questionnaires, 342
STATA software
    commands for covariate adjustment, 272
    example ANOVA, 193–196
    example Kruskal-Wallis test, 215–218
    example linear regression, 196–198
    example Mann-Whitney test/Wilcoxon Rank Sum test, 210–212
    example t-tests, 188–191, 191–193
    example Wilcoxon Sign Rank test, 213–215
    online resources, 179
statistical analysis. *See also* analysis
    in case reports and case series, 327
    case study, 301–302
    in case-control studies, 331–332
    in cohort studies, 333–337
    in cross-sectional studies, 328–330
    methods, 70
    plans for analysis of parallel group designs, 72, 72t

reporting guidelines for, 479, 480
STROBE checklist for, 480
statistical errors, 183–184. *See also* errors
statistical modeling, 346
statistical power, 155, 392
statistical questions (case study), 200–203
statistical significance, 182, 185, 186f
statistical tests. *See also* tests and testing;
specific tests
  non-parametric tests, 172, 206–224
    case studies, 173–179, 219–223, 280
  online tests, 281
  options, 184, 184t
  outcome possibilities, 183
  parametric tests, 181–205
    case studies, 173–179, 201–202
  selection of, 154–155
statisticians, 106
statistics
  basics, 151–180
  biostatistics, 151
  case study, 173–179
  descriptive, 151–152, 155
  further reading, 179–180
  inferential, 151–152
  summary, 161–168
stochastic regression imputation, 264–265
strata, 345, 364
stratification, 345–346, 363–364
  with propensity scores, 367
stratification factors, 56, 310
stratified randomization, 91–92
  with blocks, 90f, 92
  case study, 101
stratified sampling, 55–56
STROBE (STrengthening the Reporting
  of OBservational studies in
  Epidemiology), 478–479, 479–480
  checklist for observational studies,
    479–480
  further reading, 489–490
STTR (Small Business Technology Transfer)
  program, 423–424
study design(s), 68–70
  according to study phase, 77–79, 78b
  adaptive trials, 377–393
  between-subjects, 74–75

case study, 80–84, 84–85
challenging for blinding, 117
classic, for observational
  studies, 326–338
core guiding principles, 12
cross-over design, 74–75
in dermatology (case study), 80–84, 85
double-dummy design, 112, 113f
  case study, 122–123, 124
exprimental designs, 69, 69f
factorial designs, 72–73, 73f
for interventional studies, 70–76, 70f
longitudinal studies, 74–75
multifactor design with two repeated
  measures, 75
multigroup design, 72
N-of-1 trials, 75–76
non-equivalent control
  group design, 75
non-inferiority, 307–323
non-parallel, 74–75
with non-random allocation, 75
for observational studies, 326–338
one-group design, 75
parallel group designs, 70–73, 70f, 71b
for phase I studies, 77, 78b
for phase II studies, 77, 78b
for phase III studies, 77, 78b
for phase IV studies, 77, 78b
planning, 138f
possible prospective modifications, 383
quasi-experimental, 75
for rare diseases, 76
  example, 76–77
  options, 77b
and safety assessment, 458
and sample size estimation, 231
strategies to minimize
  missing data, 259
for survey studies, 435–443
three-arm (case study), 82–83
two-arm (case study), 81, 82
two-group crossover studies, 77b
types of, 68–69, 69f, 76
within-subjects, 74–75
study population, 31, 40, 45–67, 46f
  case study, 61–64, 64–66

study population (cont.)
  example, 50, 50f
  further reading, 66
  overview, 45–46
  recruitment of subjects, 63–64
  vs response to treatment, 48
  vs safety, 48
  vs study phases, 47–48
  validity and, 49, 49f
study power, 155, 231
sub-classification, 364
subgroup(s), 364
subgroup analysis, 284–286, 285f, 287
  Bonferroni correction method, 286
  example, 284, 379–380
  methods for, 287
  unexpected results, 287–288
subjects
  non-random allocation of, 75
  participant. See participants
  recruitment of. See recruitment
subscription journals, 480
sulfanilamide cold syrup, 7–8
summary statistics, 161–168
superiority, 76
superiority trials, 307–309
  vs equivalence trials, 307, 308f, 308t
  interim analysis in, 313–314
  missing data in, 314
  vs non-inferiority trials, 307, 308f, 308t
  switching to/from non-inferiority design, 314, 315f
supply costs, 422, 423t
Surgeon General's Advisory Committee on Smoking and Health, 461
surgical medicine, 350
surgical studies, 349
  blinding in, 350
  case study, 298–302
  controls for, 36–37
  example from the literature, 350–351
  further reading, 358
  interpretation of data from, 349–350
  observational studies, 348–350
  performance bias in, 350

  RCTs, 348
  recommendations for, 349
  selection of subjects, 349–350
surrogates, 39
  endpoints and outcomes, 34–35, 42–43
  further reading, 42–43
survey studies, 435–443
  aims, 435
  examples, 435
  stages of, 434–435
surveys, 30, 434–456
  administration, 448–449
  administration methods, 441, 442t
  answer types, 438
  bias in, 444
  case study, 446–450, 450–453, 453–454
  data analysis, 443
  data capture, 443
  data collection, 443
  development of, 435–438, 439
  ethical issues, 444–445
  further reading, 454–455
  instrument design, 435–441
  legal issues, 444–445
  missing data, 443
  phase IV post-marketing, 16, 458
  planning, 435–438, 439–441
  pre-test, 438–439
  questions, 436, 437–438
  report of results from, 444
  response rates, 450
  sample design for, 440
  structure of, 438
  types of questions, 437–438
  validation of, 438–439
survival analysis, 243–256
  case study, 249–251, 252–254, 254–255
  covariate adjustment for, 272
  Kaplan-Meier probability estimates, 245, 254
  missing data in, 270
  tables for, 243–244
survival time, median, 244–245
survivor bias, 339
systematic bias, 51
systematic sampling, 55

tables, 155–156, 156t
target enrollment, 143–144
target population, 31, 45, 46f, 130–134
  case study, 62–63
  definition of, 46–50, 130
  example, 50, 50f
  selection of, 62–63
teams, 30
tech industry, 417–421
technical expertise, 29
technology transfer, 423–424
telephone interviews, 441, 442t, 445
telephone randomization, 103
termination, early, 382–383
terminology, 107–109, 108f
test-dosing, 137
tests and testing. *See also specific tests*
  animal testing, 15
  diagnostic tests, 342
  hypothesis testing, 181–199
  of new interventions, 15–16
  non-parametric tests, 172, 206–224
    case studies, 173–179, 219–223, 280
    vs parametric tests, 188
  online tests, 281
  parametric tests, 181–205
    case studies, 173–179, 200–203, 204
    vs non-parametric tests, 188
  "So What?" test for research
    questions, 38–39
  t-test, 154–155, 184, 184t, 186–187
    examples, 188–191, 191–193
therapeutic misconception, 21
three-arm design (case study), 82–83
ties: adjustment for, 212
time, 32
title, manuscript, 472
trademarks, 428b
training costs, 422, 422t
transformation
  of data, 172
    case study, 177–178
  variable, 154
translational research, 17
travel costs, 422, 423t
triple-blind trials, 108, 108f, 109
  case study, 123

t-test, 154–155, 184, 184t, 186–187
  case study, 202
  paired
    SPSS commands, 199
    STATA example, 191–193
  summary of how to use, 187
  unpaired
    SPSS commands, 199
    STATA example, 188–191
Tukey's Honestly Significant Difference
  (Tukey's HSD), 287
two-arm designs (case study), 81, 82
two-group crossover studies, 77b
two-way scatter plots, 160, 160f
type I errors (false positives), 183, 227–228,
  227f, 286
type II errors (false negatives), 183–184,
  227f, 228, 286

unblinding, 110, 111f
United States Public Health Service
  (USPHS), 10–12, 404–405
unmasking (signal detection) bias, 341

vaccine safety research, 79
validation, 438–439
validity, 33, 48–50, 49f, 436–437
  external, 49–50, 49f, 53f, 458
    vs internal, 62–63
  internal, 49, 49f, 53f, 436
    vs external, 62–63
  low adherence threats to, 138f
  vs reliability, 437, 437f
  survey, 438–439
variability, random, 265
variables, 33–35, 173–174
  binary, 174
  categorical, 40, 174
  classification of, 221n3
  clinical, 34–35
  continuous, 34, 40, 154, 173
  dependent, 33
  dichotomous, 174
  discrete, 34
  format of, 155
  independent, 31–32, 33
    case study, 202–203

variables (cont.)
  multiple, 34
  nominal, 34
  ordinal, 34, 173–174, 221n3
  patient, 363
  reporting guidelines, 480
  single, 34
  surrogate, 34–35
  transformation of, 154
variance, 166–167, 212
variation, 228–229
Venereal Disease Research Laboratory
    (VDRL) test, 11
voluntary response sample, 52
volunteer bias, 339
volunteers
  participant. See participants
  recruitment of. See recruitment

weighted complete-case analysis, 263
  example, 263
  by inverse of propensity score, 368
weighted means, 295
weights, propensity score, 368
WHO (World Health Organization), 154
Wilcoxon Rank Sum (Mann-Whitney) test,
    184, 184t, 207, 209, 222, 231t
  rationale behind, 212
  SPSS commands, 218
  STATA example, 210–212
Wilcoxon Sign Rank test, 207, 209, 231t
  SPSS commands, 218
  STATA example, 213–215
Wilcoxon Two-Group Rank Sum test, 222
Wilde, Oscar, 105
within-subjects design, 74–75
World Health Organization (WHO), 154
World Medical Association
    (WMA): Declaration of Helsinki, 6,
    11, 15, 405, 465
worst-case scenario carried forward, 266,
    278–279
writing
  blinding writers, 106
  further reading, 489–490
  ghost writing, 399, 399t, 400, 481
  manuscript, 470–471, 485
  scientific, 471–476

youth
  example study designs for rare diseases in
    juvenile patients, 76–77
  recommendations for research with
    minors, 139

Z scores, 292